PA	Pulmonary artery
PAD	Pulmonary artery diastolic
Pao_2	Arterial oxygen tension or partial pressure
Pao_2	Alveolar oxygen tension or partial pressure
$P(A-a)o_2$	Alveolar arterial O_2 tension difference
$P(a/A)o_2$	Arterial alveolar tension ratio or oxygen exchange index
PAM	Pulmonary artery mean
PAP	Pulmonary artery pressure
PAS	Pulmonary artery systolic
PAWP	Pulmonary artery wedge pressure
$Petco_2$	End tidal carbon dioxide
PP	Pulse pressure
PT	Prothrombin
PTT	Partial thromboplastin time
PVR	Pulmonary vascular resistance
PVRI	Pulmonary vascular resistance index
Qs/Qt	Physiological shunt
RPP	Rate pressure product
RQ	Respiratory quotient
RR	Respiratory rate
RVSWI	Right ventricular stroke work index
Sao_2	Oxygen saturation of the hemoglobin of arterial blood
SBP	Systolic blood pressure
SI	Stroke index
SOB	Shortness of breath
Spo_2	Oxygen saturation measured by pulse oximetry
SV	Stroke volume
SVI	Stroke volume index
Svo_2	Mixed venous oxygen saturation
SVR	Systemic vascular resistance
SVRI	Systemic vascular resistance index
VC	Vital capacity
$\dot{V}o_2$	Oxygen consumption
$\dot{V}o_2I$	Oxygen consumption index
VS	Vital signs
V_T	Tidal volume
WNL	Within normal limits

WARDEN WOODS CAMPUS

**Resource Center
Centennial College of
Applied Arts and Technology
651 Warden Avenue
Scarborough, Ontario
M1L 3Z6**

2002 02 26

ADD   2 2002

DATE DUE

JUL 09 2004	
JUL 09 2004	

BRODART, CO.   Cat. No. 23-221-003

Mosby's
Critical Care Nursing Reference

Susan B. Stillwell, MSN, RN

Adjunct Faculty
Ursuline College
Division of Nursing
Pepper Pike, Ohio

SECOND EDITION

with 74 illustrations

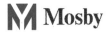 Mosby

A *Harcourt Health Sciences Company*
St. Louis   Philadelphia   London   Sydney   Toronto

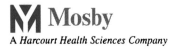

M Mosby

A Harcourt Health Sciences Company

A NOTE TO THE READER

The author and publisher have made every attempt to check dosages and nursing content for accuracy. Because the science of pharmacology is continually advancing, our knowledge base continues to expand. Therefore we recommend that the reader always check product information for changes in dosage or administration before administering any medication. This is particularly important with new or rarely used drugs.

SECOND EDITION

Printed in the United States of America

Mosby, Inc.
11830 Westline Industrial Drive
St. Louis, Missouri 63146

ISBN 0-8151-8241-4
00 / 9 8 7 6 5 4

Contributors

Catherine L. Headrick, MS, RN
Clinical Nurse Specialist, PICU
Children's Medical Center of Dallas
Dallas, Texas
Chapter 4

Adele A. Large, MSN, RN, CCRN
Case Manager, Medicine
University of Pittsburgh Medical Center
Pittsburgh, Pennsylvania
Chapters 2, 5, 6, 7

Edith McCarter Randall, MS, RN, CS
Cardiovascular/Critical Care Clinical Nurse Specialist
St. Luke's Medical Center
Phoenix, Arizona
Chapters 2, 5, 6, 7

Sharon L. Roberts, PhD, RN, FAAN
Professor, Department of Nursing
California State University—Long Beach
Long Beach, California
Chapter 3

Kerri Schneider, MSN, RN, CCRN
Staff RN/Intensive Care
St. Mary's Medical Center
Racine, Wisconsin
Adjunct Clinical Instructor, Nursing
Alverno College
Milwaukee, Wisconsin
Chapters 2, 5, 6, 7

Susan B. Stillwell, MSN, RN
Adjunct Faculty
Ursuline College Division of Nursing
Pepper Pike, Ohio
Chapters 1, 2, 7, 8, Appendices

Linda G. Waite, MN, RN, CCRN
Clinical Nurse Specialist
Fairview Southdale Hospital
Edina, Minnesota
Chapters 2, 5, 7

Marla J. Weston, MS, RN, CCRN
Director/Patient Care Systems
Samaritan Health System
Mesa, Arizona
Chapters 2, 5, 7

Acknowledgments for Previous Contributions

Bonnie M. Cegles, MS, RN, CCRN

Kerry H. Cheever, MSN, RN, CCRN, CEN

Kathie Clarke, MSN, RN, CVNS, CCRN

Colleen Counsell, MSN, RN, CCRN

Mary Ann Cammy House, MSN, RN, CCRN, CS

Dianne Lepley-Frey, MS, RN, CCRN

Ronald J. Lynch, MSN, RN, CCRN

Patricia A. Moloney-Harmon, MS, RN, CCRN

Virginia Prendergast, MSN, RN, CNRN

Cathy H. Rosenthal, MN, RN, CCRN

Laura A. Talbot, PhD, RNC

Reviewers

Alinthia Allwood-Gallagher, MA, RN, CCRN, CNAA
Montefiore Medical Center
Bronx, New York

Sara Angermuller, MEd, MSN, RN, CCRN, CEN, CNRN
Columbus College
Columbus, Georgia

Nancy Bittner, MSN, RN, CCRN
Regis College, Weston, Massachusetts
Norwood Hospital, Norwood, Massachusetts

Nicolee Fode, MS, RN
Mayo Clinic
Rochester, Minnesota

Ann Costello Galligan, EdD, RN, CS
Boston Children's Services
Boston, Massachusetts

Cindy Hermey, MN, RN, CCRN
Oconee Memorial Hospital
Seneca, South Carolina

Rosemary Hoffman, MSN, RN
University of Pittsburgh School of Nursing
Pittsburgh, Pennsylvania

Susan Ann Kaiser, BSN, RN, CCRN
Georgetown University Hospital
Washington, District of Columbia

Debbie Lammert, MSN, RN, CCRN-P
St. Francis Hospital
Tulsa, Oklahoma

Barbara McLean, MN, RN, CCRN
Nell Hodgson Woodruff School of Nursing, Emory University
Emory University School of Medicine
Atlanta, Georgia

Patricia Murphy, EdD, RN, CCRN, CRRN
Health Force
Danvers, Massachusetts

Gael Taylor, MSN, RN, CCRN, CS
James A. Haley Veteran's Hospital
Tampa, Florida

Joy Thompson, MSN-R, RN, CCRN
St. Louis University Health Sciences Center
St. Louis, Missouri

Preface

Mosby's Critical Care Nursing Reference was developed to provide the nurse clinician with a resource for accessing information about the acute care management of a patient hospitalized in the adult critical care unit. The reference is not intended to be a critical care textbook or a procedure manual and assumes that the clinician is familiar with critical care technology and the pathophysiology associated with life-threatening illness.

The second edition features the same general aspects as the first edition; however, the chapters have been reorganized, information has been updated, and additions have been made. Critical Care Patient Assessment Guides includes a figure on physiological changes in the elderly; the Critically Ill Patient has been expanded to include Acute Pain, Oxygenation in the Critically Ill, and Transport of the Critically Ill Patient. In addition, the section on Septic Shock includes the manifestations of SIRS, sepsis, and septic shock. Signal averaged electrocardiography, transesophageal echocardiography, and laparoscopy are additional diagnostic tests, and additional therapeutic modalities include transjugular intrahepatic portosystemic shunt, and lung, pancreas, and liver transplantation. A section has also been devoted to Sedation as well as Neuromuscular Blockade.

Mosby's Critical Care Nursing Reference has retained, as a separate chapter, Behavioral Manifestations in the Critically Ill Patient. This provides easy access to the information and reduces the redundancy of listing this information with every disorder, since any of these manifestations can occur regardless of the medical diagnosis. Thus the absence of the psychological component within Chapter 2 should not be mistaken for a lack of nursing care.

The pediatric component has been expanded and includes the assessment and management of pain in the child. Care of the Child in the Adult ICU remains a unique chapter and is more like a "minibook" of caring for the pediatric patient in that it covers a variety of topics and practical hints in approaching the child in the adult ICU.

Other tools that have continued to make this reference useful include the chapter on Emergency Drugs in the Adult, ACLS Algorithms, Organ Donation Guidelines, Cardiopulmonary Formulas, and Drug Dosage Charts and Conversion Factors.

Novice critical care nurses, students, and seasoned nurses who "float" to various critical care units will find the second edition of *Mosby's Critical Care Nursing Reference* a valuable resource.

Susan B. Stillwell

No
difficulty —————— Extreme
breathing   difficulty
                       breathing

No ——————————— Intolerable
pain   pain

Sample visual analogue scales. Patient places an X on the
licates the severity of the symptom.

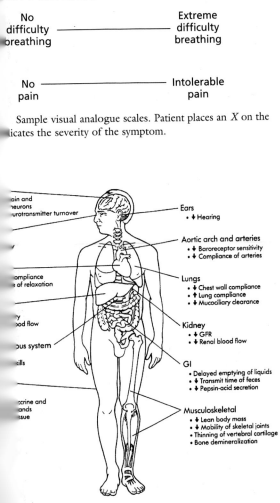

Physiological changes that occur with aging (MEOS,
nzyme oxidative system). (From Thelan LA et al: *Critical
diagnosis and management,* ed 2, St Louis, 1994, Mosby.)

Table of Contents

Critical Care
Assessment

Figure 1-1
line that in

Brain
• ↓ In size of
   number c
• Changes in

Eyes
• ↓ Visual acu

Heart
• ↓ Ventricula
• Prolonged ro

Liver
• ↓ MEOS acti
• ↓ Total liver

Peripheral ner
• ↑ Tremor
• ↓ Fine motor

Integumentar
• ↓ SQ tissue
• ↓ Number of
   sebaceous
• ↓ Connective
• ↓ Turgor

PATIENT ASSESSMENT GUIDES

Analyzing a Symptom

A positive finding can be analyzed
It is equally important to obtain p
tion about the patient's health stat
Location: Site, including any radiat
Timing: Onset, progression, and d
Setting: Place the symptom began
Quality: Characteristics or propert
Quantity: Degree of symptom—a
Alleviating factors: Factors that in
   symptom
Aggravating factors: Factors that
Associated factors: Concomitant s

Self-Report Scales

A visual analogue scale or a modifi
instruments that can be used to
such as pain and dyspnea (Figure

Head-to-Toe Survey

When a critically ill patient is adi
assessment should be performed
hours thereafter. A more frequ
detailed assessment may be n
patient's clinical disorder and/o
dition. Keep in mind the physiol
occur with aging (Figure 1-2).

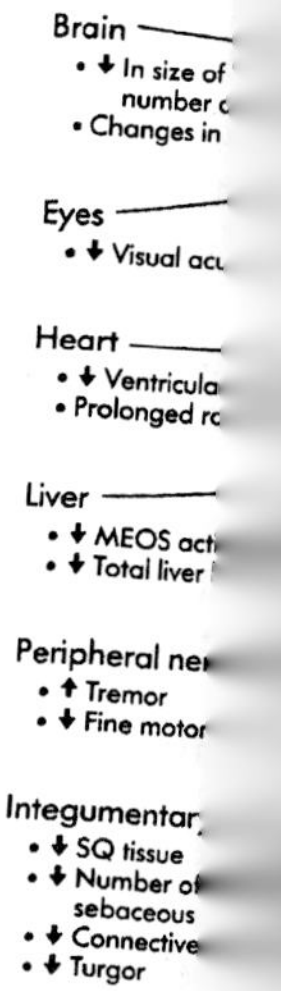

Figure 1-2
Microsomal
care nursing

Table of Contents

CHAPTER 1

Critical Care Patient Assessment Guides

PATIENT ASSESSMENT GUIDES

Analyzing a Symptom

A positive finding can be analyzed using the following guide. It is equally important to obtain pertinent negative information about the patient's health status.

Location: Site, including any radiation of the symptom

Timing: Onset, progression, and duration of the symptom

Setting: Place the symptom began

Quality: Characteristics or properties of the symptom

Quantity: Degree of symptom—amount, extent, and size

Alleviating factors: Factors that improve/relieve the symptom

Aggravating factors: Factors that make the symptom worse

Associated factors: Concomitant symptoms

Self-Report Scales

A visual analogue scale or a modified Borg Scale are self-report instruments that can be used to assess subjective sensations such as pain and dyspnea (Figure 1-1 and box on p. 3).

Head-to-Toe Survey

When a critically ill patient is admitted to the unit, a routine assessment should be performed and repeated at least every 4 hours thereafter. A more frequent and more selective or detailed assessment may be necessary, depending on the patient's clinical disorder and/or a change in his or her condition. Keep in mind the physiological changes that normally occur with aging (Figure 1-2).

No
difficulty ———————— difficulty
breathing

Extreme
difficulty
breathing

No ———————— Intolerable
pain

Intolerable
pain

Figure 1-1   Sample visual analogue scales. Patient places an X on the
line that indicates the severity of the symptom.

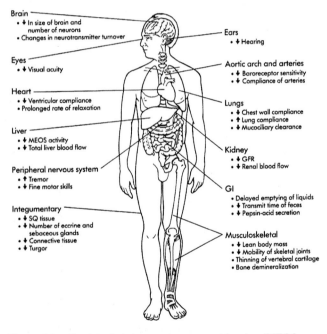

Brain
• ↓ In size of brain and
  number of neurons
• Changes in neurotransmitter turnover

Eyes
• ↓ Visual acuity

Heart
• ↓ Ventricular compliance
• Prolonged rate of relaxation

Liver
• ↓ MEOS activity
• ↓ Total liver blood flow

Peripheral nervous system
• ↑ Tremor
• ↓ Fine motor skills

Integumentary
• ↓ SQ tissue
• ↓ Number of eccrine and
  sebaceous glands
• ↓ Connective tissue
• ↓ Turgor

Ears
• ↓ Hearing

Aortic arch and arteries
• ↓ Baroreceptor sensitivity
• ↓ Compliance of arteries

Lungs
• ↓ Chest wall compliance
• ↑ Lung compliance
• ↓ Mucociliary clearance

Kidney
• ↓ GFR
• ↓ Renal blood flow

GI
• Delayed emptying of liquids
• ↓ Transmit time of feces
• ↓ Pepsin-acid secretion

Musculoskeletal
• ↓ Lean body mass
• ↓ Mobility of skeletal joints
• Thinning of vertebral cartilage
• Bone demineralization

Figure 1-2   Physiological changes that occur with aging (MEOS,
Microsomal enzyme oxidative system). (From Thelan LA et al: *Critical
care nursing: diagnosis and management,* ed 2, St Louis, 1994, Mosby.)

Modified Borg Scale

0	None/nothing at all
0.5	Very, very _____* (just noticeable)
1	Very _____
2	_____
3	Moderate
4	Somewhat severe
5	Severe
6	
7	Very severe
8	
9	Very, very severe (almost maximal)
10	Maximal

*Descriptors such as mild, weak, or slight can be inserted to assess symptoms such as pain, exertion, or breathlessness. Patients rate the symptom on a scale of 1 to 10 according to the descriptor that best indicates the severity of the symptom.
Modified from Borg GAV: Psychological bases of perceived exertion, *Med Sci Sports Exercise* 14(5):377-381, 1982.

Neurological Assessment

Level of consciousness (LOC)

Note the patient's state of wakefulness and awareness. First, observe the patient for spontaneous activity; if none is noted, verbally stimulate the patient. If the patient is unresponsive to verbal stimuli, use noxious stimuli such as applying pressure to the nail bed, pinching the trapezius muscle, or pinching the inner aspect of the arm or thigh. Avoid rubbing the sternum with knuckles, applying pressure to the supraorbital area, and pinching the nipples or testicles.

The Glasgow coma scale (GCS) is a tool for assessing consciousness (Table 1-1). The best or highest response is recorded for the purpose of assessing the degree of altered consciousness. If a patient's abilities cannot be evaluated, a notation of the condition should be documented, and the subscore should be labeled untestable.

Pupillary reaction and reflexes

Check position, size, shape, and response of the pupils. Photophobia may be associated with increased intracranial pressure or meningeal irritation. No direct pupillary response will occur in a blind eye; however, a consensual response can

TABLE 1-1 Glasgow Coma Scale

Ability	Response	Score*
Best eye response	Spontaneously (as nurse approaches)	4
	To verbal stimulus (nurse speaks/shouts)	3
	To painful stimulus (pressure on nail bed)	2
	No response to painful stimulus	1
Best motor response	Obeys simple command	6
	Localizes pain (locates and attempts to remove pain source)	5
	Withdrawal (attempts to withdraw from pain source)	4
	Flexion (Figure 1-3)	3
	Extension (Figure 1-3)	2
	No response to painful stimulus	1
Best verbal response	Oriented to time, person, place	5
	Confused, but able to converse	4
	Inappropriate words—makes little or no sense; words are recognizable	3
	Incomprehensible sounds—groans or moans; words are not recognizable	2
	No verbal response	1

*Possible score ranges between 3 and 15. 15 = alert and oriented; less than 8 = coma.

occur in the blind eye when the light is shined in the normal eye. Pinpoint pupils can result from miotic drugs, opiate drugs, or a pontine hemorrhage. Dilated pupils may result from use of cycloplegic drugs (atropine) or pressure on cranial nerve III (e.g., from a tumor or clot). Fixed pupils may be the result of barbiturate coma or hypothermia. Irregularly shaped pupils may occur as a result of cataract surgery.
Position: Pupils should be midposition.
Size: Note size in millimeters (Figure 1-4).
Shape: Pupils are normally round.
Direct light reflex: The tested pupil should constrict briskly.

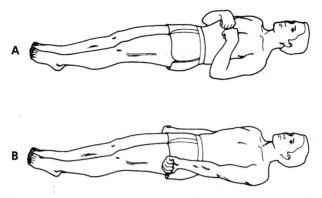

Figure 1-3   Flexion and extension. **A,** Flexion or decorticate rigidity.
B, Extension or decerebrate rigidity. (From Sheehy SB: *Mosby's manual of emergency care*, ed 4, St Louis, 1994, Mosby.)

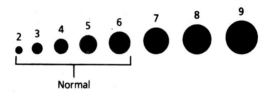

Normal

Figure 1-4   Pupil gauge in millimeters.

Consensual light reflex: Nontested pupil constricts as light is
    shined in other eye.
Accommodation: Pupils constrict and eyes converge as the
    patient focuses on an object moved toward the nose.
Corneal reflex: An absent reflex (lack of blinking or eyelid
    closure) indicates trigeminal or facial nerve damage,
    necessitating eye protection with artificial tears and eye
    shields.

Cranial nerve assessment
Table 1-2 lists the cranial nerves and components to test.

Motor function
Observe the patient's resting posture and note any spontaneous or involuntary movement; also note any rigidity, spasticity, and flaccidity. Test gross muscle strength by assessing
hand grasp and testing dorsiflexion and plantar flexion of the

TABLE 1-2   Cranial Nerves

Nerve	Evaluate
Olfactory (I)	Sense of smell
Optic (II)	Vision: visual fields and acuity
Oculomotor (III), trochlear (IV), and abducens (VI)	Pupil reactions, EOMs: III—evaluate eye movement up and outward, down and outward, and up and inward; IV—evaluate eye movement down and inward; VI—evaluate eye movement outward
Trigeminal (V)	Sensation on both sides of face, opening and closing of jaw, corneal reflex
Facial (VII)	Facial muscle movement: eye brows, smile, frown, eyelid closing; taste sensation
Acoustic (VIII)	Hearing
Glossopharyngeal (IX), vagus (X)	Gag reflex, swallowing, soft palate elevation
Spinal accessory (XI)	Shoulder shrug and head movement
Hypoglossal (XII)	Tongue position, movement, and strength

lower extremities. Compare both sides of the body and note any lateralizing signs (unilateral deterioration). A quick screening for weakness would include lifting the patient's arms off the bed and releasing them simultaneously. Observe for arm drifting, which indicates a weakness on one side of the body. A hemiparetic side falls more quickly and limply than the normal side.

Sensory function

A gross evaluation of sensory function would include light touch to the forehead, cheeks, hands, lower arms, abdomen, lower legs, and feet. Other types of sensations can be used (e.g., pain, heat/cold, vibration, position changes, and deep pressure pain). Compare both sides of the body.

Spinal cord assessment

The motor strength of each muscle group should be evaluated in patients with spinal cord dysfunction (Table 1-3). A 5-point system can be used to assess overall muscle strength

TABLE 1-3   Spinal Cord Assessment

Level of innervation	Function	Reflex
C4	Neck movement, diaphragmatic breathing	
C5	Abduction of the shoulder	Biceps (C5)
C5-6	Elbow flexion	Brachioradialis (C6)
C7-8	Elbow extension	Triceps (C7)
C6,7,8	Wrist dorsiflexion	
C8	Hand grip	
C6-8,T1	Finger extension and flexion	
L2-4	Hip flexion	
L4,5,S1	Hip extension	
L2-4	Knee extension	
L4,5-S1	Knee flexion	Patellar (L4)
L5	Dorsiflexion of the foot	
S1	Plantar flexion of the foot	

TABLE 1-4   Muscle Strength Scale

Description	Score
Normal power or muscle strength in extremities	5
Weak extremities, but patient can overcome resistance applied by examiner	4
Patient can overcome gravity (can lift extremities) but cannot overcome resistance applied by examiner	3
Weak muscle contraction, but not enough to overcome gravity (movement, but cannot lift extremities)	2
Palpable or visible muscle flicker or twitch, but no movement	1
No response to stimulus, complete paralysis	0

of the extremities (Table 1-4). A less complex system such as 0 = absent, 1 = weak, and 2 = strong may be used.

Specific dermatomal areas (Figure 1-5) should be evaluated in the patient with a spinal cord dysfunction. Terms used to describe sensory dysfunction can be found on p. 8.

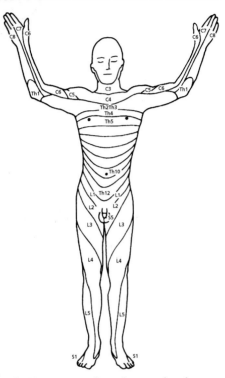

The dermatomes from the anterior view.

Figure 1-5 Dermatomes. Landmarks are: clavicle—C4; deltoid—C5; nipples—T4; navel—T10; knee—L3-L4; great toe—L5; little toe—S1; sole of foot—S1.

Analgesia: Loss of pain
Anesthesia: Complete loss of sensation
Dysesthesia: Impaired sensation
Hyperesthesia: Increased sensation
Hypesthesia: Decreased sensation
Paresthesia: Burning, tingling sensation

Peripheral neurovascular assessment

Peripheral nerves and circulation should be evaluated in patients with injury (e.g., fractures, burns) to upper or lower

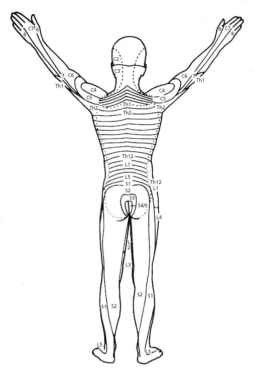

The dermatomes from the posterior view.

Figure 1-5 (cont'd)   Dermatomes. Landmarks are: clavicle—C4; deltoid—C5; nipples—T4; navel—T10; knee—L3-L4; great toe—L5; little toe—S1; sole of foot—S1. (From Thelan LA et al: *Critical care nursing: diagnosis and management,* ed 2, St Louis, 1994, Mosby.)

extremities. Both sensory and motor function of the ulnar, radial, median, and peroneal nerves should be assessed.

5 Ps: Pain, paresthesia, paralysis, pulse, and pallor.

Circulation: Check presence and amplitude of pulses, capillary refill, and skin temperature.

Movement: Upper extremities—have patient hyperextend the thumb or wrist (radial), oppose the thumb and little finger (median), and abduct all fingers (ulnar).

Lower extremities: have patient dorsiflex the foot (peroneal) and plantarflex the foot (tibial).

Sensation: Upper extremities—use a pin to prick the webbed space between the thumb and index finger (radial), distal fat pad of small finger (ulnar), and distal fat pad of index/middle finger (median).

Lower extremities: use a pin to prick the dorsal surface of the foot near the webbed space between the great and second toes.

Reflexes

Abnormal reflexes may be early signs of upper motor neuron disease, lower motor neuron disease, or disease of the afferent sensory component of muscles.

Deep tendon reflexes: Jaw, biceps, brachioradialis, triceps, patellar, and achilles reflexes can be assessed on a scale from 0 to 4+ (Table 1-5).

Pathological reflexes: Positive Babinski sign—great toe pointing upward (extension) and fanning of the other toes. Grasp reflex—patient does not release an object that has been placed in the patient's hand. Snout reflex—pursing of lips when the mouth is tapped above or below the midline.

Brainstem function

An alteration in brainstem function can affect the state of consciousness, respiratory, circulatory, and vasomotor activities, and a number of reflexes.

DERM mnemonic: The mnemonic device *DERM* can be used to assess brainstem functioning; *D* = Depth of coma; *E* = Eye assessment; *R* = Respiration assessment; *M* = Movement assessment (Table 1-6).

Oculocephalic reflex—doll's eye maneuver: Tested in the comatose patient to assess brainstem function. Positive

TABLE 1-5   Scale for Deep Tendon Reflexes

Score	Description
0	Absent
1+	Diminished
2+	Normal
3+	Increased, more brisk than average
4+	Hyperactive, clonus

TABLE 1-6   Assessing Brainstem Function Using the DERM Mnemonic

Brainstem	Herniation levels	D = Depth of coma	E = Eyes	R = Respirations	M = Motor function	Posturing
	None	Aware, alert, oriented	Equal and reactive	Eupnea	Normal	None
	Thalamus	Painful stimulus causes nonpurposeful response	Small; react to light	Cheyne-Stokes respirations	Hyperactive deep tendon reflexes	Abnormal flexion (decorticate)
	Midbrain	Painful stimulus causes nonpurposeful response	Midpoint to dilated; fixed; no reaction to light	Central neurogenic breathing	Decreased deep tendon reflexes	Abnormal extension (decerebrate)
	Pons and cerebellum	Painful stimulus causes no response	Pinpoint; fixed; no reaction to light	Biot's respirations	Flaccid	No tone
	Medulla	Painful stimulus causes no response	Midpoint to dilated; fixed; no reaction to light	Ataxia; apneusis	Flaccid	No tone

From Budassi SA, Barber J: *Mosby's manual of emergency care*, ed 3, St Louis, 1989, Mosby.

doll's eyes sign (both eyes move in the direction opposite to the head rotation) is normal and indicates an intact brainstem. If this response is absent, the patient's airway may not be protected by gag and cough reflexes.

Oculovestibular reflex—caloric testing: Usually tested in the comatose patient to assess brainstem function. With an intact brainstem, eyes deviate with nystagmus toward the ear that is irrigated with cold water. An absent reflex (both eyes remain fixed in midline position) may indicate impending brain death. Neuromuscular blocking agents, barbiturates, and antibiotic agents can inhibit this reflex.

Determining brain death

Reversible conditions such as sedation, neuromuscular blockade, shock, hypothermia, and metabolic imbalances must be excluded. The clinical examination is most important; however, laboratory tests may be used in conjunction with the clinical examination to confirm brain death. The absence of recordable brain waves on the electroencephalogram (EEG) is associated with brain death. However, EEGs may produce false positive and false negative results. A cerebral blood flow (CBF) study is more useful than the EEG. The absence of cerebral circulation is diagnostic of brain death regardless of cause.

Clinical examination: The following findings must be present:
- Patient must be comatose.
- Pupils must be nonreactive.
- Corneal reflex must be absent.
- Gag reflex must be absent.
- Cough reflex must be absent.
- Oculocephalic reflex must be absent.
- Oculovestibular reflex must be absent.
- Spontaneous respirations must be absent. (See Apnea testing.)

Apnea testing: To test for the presence of apnea, 100% oxygen is administered to the patient for 10 to 20 minutes. The ventilator is withdrawn while the patient receives passive flow of 100% oxygen. Lack of spontaneous respirations in the presence of adequate carbon dioxide stimulus ($Paco_2$ >60 mm Hg or >20 mm Hg from baseline and respiratory acidosis) indicates that the brainstem is nonfunctioning.

Incisions, drainage, and equipment

Assess the condition of incisional sites from neurosurgical surgeries and procedures. Assess for the presence of cerebral spinal fluid drainage (e.g., rhinorrhea or otorrhea). Assess the ventriculostomy site and other equipment and devices for proper functioning and complications.

Intracranial monitoring

Obtain ICP and calculate CPP. (See ICP monitoring on p. 511 and formula on p. 757.)

Pulmonary Assessment

Respirations

Determine respiratory rate and rhythm (Figure 1-6). Assess chest for depth of respirations, paradoxical movement, and symmetry of respirations. Note use of accessory muscles, nasal flaring, tracheal deviation, and cough.

Breath sounds

Auscultate all lung fields (Figures 1-7 and 1-8 for location of lobes and normal breath sounds).

Bronchial sounds: High-pitched and normally heard over the trachea. Timing includes an inspiration phase less than the expiration phase. If heard in lung fields, this usually indicates consolidation.

Vesicular sounds: Low-pitched and normally heard in the periphery of the lungs. Timing includes an inspiration phase greater than the expiration phase.

Bronchovesicular sounds: Medium-pitched, with a muffled quality. Timing includes an inspiration phase equal to the expiration phase.

Adventitious sounds

Assess breath and voice sounds.

Crackles: Discontinuous sounds heard during inspiration that can be classified as "fine" (similar to rubbing strands of hair together next to the ear) or "coarse" (bubbling quality similar to carbonated soda). Generally not cleared with coughing.

Wheezes: High-pitched sounds that may be heard during inspiration or expiration.

Rhonchi: Low, coarse sounds of a "snoring" quality. Generally clears with coughing.

Pleural friction rub: Grating, harsh sound, located in an area of intense chest wall pain.

Pattern		Description
Eupnea		Rhythm is smooth and even with expiration longer than inspiration.
Tachypnea		Rapid superficial breathing; regular or irregular rhythm.
Bradypnea		Slow respiratory rate; deeper than usual depth; regular rhythm.
Apnea		Cessation of breathing.
Hyperpnea		Increased depth of respiration with a normal to increased rate and regular rhythm.
Cheyne-Stokes respiration		Periodic breathing associated with periods of apnea, alternating regularly with a series of respiratory cycles; the respiratory cycle gradually increases, then decreases in rate and depth.
Ataxic breathing		Periods of apnea alternating irregularly with a series of shallow breaths of equal depth.
Kussmaul's respiration		Deep regular sighing respirations with an increase in respiratory rate.
Apneusis		Long, gasping inspiratory phase followed by a short, inadequate expiratory phase.
Obstructed breathing		Long, ineffective expiratory phase with shallow, increased respirations.

Figure 1-6 Respiratory patterns. (Modified from Talbot L, Meyers-Marquardt M: *Pocket guide to critical care assessment*, ed 2, St Louis, 1993, Mosby.)

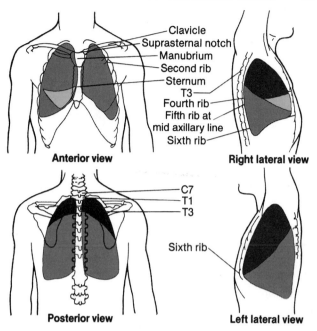

Figure 1-7   Location of lobes of the lung using anatomical landmarks. (From Talbot J, Meyers-Marquardt M: *Pocket guide to critical care assessment,* ed 2, St Louis, 1993, Mosby.)

Bronchophony: Spoken words (have patient say "99") that are heard clearly and distinctly are indicative of lung consolidation.

Whispered pectoriloguy: Extreme bronchophony, such that a voice sound (have patient whisper "99") is heard clearly and distinctly.

Egophony: Spoken word assumes a nasal quality (have patient say "E"; it is heard as "A") indicative of consolidation or pleural effusion.

Artificial airway

Check placement and patency of artificial airway (e.g., oral/nasal airway or endotracheal tube or tracheostomy). Determine cuff pressure of endotracheal tube or tracheostomy.

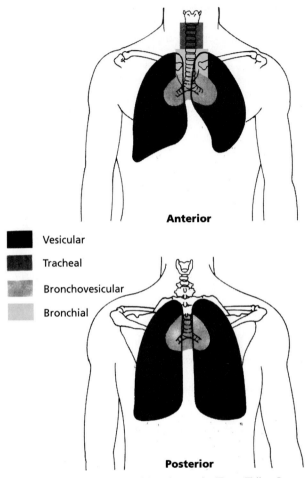

Figure 1-8 Location of normal breath sounds. (From Talbot L, Meyers-Marquardt M: *Pocket guide to critical care assessment,* ed 2, St Louis, 1993, Mosby.)

Oxygenation/ventilation

Check the oxygen delivery system, ventilator settings, and alarms. Obtain oxygen saturation and carbon dioxide readings.

Chest drainage

Assess system for proper functioning and note the amount, color, and character of chest drainage.

Oxygenation calculations

Monitor relevant parameters. (See Cardiopulmonary parameters, p. 751.)

Cardiovascular Assessment

Heart rate and rhythm

Note monitor lead placement and obtain a rhythm strip to determine rate and rhythm. (See Rhythm strip analysis, p. 499.)

Integument

Note color, temperature, and moisture. Check anterior chest wall for capillary refill (>3 sec reflects poor tissue perfusion). Evaluate severity of edema (Table 1-7).

Central venous pressure (CVP)

Check neck veins to estimate CVP (Figure 1-9). Note presence of Kussmaul's sign (level of pulsation in internal jugular increases on inspiration). If right ventricular failure is suspected, test hepatojugular reflex (HJR) by applying firm pressure with the palm of the hand to the upper quadrant of the patient's abdomen for 30 to 60 seconds. An increase in venous level >3 cm = positive HJR.

Pulses

Check pulses bilaterally *except* for carotids. Note rate, rhythm, equality, and amplitude. Figure 1-10 shows variations in arterial pulses. The following scale can be used to describe pulses: 0 = absent, +1 = weak, +2 = normal, +3 = bounding.

TABLE 1-7   Grading Scale for Edema

Depth of pitting edema	Score
<¼ in	+1
¼-½ in	+2
½-1 in	+3
>1 in	+4

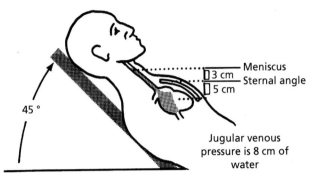

Figure 1-9   Estimation of central venous pressure. Identify the highest level of pulsations in the internal jugular vein (meniscus). Determine the vertical distance between the sternal angle and meniscus. Add that distance to the constant 5 cm (sternal angle is 5 cm above mid-RA level).

Heart sounds
Systematically auscultate each area of the precordium (Figure 1-11), concentrating on one component of the cardiac cycle at a time. The bell of the stethoscope accentuates lower frequency sounds (e.g., S_3, S_4). The diaphragm of the stethoscope accentuates high-pitched sounds (e.g., S_1, S_2). Figure 1-12 illustrates heart sounds in relation to electrocardiogram (ECG). Table 1-8 lists the various heart sounds and differentiating components.

Heart murmurs
Describe murmurs according to location (e.g., distance from midsternal, midclavicular, or axillary lines); radiation—where the sound is transmitted; loudness—grades I to VI (Table 1-9); pitch—high or low; shape—crescendo, decrescendo, crescendo-decrescendo, plateau; and quality—harsh, rumbling, musical, blowing.

Blood pressure
Assess blood pressure on both arms. Use a blood pressure cuff 20% wider than the diameter of the limb to avoid false high or low pressures.

AUSCULTATORY GAP
Determine the presence of an auscultatory gap (Figure 1-13).

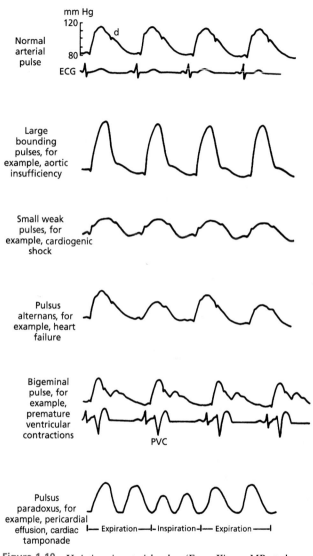

Figure 1-10   Variations in arterial pulse. (From Kinney MR et al: *Comprehensive cardiac care,* ed 8, St Louis, 1995, Mosby.)

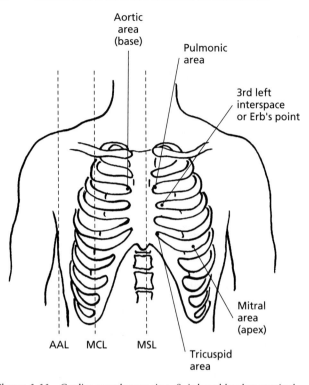

Figure 1-11 Cardiac auscultatory sites. S$_1$ is heard loudest at mitral and tricuspid areas. S$_2$ is heard loudest at aortic and pulmonic areas. S$_3$ and S$_4$ are heard best at the mitral area. *AAL,* Anterior axillary line; *MCL,* midclavicular line; *MSL,* midsternal line.

PULSUS PARADOXUS

Determine the presence of pulsus paradoxus. Slowly deflate the BP cuff (1 mm Hg per respiratory cycle); note when the first sound is heard, which will be on expiration. Note when sounds begin again and are heard continuously (during inspiration and expiration). If the difference between the first sound and the continuous sound is >10 mm Hg, pulsus paradoxus is present.

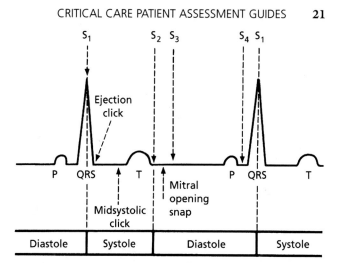

Figure 1-12   Heart sounds in relation to the ECG.

TABLE 1-8   Differentiating Heart Sounds

Heart sound	Best area to auscultate	Timing
S_1	Apex	Systole
S_2	Base	Diastole
S_3	Apex, LSB	Early diastole, after S_2
S_4	Apex, LSB	Late diastole, before S_1
Split S_1	4ICS, LSB	Systole
Split S_2	2ICS, LSB	End of systole
Aortic ejection sound	2ICS, RSB; apex	Early systole
Pulmonic ejection sound	2ICS, LSB	Early systole
Midsystolic click	Apex	Mid to late systole
Opening snap	Lower LSB, 4ICS	Early diastole
Pericardial friction rub	Loudest along LSB	Systole and diastole

ICS, Intercostal space; LSB, left sternal border; RSB, right sternal border.

TABLE 1-9 Murmur Grading Scale

Grade	Description
I/VI	Faint, barely audible
II/VI	Quiet, heard immediately on auscultation
III/VI	Moderately loud, no thrill
IV/VI	Loud, thrill
V/VI	Very loud, requires a stethoscope; thrill present
VI/VI	Same as V/VI but can be heard with stethoscope off the chest

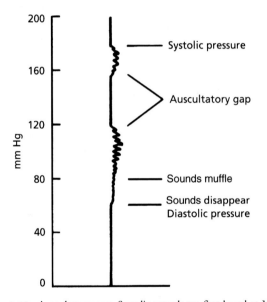

Figure 1-13 Auscultatory gap. Systolic sounds are first heard at 180 mm Hg. They disappear at 160 mm Hg and reappear at 120 mm Hg; the silent interval is known as the *auscultatory gap*. Korotkoff sounds muffle at 80 mm Hg and disappear at 60 mm Hg. Blood pressure is recorded at 180/80/60 with auscultatory gap. If the cuff was inflated to 150 mm Hg, the reading may have been interpreted as normotensive. (From Kinney MR et al: *Comprehensive cardiac care,* ed 8, St Louis, 1995, Mosby.)

Hemodynamic monitoring

Obtain readings and calculate cardiopulmonary parameters. (See Hemodynamic monitoring on pp. 483, 492, 518 and Cardiopulmonary formulas on p. 751.)

Pacemaker

Validate settings. Assess for failure to capture and failure to sense. Assess what percentage of the patient's rhythm is paced.

Gastrointestinal Assessment

Bowel sounds

Auscultate all quadrants (Figure 1-14).

Absent sounds: May be associated with intestinal obstruction, paralytic ileus, or peritonitis. Listen for a least 5 minutes.

Intensified or gurgling sounds: May be associated with early intestinal obstruction, increased peristalsis, or diarrhea.

Abdomen

Note size, shape, and symmetry. Measure abdominal girth. Palpate for tenderness or masses.

Bowel elimination

Note characteristics of stool; guaiac stool for occult blood.

Nasogastric tube

Check placement, patency, drainage, and amount of suction. Check pH of gastric secretions, guaiac secretions. If the NG tube is used for enteral feeding, check placement and residual. Note skin condition at tube insertion site.

Drains

Note type and location of drain. Check for proper functioning of drainage system and the characteristics and amount of drainage. Assess skin condition.

Incisions and stomas

Assess color, approximation and presence of any swelling or drainage of incisions. Assess color and moisture of stoma, note if stoma is flush, retracted or prolapsed. Assess condition of periostomal skin.

Genitourinary Assessment

Genitalia

Check external genitalia for any drainage, inflammation, or lesions.

Fluid status

Check weight daily. An increase of 0.5 kg/day suggests fluid retention. Measure I & O; 1 L fluid ~1 kg of body weight. Table 1-10 lists findings associated with volume excess or deficit.

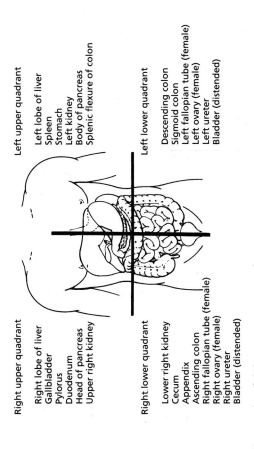

Right upper quadrant

Right lobe of liver
Gallbladder
Pylorus
Duodenum
Head of pancreas
Upper right kidney

Left upper quadrant

Left lobe of liver
Spleen
Stomach
Left kidney
Body of pancreas
Splenic flexure of colon

Right lower quadrant

Lower right kidney
Cecum
Appendix
Ascending colon
Right fallopian tube (female)
Right ovary (female)
Right ureter
Bladder (distended)

Left lower quadrant

Descending colon
Sigmoid colon
Left fallopian tube (female)
Left ovary (female)
Left ureter
Bladder (distended)

Figure 1-14   Topography of abdomen.

TABLE 1-10 Signs and Symptoms Associated with Volume Disturbances

	Hypovolemia	Hypervolemia
Weight	Acute loss	Acute gain
Pulse	Decrease pulse pressure Tachycardia	Bounding
Blood pressure	Postural hypotension	Hypertension
Mucous membranes	Dry	Moist
Turgor	Decreased skin elasticity	Pitting edema
Peripheral veins	JVP flat when supine Slow filling hand veins	JVP elevated
Hemodynamics	CVP <2 mm Hg Decreased PAWP	CVP >6 mm Hg Increased PAWP
Other	Thirst Urine output <30 ml/hr	Cough Dyspnea Crackles S_3
Laboratory data	Increased hemoglobin Increased hematocrit Increased serum osmolality Increased specific gravity Increased BUN/ creatinine ratio	Decreased hemoglobin Decreased hematocrit Decreased serum osmolality Decreased specific gravity

JVP, Jugular venous pressure; CVP, central venous pressure; PAWP, pulmonary artery wedge pressure.

Bladder

Percuss the abdomen for bladder distention.

Urine

Identify type of urinary drainage tube and assess proper functioning. Measure urinary output. Note color and consistency.

Anuria: <100 ml/24 hr

Oliguria: 100 to 400 ml/24 hr

SCORING SYSTEMS FOR THE ICU PATIENT

Apache III

The Acute Physiology and Chronic Health Evaluation (APACHE III) is a prognostic scoring system[9] (see p. 746).

The score, which can range from 0 to 299, is determined from physiological values, age, and the presence of chronic illness. The APACHE III risk equation can be used to calculate a predicted risk of hospital mortality and takes into account the patient's APACHE III score, major disease category, and treatment location before the ICU admission.

Trauma Score

The trauma score (see p. 742) is a system for estimating the severity of patient injury.[4,5] The patient's LOC and cardiopulmonary function are assessed. A numerical value is assigned to each of the assessment parameters. The total score reflects the severity of the injury and a survival estimate for the patient can be projected from the score.

Therapeutic Intervention Scoring System (TISS)

TISS has been used to determine severity of illness, establish nurse/patient ratios, and assess current bed utilization and need.[8] Patient classification of severity of illness is based on points: class I, under 10 points; class II, 10 to 19 points; class III, 20 to 39 points; and class IV, 40 or more points. (See p. 743.)

It has been proposed that class IV patients receive a 1:1 nurse/patient ratio and that an accomplished critical care nurse should be capable of managing 40 to 50 patient TISS points.

REFERENCES

1. Albert P: Overview of the organ donation process, *Crit Care Nurs Clin North Am* 6(3):553-65, 1994.
2. Borg G: Psychophysical bases of perceived exertion, *Med Sci Sports Exercise* 14(5):377-381, 1982.
3. Budassi SA, Barber J: *Mosby's manual of emergency care,* ed 3, St Louis, 1989, Mosby.
4. Champion HR et al: Trauma score, *Crit Care Med* 9(9):672-676, 1981.
5. Champion HR, Gainer PS, Yackee E: A progress report on the trauma score in predicting a fatal outcome, *J Trauma* 26(10):927-931, 1986.
6. Daily E, Schroeder J: *Techniques in bedside hemodynamic monitoring,* St Louis, 1994, Mosby.
7. Guidelines for the determination of death: Report of the Medical Consultants in the Diagnosis of Death to the President's Commission for the Study of Ethical Problems in Medicine and Biomedical and Behavioral Research, *JAMA* 246:2184-2186, 1981.

8. Keene R, Cullen D: Therapeutic intervention scoring system: update 1983, *Crit Care Med* 11(1):1-3, 1983.
9. Knaus WA et al: APACHE III prognostic system, *Chest* 100:1619-1636, 1991.
10. Parrillo JE, Bone RC: *Critical care medicine: principles of diagnosis and management,* St Louis, 1995, Mosby.
11. Stillwell S, Randall E: *Pocket guide to cardiovascular care,* ed 2, St Louis, 1994, Mosby.
12. Talbot L, Meyers-Marquardt M: *Pocket guide to critical care assessment,* ed 2, St Louis, 1993, Mosby.
13. Teasdale G, Jennett B: Glasgow coma scale, *Lancet* 2:81-83, 1974.
14. Thelan LA et al: *Critical care nursing: diagnosis and management,* ed 2, St Louis, 1994, Mosby.

The Critically Ill Patient

Aspects of Nursing Common to All Critically Ill Patients

ELECTRICAL SAFETY

In the critical care environment, the increased complexity of technology has also increased the potential for patient injury from electrical shock. Electrical systems should be designed to provide a grounding system that protects the patient and staff from becoming part of an electrical circuit and to protect critical care patients, who are electrically sensitive, from current leakage that may disrupt the electrical conduction system of the heart.

Conductors of electricity include all metals (for example, copper, silver, and iron) and ionic fluids. Insulators, which are highly resistant to the flow of electricity, include such items as rubber, glass, plastic, cotton, and intact dry skin. A ground is a low-resistance electrical pathway that is used to return stray current to the ground and is an important concept in electrical safety.

▶ **Nursing Diagnosis:** Risk for injury: electrical shock

OUTCOME CRITERION
- Patient will not experience electrical shock.

INTERVENTIONS
1. Wear rubber gloves when handling uninsulated pacemaker wires or when adjusting pacemaker settings.
2. Place plastic caps or rubber sleeving over uninsulated wires and terminals.
3. Cover external pacemaker battery with a rubber glove.
4. Examine patient-owned equipment. Only battery-powered appliances should be allowed.

5. Inspect metal beds for adequate grounding.
6. Keep wet items (drinking water, saline, ice chips) off monitors and other electrical equipment.
7. Change wet bed linens and wipe up spills immediately.
8. Do not touch the patient and an electrical device simultaneously; touch the bed rails before touching the patient.
9. Observe the ECG tracing for 60-cycle interference, an indicator of current leakage. Replace patient cable or electrode pads. If these measures do not relieve the problem, identify and remove the offending equipment for repair.
10. Check all electrical equipment for a current safety inspection tag.
11. Inspect the plugs and cords of electrical devices because these parts are the most susceptible to damage. Plugs should be three-prong and damage-free; cord line should be free from frayed wires or cracked insulation. Remove a plug from an outlet by grasping the plug, not pulling on the cord.
12. Turn equipment off before unplugging it.
13. Avoid using extension cords and connectors that allow three-prong plugs to be used in two-prong outlets.
14. Report malfunctioning or damaged equipment to the biomedical engineering department. Dropped equipment should be serviced by the biomedical engineering department before use, since the equipment may malfunction without visible signs of damage.

FAMILY

The hospitalization of a family member can be very stressful and create specific needs for the family. If these needs go unmet, tension may mount, leading to major disorganization and ineffective coping. Although the critical care nurse intervenes to resolve life-threatening problems, a holistic approach to the patient, which includes the family, is essential to the well-being of the patient.

▶ **Nursing Diagnosis:**   Risk for altered family process
OUTCOME CRITERIA
• Family will state that their needs are met.
• Family will demonstrate adequate coping behaviors.
INTERVENTIONS
1. Introduce yourself to the family. Display competence in caring for their relative.
2. Provide continuity of caregivers whenever possible.

3. Approach the family with a relaxed and humanistic attitude and volunteer information frequently without waiting to be asked. Listen to their expressions of fear, anger, or anxiety. Avoid defensive retorts. Provide the family a time away from the bedside to ventilate their concerns. Answer questions honestly and provide facts frequently regarding their relative's condition. Anticipate repeating information and allowing time for them to digest the information during this crisis period.

4. Assess critical junctures or risk points that may impact family expectations and satisfaction (e.g., family expressing anger, patient awaiting surgery or near discharge).

5. Provide the family with written information about the unit policies and services available. Information should include the phone number of the unit as well as location of the waiting room.

6. Obtain the family contact phone number and contact the family spokesperson at least daily with information about the patient's condition and any changes in medical or nursing care.

7. Clarify the family's perception of their relative's illness and validate their understanding of the situation. Let them know the staff cares for their relative and that the best care is being given.

8. Individualize visiting hours; explain the equipment being used and why things are being done; assess family members' need to participate in their relative's care and allow as much participation as is reasonably possible. Be sensitive to the family's need to be left alone with their relative. Arrange equipment so that family members can touch their relative.

9. Reassure the family that they will be contacted if the relative's condition worsens.

10. Offer the family an opportunity to meet with the hospital chaplain or social worker.

11. Encourage the family to meet their own physical and personal needs, such as eating and sleeping.

ACUTE PAIN

Pain is a subjective and personal experience. Alert and awake patients can indicate if they are experiencing pain. However, nurses must be aware of the patients who are mechanically ventilated or who have an alteration in mental status and cannot vocalize or adequately indicate their pain. Careful pain assessment and evaluation of pain relief following the administration of analgesic agents as well as nonpharmacological therapies are critical. Patients have a right to have their pain controlled, and we have an ethical obligation to ensure successful pain management.

Critically ill patients can experience pain from their disease process or procedures such as chest tube removal or endotracheal suctioning. Other factors that can aggravate pain include anxiety or the inability to communicate. Pain can cause an increase in the sympathetic nervous system and in myocardial oxygen consumption. In addition, the metabolic-endocrine stress response is activated, which can possibly deplete energy substrates necessary for healing.

Risks of respiratory depression, addiction, tolerance, and physical dependence with narcotic administration exist. However, the patient should be treated individually; these concerns should not deter from the decision to medicate the patient. The incidence of addiction and respiratory depression as a result of narcotic use is less than 1% and physical dependence and tolerance on narcotics is unusual in short-term use.

Misperceptions of pharmacologic agents that do not relieve pain include neuromuscular blocking agents (e.g., vecuronium, tracrium) and sedatives (e.g., midazolam, propofol, versed). Patients who have pain and are receiving a neuromuscular blocking agent or sedative must receive an analgesic agent to control the pain.

▶ **Nursing Diagnosis:**   Pain
OUTCOME CRITERION
• Patient will communicate adequate pain relief.
INTERVENTIONS
1. Be alert to cues such as grimacing, groaning, grunting, sobbing, crying, irritability, withdrawing, or hostility that may signal pain in the critically ill.
2. Observe for sympathetic nervous system stimulation, which may signal pain in the critically ill patient (i.e., increased respiratory rate, increased heart rate, increased blood pressure, dilated pupils, and pallor). Note that some of these symptoms can also indicate other conditions such as hypoxia.
3. Ask direct questions as to the location, intensity, and quality of pain. Visual analogue scales, verbal rating scales,

and body diagrams can be used to monitor the patient's pain intensity in both intubated and nonintubated patients.

4. Assess the patient's pain medication history, since taking narcotics prior to the hospitalization may increase the patient's tolerance to narcotics, requiring a higher-than-average dose.

5. Note anesthetic agents used in the immediate postoperative patient. Enflurane, halothane, and isoflurane are short-acting and provide little analgesia postoperatively. If narcotics have been used, some residual analgesia may be present, however; check if any narcotic antagonists have been administered at the end of surgery.

6. Determine if the patient has any impaired renal or liver function, which could affect the uptake and removal of analgesic drugs.

7. Be aware that conditions such as myasthenia gravis and COPD may require that patients receive an initial reduction in narcotic dose.

8. Reduce or eliminate aggravating factors such as nausea and anxiety. Administer sedatives as ordered for anxiety and antiemetics for nausea. Provide comfort by positioning patient and readjusting various invasive tubes and equipment, as well as keeping the patient warm and dry.

9. Explain to the patient that preventing pain is easier than trying to reduce it once it becomes severe.

10. Assure the patient that addiction potential is negligible and explain that pain control/relief is beneficial and necessary for healing.

11. Collaborate with the physician regarding around-the-clock administration of analgesics since a steady state blood level is required for the drug to be continuously effective.

12. If patient controlled analgesia (PCA) is used, instruct the patient on its use.

13. Medicate the patient prior to procedures or treatments such as chest tube removal or insertion, coughing, and deep breathing.

14. Provide a calm and nurturing atmosphere; nonpharmacologic therapies such as progressive relaxation, music, or imagery may also be employed.

15. Be sensitive to the need for analgesics in the patient receiving neuromuscular blocking agents since neuromuscular blocking agents do not relieve pain.

16. Be sensitive to the need for analgesics in patients receiving sedatives since sedatives alone do not relieve pain and may increase the patient's sensitivity to pain.

17. Evaluate if the therapies have alleviated the pain; increase the frequency of assessment if the pain is poorly controlled. Collaborate with the physician to revise the pain management plan if pain is not adequately controlled. Evaluate the presence of adverse effects such as a respiratory rate that is less than 10/min.

18. See epidural analgesia—see p. 539.

INFECTION CONTROL

Critically ill patients are exposed to many factors in addition to their underlying illness that depress the immune system and lower the body's defenses. The patient's own organisms, as well as environmental sources of organisms or cross-contamination can cause infection. The first, second, and third lines of defense can be adversely affected by therapeutic interventions, thus placing the patient at risk for infection.

The patient's first line of defense includes epithelial surfaces and secretions that provide a barrier between the internal and external environments. Table 2-1 lists a patient's first line of defense and examples that interrupt the system.

The patient's second line of defense involves the inflammatory response, which occurs when the first line of defense fails, or as a result of the patient's condition (for example, cancer, myocardial infarction). The response can be localized (red, edematous, warm, painful) or systemic (fever, malaise, leukocytosis, neutrophilia). The inflammatory response always accompanies an infection; however, it can also occur without an infection (e.g., trauma, burns). Factors that impair the inflammatory response include stress and pharmacological agents such as corticosteroids, immunosuppressants, and aspirin.

The patient's third line of defense involves acquired immunity. Malnutrition, age, anesthesia, radiation, and chemotherapy can adversely affect the third line of defense.

▶ **Nursing Diagnoses:** Risk for infection; Risk for altered protection
OUTCOME CRITERIA
- Temperature 36.5° C (97.7° F) to 38° C (100.4° F)
- Absence of chills, diaphoresis
- Skin without redness and exudate

TABLE 2-1   First Line of Defense

Body system	Protective barrier	Conditions disrupting protective barriers
Integument	Skin	Pressure ulcers
		Surgical incisions
		Invasive lines
		Invasive procedures
		Burns
		Steroids
Pulmonary	Mucociliary escalator	Intubation
		Endoscopic procedures
	Reflexes: sneeze, cough, gag	Sedation ($\downarrow$ LOC)
		Cranial nerve impairment
	Normal flora	Antibiotics
Gastrointestinal	Gastric pH	NG/NI intubation
	Motility	H_2 antagonists
	Intact mucosal epithelium	Antacids
		Endoscopic procedures
	Normal flora	Antibiotics
		Electrolyte imbalance
Genitourinary	Micturation	Urinary catheterization
	Urine pH	Incontinence
	Bladder mucosa	Glycosuria
	Vaginal pH	Antibiotics
	Normal flora	

- Mucous membranes intact
- Clear breath sounds
- Absence of dysuria
- Urine clear yellow
- WBC 5-10 $\times$ 10^3/µl

INTERVENTIONS

1. Avoid cross-contamination: wash hands, avoid sharing equipment, use sterile equipment, avoid "dirty" to "clean" activities.
2. Obtain temperature q4h and assess for diaphoresis and chills. Monitor serial WBC counts.
3. Maintain ICU environmental temperature ~75° F (23.8° C).

INTEGUMENT

1. Provide meticulous skin care.
   a. Assess pressure points (Figure 2-1). Nonblanchable erythema of intact skin is a sign of a pressure ulcer.

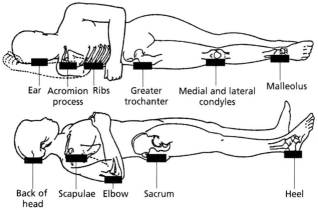

Ear Acromion Ribs   Greater   Medial and lateral   Malleolus
     process   trochanter   condyles

Back of Scapulae Elbow   Sacrum   Heel
head

Figure 2-1   Pressure points.

Hardness, discoloration, or warmth of the skin may
also indicate skin ulceration.

b. Turn and reposition the patient frequently since continued pressure can result in ischemia; provide ROM
q2-4h to increase circulation.

c. Use pressure-relieving or pressure-reducing devices,
such as an air mattress or specialty bed. Avoid "dough-
nuts," since these devices may increase pressure.

d. Moisturize skin sparingly, because too much moisture
can macerate skin. Avoid vigorous massaging, since
further damage to underlying tissue can occur.

e. Clean skin of feces or urine immediately. Apply petro-
latum ointment or a spray that protects against moisture to perianal area.

f. Avoid skin stripping by using gauze or a stockinette to
secure dressings if at all possible or Montgomery straps
to avoid multiple tape applications.

2. Consult with nutritionist regarding the dietary needs of the
patient. Patient should be hydrated and in positive nitrogen balance.

3. Avoid shearing forces by limiting HOB to no greater than
30 degrees. Use sheepskin elbow and heel protectors to
prevent friction. Keep sheets loose and lift patients to reposition them. Turning sheets can decrease shear and friction.

4. Assess nares for pressure areas associated with NG or ET
tubes; assess periostomal skin for chemical irritation;

assess mouth and lips for dryness associated with NPO status.

5. Closely monitor patient receiving vasopressors for tissue ischemia.
6. Use sterile technique with invasive lines, incisions, tubings, drains, and so on. Keep stopcocks covered with sterile caps. Change wet or soiled dressings immediately.
7. Follow infection control protocol for changing IV sites, dressings, tubing, and solutions.

PULMONARY

1. Assess cough and gag reflexes to evaluate presence of protective reflexes.
2. Assess lungs for adventitious sounds.
3. Provide pulmonary hygiene: C & DB, chest physiotherapy, incentive spirometry.
4. Position the patient to facilitate chest excursion. Mobilize patient as soon as possible.
5. Keep HOB elevated or place the patient in sidelying position if LOC is decreased or the patient is receiving tube feedings. Turn tube feedings off during chest physiotherapy and bedscale weighing to prevent aspiration.
6. If the patient is intubated, check cuff pressure to prevent mucosal injury; drain respiratory circuit of water accumulation.
7. Use sterile technique when suctioning.
8. Ensure that respiratory equipment is replaced periodically.

GASTROINTESTINAL

1. Assess the patient's abdomen for distention or change in bowel sounds.
2. Prevent GI contamination by changing tube feeding containers q24h. Rinse container before adding new feeding to the bag. Fill container with enough tube feeding for 4 hours. Refrigerate unused feeding.
3. Assess for tube feeding residual q4h.

GENITOURINARY

1. Inspect urinary meatus for any drainage.
2. Assess urine for cloudiness, presence of glucose, or foul odor.
3. If the patient is incontinent of stool, clean the patient and the catheter tubing; avoid a back-and-forth motion on tubing, which could lead to fecal contamination of the urinary meatus.

4. Check indwelling urinary catheter tubing for any kinks that may obstruct urine flow. Do not irrigate the catheter unless an obstruction is suspected. Keep the drainage bag lower than the patient's bladder. Secure the catheter to the patient's leg and avoid excessive manipulation of the catheter. Provide individual patient-labeled containers for emptying the drainage bags.
5. Remove the urinary catheter as soon as possible.
6. When the urinary catheter is removed, assess the patient for dysuria, frequency, urgency, and flank or labial pain.

OXYGENATION IN THE CRITICALLY ILL

The critically ill patient is at risk for tissue hypoxia, the underlying event that results in cellular dysfunction, organ failure, and death. Thus it is important to understand the concepts of oxygenation and the relevant parameters that can be monitored in the critically ill. Concepts of oxygenation include (1) oxygen transport or delivery (DO_2), (2) oxygen consumption (VO_2), (3) oxygen extraction, (4) cardiac output/index (CO/CI), (5) hemoglobin (Hgb), (6) hemoglobin saturation (SO_2), and (7) partial pressure of oxygen (PO_2).

Tissue oxygen consumption is independent of oxygen delivery during steady states. The amount of oxygen utilized by the cells (oxygen consumption) determines the amount of oxygen delivered to the cells. If tissue oxygen demand increases, more oxygen is extracted from the blood without requiring additional blood flow (e.g., CO/CI). As the demand increases, however, an increase in blood flow will be necessary to provide adequate supply. The more blood flow, the more oxygen is extracted, up to a point. The point at which oxygen consumption becomes dependent upon oxygen delivery is referred to as "critical oxygen delivery." If there is a further increase in metabolic demand, these compensatory mechanisms may not be adequate and an oxygen debt results.

In addition to cardiac function, the lungs also play a role in tissue oxygenation. Conditions such as atelectasis, pneumonia, and pulmonary edema may cause arterial hypoxemia (decreased PaO_2 and SaO_2). To assess the extent to which the pulmonary system contributes to inadequate tissue oxygenation, intrapulmonary shunting can be evaluated. Intrapulmonary shunting is an oxygen content index that can be estimated with a number of equations (e.g., Qs/Qt, $P(A-a)O_2$, $P(a/A)O_2$ ratio, or the PaO_2/FIO_2 ratio).

Oxygen extraction ratio (ERO_2) is a fractional comparison of oxygen consumption to oxygen delivery. It is an index of the efficiency of total tissue extraction of oxygen from the extracellular environment. Normally 22 to 28% of all oxygen that is transported to the cells is removed from the hemoglobin by the cells. An increased extraction ratio ≥ 0.60 reflects either an inadequate cardiac output or inadequate arterial oxygen content (SaO_2, PaO_2, Hgb) to meet oxygen demands and is thought to be associated with anaerobic metabolism. Oxygen extraction can be estimated with SvO_2 monitoring and analysis (see p. 528). Some conditions (e.g., septic shock, cyanide poisoning and ARDS), interfere with oxygen extraction. Adequate levels of $\dot{D}O_2$ may exist, yet tissue ischemia may occur. These conditions may benefit from supranormal levels of $\dot{D}O_2$ to optimize $\dot{V}O_2$.

When oxygen content, delivery, and extraction are inadequate, the cells depend on anaerobic metabolism. This results in lactic acidosis. A serum lactate level can provide information about cellular oxygenation; however, a single value does not necessarily reflect immediate changes and is not always reliable. There is a lag time between the generation of lactate in the cells and the accumulation of lactate in the serum. Thus the absence of lactate does not reflect the absence of anerobic metabolism. Serial lactate levels may provide more helpful information.

When the patient's cellular oxygenation is being threatened, efforts to increase oxygen content and oxygen transport or to decrease oxygen consumption should be made. See Table 2-2 for factors interfering with oxygen delivery and oxygen consumption.

▶ **Nursing Diagnosis:** Risk for altered tissue perfusion
OUTCOME CRITERIA
- CI   2.5-4.0 L/min/m²
- $\dot{D}O_2I$ 500-650 ml/min/m²
- $\dot{V}O_2I$ 115-165 ml/min/m²
- SvO_2 60-80%
- PaO_2 80-100 mm Hg
- O_2 sat $\geq 95\%$
- ERO_2 22-28%
- Qs/Qt   0-8%
- PaO_2/FIO_2 >250
- $P(a/A)O_2$ ≥ 0.75
- Hct   37-47% (females)
                 40-54% (males)

TABLE 2-2   Some Factors Affecting Oxygen Delivery and Consumption

Factors that impede $\dot{D}o_2$	
HR:	Dysrhythmias
SV:	MI, HF, hypovolemia, elevated SVR
O_2 content:	Hypoxic anemia, intrapulmonary shunt, histotoxic anemia

Factors that increase $\dot{V}o_2$	
Anxiety	Shivering
Fever	Increased WOB
Pain	Hypermetabolism

Conditions that impair ERo_2	
Septic shock	ARDS
Cyanide poisoning	Edema

HR, heart rate; SV, stroke volume; O_2, oxygen; MI, myocardial infarction; HF, heart failure; SVR, systemic vascular resistance; WOB, work of breathing; ARDS, acute respiratory distress syndrome

INTERVENTIONS

1. Correct hypoxemia and increase oxygen saturation. Administer supplemental oxygen as ordered; intubation and mechanical ventilation may be needed.
2. Increase cardiac output by manipulating heart rate or stroke volume: optimize preload, contractility, and afterload. Administer antidysrhythmic agents as ordered. Administer fluids or diuretics as ordered to maintain effective blood volume, generally not to exceed a PAWP of 15 mm Hg. Fluid volume overload can potentially impair oxygen diffusion. Administer electrolytes as ordered to correct imbalances, administer inotropes (dobutamine) and titrate vasopressors (dopamine or norepinephrine) as ordered. Vasodilators (nitroprusside) may be needed in some cases to decrease SVR.
3. Administer blood products/blood substitutes as ordered to improve oxygen carrying capacity.

4. Decrease metabolic demands: relieve pain, keep patient warm and dry, relieve/reduce anxiety, maintain bedrest, and allow for periods of uninterrupted rest; suction if patient unable to handle secretions; prevent infection. Anticipate sedation and possible neuromuscular blockade.

5. Monitor intramucosal pH (if available) to assess tissue oxygenation of the gut.

6. Anticipate supranormal levels of $\dot{D}o_2$ to optimize $\dot{V}o_2$ in some patients.

7. Monitor CI, Spo_2 and Svo_2. Note trends and patient response to therapy and activities/nursing interventions.

8. Calculate $\dot{D}o_2I$, $\dot{V}o_2I$, ERo_2 and estimate intrapulmonary shunt. Note trends and patient response to therapy.

9. Monitor ABGs, Hgb and Hct levels.

10. Monitor patient's mentation, urine output, skin temperature, and capillary refill in addition to BP and trends in arterial lactate levels.

11. See Svo_2 monitoring—p. 528.

NUTRITION

Adequate nutrition is essential in critically ill persons to decrease the risks of malnutrition-associated complications. Patients with fevers, burns, or trauma may require as much as 8000 to 10,000 kcal a day to meet their metabolic needs. Inability to ingest food orally because of unconsciousness, weakness, dysphagia, intubation, vomiting, or trauma rapidly results in muscle catabolism. Not only can fluid and electrolyte imbalance cause severe cardiopulmonary problems, but protein and mineral loss can also delay healing and recovery, as well as lead to shock.

To supply the calories needed for seriously ill persons to regain their strength, most patients in the intensive care unit receive nutritional support either by enteral or parenteral routes. Enteral nutrition is considered superior to parenteral nutrition, since it is physiological and maintains the integrity of the GI tract. (Disruption of intestinal mucosa may lead to hypermetabolism and multiple organ failure.) Parenteral nutrition is instituted when the GI tract is not functioning properly. Ongoing nutritional assessments are required and adjustments made based on the patient's response and changing caloric needs.

▶ **Nursing Diagnosis:**   Altered nutrition: less than body requirements

OUTCOME CRITERIA
- Stabilized target weight
- Serum albumin 3.5-5 g/dl
- Serum transferrin >200 mg/dl
- Lymphocytes >1500 cells/mm^3
- Positive nitrogen balance

INTERVENTIONS

1. Assess energy needs using the Harris-Benedict equation (p. 758) or assist with indirect calorimetry. An estimate of caloric needs for the critically ill patient is 40 to 50 kcal/kg.
2. Estimate ideal body weight with the following formula: 50 kg (males) or 45 kg (females) + 2.3 (for each inch above 5 feet) ± 10%.
3. Compare serial weights; rapid (0.5 to 1.0 kg/day) changes indicate fluid imbalance and not an imbalance between nutritional needs and intake.
4. Assess GI status: bowel sounds, vomiting, diarrhea, or abdominal pain may interfere with nutritional absorption.
5. Review nutritional profile to evaluate patient response to therapy.
6. Consult with the nutritionist for formal nutritional evaluation.
7. Provide mouth care to prevent stomatitis, which can adversely affect the patient's ability to eat.
8. Create a pleasing environment to improve patient's appetite; avoid offensive sights at the bedside; prepare the patient by making certain that hands and face have been washed.
9. Assist the patient as necessary, since fatigue and weakness or the presence of invasive equipment may discourage the patient from feeding self.
10. Administer enteral nutrition as prescribed. (See p. 635.)
11. Administer parenteral nutrition as prescribed. (See p. 639.)

TRANSPORT OF THE CRITICALLY ILL

Moving the critically ill patients for diagnostic tests or procedures, or to another facility for treatment, can involve some risks to the patient. Risks should be weighed against the benefits before a decision to transport the patient is made. Hospitals should have policies and protocols for inter- and intrahospital patient transfers. Critical elements for transporting the patient include: pretransport coordination and communication, competent personnel to accompany the patient, appropriate level of monitoring for the patient's condition including appropriate equipment, and patient/family preparation. The following information is from Guidelines for the Transfer of Critically Ill Patients.

▶ **Nursing Diagnosis:**   Risk for injury
OUTCOME CRITERION
• Patient's condition will not deteriorate.
INTERVENTIONS
1. Stabilize the patient before transport.
2. Consider: intubation prior to the transport, insertion of nasogastric tube to prevent aspiration and stopping enteral feedings.
3. Secure all tubes, catheters, and monitoring lines, etc.
4. Anticipate potential emergencies (e.g., chest tube removal, accidental extubation) and include necessary replacement equipment with transport.
5. Communicate the patient's condition to the receiving end; confirm that the receiving end is ready.
6. Contact ancillary services to assist in transport and notify the responsible physician of the transfer.
7. For interhospital transport, select the mode of transportation and send a copy of the current medical record.
8. One critical care nurse plus one additional health care member, generally a respiratory therapist if patient is mechanically ventilated, should accompany the patient. If the patient is physiologically unstable and may require interventions beyond the scope of standing orders or nursing practice, a physician should accompany the transport.
9. For interhospital transport, select personnel with the appropriate competencies and qualifications (e.g., able to intubate) to accompany the patient.
10. Continually monitor the cardiac rate and rhythm, and oxygenation status with pulse oximetry.
11. When appropriate, monitor hemodynamic measurements including PA pressures, PAWP, CVP, and cardiac output, and other measurements such as ICP, capnography, and airway pressures in patients who are intubated and receiving mechanical ventilation.

12. Standard resuscitation drugs, defibrillator, oxygen source and airway management equipment, and blood pressure cuff should accompany the patient. Battery operated infusion pumps should be used for IV fluids and medications during the transport.

13. Scheduled medications should be administered during the transport.

14. A plan to access a resuscitation cart and suction equipment (within 4 minutes) should be made.

15. Meet the needs of the patient and family; explain the reason for moving the patient and answer any questions they may have.

16. For interhospital transport, explain the reason for transfer and give the location of the receiving facility to family.

TEACHING-LEARNING

The critically ill patient requires constant intensive nursing care of life-threatening physiological problems. However, critical care nursing also focuses on supporting psychological and social integrity and restoring health. Teaching is an independent nursing activity that can assist the patient and family in understanding the disease process and prescribed therapies so that the patient and family are provided the necessary information and resources to maintain optimal health.

Questions should be answered honestly and procedures explained; however, teaching should not be initiated when the patient and family are feeling the impact of the illness and expressing feelings of dying, loss of control, and hopelessness. Once the patient and family express the need for explanations or discuss the events that led to the ICU hospitalization, the patient and family may be ready to learn. Learning everything one needs to know will not occur during the ICU hospitalization; however, the process can be initiated in the ICU.

▶ **Nursing Diagnosis:**   Knowledge deficit
OUTCOME CRITERIA
- Patient/family will verbalize accurate understanding of illness and treatment plan.
- Patient will demonstrate self-management skills.
INTERVENTIONS
1. Assess the patient's and family's perception of the illness. Be sensitive to questions asked about the illness or a

demonstrated interest in what is being done for them. Validate the learning need.

2. Provide information by answering questions immediately or, if possible, schedule a time to include the family and discuss the disease process, medications, dietary restrictions, activity level, signs and symptoms to report to a health care professional, or any procedure or therapeutic measure the patient is interested in. Include other health care team members as needed to meet the learning needs of the patient and family.

3. Tailor the teaching to the patient's strengths. Take into account that fever, pain, fatigue, lack of sleep, fear, and some medications may interfere with the patient's learning. "Teaching sessions" may be incidental, but an overall plan should be developed based on the assessed needs. The plan should include outcomes, content to be learned, and strategies to facilitate learning.

4. Provide printed materials and written information as appropriate. Allow opportunities for answering questions and clarifying misconceptions.

5. Discuss available support services and resources; offer to contact the service if the patient or family request it (e.g., social worker, dietician).

6. Forward a copy of the teaching-learning plan to the nursing staff when the patient is transferred from the ICU. Communicate the degree of learning (outcome achievement) to the staff and document the information in the chart.

7. If the patient is undergoing surgery, provide information about the surgical experience: preoperative expectations, including NPO status, breathing exercises, surgical preparation, and preoperative medications. Include specifics regarding the surgical procedure. Discuss the postoperative experience: nurse availability, pain control, ET tube and communication, IV lines, tubes and equipment, C & DB and early mobilization, as well as any specifics on the surgical procedure.

ICU DISCHARGE

When the critically ill patient is physiologically stable and is to be discharged from the ICU, anxiety similar to separation anxiety may be experienced. Physically the patient is ready, but psychologically may not feel secure about the move to the new environment. New nurse-patient relationships must be developed as trusting ICU nurse-patient relationships are terminated and family members decide to terminate their all-night vigils, thinking their relative is "out of danger." Thus the patient's anxiety may be heightened during a time when support systems are needed yet less available.

▶ **Nursing Diagnosis:**   Risk for relocation stress syndrome

OUTCOME CRITERIA
- Patient will recognize own anxiety and verbalize anxious feelings.
- Patient will use appropriate coping mechanisms in controlling anxiety.

INTERVENTIONS
1. Discuss transfer plans early in an ICU hospitalization.
2. Keep the patient and family informed of any improvement and present the transfer in a positive manner; emphasize the recovery and not the need for a bed.
3. Explain what is expected of the patient and family in the new environment, such as what is restricted and what is not, and the floor routine.
4. During the ICU stay, identify patient and family learning needs about the illness, medications, and signs and symptoms to report.
5. Allow the patient and family to verbalize their feelings and acknowledge these feelings. Ideally, have the patient meet the new staff members before the actual transfer. Ensure a bedside introduction to the nurses on the receiving unit.
6. Reassure the patient about the skill and expertise of the nurses on the unit to which the patient is to be transferred.
7. Complete the transfer form or ICU summary form to facilitate continuity of care.
8. Transfer the patient during the day if at all possible so that the patient has time to become oriented to the new environment.
9. If the family is not present during the transfer, contact the family and inform them that their relative has been transferred.

Neurological Disorders

ACUTE SPINAL CORD INJURY

Clinical Brief

Most injuries to the spinal cord result from trauma and are usually associated with complete loss of function below the level of injury. The etiologies include motor vehicle accidents, falls, acts of violence, and sports injuries. Damage to the cord may also be related to tumors, abscesses, or other pathological conditions of the spine, such as congenital malformations or arthritis.

A *complete* spinal cord injury implies transection, compression, or infarction of the spinal cord. Complete injuries are associated with total loss of all motor and sensory functions below the level of the injury and represent irreversible spinal cord damage. Cervical cord injury is associated with a loss of motor function in the upper and lower extremities (quadriplegia), whereas injuries below the cervicothoracic junction affect only the lower extremities (paraplegia).

Incomplete spinal cord injuries can result from partial cord transection, compression, or contusion. There is some sparing of motor and/or sensory function below the level of injury. The box on pp. 49-50 list various syndromes associated with incomplete injuries.

Spinal shock is a state characterized by areflexia and flaccid paralysis that occurs immediately after the injury. The loss of reflexes and sensorimotor and autonomic function below the level of injury is temporary and may last a few hours to several weeks. The appearance of involuntary spastic movement indicates that spinal shock has ended.

Neurogenic shock is a syndrome characterized by hypotension resulting from the vasodilation of the vascular beds below the level of injury, bradycardia secondary to the suppression of the cardiac accelerator reflex, and loss of the ability to sweat below the level of injury due to the lack of innervation of the sweat glands. Neurogenic shock can occur in patients with cervical cord injury.

Presenting signs and symptoms

The signs and symptoms depend on the level and degree of injury (see the box on pp. 49-50 and Table 2-3).

Physical examination

The box on pp. 49-50 and Table 2-3 describe spinal cord injuries and corresponding functional losses.

Vital signs:

Neurogenic shock

BP: Hypotension

HR: Bradycardia

Temperature: Hypothermia—35.5° C (96° F) to 36.6° C (98° F)

Diagnostic findings

No one diagnostic test is used; a combination of tests and clinical presentation confirms the diagnosis of vertebral and/or spinal cord injury.

SPINAL RADIOGRAPHY

- Multiple spinal radiographs confirm the type and location of vertebral fracture.
- Fractures and/or dislocations can occur in different segments in 20% of severe trauma patients.
- Tumors, arthritic changes, and congenital abnormalities may also be visualized.

COMPUTED TOMOGRAPHY (CT SCAN)

- Visualizes fractures not detected on radiographs.
- Reflects compromise of the spinal canal or nerve roots by bony fragments or extensive fractures.

MAGNETIC RESONANCE IMAGING (MRI)

- Identifies extent of spinal cord damage, degree of cord contusion.
- Demonstrates presence of blood, edema, necrotic tissue, disk herniation, or tumor growth.

Acute Care Patient Management

Goals of treatment

Stabilize the spine and prevent secondary injury to the cord

Cervical collar or brace

Cervical traction with tongs

Halo brace

Kinetic bed

Corticosteroids, such as methylprednisolone

Osmotic diuretics, such as mannitol (controversial)

Text continued on p. 54.

Incomplete Spinal Cord Lesion and Corresponding Acute Functional Loss

Anterior cord syndrome

Anterior cord syndrome is caused by damage to or an infarction of the anterior two thirds of the spinal cord. A hyperflexion injury of the cervical spine may cause bone fragments or disk material to collapse or press on the anterior spinal artery, which supplies two thirds of the anterior cord, while the posterior portion of the spinal cord is spared.

Patient presentation

- Loss of spinothalamic function (pain and temperature) below the level of the lesion.
- Complete paralysis below the level of the lesion.
- Spared posterior column function (position, pressure, vibration and light touch sensations).
- Hyperesthesia (unusual sensitivity to sensory stimuli) and hypalgesia (lessened sensitivity to pain) below the level of the lesion.

Central cord syndrome

This syndrome is caused by damage or edema to the center portion of the spinal cord in the cervical region. There is central squeezing of the cord, while the periphery of the cord is spared. This pattern is usually associated with degenerative arthritis or osteophytic changes in the cervical vertebrae. A hyperextension injury can cause buckling of the ligamentum flavum, which in turn puts a "squeeze" on the cord as the column bends, interrupting the blood supply.

Patient presentation

- Motor loss in the upper extremities is greater than in the lower extremities, more profound in hands and fingers.
- Leg function is usually intact but may be weak.
- Sensory loss in upper extremities is greater than lower extremities and more profound in hands and fingers.
- Bowel and bladder problems may or may not be present; some saddle sensation is retained.

Posterior cord syndrome

Posterior cord syndrome is a very rare condition in which the posterior third of the spinal cord is affected. It is usually caused by a hyperextension injury or a direct penetrating mechanism, such as a knife wound.

Continued.

Incomplete Spinal Cord Lesion and Corresponding Acute Functional Loss—cont'd

Patient presentation

- Loss of positional sense, vibration, and light touch below the level of the lesion.
- Motor function, pain, and temperature sense are usually intact.

Brown-Sequard syndrome

Brown-Sequard syndrome is usually caused by a transverse hemisection of the cord. Damage is to one side of the cord only and is usually associated with a penetrating injury, herniated disk, or bone fragment.

Patient presentation

- Loss of position, vibration, and light touch sensation on the same side of the body (ipsilateral) below the level of the lesion.
- Loss of motor function on the same side of the body (ipsilateral) below the level of the lesion.
- Loss of pain and temperature sensation on the opposite side of the body (contralateral) below the level of the lesion.

Horner's syndrome

This syndrome is caused by a partial cord transection at T1 or above. A lesion of either the preganglionic sympathetic trunk or the postganglionic sympathetic neurons of the superior cervical ganglion will result in this syndrome.

Patient presentation

- The pupil on the same side (ipsilateral) of the injury is smaller (miosis) than the opposite pupil.
- The ipsilateral eyeball sinks (enophthalmus) and the affected eyelid droops (ptosis).
- The ipsilateral side of the face does not sweat (anhidrosis).
- Difficulty in speaking or hoarseness (dysphonia) may occur with hyperextension injury to the cervical cord that also causes injury to the laryngeal nerve.

TABLE 2-3 Complete Spinal Cord Segmental Lesion and Corresponding Acute Functional Loss

Spinal level	Muscles	Dermatome	Acute dysfunction	At risk for
C1-C2	All muscles below trapezius, sterno-cleidomastoid	Back of head	Quadriplegia (complete); total loss of independent respiratory function; total loss of motor and sensory function from neck down	Death, hypotension, bradycardia, dysrhythmias, hypothermia, ileus, atonic bladder, skin breakdown
C3-C5 C5	Diaphragm Trapezius	Ear, neckline from clavicle to wrist	Quadriplegia (complete); minimal or absent diaphragmatic function; absent intercostal respiratory effort; loss of all motor function below shoulders and sensation below clavicles	Hypotension, bradycardia, dysrhythmias, hypothermia, ileus, atonic bladder, skin breakdown
C6	Deltoid, biceps and external rotator muscles of shoulders	Lateral third of arm, shoulder to thumb and index finger	Quadriplegia (complete); decreased respiratory function: absent intercostal respiratory effort (diaphragm intact); can move head, shoulders, with some gross arm flexion	Same as above

Continued.

TABLE 2-3 Complete Spinal Cord Segmental Lesion and Corresponding Acute Functional Loss—cont'd

Spinal level	Muscles	Dermatome	Acute dysfunction	At risk for
C7	Latissimus, serratus, pectoralis, radial wrist extensors	Dorsal and palmar midarm to first two digits	Quadriplegia (incomplete); decreased respiratory function: absent intercostal effort (diaphragm intact); can flex and extend elbow	Same as above
C8	Triceps, finger extensors and flexors	Medial third of arm, including digits three and four	Quadriplegia (incomplete); decreased respiratory function: decreased intercostal effort (diaphragm intact); some intrinsic hand function, thumb and index pincher movement present	Same as above
T1	Hand intrinsics, ulnar, wrist, and fingers	Medial arm, axilla	Paraplegia; decreased respiratory function with diaphragmatic breathing; arm function intact; finger spreading, grip and wrist flexion present	Same as above

T2-T6	Upper intercostals, upper back	T4 is at nipple line	Paraplegia; some use of intercostal muscles; good upper body strength; loss of bowel and bladder function; can stand with braces	Ileus, atonic bladder, skin breakdown
T6-T12	Abdominals, thoracic extensors	T10 is at umbilicus; T12 is at groin	Paraplegia; no interference with respiratory function; loss of bowel and bladder function; paralysis of legs; can ambulate with braces	Atonic bladder, fecal retention
L1-L4 L2-L4	Iliopsoas Quadriceps	Groin, upper thigh and knee Anterior thigh, knee and lower leg	With injuries below L2, a loss in sensorimotor, bowel, bladder, and sexual function may result, depending on nerve root damage in the acute phase	
L5-S2	Hamstrings, extensor digitorum, gluteus maximus, gastrocnemius	Great toe, lateral foot, sole, achilles, posterior thigh	Injuries above the sacrum convert to reflex, and bowel and bladder are uninhibited when reflexes return; with sacral injuries they are likely to retain atonic bowel and bladder secondary to absent reflexes	
S3-S5	Bowel and bladder sphincters	Genitals, saddle area		

Surgery: decompression laminectomy, spinal fusion, and
   spinal instrumentation
Support cardiopulmonary function
   Supplemental oxygen
   Intubation and mechanical ventilation
   Kinetic bed
   Crystalloid infusions
   Inotropic and/or vasopressor agents
   Atropine for bradycardia
Decrease/alleviate pain and muscle spasms
   Analgesics (e.g., acetaminophen, codeine, morphine)
   Muscle relaxants (e.g., diazepam, baclofen, dantrolene
   sodium)
Detect/prevent clinical sequelae (Table 2-4)

▶ **Priority Nursing Diagnoses**
Risk for injury
Impaired gas exchange
Decreased cardiac output
Ineffective breathing pattern
Ineffective airway clearance
Risk for altered protection (see p. 33)
Altered nutrition: less than body requirements
(see p. 41)
Risk for altered family process (see p. 29)

▶ **Nursing Diagnosis:**   Risk for injury related to displace-
ment of fracture, spinal shock, or ascending cord edema
   OUTCOME CRITERIA
   • Absence of progressive neurological dysfunction
   • Improved sensory, motor, and reflex functions
   PATIENT MONITORING
   1. CVP and PA pressures (if available) may be used to
      evaluate fluid volume status; both overhydration and
      dehydration can adversely affect spinal cord circulation.
   PHYSICAL ASSESSMENT
   1. Determine baseline motor function (strength and tone)
      and conduct ongoing assessments for changes that may
      indicate increasing cord edema. (See the box on pp. 49-
      50 and Table 2-3.)
   2. Assess baseline sensory level (pain, light touch, and posi-
      tional sense) and mark level of sensation on the patient's
      body. (See Figure 1-5.) Conduct ongoing assessments to
      determine improvement or deterioration. Also note the

TABLE 2-4 Clinical Sequelae of Acute Spinal Cord Injuries*

Complication	Signs and symptoms
Respiratory insufficiency or arrest	Increasing work of breathing, NIF >–30, VC <15ml/kg, shallow and rapid respirations, cessation of breathing
Spinal shock	Flaccid, total paralysis of all skeletal muscles, loss of spinal reflexes, loss of sensation (pain, proprioception, touch, temperature, and pressure) below the level of injury; bowel and bladder dysfunction and possible priapism
Neurogenic shock	Symptomatic hypotension: SBP <90 mm Hg Bradycardia: HR <50 beats/min Hypothermia: Temperature <37° C (<98.6° F)
Autonomic dysreflexia (hyperreflexia)	Occurs only in patients with injuries above the T6 level once recovered from spinal shock and reflex activity has returned; paroxysmal hypertension (SBP 240 to 300 mm Hg), with bradycardia, pounding headache, blurred vision, vasodilation, flushing, profuse sweating, piloerection (gooseflesh) above the level of lesion, nasal congestion, nausea, possible chest pain; if not controlled, status epilepticus, stroke, and death are possible
Orthostatic hypotension	Dizziness, lightheadedness, loss of consciousness, drop in SBP when assuming an upright position
Immobility	Contractures, skin impairment, deep-vein thrombosis, emboli, pneumonia, atelectasis

*Above T6 level.

NEURO

patient's reports of paresthesia (numbness or tingling) in extremities.

3. Observe for priapism, assess rectal tone, and note reflexive activity to evaluate course of spinal shock and/or return of neurological function.

4. Assess the patient for development of clinical sequelae. (See Table 2-4.)

DIAGNOSTICS ASSESSMENT
1. Review serial radiographs for proper spinal alignment.

PATIENT MANAGEMENT
1. Maintain the patient's neck in alignment until tongs or a halo ring is applied; avoid neck flexion, extension, or rotation.
2. Record the amount of weights necessary to achieve realignment. Ensure that the weights hang free and that the body is in proper alignment for optimal traction. If vertebral alignment of the neck is incorrect, additional weights will be applied to the tongs and follow-up lateral cervical radiographs will be taken until realignment is reached. Proper body alignment should be ensured, especially if a kinetic bed is used.
3. Corticosteroid therapy (e.g., methylprednisolone) may be ordered. Generally, within the first 8 hours after injury, administer a bolus dose of 30 mg/kg IV over 15 minutes, wait 45 minutes, then start a maintenance infusion of 5.4 mg/kg per hour for the next 23 hours. An osmotic diuretic (e.g., mannitol) may be ordered to decrease edema at the site of injury. Muscle relaxants (e.g., diazepam, baclofen) and analgesics (e.g., acetaminophen, codeine, or morphine) may be ordered to decrease pain and/or muscle spasms to facilitate spinal realignment.
4. Anticipate surgical management in patients with spinal cord compression.

▶ **Nursing Diagnoses:** **Impaired gas exchange** related to alveolar hypoventilation; **Ineffective breathing pattern** secondary to paresis or paralysis of respiratory muscles; **Ineffective airway clearance** related to bronchial secretions and impaired cough

OUTCOME CRITERIA
- Alert and oriented
- O_2 sat   ≥95%
- PaO_2 80-100 mm Hg
- $PaCO_2$ 35-45 mm Hg
- Vital capacity 15 ml/kg
- NIF   >−30 cm H_2O
- V_T >5 ml/kg
- RR   12-20, eupnea
- HR   60-100 beats/min
- SBP   90-140 mm Hg
- Lungs clear to auscultation

PATIENT MONITORING

1. Continuously monitor ECG, since hypoxemia is a risk factor for dysrhythmias.
2. Continuously monitor oxygen saturation with pulse oximetry (SpO_2). Monitor interventions and patient activities that may adversely affect oxygen saturation.
3. Monitor spontaneous ventilation, negative inspiratory force, tidal volume, and vital capacity every 4 to 8 hours. Decreasing values suggest loss of intercostal and abdominal muscle motion and strength, and are parameters for predicting impending respiratory failure requiring intubation and mechanical ventilation. (Hypoxemia and hypercapnia may be late findings.)

PHYSICAL ASSESSMENT

1. Assess respiratory rate, pattern, use of accessory muscles, and the ability to and strength of cough hourly (or more frequently if indicated) for the first 24 to 48 hours, then every 4 hours if the patient's condition remains stable. Inspect chest expansion for symmetry and to assess intercostal muscle strength and observe epigastric area to assess diaphragmatic function. Increasing difficulty swallowing or coughing may indicate ascending cord edema. If halo traction has been placed, check to see that the fiberglass vest does not restrict ventilatory efforts.
2. Auscultate all lung fields and record breath sounds every 2 to 4 hours. Be alert to areas of absent or decreasing breath sounds or the development of adventitious sounds (i.e., crackles, rhonchi). Hypoventilation is common and leads to accumulation of secretions, atelectasis, and possible pneumonia.
3. Assess for signs of respiratory distress (e.g., patient's complaints of SOB, shallow and rapid respirations, vital capacity <15 ml/kg, and changes in sensorium).
4. Auscultate abdomen in all four quadrants for the presence of bowel sounds. Measure and record abdominal girth every 4 to 8 hours, since paralytic ileus and abdominal distention can interfere with respirations and potentiate the risk for aspiration.
5. Assess the patient for development of clinical sequelae. (See Table 2-4.)

DIAGNOSTICS ASSESSMENT

1. Review serial ABGs for adequacy of gas exchange.

NEURO

2. Review serial chest radiographs to evaluate pulmonary congestion and possible development of atelectasis, consolidation, or pneumonia.

3. Review a flat plate of the abdomen (as available) if distention persists.

4. Review serial Hgb and Hct levels to detect possible blood loss from internal bleeding. Oxygen-carrying capability can be adversely affected with blood loss.

PATIENT MANAGEMENT

1. Decrease factors that increase oxygen demands, such as fever and anxiety.

2. If cervical injury is present, or has not been ruled out, *do not hyperextend* the patient's neck for oral intubation—use the jaw-thrust method to prevent further cervical injury.

3. Once the spinal cord injury is stabilized, promote pulmonary hygiene: incentive spirometry, C & DB, chest physiotherapy, and position changes every 2 hours. Position the patient for effective chest excursion. A kinetic bed may be used to promote mobilization of secretions. If the patient is unable to cough effectively, manually assist by placing the palm of the hand under the diaphragm (between the xiphoid and umbilicus) and pushing up on the abdominal muscles as the patient exhales.

4. Administer oxygen as ordered. Mechanical ventilation may be required. (See p. 577 for information on mechanical ventilation.)

5. Suction the patient's secretions if needed. Hyperoxygenate the patient's lungs before suctioning and limit passes of the suction catheter to 15 seconds or less to avoid periods of desaturation and bradycardia. Document the quality and quantity of secretions.

6. Check patency and functioning of the nasogastric tube every 2 to 4 hours, since abdominal distention can impair diaphragmatic breathing.

7. Conduct passive range of motion exercises and apply antiembolism stockings to promote venous return and decrease the risk for deep-vein thrombosis (DVT) and pulmonary embolus. Sequential compression devices may be used. Measure thigh and calf circumference to detect any increase in size that may suggest DVT. Prophylactic subcutaneous heparin may be ordered, but is contraindicated if internal bleeding or splenic injury is suspected.

▶ **Nursing Diagnosis:**   Decreased cardiac output related to relative hypovolemia and bradycardia secondary to neurogenic shock

OUTCOME CRITERIA
- Alert and oriented
- SBP   90-140 mm Hg
- HR   60-100 beats/min
- CVP   2-6 mm Hg
- PAS   15-30 mm Hg
- PAD   5-15 mm Hg
- PAWP   4-12 mm Hg
- CI   2.5-4 L/min/m^2
- SVRI   1700-2600 dynes/sec/cm^{-5}/m^2
- Peripheral pulses strong and equal
- Urine output 30 ml/hr or 0.5-1 ml/kg/hr

PATIENT MONITORING
1. Monitor ECG rhythm and rate for dysrhythmia development. Bradycardia and sinus pauses are common complications in acute cervical injuries. Hypothermia may aggravate bradycardia.
2. Continuously monitor blood pressure (via arterial catheter if possible) since neurogenic shock or autonomic dysreflexia can cause fluctuations in BP. Note adverse changes in blood pressure that may be related to patient position.
3. CVP and PA pressure monitoring (if available) may be used to evaluate fluid volume status. Fluid volume overload may lead to pulmonary edema. Obtain CO/CI; monitor SVRI.
4. Measure intake and output hourly and determine fluid volume balance every shift. Urinary output <30 ml/hr for 2 consecutive hours may signal decreased renal perfusion secondary to decreased CO.

PHYSICAL ASSESSMENT
1. Assess skin temperature and color, capillary refill, and peripheral pulses as indicators of CO.
2. Assess LOC to evaluate cerebral perfusion; lightheadedness, fainting, or dizziness may occur with a change in patient position (orthostatic hypotension).
3. Assess patient for development of clinical sequelae. (See Table 2-4.)

DIAGNOSTICS ASSESSMENT
None

PATIENT MANAGEMENT

1. Optimize venous return or decrease risk of hypotension by changing patient's position slowly and performing passive range of motion exercises every 2 hours. If necessary, elevate lower extremities to support blood pressure. Use antiembolism hose, ace wraps to legs, and/or abdominal binder when getting the patient out of bed.
2. Administer intravenous crystalloids (Lactated Ringer's, $D_5.45NS$) as ordered to maintain hydration and circulatory volume and to control mild hypotension. Monitor for mild dehydration or overhydration, since both conditions can compromise spinal circulation.
3. Dopamine or dobutamine may be ordered to support BP related to compromised sympathetic outflow. Titrate infusions to desired effect.
4. Administer atropine as ordered to treat bradydysrhythmias.

▶ **Nursing Diagnosis:** Autonomic dysreflexia (AD) related to excessive, uninhibited sympathetic response to certain noxious stimuli (e.g., distended bowel and/or bladder, skin irritation) in patients with T6 or above spinal cord injury.

OUTCOME CRITERIA

- SBP   90-140 mm Hg
- DBP   60-80 mm Hg
- HR   60-100 beats/min
- No complaint of headache
- Absence of apprehension, chills and nasal stuffiness
- Absence of flushing and diaphoresis above the level of injury
- Absence of pilomotor erection (goose bumps), pallor and coolness below the level of injury

PATIENT MONITORING

1. Monitor blood pressure for changes signaling excessive sympathetic response. Hypertension may be severe, resulting in cerebral hemorrhage and/or myocardial infarction.
2. Monitor ECG continuously for changes in rate and rhythm; bradycardia or tachycardia can occur.
3. Monitor urine color and characteristics since urinary tract infections or occlusion of catheter tubing can cause autonomic dysreflexia.

PHYSICAL ASSESSMENT

1. Assess for severe, pounding headache and perspiration to face, neck, and upper chest.
2. Assess abdomen and bowel pattern since constipation/fecal impaction are common causes of autonomic dysreflexia.

3. Assess skin for lesions, redness, pressure ulcers since skin irritation can precipitate autonomic dysreflexia.
4. Assess for other risk factors for developing autonomic dysreflexia: pain or sudden changes in environmental temperature.

DIAGNOSTICS ASSESSMENT
None

PATIENT MANAGEMENT
1. Reduce risk factors.
   a. Institute bowel program to prevent fecal impaction.
   b. Keep bladder drained with indwelling urinary catheter and start intermittent catheterization program as quickly as possible. Keep catheter tubing patent and avoid kinks in tubing.
   c. Keep sheets and bed linens clean, dry, and wrinkle-free.
   d. Initiate meticulous skin care.
   e. Maintain a constant environmental temperature.
   f. Maintain aseptic technique with invasive procedures/equipment.
2. If patient is symptomatic,
   a. elevate the head of the bed to promote cerebral venous return and decrease BP; stay with the patient and monitor VS q3 to 5 minutes.
   b. check for bladder distention; catheterize the patient and drain 500 ml of urine and recheck BP; if BP is still elevated drain another 500 ml of urine. Continue to monitor BP since the bladder can go into severe contractions, causing hypertension. Tetracaine may be ordered to decrease the flow of impulses from the bladder. If patient has an indwelling catheter, check for kinks or sediment. Irrigate the catheter, if an occlusion is suspected, with no more than 30 ml of sterile normal saline. If the bladder is in tetany, the fluid will enter but not drain out.
   c. check the rectum for fecal impaction using a glove lubricated with anesthetic ointment. If impaction is felt, insert anesthetic ointment into rectum 10 minutes before manually removing the impaction; this will decrease the flow of impulses from the bowel. A low hypertonic enema or a suppository may be given to assist bowel evacuation.
   d. remove any objects under the patient, loosen the patient's clothing, and smooth out wrinkled bed linens.
3. If symptoms do not subside, antihypertensive agents such as hydralazine 5 to 10 mg IV, nifedipine 10 mg SL,

NEURO

and/or nitropaste 1 to 2 inches may be ordered. Avoid abrupt lowering of blood pressure.

ARTERIOVENOUS MALFORMATION (AVM)

Clinical Brief

AVMs are malformations of the cerebral vascular system in which tortuous, tangled, and malformed arterial channels drain directly into the venous system without an intervening capillary bed. Because there is a direct communication of arteries to veins, blood flow increases and leads to increased venous pressure.

The arteries supplying the AVM tend to dilate with time as a result of increased flow through the lesion. Likewise, the veins enlarge as the flow increases, creating a vicious cycle that can make these lesions increase in size. This large flow or shunting of blood through the AVM can render adjacent areas (and sometimes distal areas) of the brain ischemic.

Presenting signs and symptoms

Headache, seizures, syncope, and progressive neurological deficits may be present. A devastating hemorrhage can result in a comatose, moribund state.

Physical examination

Vital signs:

BP: Normotensive or hypertensive

HR: Mild tachycardia may be present

RR: Eupnea

Neurological: Depending on the area of the brain in which the AVM is located, there may be speech, motor, or sensory deficits. There also may be problems with vision, memory, and coordination.

Diagnostic findings

CT scan without contrast: identifies the location of the AVM and presence of hemorrhage or hydrocephalus.

CT scan with contrast: visualizes the extent and location of the AVM, and possible feeding arteries.

MRI: confirms relationship of the vascular channels to the surrounding brain and the degree of surrounding hemorrhage or edema. Aids in the planning of the surgical approach.

Cerebral angiography: the definitive diagnostic procedure, and is essential in planning for resection of AVM. Will include the carotid and vertebral circulations to assess all possible areas of vascular supply. Essential for determining the flow dynamics of the AVM and possibility for embolization.

Acute Care Patient Management

Goals of treatment

Obliterate/excise malformation

Embolization: silastic beads, balloons, or gluing for thrombosis and destruction of lesions

Surgical: craniotomy for complete removal, clipping, or ligation of feeding vessels

Radiotherapy: proton-beam radiation, gamma knife therapy, and linear accelerator

Prevent cerebral vascular bleed

Subarachnoid precautions

Antihypertensives (e.g., labetalol, hydralazine hydrochloride, methyldopa, propranolol, sodium nitroprusside)

Stool softeners or mild laxatives

Sedatives (e.g., phenobarbital)

Control symptoms

Antipyretics (e.g., acetaminophen)

Anticonvulsants (e.g., phenytoin, phenobarbital)

Analgesics (e.g., acetaminophen, Tylenol with codeine, morphine)

Detect/prevent clinical sequelae (Table 2-5)

▶ **Priority Nursing Diagnoses**

Altered tissue perfusion: cerebral

Risk for injury

Risk for altered protection (see p. 33)

Altered nutrition: less than body requirements (see p. 41)

Risk for altered family process (see p. 29)

See also CVA (p. 72)

▶ **Nursing Diagnosis:** Altered tissue perfusion: cerebral related to shunting of blood from cerebral tissue and/or intracerebral hemorrhage

OUTCOME CRITERIA

• Alert and oriented
• Pupils equal and normoreactive
• SBP   90-140 mm Hg
• HR   60-100 beats/min
• RR   12-20, eupnea
• Motor function equal bilaterally

NEURO

TABLE 2-5 Clinical Sequelae of AVM

Complication	Signs and symptoms
Intracerebral bleeding	Clinical signs vary, depending on the area involved. In general there is deterioration in consciousness, worsening headache, unilateral motor weakness, decreased EOMs, visual deficits, and changes in vital signs, particularly the respiratory pattern. There may be speech deficits (e.g., slurring, or receptive or expressive aphasia).
	Meningeal signs may be present (e.g., severe headache, nuchal rigidity, fever, photophobia, lethargy, nausea, and vomiting).

- Absence of headache, nystagmus, and nausea
- ICP   <15 mm Hg
- CPP   60-100 mm Hg

PATIENT MONITORING
1. Monitor ECG continuously, since hypoxemia and cerebral bleeding are risk factors for pronounced ST segment and T-wave changes, and life-threatening dysrhythmias.
2. Monitor ICP, analyze the ICP waveform, and calculate cerebral perfusion pressure (CPP) every hour. (See p. 511 for ICP monitoring.)
3. Monitor BP, P every 15 to 30" initially; obtain CVP and/or PA pressures (if available) every hour or more frequently if indicated.

PHYSICAL ASSESSMENT
1. Assess neurological status using Glasgow coma scale and assess for changes suggesting increased ICP and herniation. Be alert for subtle changes and new focal deficits.
2. Assess for factors that can cause increased ICP; evaluate patient for restlessness, distended bladder, constipation, hypoxemia, headache, fear, or anxiety.
3. Assess patient for development of clinical sequelae. (See Table 2-5.)

DIAGNOSTICS ASSESSMENT

1. Review serial ABGs for decreasing Pao_2 (<60 mm Hg) or increasing $Paco_2$ (>45 mm Hg) because these disturbances can increase ICP.

PATIENT MANAGEMENT

1. Maintain patient airway and administer oxygen as ordered to prevent hypoxemia.
2. Institute measures to minimize external stimuli and maintain BP (see the box on p. 68).
3. Administer antihypertensives as ordered (e.g., labetalol hydrochloride [Trandate], hydralazine hydrochloride [Apresoline], methyldopa [Aldomet], propranolol [Inderal], or sodium nitroprusside [Nipride]) to control blood pressure. Monitor drug's effect on MAP and CPP.
4. Sedatives and stool softeners may be ordered to reduce agitation and straining.
5. Anticipate interventions such as embolization, resection, clipping, ligation of feeding vessels, proton-beam therapy, or gamma radiation.

▶ **Nursing Diagnosis:** Risk for injury: seizure

OUTCOME CRITERIA

- Patient will be seizure free.
- Patient will not injure self.

PATIENT MONITORING

None

PHYSICAL ASSESSMENT

1. Observe clinical presentation during seizure activity. Note time of onset, body parts involved, and characteristics of movement; observe respiratory pattern; note pupil size, deviation, and nystagmus; note duration of seizure activity.
2. Evaluate neurological status during postictal state and examine patient for any injuries.
3. Assess patient for development of clinical sequelae. (See Table 2-5.)

DIAGNOSTICS ASSESSMENT

1. Review serum anticonvulsant drug levels (if available) for therapeutic range.

PATIENT MANAGEMENT

1. Institute seizure precautions: pad side rails, maintain the bed in low position; keep an airway at bedside. Have suction and oxygen available.
2. Protect the patient during seizure activity: protect head from injury, avoid restraining the patient; do not force any airway into the mouth once a seizure has begun.

3. Suction the patient's secretions if necessary and maintain an adequate airway during postictal state.
4. Administer anticonvulsant medications as prescribed.

CEREBRAL ANEURYSM AND SUBARACHNOID HEMORRHAGE

Clinical Brief

An aneurysm is a thin-walled, round or saccular dilation arising from a cerebral artery. The most common site is at the bifurcation of the main cerebral vessels that make up the circle of Willis. Large aneurysms may produce focal neurological deficits from compressing brain tissue or lead to a stroke secondary to thrombus formation and embolization. Cerebral aneurysms are the most common source of subarachnoid hemorrhage. When a cerebral aneurysm ruptures, blood enters the subarachnoid space, ventricular system, and surrounding brain tissue. The blood acts as an irritant and causes vasospasm, a constriction of cerebral arteries. Vasospasm impairs cerebral blood flow, which can result in cerebral ischemia and infarction.

Presenting signs and symptoms

Often the patient will report the sudden onset of a violent headache—"the worst headache of my life"—at the time of bleeding. This usually continues as a severe headache accompanied by nausea and vomiting, photophobia, and nuchal rigidity. Specific neurological deficits are related to the site and extent of the hemorrhage and may include a deteriorating level of consciousness, oculomotor nerve dysfunction, paralysis of extraocular muscles, and sensorimotor deficits in the patient.

Physical examination

Vital signs:

    BP: Generally hypertensive or very labile, depending on extent of hemorrhage and level of ICP

    HR: Mild tachycardia, dysrhythmias

    RR: Tachypnea

    Temperature: Low-grade fever 24 hours after initial rupture as a result of meningeal irritation

Pulmonary: Respiratory pattern changes may be present, depending on the level of ICP and area of hemorrhage (see Table 1-6)

Neurological: As the severity of the hemorrhage increases, the level of consciousness generally decreases with corresponding severity of neurological deficits; signs of

TABLE 2-6   Classification of Cerebral Aneurysm Hemorrhage

Category	Criteria
Grade I	Asymptomatic or minimal headache and slight nuchal rigidity
Grade II	Moderate to severe headache
	Nuchal rigidity, no neurological deficit other than cranial nerve palsy
Grade III	Drowsiness, confusion or mild focal deficit
Grade IV	Stupor, moderate to severe hemiparesis, possibly early decerebrate rigidity and vegetative disturbances
Grade V	Deep coma, decerebrate rigidity, moribund appearance

From Hunt W, Hess R: Surgical risk as related to time of intervention in the repair of intracranial aneurysms, *J Neurosurg* 28:14, 1968.

NEURO

meningeal irritation: stiff neck, and positive Kernig's and Brudzinski's signs may be present (see Table 2-6 for a classification of cerebral aneurysm hemorrhage)

Diagnostic findings

COMPUTED TOMOGRAPHY (CT) SCAN
- Identifies large aneurysms (larger than 10mm) and extent of subarachnoid or intracerebral hemorrhage.
- Detects the presence of hydrocephalus.

CEREBRAL ANGIOGRAPHY
- Anterior and posterior circulations are studied to document presence of aneurysm(s) and possible vasospasm. The gold standard for visualizing aneurysms.

MAGNETIC RESONANCE IMAGING (MRI)
- Reveals small aneurysms not visualized with CT scan.

TRANSCRANIAL DOPPLER (TCD)
- Noninvasive cerebral blood flow studies to aid in diagnosing vasospasm.

MAGNETIC RESONANCE ANGIOGRAPHY (MRA)
- Aids in the diagnosis of large intracranial aneurysms and AVMs. Magnetic resonance angiography can yield information about the size, shape, and orientation of an aneurysm's orifice (the part of the vessel that communicates with the parent vessel).

CSF STUDIES

- Confirms blood in CSF in cases where CT scan has been negative.
- Lumbar puncture opening pressure can be as high as 250 cm H_2O (normal is 90 to 180 cm H_2O or 5 to 15 mm Hg).

Acute Care Patient Management

Goals of treatment

Secure the aneurysm
    Surgery: aneurysm clipping or ligation
    Endovascular balloon occlusion
Prevent rebleeding
    Subarachnoid precautions (see the box below)
    Antihypertensives (e.g., labetalol, hydralazine hydrochloride, propranolol, sodium nitroprusside)
    Stool softeners
    Anticonvulsants (e.g., phenytoin, phenobarbital)

Subarachnoid Precautions

- Place the patient in a quiet, dimly lit private room. Television, telephone, radio, and reading may be restricted.
- Complete bed rest is required, and the patient should be positioned with the HOB elevated 30 to 45 degrees.
- Instruct the patient to avoid a Valsalva maneuver or straining of any kind, since these activities can increase ICP. Have the patient exhale while being turned. Caution the patient against coughing, sneezing, and straining during a bowel movement. Stool softeners may be ordered.
- Obtain BP, P, RR, and assess neurological signs at least every 30" initially (may be as frequently as every 5" to 15"). This schedule may be altered, depending on patient condition.
- Perform activities for the patient (e.g., feeding, bathing, or shaving) that could cause the patient to overexert and raise the blood pressure. Keep activities at a minimum, pace interventions, and provide uninterrupted rest periods.
- Caution visitors against upsetting the patient in any way, because excitement or anger could increase blood pressure and intracranial pressure. The number of visitors as well as the duration of their visits may need to be limited.
- Provide analgesics for headache, since pain can cause restlessness and elevated BP. Sedatives may also be required.

Control cerebral vasospasm
  Ensure hydration and normalize BP
    (hypervolemic/hypertension therapy)
  Calcium channel blocking agents (e.g., nimodipine,
    nicardipine)
Detect/prevent clinical sequelae (Table 2-7)

TABLE 2-7   Clinical Sequelae of Cerebral Aneurysm Rupture

Complication	Signs and symptoms
SIADH	Low serum osmolality (<280mOsm/L), dilutional hyponatremia, decreased urinary output (400-500ml/24hrs), generalized weight gain
Seizures	Tonic-clonic movements
Cerebral vasospasm	In general there is progressive deterioration in consciousness, mental confusion, motor and sensory deficits; visual and speech deficits may also be present
Rebleeding	Sudden, severe headache; nausea and vomiting; deterioration in LOC or comatose; new neurological deficits
Increased intracranial pressure (IICP)	Decreasing LOC, severe headache, nausea, vomiting, motor dysfunction, seizures, irregular breathing pattern (e.g., Cheyne-Stokes, central neurogenic hyperventilation, ataxia, apneustic), positive Babinski's sign, contralateral sensorimotor changes; changes in pupillary size, shape, and reaction; other cranial nerve involvement dependent upon the severity
Herniation	Comatose with no response to painful stimuli; VS changes: bradycardia, increasing systolic BP with a widening pulse pressure, cessation of respirations, absent brainstem reflexes (e.g., corneal, gag, swallow, oculocephalic, and oculovestibular), ipsilateral or bilateral pupillary dilation

▶ **Priority Nursing Diagnoses**
Altered tissue perfusion: cerebral
Risk for altered protection (see p. 33)
Altered nutrition: less than body requirements
(see p. 41)
Risk for altered family process (see p. 29)
See also CVA (p. 72)

▶ **Nursing Diagnosis:** Altered tissue perfusion: cerebral
related to bleeding and cerebral vasospasm

OUTCOME CRITERIA
• Patient will be alert and oriented
• Pupils equal and normoreactive
• MAP   >70 mm Hg
• HR   60-100 beats/min
• RR   12-20, eupnea
• Motor function equal bilaterally
• Absence of headache, papilledema, nystagmus, nausea,
  and seizures
• ICP   <15 mm Hg
• CPP   60-100 mm Hg

PATIENT MONITORING
1. Continuously monitor BP and MAP. Fluctuations in BP
   may increase risk of aneurysm rebleeding, cerebral
   ischemia, or stroke.
2. Continuously monitor ECG, since hypoxemia and cerebral bleeding are risk factors for pronounced ST segment
   and T-wave changes, and life-threatening dysrhythmias.
3. Monitor ICP; analyze ICP waveform and calculate cerebral perfusion pressure (CPP) every hour. (See p. 511 for
   ICP monitoring.)
4. Monitor vital signs q15 to 30" initially and evaluate
   patient response to therapy.
5. Monitor intake and output hourly and calculate hourly
   running totals to determine fluid volume balance.

PHYSICAL ASSESSMENT
1. Assess neurological status for signs/symptoms that may
   indicate rebleed, cerebral vasospasm, and increased ICP.
   (See Table 2-7.) Be alert for subtle changes and new
   focal deficits. Cerebral vasospasms generally occur 4 to
   12 days after SAH; rebleeding generally occurs within
   the first 48 hours.
2. Assess temperature every 2-4 hours. Because of the concern
   of possible seizure activity, avoid oral temperature taking.

3. Assess for factors that can cause increased ICP: distended bladder, constipation, hypoxemia, hypercapnia, headache, fear, or anxiety.

4. Assess patient for development of clinical sequelae. (See Table 2-7.)

DIAGNOSTICS ASSESSMENT

1. Review serial ABGs for decreasing Pao_2 (<60 mm Hg) or increasing $Paco_2$ (>45 mm Hg), since these disturbances can increase ICP.

2. Review serial electrolytes for hyponatremia, which may contribute to an altered mental state.

3. Note trends on transcranial doppler (TCD) studies; an increasing mean value may reflect vasospasm.

PATIENT MANAGEMENT

1. Maintain patient airway and administer oxygen as ordered. If patient is intubated and mechanically ventilated, see p. 577 for information on mechanical ventilation.

2. Institute subarachnoid precautions. (See the box on p. 68.)

3. Administer antihypertensives as ordered to control sustained elevated BP (e.g., labetalol, hydralazine hydrochloride, propranolol, or sodium nitroprusside). Monitor MAP and CPP closely since a drastic reduction in BP can cause ischemia and possibly central infarction.

4. To optimize cerebral blood flow during symptomatic vasospasm, hypervolemic therapy may be ordered. Five % serum albumin is administered to maintain a CVP of 10 to 12 mm Hg and PA diastolic of 14 to 16 mm Hg. If neurological deficits continue, arterial hypertension may be induced with pharmacological agents such as phenylephrine, dopamine, or dobutamine to raise SBP no greater than 240 mm Hg in patients with obliterated aneurysms or above 160 mm Hg in patients with untreated aneurysms. Monitor BP, MAP, and CPP closely and monitor for pulmonary and cardiac congestion.

5. Calcium channel blocking agents may be ordered to reduce the severity of cerebral inchemia associated with cerebral vasospasm. Monitor the drug's effect on BP and HR.

6. Other pharmacological agents to prevent rebleeding and increased ICP include antipyretics (e.g., acetaminophen) to keep patient normothermic; anticonvulsants (e.g., phenytoin, phenobarbital) to prevent or control seizures; analgesics (e.g., acetaminophen or Tylenol with codeine, morphine sulfate) for headaches; stool softeners or mild

laxatives, to prevent constipation and straining; and sedatives (e.g., phenobarbital) to decrease agitation.
7. Anticipate early surgical intervention for clipping or ligation of the aneurysm.
8. Endovascular balloon occlusion (inflation of a balloon, using a liquid polymerizing agent that hardens, inside the aneurysm) may be an option for aneurysms that are anatomically inoperable.

CEREBROVASCULAR ACCIDENT (CVA) OR STROKE

Clinical Brief

A CVA is an interruption of blood supply to brain tissue causing ischemia or infarction and resulting in temporary or permanent focal neurological deficits. The neurological deficits exhibited depend on the severity of the interruption and the cerebral artery involved. Temporary deficits or transient ischemic attacks (TIAs) produce slight symptoms that disappear in a few minutes to hours; these may be warning signs of an impending stroke, whereas a major stroke is more severe, symptoms persist longer than 24 hours, and permanent deficits occur. CVAs are classified as thrombotic, embolic, and hemorrhagic.

Thrombotic stroke

A thrombotic stroke, the most common type, is associated with atherosclerosis and narrowing of the lumen of the cerebral artery. The progression of occlusion may take several hours or days, and the evolution of symptoms are referred to as a "stroke in evolution." A stroke is complete when symptoms have stabilized and the neurological deficits are permanent.

Embolic stroke

An embolic stroke is most often associated with heart disease (e.g., rheumatic heart disease with mitral stenosis, subacute bacterial endocarditis), atrial fibrillation, and cardiac or vascular surgery. Embolic strokes evolve rapidly over a few seconds or minutes and are usually without warning signs.

Hemorrhagic stroke

A hemorrhagic stroke is most commonly associated with severe hypertension, ruptured cerebral aneurysm, or cerebral AVM, or it is precipitated by bleeding disorders that result in intracerebral hemorrhage. The onset of symptoms develops suddenly, with rapid progression of neurological deficits.

Risk factors for stroke are many and varied but include a history of hypertension, heart disease (especially valvular), cardiac dysrhythmias, cigarette smoking, diabetes mellitus, and obesity. In addition, patients with a strong family history of ischemic heart disease and stroke, as well as those with hyperlipidemia, appear at greater risk. Medications such as oral contraceptives, aspirin, and anticoagulants may also place patients at risk.

Presenting signs and symptoms

Signs and symptoms are directly related to the cerebral artery affected and the function of the portion of the brain that it supplies. A list of major cerebral vessels and their common correlating manifestations are listed in the box on pp. 74-75.

Physical examination

Vital signs: may be normal, or the following may be found:
  BP: With preexisting hypertension, BP may exceed 200/100 mm Hg
  HR: Mild tachycardia may be present or the rhythm irregular if associated with atrial fibrillation
  RR: Eupnea or Cheyne-Stokes respirations may be present
  Temperature: Afebrile, or elevated if the thermoregulation center is involved
Cardiovascular: Peripheral pulses may be diminished or weak in the presence of atrial fibrillation; jugular bruits may be present with atherosclerosis
Pulmonary: Chest is clear to auscultation; some rhonchi may be present if there is a history of smoking
Neurological: See the box on pp. 74-75

Diagnostic findings

CT SCAN
- Visualizes areas of ischemia or infarction.

CEREBRAL ANGIOGRAM
- Usually postponed until patient's condition is stabilized; evaluates and identifies areas of ulceration, stenosis, thrombus, and occlusion and patterns of collateral flow.
- Demonstrates presence of an aneurysm or AVM and any avascular zones and displaced arteries and veins from hemorrhage.
- Areas studies include aortic arch, carotids, and cerebral blood vessels.

LUMBAR PUNCTURE
- Normal pressure will be seen in cerebral thrombosis, embolus, and TIA; fluid is usually clear.
- In subarachnoid and intracerebral hemorrhage, the pressure is usually elevated and fluid is grossly bloody.

Correlation of Cerebral Artery Involvement and Common Manifestations

Internal carotid artery

Contralateral paresthesia (abnormal sensations) and hemiparesis (weakness) of arm, face, and leg

Eventually complete contralateral hemiplegia (paralysis) and hemianesthesia (loss of sensation)

Visual blurring or changes, hemianopsia (loss of half of visual field), repeated attacks of blindness in the ipsilateral eye

Dysphasia with dominant hemisphere involvement

Anterior cerebral artery

Mental impairment such as perseveration, confusion, amnesia, and personality changes

Contralateral hemiparesis or hemiplegia with leg loss > than arm

Sensory loss over toes, foot, and leg

Ataxia (motor incoordination), impaired gait, incontinence, and akinetic mutism

Middle cerebral artery

LOC varies from confusion to coma

Contralateral hemiparesis or hemiplegia with face and arm loss > than leg

Sensory impairment over same areas of hemiplegia

Aphasia (inability to express or interpret speech) or dysphasia (impaired speech) with dominant hemisphere involvement

Homonymous hemianopsia (loss of vision on the same side of both visual fields), inability to turn eyes toward the paralyzed side

Posterior cerebral artery

Contralateral hemiplegia with sensory loss

Confusion, memory involvement, and receptive speech deficits with dominant hemisphere involvement

Homonymous hemianopsia

Vertebrobasilar artery

Dizziness, vertigo, nausea, ataxia, and syncope

Visual disturbances, nystagmus, diplopia, field deficits, and blindness

Correlation of Cerebral Artery Involvement and Common Manifestations—cont'd

Numbness and paresis (face, tongue, mouth, one or more limbs), dysphagia (inability to swallow), and dysarthria (difficulty in articulation)

Symptoms related to left versus right hemisphere involvement

Left hemisphere	Right hemisphere
Right-sided hemiplegia or hemiparesis	Left-sided hemiplegia or hemiparesis
Expressive, receptive, or global aphasia	Spatial, perceptual deficits
Decreased performance on verbal and math testing	Denial of the disability on affected side
Slow and cautious behavior	Distractibility, impulsive behavior and poor judgment
Defects in right visual field	
Difficulty in distinguishing left from right	Defects in left visual field

- Total protein level may be elevated in cases of thrombosis as a result of the inflammatory process.

ECHOCARDIOGRAM
- Rules out a cardiac source of emboli.

ECG
- Rules out the presence of a silent myocardial infarction.
- Determines the presence of dysrhythmias as a source of emboli.

MRI
- Reflects areas of infarction as early as 8 hours after the ischemic insult.

MRA
- Images the entire carotid artery from the aortic arch through the circle of Wellis and provides information determining the need for carotid endarterectomy.

Acute Care Patient Management

Goals of treatment
Augment blood flow
    Hemodilution
    Thrombolytics, Endarterectomy

Prevent thrombotic events
  Anticoagulation
  Antiplatelet agents
Protect neurons
  Calcium channel blocking agents
Prevent further hemorrhagic events
  Treat the cause: cerebral AVM, cerebral aneurysm, or
    hypertension
Reduce increased intracranial pressure
  Ventriculostomy for ICP monitoring and CSF drainage
  Corticosteroids (e.g., dexamethasone [Decadron])
  Osmotic diuretics (e.g., mannitol, urea)
  Loop diuretics (e.g., furosemide [Lasix])
Detect/prevent clinical sequelae (Table 2-8)

▶ **Priority Nursing Diagnoses**
Altered tissue perfusion: cerebral
Ineffective airway clearance
Risk for aspiration
Impaired communication
Risk for altered protection (see p. 33)
Altered nutrition: less than body requirements
(see p. 41)
Risk for altered family process (see p. 29)

▶ **Nursing Diagnosis:** Altered tissue perfusion: cerebral
related to increased intracranial pressure secondary to cerebral ischemia, edema, or hemorrhage

OUTCOME CRITERIA
• Patient will be alert and oriented
• Pupils equal and normoreactive
• Improvement in presenting neurological deficits and/or
  the absence of any new focal deficits
• ICP   <15 mm Hg
• CPP   60-100 mm Hg

PATIENT MONITORING
1. Continuously monitor ECG for changes (e.g., ventricular
   ectopy is common).
2. Continuously monitor oxygen saturation with pulse
   oximetry (SpO_2). Monitor interventions and patient
   activities that may adversely affect oxygen saturation.
3. If ICP monitoring is being used, calculate CPP to evaluate the patient's response to therapy. (See p. 511 for ICP
   monitoring.)
4. Monitor blood pressure q15 to 30" initially and if titrating vasoactive agents.

TABLE 2-8   Clinical Sequelae of Stroke

Complication	Signs and symptoms
Seizures	Tonic-clonic movements
Dysrhythmias/ECG changes	Change in rate and rhythm; QT prolongation, ST segment depression, T-wave inversion
Respiratory insufficiency or arrest	Shallow respirations, cessation of breathing
Increased intracranial pressure (IICP)	Decreasing LOC, severe headache, nausea, vomiting, motor dysfunction, seizures, irregular breathing pattern (e.g., Cheyne-Stokes, central neurogenic hyperventilation, ataxia, apneustic), positive Babinski's sign, contralateral sensorimotor changes; changes in pupillary size, shape, and reaction; other cranial nerve involvement dependent upon the severity
Herniation	Comatose with no response to painful stimuli; VS changes: bradycardia, increasing systolic BP with a widening pulse pressure, cessation of respirations, absent brainstem reflexes (e.g., corneal, gag, swallow, oculocephalic, and oculovestibular), ipsilateral or bilateral pupillary dilation

NEURO

5. Monitor CVP and PA pressures (if available). Increasing pressures may signal the onset of fluid overload, which may increase cerebral edema.
6. Monitor intake and output hourly and calculate fluid balance every shift to evaluate fluid volume status. Fluid overload can increase cerebral edema and further increase ICP.

PHYSICAL ASSESSMENT

1. Establish a neurological baseline with the Glasgow coma scale and perform ongoing assessments. Assess for signs and symptoms of increased ICP: headache, nausea, vomiting, altered LOC, pupillary changes, visual defects, and sensorimotor dysfunction. Test protective reflexes (e.g., cough, gag, corneal).

2. Assess for factors that can increase ICP: hypoxemia, hypercapnia, fever, anxiety, constipation, and bladder distention.
3. Assess patient for development of clinical sequelae. (See Table 2-8.)

DIAGNOSTICS ASSESSMENT

1. Review serial PT, INR, and PTT for therapeutic levels if the patient is receiving anticoagulant therapy. Generally 1.5 × control is the goal of therapy.
2. Review serial electrolytes levels, especially if diuretic therapy is employed.
3. Review serial ABGs to identify hypoxemia (Pao_2 <60 mm Hg) and hypercapnia ($Paco_2$ >45mm Hg), since these disturbances can cause increased ICP.

PATIENT MANAGEMENT

1. Maintain the head of the bed at 30 degrees for patients with hemorrhagic stroke, or as ordered. Keep the patient's head in straight alignment and prevent extreme hip flexion. Pace nursing activities to allow the patient uninterrupted rest periods. Turn the patient to the lateral recumbent position to decrease the chances of aspiration. Instruct the patient to exhale while being turned or repositioned.
2. Elevated BP is generally not treated unless MAP >130 mm Hg or SBP >220 mm Hg. Monitor BP cautiously and avoid a precipitous drop in BP.
3. Osmotic diuretics (e.g., mannitol or urea) may be ordered to decrease cerebral edema. Carefully monitor CPP, ICP, urine output, and blood pressure.
4. Anticoagulation medications (e.g., heparin, coumadin) may be ordered for patients who have had an embolic stroke. Antiplatelet drugs (e.g., aspirin, ticlopidine, and dipyridamole) may also be ordered. Monitor for bruising and guaiac-test urine, stool, and NG aspirate for occult blood. Protect the patient from injury (e.g., use soft toothbrush for oral hygiene and use electric razor).
5. Prevent constipation by establishing a bowel regimen as individually warranted.
6. Provide the patient and family with realistic information and a rationale for frequent assessments, the relationship between the patient's condition and clinical symptoms, and the treatment/care plan.
7. Maintain ventriculostomy (if present) and drain CSF according to established parameters.

▶ **Nursing Diagnoses:** **Ineffective airway clearance** and **Risk for aspiration** related to altered consciousness or cough reflex dysfunction

OUTCOME CRITERIA
- Patient will maintain a patent airway
- Absence of aspiration
- RR   12-20, eupnea
- Lungs clear to auscultation
- O_2 sat   ≥95%
- Pao_2 80-100 mm Hg
- $Paco_2$ 35-45 mm Hg
- pH   7.35-7.45

PATIENT MONITORING
1. Continuously monitor oxygen saturation with pulse oximetry (Spo_2). Monitor interventions and patient activities that may adversely affect oxygen saturation.

PHYSICAL ASSESSMENT
1. Ongoing assessment of respiratory status should be done. Note the rate, quality, and pattern; the patency of the upper airway and the patient's ability to handle oral secretions; skin color, nail beds, peripheral pulses, and skin temperature; and the presence and strength of gag, cough, and swallow reflexes.
2. Assess the lungs and note the presence of adventitious sounds. Note any restlessness or change in LOC that may suggest hypoxia.

DIAGNOSTICS ASSESSMENT
1. Review serial ABGs for hypoxemia and hypercapnia, since these disturbances can increase ICP.
2. Review serial chest radiographs to evaluate for possible aspiration or pulmonary congestion.

PATIENT MANAGEMENT
1. Maintain a patent airway by turning and positioning the patient to facilitate drainage of oropharyngeal secretions, providing an oral airway if necessary and suctioning secretions.
2. Once the patient's breathing is stabilized, provide pulmonary hygiene: C & DB therapy every hour and prn; provide chest physiotherapy and postural drainage if warranted and not contraindicated by increased ICP.
3. Administer oxygen with adequate humidification as ordered.
4. An NG tube may be required to prevent gastric distention and potential aspiration; check placement and patency.

5. Assist the patient with feedings if the gag and cough reflexes are intact; place the patient in an upright position and offer semisoft foods to avoid the risk of aspiration. Contact the speech therapist for swallowing evaluation if necessary.

▶ **Nursing Diagnosis:** Impaired communication: dysarthria (impaired muscle involvement), expressive aphasia (inability to express thoughts verbally or in writing), receptive aphasia (inability to understand the spoken or written word), or dysphasia (impaired speech) related to cerebral ischemia or injury

OUTCOME CRITERION
• Patient will be able to communicate needs.

PATIENT MONITORING
None

PHYSICAL ASSESSMENT
1. Assess for any deficits/decreases in communication skills/ability, articulation, comprehension/verbalization.
2. Record the following characteristics of the patient's speech: spontaneity, fluency, and context.
3. Examine the muscles used for speech, testing cranial nerves VII, IX, X, and XII. (See Table 1-2.)
4. Ask the patient to follow verbal, then demonstrated, commands.
5. Ask the patient to repeat simple phrases and sentences; test the patient for the ability to follow written commands.
6. Ask the patient to identify common objects, such as pen, scissors, pin.

DIAGNOSTICS ASSESSMENT
None

PATIENT MANAGEMENT
1. Limit the amount of environmental stimuli to decrease distractions and reduce confusion for the patient.
2. Encourage the patient to focus on one task at a time; speak in a clear, calm voice. Focus on simple, basic words and short sentences, allowing time for the patient to respond. Repeat or rephrase sentences as necessary.
3. Avoid appearing rushed; anticipate the patient's needs and encourage patience when the patient is frustrated by attempts at communication.
4. Try to assign consistent caregivers.
5. Instruct the family about limiting stimuli to prevent confusion for the patient. Keep the family informed and involved in the plan of care.
6. For expressive aphasia, encourage the patient's present speech and encourage spontaneous attempts at speech;

allow sufficient time for the patient to respond to questions and words; cue with the first syllable or give a choice of words; provide alternate means, such as picture cards, word cards, or writing table.

7. For receptive aphasia, use concrete words to communicate nouns and verbs; use gestures and pictures and write messages; use word and phrase cards. Begin introducing words to the patient in the following order: noun, verb, pronoun.

8. Refer the patient to a speech therapist or pathologist for formal evaluation.

NEURO

HEAD INJURY

Clinical Brief

Head injury involves trauma to the scalp, skull (cranium and facial bones), or brain. The severity of the injury is related to the degree of initial brain damage and associated secondary changes.

Primary injury occurs with an impact from an acceleration-deceleration or rotational force, and includes fracture, concussion, contusion, and laceration. The effects of injury on cerebral tissue can be focal or diffuse. Secondary injuries such as hematomas, intracranial hypertension, CNS infections, hypotension, hypoxemia, and hypercapnia often follow the primary injury. The clinician has no control over the primary injury; however, every attempt must be made to prevent or control secondary injuries, which can increase morbidity and mortality.

Classification of head injuries according to location and effect on the brain, as well as presenting signs and symptoms and diagnostic tests, are covered in Table 2-9.

Presenting signs and symptoms

Depending on the extent, degree, and location of brain injury, patients may have varying levels of consciousness and neurological deficits (Table 2-9).

Physical examination

Vital signs:

BP:

Wide fluctuations may be seen; commonly patient is hypertensive, which may reflect increased ICP or may also be a preexisting condition

When hypertension is present with bradycardia, a widened pulse pressure, and irregular respirations (Cushing's triad), it reflects a late and possibly terminal sign of increased ICP indicative of loss of autoregulation

Text continued on p. 87.

TABLE 2-9 Classification of Head Injury According to Location and Effect on the Brain

Location	Description and presenting signs and symptoms	Diagnostic findings
Scalp injuries		
Contusion	Bruise injury to the tissue of the scalp, with possible effusion of blood into the subcutaneous space without a break in the skin	Objective observation
Abrasion	Scraping away of part of the top layer of skin on the scalp	
Laceration	Wound or tear in the tissue of the scalp that tends to bleed profusely	
Skull fracture injuries		Diagnosis is primarily based on skull radiographs; these are viewed carefully to note air in the paranasal sinuses or other areas that may indicate a basilar skull fracture
Linear	Nondisplaced fracture of the skull at point of injury; swelling, ecchymosis, or tenderness is noted on the scalp; scalp contusion or laceration may also be present	
Comminuted	Multiple fragmented linear fractures	
Depressed	Displacement of comminuted fragments, associated with dural laceration and brain injury; look for cerebrospinal fluid leakage from the ear (otorrhea) or nose (rhinorrhea); swelling, ecchymosis, and other scalp injuries are common	
Compound	May be linear, comminuted, or depressed; external opening through scalp, mucous membranes of sinuses, or the tympanum (also see s/s for depressed fracture)	

Basilar skull	Linear fracture from base of temporal or frontal bone extending into the anterior, middle, or posterior fossa; produces characteristic clinical features, depending on site of fracture (e.g., raccoon's eyes [periorbital ecchymosis], Battle's sign [mastoidal ecchymosis], otorrhea, rhinorrhea, and anosmia [impairment of the sense of smell])	Radiograph may or may not reveal basilar fracture; CT scan and/or clinical features confirm the diagnosis; skull radiographs and CT scan confirm location and extent
Facial	Fractures of the facial bones produce disfigurement and facial motor and sensory dysfunction	
Meningeal tears	Dural laceration from compound or depressed fractures or from penetrating objects; s/s of meningitis (elevated temperature, stiff neck, pain on flexion of neck, deterioration of neurological signs, elevated WBC)	Leakage of CSF may be observed and will test positive for glucose; blood with CSF produces halo sign; CSF leak confirmed by cisternography
Diffuse cerebral injuries Concussion	Violent jarring or shaking of the brain; transient loss of consciousness, memory loss, nausea, vomiting, dizziness, unsteady gait, headache	Diagnosis made by clinical findings in the absence of focal lesion on CT; CT scan without contrast or MRI detects presence of contusion, hematoma, hemorrhage, hydrocephalus, edema, or midline shift; echo shows size of hematoma judged by midline shift

Continued.

NEURO

TABLE 2-9 Classification of Head Injury According to Location and Effect on the Brain—cont'd

Location	Description and presenting signs and symptoms	Diagnostic findings
Diffuse axonal injury	Stretching and tearing of axons that occur with high speed acceleration—deceleration (motor vehicle accidents); immediate coma, decerebration, initially low ICP, vegetative state and death	
Hypoxic brain injury	Brain deprived of an adequate oxygen supply resulting from cardiac arrest or a nonpenetrating head injury; varying degrees of elevated ICP, mild cognitive deficits to a vegetative state	
Focal cerebral injuries		
Contusion	Bruising of the brain with perivascular hemorrhage; loss of consciousness, speech, sensory or motor disturbances, depending on site involved; anterograde or retrograde memory loss	
Laceration	Tearing of brain tissue accompanied by focal swelling; can lead to intracranial bleeding, brain displacement, and death	
	Decreased LOC, sensorimotor dysfunction, abnormal size and reaction in pupils, extraocular paralysis, other cranial nerve dysfunctions, seizures, and aphasia	

Brainstem injury	Primary—results from direct trauma, fracture, or torsion injury; secondary—may occur as a result of compression from increased ICP and herniation of temporal lobe; decreased LOC, abnormal breathing patterns, abnormal size and reaction in pupils, abnormal eye movement, motor deficits, and abnormal reflexes	Same as cerebral injuries
Hemorrhage Subdural hematoma	Bleeding occurs into the subdural space (between the dura mater and above the arachnoid layer); hematoma caused by slow bleeding usually from venous vessels; s/s usually slower than epidural hematoma; altered LOC, headache, personality changes, ipsilateral dilated pupil, and contralateral weakness	Same as cerebral injuries
Intracerebral hematoma	Bleeding is located within the brain tissue and may involve small arteries or veins; mortality is high; s/s depend on the location and size and are frequently indistinguishable from those of contusion; sudden onset of headache may be accompanied with nausea and vomiting; rapid deterioration with respiratory distress and coma	Same as cerebral injuries; CT with contrast will demonstrate presence of aneurysm, AVM, or tumor

Continued.

TABLE 2-9 Classification of Head Injury According to Location and Effect on the Brain—cont'd

Location	Description and presenting signs and symptoms	Diagnostic findings
Epidural hematoma	Extradural bleeding above the dura mater (between the periosteal lining of the skull and dura mater); usually caused by arterial bleeding from a torn middle meningeal artery and often associated with a fracture of the temporal bone; clot presses on brain and can cause rapid herniation and death; brief loss of consciousness followed by lucid period; severe vomiting, headache, rapid deterioration with decreased LOC, ipsilateral dilated pupil, contralateral hemiparesis, and seizures may occur	Same as cerebral injuries; brain scan is helpful with isodense hematomas; MRI may differentiate hemorrhages that occurred at different times
Subarachnoid hemorrhage and intraventricular hemorrhage	Bleeding is usually associated with ruptured aneurysm or AVM; s/s of restlessness, severe headache, nuchal rigidity, elevated temperature, positive Kernig's sign (loss of ability to extend leg when thigh is flexed on abdomen), photophobia	Same as cerebral injuries; CSF studies will reflect blood and elevated protein and pressure

Hypotension from head injury alone is rare but may also indicate a terminal event

HR:
Bradycardia, associated with increased ICP
Tachycardia, seen with occult hemorrhage or as a terminal event

RR: Pathological respiratory pattern will roughly correlate with the level of neurological injury, ranging from Cheyne-Stokes, central neurogenic hyperventilation, apneustic to ataxic breathing (see Table 1-6)

Temperature:
Will vary widely with hypothalamic injuries
Hyperthermic with subarachnoid hemorrhage or infections

Pulmonary: Adventitious sounds may be present

Cardiovascular: Cardiac dysrhythmias are not uncommon and may be life threatening

Neurological: see Table 2-9

Diagnostic findings
See Table 2-9

Acute Care Patient Management

Goals of treatment
Optimize oxygenation
Ensure patent airway
Supplemental oxygen
Intubation and mechanical ventilation
IV fluids, blood replacement
Vasopressor, antihypertensive, and vasodilator agents
Control and/or reduce increased ICP
CSF drainage
Osmotic diuretics
Glucocorticoids (controversial)
Evacuation of hematoma via burr hole or craniotomy
Hyperventilation therapy
Barbiturate coma
Detect/prevent clinical sequelae (Table 2-10)

▶ **Priority Nursing Diagnoses**
Impaired gas exchange
Altered tissue perfusion: cerebral
Risk for altered protection (see p. 33)
Altered nutrition: less than body requirements (see p. 41)
Risk for altered family process (see p. 29)

NEURO

TABLE 2-10 Clinical Sequelae of Head Injury

Complication	Signs and symptoms
Neurogenic pulmonary edema	Severe restlessness, anxiety, confusion, diaphoresis, cyanosis, distended neck veins, moist, rapid, and shallow respirations, crackles, rhonchi, elevated BP, thready pulse, frothy and bloody sputum
ARDS	Dyspnea, RR >30, labored breathing, decreased compliance (30-40 cm H_2O), PAWP <18 mm Hg, hypoxemia refractory to increase in FIO_2
DIC	Bleeding from areas of injury, puncture sites, mucous membranes; hematuria, ecchymoses, prolonged PT and PTT; decreased fibrinogen, platelets, factors V, VIII, XIII, II; increased FSP
DI	Serum osmolality >300 mOsm/kg, serum sodium >145mEq/L, urine osmolality <300 mOsm/L, urine specific gravity <1.005, urine output >200 ml/hr for 2 consecutive hours
SIADH	Low serum osmolality (<275 mOsm/L), serum sodium <130 mEq/L, decreased urinary output (400 to 500 ml/24 hrs), generalized weight gain, urine osm > serum osm
Myocardial ischemia	Dysrhythmias, electrographic changes

▶ **Nursing Diagnoses:** **Impaired gas exchange** related to hypoventilation secondary to altered level of consciousness or interstitial fluid secondary to neurogenic pulmonary edema; **Ineffective breathing pattern** secondary to injury to respiratory center

OUTCOME CRITERIA
- Patient will be alert and oriented
- PaO_2 80-100 mm Hg
- O_2 sat   ≥95%
- $PaCO_2$ in low limits of normal range (28-30 mm Hg)
- pH   7.35-7.45
- RR   12-20, eupnea
- Absence of adventitious breath sounds
- PAWP   4-12 mm Hg

PATIENT MONITORING

1. Continuously monitor oxygen saturation with pulse oximetry (SpO_2). Monitor interventions and patient activities that may adversely affect oxygen saturation.

2. Monitor CVP and PA pressures, including PAWP (if available) to monitor fluid volume status. Increasing wedge pressure may indicate development of neurogenic pulmonary edema. Calculate PVRI; hypoxemia can increase sympathetic tone and increase pulmonary vaso-constriction.

PHYSICAL ASSESSMENT

1. Assess the patient's ability to handle oral secretions. Assess respiratory rate, depth, and rhythm frequently. Auscultate breath sounds q1 to 2h and prn.

2. Assess for signs and symptoms of hypoxia: change in LOC, increased restlessness, and irritability. Assess nailbeds, capillary refill, and skin temperature. Cyanosis is a late sign.

3. Assess integrity of the gag and cough reflexes; the patient may need to be intubated if reflexes are not intact.

4. Assess patient for the development of clinical sequelae. (See Table 2-10.)

DIAGNOSTICS ASSESSMENT

1. Review serial ABGs for hypoxemia (PaO_2 <60 mm Hg) and hypercapnia ($PaCO_2$ >45 mm Hg); these disturbances can increase ICP.

2. Review serial chest radiographs for pulmonary congestion.

PATIENT MANAGEMENT

1. Administer oxygen as ordered. Ensure airway patency by proper positioning of the head and neck. Keep HOB elevated at 30 degrees to enhance chest excursion. If cervical injury has not been ruled out, *do not hyperex-tend the neck* for oral intubation; use the jaw-thrust method. Because of the risk of direct brain trauma or infection during insertion, nasopharyngeal airways should be avoided in the presence of rhinorrhea (a sign that may reflect a break in the integrity of the skull). An oral airway or bite block can prevent the patient from biting an endotracheal tube if orally intubated.

2. Provide pulmonary hygiene to reduce the risk of pul-monary complications (e.g., pneumonia, atelectasis). Ini-tiate C & DB therapy and reposition the patient to mobilize secretions, carefully monitoring for increased

NEURO

ICP. *Avoid* coughing exercises for a patient at risk of increased ICP.

3. Suction secretions only as needed. Before suctioning instill lidocaine 1 mg/kg into the endotracheal tube to suppress the patient's cough reflex and blunt increases in ICP. Hyperoxygenate before and after suctioning and limit passes of suction catheter to 15 seconds or less to avoid hypoxia. Document quality and quantity of secretions. *Never* use nasotracheal suctioning in the presence of rhinorrhea because of the risk of direct brain trauma or infection.

▶ **Nursing Diagnoses:** Altered tissue perfusion: cerebral related to **Decreased adaptive capacity** secondary to space-occupying lesion or cerebral edema

OUTCOME CRITERIA
- Patient will be alert and oriented
- Pupils equal and normoreactive
- Motor strength equal bilaterally
- RR   12-20, eupnea
- HR   60-100 beats/min
- ICP   0-15 mm Hg
- CPP   60-100 mm Hg
- Absence of headache, vomiting, seizures

PATIENT MONITORING
1. Continuously monitor ECG for changes in rate and rhythm and nonspecific ST and T-wave changes.

2. Monitor ICP trends every hour, or more often if patient's condition warrants. Analyze the ICP waveform and calculate cerebral perfusion pressure (CPP) q30 to 60". CPP less than 60 mm Hg leads to decreased cerebral blood flow (CBF), resulting in cerebral ischemia. (See ICP monitoring, p. 511.)

3. Monitor blood pressure frequently, since hypotension and hypertension can increase ICP, and vasopressor or vasodilator therapy may be used.

4. Monitor CVP and/or PA pressure (if available) every hour, since both parameters reflect the capacity of the vascular system to accept volume and can be used to monitor for imbalances that can compromise CPP.

5. Monitor I & O hourly and calculate hourly running totals. Polyuria (5 to 10 L/day) or oliguria (400 to 500 ml/day) may signal onset of diabetes insipidus or SIADH.

6. Monitor urine specific gravity q2h. Urine specific gravity will be increased in SIADH and decreased with diuretic administration; urine specific gravity will be decreased with the diuresis associated with DI.

PHYSICAL ASSESSMENT

1. Assess neurological status for signs and symptoms of herniation: progressive deterioration in LOC and motor function; changes in respiratory patterns (deep sighing and yawning may signal impending herniation); ipsilateral pupil dilation, pupils sluggish or nonreactive to light. (See Table 1-6.)

2. Assess for factors that can cause increased ICP, such as a distended bladder, hypoxemia, hypercapnia, headache, fear, or anxiety.

3. Assess temperature; fever may reflect damage to the hypothalamus and increase metabolic demands and oxygen consumption. Because of the concern of possible seizure activity, avoid oral temperature taking.

4. Assess respiratory rate and rhythm. Central neurogenic hyperventilation may occur as a compensatory mechanism to increased ICP; Cheyne-Stokes respiratory pattern often precedes herniation; ataxic or agonal respirations are associated with damage to the medulla.

5. Test cranial nerve function, since nerve damage can result from craniocerebral trauma. (See Table 1-2.) Table 2-11 identifies conditions that may have cranial nerve involvement.

6. Assess patient for development of clinical sequelae. (See Table 2-10.)

DIAGNOSTICS ASSESSMENT

1. Review serial ABGs for hypoxemia (Pao_2 <60 mm Hg) and hypercapnia ($Paco_2$ >45 mm Hg); these disturbances can increase ICP.

2. Review serial electrolyte studies, serum and urine osmolality, and specific gravity for imbalances secondary to diuretic use and/or development of diabetes insipidus (DI) or SIADH.

3. Review serial Hgb and Hct levels for anemic states; WBC counts to evaluate the inflammatory process; FDP, PT, and PTT to identify coagulation deficiencies; and glucose levels for hyperglycemia from steroid use.

4. Review baseline and serial CT or MRI reports.

NEURO

TABLE 2-11 Cranial Nerve Functions and Clinical Correlations

Nerve	Function	Clinical correlation
I Olfactory	Smell	Anterior fossa or cribriform plate fracture, frontal lobe or pituitary lesion, tumor, or meningitis
II Optic	Vision	Anterior fossa or orbital plate fracture, direct eye trauma, vascular disruption via carotid system and cerebral lesion
III Oculomotor	Elevates lid, moves eyeball, constricts pupil	Orbital plate fracture, temporal lobe swelling, increased ICP, aneurysm compression, or damage to midbrain
IV Trochlear	Moves eyeball	Inflammation or aneurysm
V Trigeminal	Muscles of mastication, facial sensation	Fractures of skull/face, pontine tumors, trauma
VI Abducens	Moves eyeball	Trauma, increased ICP, aneurysms, inflammation
VII Facial	Muscles of facial movement and taste	Temporal bone or middle fossa fracture, tumors, stroke, Bell's palsy, pons and medulla damage
VIII Acoustic	Hearing and balance	Temporal bone or middle fossa fractures, tumors, infection
IX Glossopharyngeal	Sensation for gag, swallow	Dysfunction, usually seen with vagus nerve
X Vagus	Innervation of pharynx and thoracic/abdominal viscera	Surgery (e.g., endarterectomy); unopposed action with cervical spine injuries, medulla damage
XI Accessory	Turns head	Neck surgery or trauma
XII Hypoglossal	Tongue movement	Brainstem involvement or higher

Modified from Plum F, Posner J: 1980; Hickey J: 1986; Kinney M, Packa D, Dunbar S: 1988.

PATIENT MANAGEMENT

1. Administer oxygen as ordered to maximize cerebral perfusion.
2. Reduce or minimize fluctuations in ICP by maintaining the patient's head and neck in neutral position, elevating the HOB to 30 degrees to promote cerebral venous drainage, and avoiding extreme flexion of hips. Avoid taping the endotracheal tube around the patient's neck.
3. Space nursing activities and allow the patient to rest between activities to decrease possible increased ICP. Calculate CPP before and after all nursing activities. If an increase in ICP is observed or the CPP falls below 60 mm Hg, stop the activity and allow the patient to rest until the ICP and CPP return to the previous reading.
4. Administer intravenous fluids carefully to minimize fluctuations in vascular load and ICP. Fluid restrictions may be imposed. Hypotonic fluids (D_5W) are usually avoided to reduce the risk of cerebral edema.
5. Antihypertensive agents and vasopressor agents may be ordered to maintain BP. Monitor BP and CPP carefully.
6. Osmotic diuretics (e.g., mannitol) may be used to reduce edema. Monitor serum osmolality closely; an increased osmolality (greater than 310 mOsm/kg) may disrupt the blood brain barrier and actually increase edema. Monitor for hypotension, which decreases CPP, and observe for increased ICP, which may occur 8 to 12 hours after osmotic diuresis. If loop diuretics are used, monitor urine output and electrolytes.
7. Glucocorticoids (controversial) such as dexamethasone may be ordered. Monitor for hyperglycemia and GI bleeding.
8. Other pharmacological agents to reduce ICP may include phenytoin (Dilantin), to treat or prevent seizure activity; acetaminophen, to maintain normothermia, since hyperthermia increases metabolic needs; morphine sulfate and versed for sedation, and paralytics to control agitation/reduce intracranial hypertension, and/or assist with optimum ventilation.
9. Hyperventilation therapy and barbiturate coma may be employed. (See pp. 559, 566.)
10. Surgical intervention may be required to evacuate the hematoma. (See p. 563.)

NEURO

INTRACEREBRAL HEMORRHAGE (ICH)

Clinical Brief

Bleeding into the brain tissue is frequently the result of sudden rupture of a blood vessel within the brain. The effects depend on the location of the rupture and actual size of the clot. Brain tissue adjacent to the clot is displaced and produces focal neurological signs. The most common site for this type of hematoma is in the basal ganglia, followed by the thalamic region.

The usual precipitating factor of a cerebral hemorrhage is hypertension. Other possible causes may include an aneurysm, AVM, tumors, trauma, or hemorrhagic disorders. In addition, illicit use of cocaine or crack may result in an intracerebral hemorrhage.

Presenting signs and symptoms

A headache of sudden onset, occasionally accompanied by nausea and vomiting, may accompany intracerebral hemorrhage. The neurological deficits that are initially seen will reflect the anatomical location of the hemorrhage. As the intracranial pressure increases there is evidence of developing uncal or central herniation with accompanying changes in pupils, respirations, and vital signs. The clinical sequelae for ICH are the same for stroke. (See Table 2-8.)

Acute Care Patient Management

The management of intracerebral hemorrhage secondary to hypertension is similar to hemorrhage associated with head trauma. Treatment is aimed toward reducing the severely elevated BP and normalizing ICP. (See Head injury, p. 81.)

SEIZURES—STATUS EPILEPTICUS

Clinical Brief

Seizures represent intermittent, sudden, massive discharge of abnormal activity from a group of neurons within the brain. The electrical discharges may remain localized within one area of the brain, spread to involve adjacent areas in the same hemisphere, or spread across the midline to affect the contralateral hemisphere. Depending on the area of the brain involved and the pattern of spread, seizures may be generalized: tonic-clonic (grand mal), absence (petite mal), and bilateral myoclonus; or partial: focal motor, focal sensory, or complex.

Status epilepticus (convulsive status) represents a neurological emergency in which recurrent abnormal discharges occur without allowing the brain time to recover between seizures. Status epilepticus should be suspected in patients who do not begin to wake up within 20 minutes after a seizure.

Causes of status epilepticus include sudden and total suppression of anticonvulsants (withdrawal), subtherapeutic levels of anticonvulsants, meningitis, encephalitis, cortical brain tumors, metabolic and toxic encephalopathies, subarachnoid and intracerebral hemorrhage, and severe head injury. Drug overdoses, hypoxia (e.g., carbon monoxide poisoning, drowning), and withdrawal from alcohol use may also potentiate status epilepticus.

NEURO

Presenting signs and symptoms
The patient is comatose, and motor activity is divided between the repetitive tonic and clonic phases of the seizure.

Physical examination
Vital signs:
  BP: Mild hypertension initially; hypotension with circulatory collapse
  HR: Tachycardia
  RR: Apnea during tonic phase; irregular gasping respiration during clonic phase
  Temperature: Mild to moderately elevated
Pulmonary: Hypoxia and cyanosis during seizure activity
Cardiovascular: With sustained seizure activity, cardiovascular collapse possible
Neurological: Recurring, generalized tonic-clonic movements without the patient regaining consciousness; incontinence, perspiration, salivation, and emesis may occur; pupils are often fixed and dilated; eyes may be deviated or dysconjugate

Diagnostic findings
Clinical manifestations are the basis for diagnosis. Diagnostic tests are performed to identify the cause of the seizure.

Acute Care Patient Management

Goals of treatment
Maintain oxygenation
  Establishment of an airway
  Supplemental oxygen
  Intubation
  Mechanical ventilation

Maintain hemodynamic stability
    IV fluids
    Vasopressor or vasodilator agents
Control seizure activity
    Fast-acting anticonvulsant therapy (e.g., intravenous
      lorazepam, diazepam)
    Long-acting anticonvulsant therapy (e.g., intravenous
      phenytoin, phenobarbital)
    Neuromuscular blockade (e.g., paraldehyde, lidocaine,
      general anesthesia)
Identify and treat cause
    Implementation of appropriate therapy
Detect/prevent clinical sequelae (Table 2-12)

▶ **Priority Nursing Diagnoses**
Risk for injury
Risk for altered protection (see p. 33)
Altered nutrition: less than body requirements
(see p. 41)
Risk for altered family process (see p. 29)

▶ **Nursing Diagnosis:** **Risk for injury** related to increased
metabolic demand secondary to continuous seizure activity
OUTCOME CRITERIA
- Patient will be alert and oriented
- Pupils equal, round, and normoreactive
- Motor strength equal in all extremities
- SBP   90-140 mm Hg
- HR   60-100 beats/min
- RR   12-20, eupnea
- Normothermic
- PaO_2 80-100 mm Hg
- $PaCO_2$ 35-45 mm Hg
- O_2 sat   ≥95%
- pH   7.35-7.45
- HCO_3 22-25 mEq/L
- Absence of musculoskeletal trauma
- Urine output 30 ml/hr or 0.5-1 ml/kg/hr

PATIENT MONITORING
1. Continuously monitor for cardiac dysrhythmias, which
   may occur as a result of hypoxemia, acidosis, or anticonvulsant drug administration.
2. Continuously monitor oxygen saturation with pulse
   oximetry (SpO_2).
3. Monitor CPP if ICP monitoring is available.

4. Monitor the compressed spectral analysis (CSA), if available, for continued EEG trends and effectiveness of medications.
5. Monitor intake and output; myoglobinuria may occur with prolonged seizure activity and lead to renal failure.

PHYSICAL ASSESSMENT

1. Assess and document information detailing seizure activity: length of tonic and clonic phases, motor characteristics and body involvement, and deviation of eyes and pupil reaction. NOTE: Use room light to assess pupils, since a direct flashing light may elicit or cause progression of seizure. Note any automatic behavior (e.g., lip smacking, chewing), incontinence, or cyanosis.
2. Assess respiratory status, including airway patency; rate, depth, and rhythm of respirations; breath sounds; use of accessory muscles; and color of skin, lips, and nail beds. Monitor ability to handle secretions, and assess gag, cough, and swallow reflexes.
3. Assess peripheral pulses, skin, and urinary output at least every hour to evaluate tissue perfusion.
4. During seizure activity and during the administration of anticonvulsant drugs, monitor VS. Respiratory depression, decreased BP, and dysrhythmias can occur with rapid infusion of diazepam, phenytoin, and phenobarbital.
5. Perform baseline and serial neurological assessments after status is interrupted. During the postictal phase of the seizure, assessment should include LOC, motor response to stimuli, and speech every 15 min × 4 then every 30 min × 4. Patient responses should improve with each assessment. Be alert to the presence of focal findings suggestive of an expanding lesion and signs of increased ICP.
6. After the seizure, assess skin integrity for bruises, lacerations, or shearing injuries. Assess tongue, lips, and mouth for evidence of bite injuries.
7. Assess IV insertion sites for patency and extravasation of anticonvulsants.
8. Assess patients for development of clinical sequelae (Table 2-12).

DIAGNOSTICS ASSESSMENT

1. Review EEG recording and maintain communication with the physician regarding the results.

NEURO

TABLE 2-12 Clinical Sequelae of Seizures

Complication	Signs and symptoms
Respiratory arrest due to obstructed airway or changes in respiratory status during a seizure	Cessation of breathing
Trauma/falls incurred during the seizure	Musculoskeletal trauma
Cardiopulmonary arrest	Nonpalpable pulse, absent respirations

2. Review electrolyte and blood glucose levels, since electrolyte imbalance and hypoglycemia may precipitate seizures or occur as a result of prolonged seizure activity.
3. Review serum anticonvulsant drug levels for therapeutic ranges.
4. Review ABGs for hypoxemia and acidosis; both abnormalities can precipitate seizures or can occur as a result of prolonged seizure activity.
5. Review lumbar puncture (LP) results if available.
6. Review chest radiographs for indications of pulmonary complications (e.g., infiltrates, aspiration).

PATIENT MANAGEMENT
1. Pad side rails and keep them up at all times; maintain the bed in its lowest position.
2. Keep an oral airway at the bedside with suction equipment.
3. Protect the patient during the seizure (e.g., do not restrain the patient, and guide extremity movement during the seizure to prevent injury and protect the patient's head.
4. Maintain airway and ventilation to ensure maximum delivery of oxygen to the brain cells. Administer an oxygen concentration of 100% during seizure activity. An oral airway may help to maintain airway patency, but *do not force an airway* during seizure activity.
5. Position the patient on one side to facilitate drainage of oral secretions, and suction as necessary. *Do not* simply turn the patient's head to the side; this position promotes aspiration of emesis or secretions, occludes the

airway, and interferes with venous return, which increases ICP. Maintain a suction setup at all times.

6. Be prepared to assist with intubation and mechanical ventilation if necessary. (See p. 577 for information on mechanical ventilation.)

7. An NG tube may be required to prevent vomiting and the risk of aspiration.

8. Maintain a large-bore IV line for fluids and medication administration. Assess IV insertion sites for patency, especially after seizure activity, and be particularly careful to avoid extravasation of anticonvulsants.

9. Administer anticonvulsants as ordered:
   - Lorazepam can be administered 1 to 2 mg slow IVP while monitoring blood pressure.
   - Diazepam can be administered 2 mg/min slow IVP. If seizure continues, diazepam per continuous drip may be required—usual dosage is 100 mg in 500 ml D_5W at 10 to 15 mg/hr. Monitor patient continuously for respiratory depression and hypotension.
   - Phenobarbital 500 to 1000 mg (10 to 20 mg/kg) IV and/or phenytoin 500 to 1000 mg (18 mg/kg) IV may be ordered. IV line must be flushed with NS before and after administration. No other medications may be infused in the same line at the same time. Monitor LOC, BP, RR.
   - Other pharmacological therapy may include paraldehyde, lidocaine, general anesthesia, or neuromuscular blockade to stop the seizure activity. If neuromuscular blocking agents are used, the tonic-clonic motor activity will stop but not the abnormal cerebral electrical activity.

10. After the seizure, stay with the patient, reassuring and reorienting the patient as necessary. Keep the patient in a side-lying position to facilitate drainage of oral secretions; suction the secretions as needed.

NEURO

Pulmonary Disorders

ACUTE RESPIRATORY FAILURE (ARF)
Clinical Brief
Respiratory failure results from the inability of the lungs to adequately oxygenate the blood to meet the metabolic needs of the body. The impaired gas exchange results in hypoxemia with or without hypoventilation. Causes of ARF (Table 2-13) involve four mechanisms.

Alveolar hypoventilation occurs in disorders of the CNS or neuromuscular system, causing less oxygen to be supplied and less carbon dioxide to be removed.

Intrapulmonary shunting occurs when oxygenated blood is shunted past the alveoli (e.g., the alveolus is fluid filled or collapsed, and the shunted blood, which is poorly oxygenated, mixes with oxygenated blood, lowering the Pao_2).

Ventilation-perfusion mismatch occurs when there is blood flow to the underventilated areas of the lung or when there is adequate ventilation but blood flow is decreased or absent in that area.

Diffusion abnormalities occur when gas exchange across the alveolar capillary membrane is disrupted, such as in pulmonary edema or pulmonary fibrosis.

Presenting signs and symptoms
The patient may have an increased respiratory rate, shallow respirations, use of accessory muscles, and an altered level of consciousness. COPD patients may exhibit increased cough and dyspnea.

Physical examination
Appearance: Diaphoretic, agitated, restless

Vital signs:
    BP: ↑ due to hypoxemia or ↓ in shock
    HR: Tachycardia
    RR: >30
    Temperature: Normal or ↑ with infectious process

Skin: Cool and dry to diaphoretic

TABLE 2-13   Causes of Respiratory Failure

System	Disorder	Example
Central nervous	Overdose	Narcotics, sedatives, anesthetics, barbiturates
	Head trauma	Brainstem injury
	Infections	Meningitis, encephalitis
Neuromuscular	Infections	Polio
	Trauma	Spinal cord injury
	Neurological condition	Myasthenia gravis Guillain-Barré syndrome
Respiratory	Airway obstruction	Epiglottitis, fractured trachea, laryngeal edema, laryngospasm, asthma
	Pulmonary	Flail chest, pneumothorax, hemothorax, COPD exacerbation, pneumonia, pulmonary edema, ARDS

Neurological: Restlessness, deteriorating mental status

Pulmonary: Shallow breathing, use of accessory muscles and paradoxical motion of abdomen. Tachypnea, progressing to respiratory arrest

Diagnostic findings

Room air arterial blood gases: PaO_2 <50 mm Hg, usually with an increased $PaCO_2$ (>50 mm Hg) and decreased pH.

The development of ARF in COPD patients reveals a low to normal pH, elevated bicarbonate level, decreased serum chloride level, an abrupt exacerbation of dyspnea, and impaired mental status.

TABLE 2-14   Clinical Sequelae of Respiratory Failure

Complication	Signs and symptoms
Tissue hypoxia	Restlessness, decreased level of consciousness, dysrhythmias, angina, myocardial infarction, right-sided heart failure
Cardiopulmonary arrest	Absence of palpable pulses, no spontaneous respirations (non-ventilated patients)

PULM

Acute Care Patient Management
Goals of treatment
Optimize oxygenation
   Oxygen therapy
   Mechanical ventilation
   Bronchodilator therapy
   Treatment of underlying problem
Detect/prevent clinical sequelae (Table 2-14)
▶ **Priority Nursing Diagnoses**
Impaired gas exchange
Altered protection (see p. 33)
Altered nutrition: less than body requirements
(see p. 41)
Risk for altered family process (see p. 29)
▶ **Nursing Diagnosis:**   Impaired gas exchange related to hypoventilation, increased pulmonary shunt, ventilation-perfusion mismatch, and diffusion disturbances
OUTCOME CRITERIA
• Patient will be alert and oriented
• Lungs clear to auscultation
• PaO_2 80-100 mm Hg (50-55 mm Hg in a COPD patient)
• pH   7.35-7.45
• $PaCO_2$ 35-45 mm Hg (baseline $PaCO_2$ for patient with COPD)
• O_2 sat   ≥95%
• SvO_2 60%-80%

- SBP   90-140 mm Hg
- MAP   70-105 mm Hg
- HR   60-100 beats/min
- RR   12-20, eupnea

PATIENT MONITORING

1. Continuously monitor oxygen saturation with pulse oximetry (SpO_2). If SvO_2 monitoring is available, continuously monitor readings. Carefully monitor nursing interventions and patient activities that may adversely affect oxygenation status.

2. Monitor PA systolic pressure (if available) since hypoxemia can increase sympathetic tone and increase pulmonary vasoconstriction.

3. Continuously monitor ECG for changes in HR, ischemic changes, and development of dysrhythmias.

4. Continuously monitor arterial BP, PA pressures, CO/CI, and CVP, since hypoxemia can produce deleterious effects on the cardiovascular system.

PHYSICAL ASSESSMENT

1. Assess LOC: If the patient becomes restless or agitated or complains of a headache, these signs may signal decreased cerebral oxygenation.

2. Assess for signs of respiratory distress, signaling the need for mechanical ventilation: intercostal retractions, RR >30/min, and paradoxical breathing.

3. Assess lung sounds: wheezes indicate bronchospasm, which may require bronchodilator treatment.

4. Assess the patient for signs of heart failure: JVD, peripheral edema, cough, crackles, S_3, tachycardia.

5. Assess the patient for development of clinical sequelae. (See Table 2-14.)

DIAGNOSTICS ASSESSMENT

1. Review ABGs for decreasing PaO_2 and acidosis. In COPD patients, $PaCO_2$ levels are normally high and are not the sole factor on which to base the decision to intubate and mechanically ventilate the patient's lungs.

2. Review Hgb and Hct levels, since inadequate hemoglobin adversely affects oxygen-carrying capacity.

PATIENT MANAGEMENT

1. Administer oxygen therapy as ordered; generally the patient with COPD will require nasal prongs or a Venturi mask.

2. Assist the patient to assume a position that improves chest excursion. Correlate the effects of position changes on oxygen saturation to determine which position improves oxygenation.

3. If the patient's lungs are mechanically ventilated, see p. 577 for more information on mechanical ventilation.

4. β Agonists (metaproterenol) may be prescribed to relieve bronchoconstriction; intravenous theophylline may be required to decrease airway reactivity, improve diaphragmatic muscle contractility, and reverse muscle fatigue.

5. Anticholinergic agents (atropine, ipratropium) may be administered by inhalation to relieve bronchoconstriction.

6. Corticosteroids may be prescribed to reduce an inflammatory response in patients with lung disease.

7. Proceed in a calm manner and reassure the anxious and fearful patient, since anxiety and fear may increase feelings of dyspnea.

8. Reduce oxygen demands by pacing activities and scheduling rest periods for the patient, relieving anxiety and fever, and sedating the patient as needed, closely monitoring respiratory function.

9. Provide pulmonary hygiene: chest physiotherapy, postural drainage, deep breathing and coughing. Suction secretions if the patient's cough is ineffective.

PULM

ACUTE RESPIRATORY DISTRESS SYNDROME (ARDS)

Clinical Brief
ARDS is a syndrome that results from an acute injury, but not all patients with an acute lung injury develop ARDS. Causes are multifactorial and may include trauma, sepsis, aspiration, shock, pancreatitis, or any condition that causes a direct or indirect lung injury. Whatever the cause, a systemic inflammatory reaction is initiated. Noncardiogenic pulmonary edema, decreased lung compliance, and hypoxemia refractory to supplemental oxygen characterize ARDS.

Presenting signs and symptoms
The patient may exhibit: dyspnea, tachypnea, tachycardia, restlessness, and anxiety. Respiratory failure progresses and the patient may exhibit multiorgan dysfunction.

Physical examination
Vital signs:
  BP: ↑ or ↓ hypoxemia or hemodynamic compromise

HR: ↑ or ↓ in response to hypoxemia

RR: >30/min

Neurological: Restlessness, agitation, decrease in sensorium

Pulmonary: Cough, fine inspiratory crackles, use of accessory muscles

Diagnostic findings

ARTERIAL BLOOD GASES

PaO_2 <50 mm Hg on FIO_2 .60

CHEST RADIOGRAPH

May be normal for the first 12 to 24 hours after the respiratory distress occurs. The earliest abnormalities seen are patchy, bilateral, interstitial, and alveolar infiltrates. If the patient improves, the radiographic appearance may return to normal. When the disease progresses, the alveolar infiltrates advance to a diffuse consolidation. (See Figure 5-3.)

PULMONARY FUNCTION

- Compliance <50 ml/cm H_2O
- Decreased FRC
- Shunt fraction (Qs/Qt) >5%
- Deadspace ventilation (VD/VT) >0.45
- Alveolar-arterial gradient ($P[A-a]O_2$) >15 mm Hg on room air or >50 mm Hg on 100% oxygen
- PaO_2/FIO_2 ≤200 mm Hg
- PAWP <18 mm Hg

Acute Care Patient Management

Goals of treatment

Optimize tissue oxygenation

    Noninvasive CPAP or BiPAP

    Intubation/PEEP

    High-frequency ventilation

    Inverse ratio ventilation

    Extracorporeal membrane oxygenation (ECMO)

    Ensure adequate CO and Hgb

    Treat underlying cause

Maintain hemodynamic stability

    Crystalloid or colloid infusion

    Diuretic agents

    Vasodilator agents

    Inotropic agents

    Prostaglandin E_1

    Nonsteroidal anti-inflammatory agents

    Corticosteroids (controversial)

In clinical trials: Surfactant replacement
N-acetylcysteine (NAC)
Inhaled nitric oxide
Detect/prevent clinical sequelae (Table 2-15)

▶ **Priority Nursing Diagnoses**
Impaired gas exchange
Ineffective breathing pattern
Altered tissue perfusion
Risk for altered protection (see p. 33)
Altered nutrition: less than body requirements
(see p. 41)
Risk for altered family process (see p. 29)

▶ **Nursing Diagnoses:** Impaired gas exchange related to interstitial and alveolar fluid accumulation; Ineffective breathing pattern related to decreased compliance

OUTCOME CRITERIA
- Patient will be alert and oriented
- O_2 sat ≥95%
- Svo_2 60%-80%
- VC 10-15 ml/kg
- RR 12-20/min
- Eupnea
- Lung sounds clear to auscultation
- HR 60-100 beats/min
- $P(a/A)o_2$ ratio >0.60
- Pao_2/Fio_2 ≥200 mm Hg

PULM

TABLE 2-15   Clinical Sequelae of Acute Respiratory Distress Syndrome

Complication	Signs and symptoms
Dysrhythmias	Changes in rate, rhythm Change in LOC or syncope
Pneumonia	Purulent sputum, fever
GI bleeding	Coffee-ground emesis, guaiac-positive emesis and stool
DIC	Bleeding from any orifice, mucous membranes; petechiae, hematuria, hematemesis; prolonged PT/PTT; ↑ fibrin split products; ↓ platelets
Renal failure	Decreased urine output; ↑ BUN and Cr
Respiratory arrest	Cessation of breathing

PATIENT MONITORING

1. Continuously monitor ECG for dysrhythmias that may be related to hypoxemia or acid-base imbalances.

2. Continuously monitor oxygen saturation with pulse oximetry (SpO_2). Carefully monitor interventions and patient activities that may adversely affect oxygen saturation.

3. Continuously monitor SvO_2 (if available); carefully monitor interventions and patient activities that may adversely affect oxygenation.

4. Monitor pulmonary function by evaluating serial vital capacities and tidal volumes. Calculate compliance q8h. (See Pulmonary function tests, p. 470.)

5. Monitor PA systolic, since hypoxia can increase sympathetic tone and increase pulmonary vasoconstriction. Calculate PVRI.

6. Obtain CO/CI readings, since oxygen delivery depends on adequate cardiac output.

7. Calculate $P(a/A)O_2$ ratio and PaO_2/FIO_2 to evaluate oxygenation.

8. Monitor fluid volume status: measure I & O q1h, determine fluid balance q8h. Compare serial weights for changes (1 kg ~ 1000 ml of fluid). Fluid excess may cause cardiogenic pulmonary edema.

9. If the patient's lungs are mechanically ventilated, see Mechanical ventilation on p. 577.

PHYSICAL ASSESSMENT

1. Assess respiratory status q2h or more often, depending on patient condition. Note respiratory rate, rhythm, depth, and use of accessory muscles. Observe for paradoxical breathing pattern, increased restlessness, increased complaints of dyspnea, and changes in level of consciousness. Cyanosis is a late sign of respiratory distress.

2. Assess the patient for development of clinical sequelae. (See Table 2-15.)

DIAGNOSTICS ASSESSMENT

1. Review serial ABGs to evaluate oxygenation and acid-base balance.

2. Review serial chest radiographs to evaluate improving or worsening condition. Chest radiographs can provide a rough estimate of extravascular lung water.

3. Review serial Hgb and Hct levels; a reduced Hgb can adversely affect oxygen-carrying capacity.

PATIENT MANAGEMENT

1. Administer oxygen as ordered; intubation and mechanical ventilation are usually required. (See p. 577 for information on mechanical ventilation.)
2. Reposition the patient to improve oxygenation and mobilize secretions. Evaluate the patient's response to position changes with ABGs to determine the best position for oxygenation.
3. Provide chest physiotherapy and postural drainage to mobilize secretions; follow with deep breathing and coughing or suctioning. Preoxygenate the patient's lungs with FIO_2 1.0 to prevent a decrease in oxygen saturation. Note the characteristics of the sputum.
4. Administer antibiotics as ordered to treat the identified organism.
5. Anticipate diuretic therapy to keep the patient "dry" without adversely affecting intravascular volume and cardiac output.
6. Decrease oxygen consumption by limiting and pacing activities, providing uninterrupted rest, limiting visitors if necessary, decreasing anxiety with distraction or relaxation therapy, and decreasing fever.
7. High-frequency ventilation, inverse-ratio ventilation, or ECMO may be used to improve gas exchange. (See pp. 511, 573.)
8. Anticipate volume therapy, inotropic agents, vasodilators, prostaglandin E_1, and steroids to decrease pulmonary vasoconstriction. Be aware that utilization of surfactant, NAC, and inhaled nitric oxide are presently in clinical studies.
9. NG intubation may be required to decompress the stomach and decrease the risk of aspiration.
10. Nutritional support will be required to prevent respiratory muscle dysfunction and to maintain immunological defense mechanisms.

▶ **Nursing Diagnoses:** Altered tissue perfusion related to hypoxia and/or **Decreased cardiac output** secondary to decreased venous return with PEEP and diuretic therapy

OUTCOME CRITERIA

- Patient will be alert and oriented
- SBP 90-140 mm Hg

PULM

- MAP   70-105 mm Hg
- CVP   2-6 mm Hg
- HR   60-100 beats/min
- SV   50-100 ml
- CI   2.5-4 L/min/m^2
- Urine output 30 ml/hr or 0.5-1 ml/kg/hr
- Peripheral pulses strong
- PAWP   4-12 mm Hg
- SVRI   1700-2600 dynes/sec/cm^{-5}/m^2
- PVRI   200-450 dynes/sec/cm^{-5}/m^2

PATIENT MONITORING

1. Obtain PA, arterial BP, and CVP readings q1h or more often if titrating pharmacological agents or increasing PEEP levels. Monitor MAP; a MAP <60 can adversely affect cerebral and renal perfusion. Obtain CO/CI and SV; pulse pressure is also an indicator of stroke volume. Monitor SVRI and PVRI.

2. Monitor fluid volume status: measure I & O hourly; determine fluid balance every 8 hours. Compare serial weights for changes (1 kg ~ 1000 ml of fluid). Decrease in urinary output may be related to decreased renal perfusion secondary to decreased CO or development of SIADH in the patient undergoing mechanical ventilation therapy.

3. Continuously monitor ECG for signs of myocardial ischemia or the onset of dysrhythmias.

PHYSICAL ASSESSMENT

1. Assess LOC, skin, peripheral pulses, and capillary refill as indicators of cardiac output and tissue perfusion.

2. Assess the patient for development of clinical sequelae. (See Table 2-15.)

DIAGNOSTICS ASSESSMENT

1. Review serial ABGs; hypoxemia and acidosis can adversely affect myocardial contractility and contribute to decreasing CO.

2. Review serial Hgb and Hct levels; adequate hemoglobin is necessary to maintain normal oxygen transport.

3. Review lactate levels, which are an indicator of anaerobic metabolism. Increased levels may signal decreased O_2 delivery.

PATIENT MANAGEMENT

1. Administer crystalloids or colloids as ordered to maintain adequate preload. Monitor fluid status carefully, since

excessive fluid can increase hydrostatic pressure and worsen pulmonary edema.

2. Titrate positive inotropic agents to improve myocardial contractility and increase CO. Vasopressor agents may be required to maintain SBP ≥90 mm Hg.

CHEST TRAUMA

Clinical Brief

Injuries to the structures of the thorax can be caused by blunt or penetrating injuries (e.g., motor vehicle accidents, falls, gunshot wounds, and stab wounds). Tissue hypoxia is a major concern, since the intrathoracic organs are highly vascular and hemorrhagic shock is common. Hypercarbia may result from hypoventilation. Respiratory acidosis may be caused by inadequate ventilation, depressed level of consciousness, or changes in intrathoracic pressure relationships. Pleural pressures can change, leading to collapsed lungs or mediastinal shift; ventilation-perfusion mismatch can also occur as a result of the injury. Dysrhythmias can occur with myocardial injury secondary to trauma to the sternum. According to the American College of Surgeons, approximately 25% of all trauma deaths are a result of chest injuries (see Table 2-16 for a summary of chest injuries).

Acute Care Patient Management

Goals of treatment

Improve ventilation and gas exchange
    Provide an airway
    Oxygen therapy
    Intubation and mechanical ventilation
    Chest tube (CT) insertion
    Hemothorax: CT, thoracotomy
    Pulmonary contusion: diuretics, methylprednisone (controversial), unilateral lung ventilation, ECMO
    Tracheobronchial tear: thoracotomy: HFJV
    Esophageal rupture: NG intubation, surgical repair
Maintain hemodynamic stability
    Crystalloid infusion
    Blood products
    Autotransfusion
    Needle decompression for tension pneumothorax
    Myocardial contusion: antidysrhythmic agents
Decrease/alleviate pain
    Narcotics

PULM

TABLE 2-16 Summary of Chest Injuries

Injury	Clinical brief	Signs and symptoms
Flail chest	Instability of chest wall as a result of multiple rib or sternal fractures Diagnostic findings: chest radiograph confirms fractures; abnormal respiratory motion and crepitus aids diagnosis	Paradoxical chest motion, labored shallow respirations, subcutaneous emphysema
Pneumothorax	Accumulation of air in the pleural space; partial or total lung collapse Diagnostic findings: chest radiograph visualizes air between visceral and parietal pleura	Dyspnea, decreased or absent breath sounds Open pneumothorax: wound present, often sucking in nature Closed pneumothorax: no opening to external environment
Tension pneumothorax	Accumulation of air without a means of escape, causing complete collapse of the lung and mediastinal shift; immediate decompression necessary Diagnostic findings: clinical, *not* radiological, findings are the basis for diagnosis	Severe dyspnea, cyanosis, restlessness, distended neck veins, absence of breath sounds on affected side, tracheal shift to the unaffected side, hypotension, distant heart sounds, tachycardia
Hemothorax	Accumulation of blood in the pleural space Diagnostic findings: chest radiograph visualizes blood accumulation	Cool, clammy skin; hypotension, decreased capillary refill, tachycardia, absent breath sounds on affected side

Pulmonary contusion	Injury to lung tissue that can cause respiratory failure, potentially lethal Diagnostic findings: chest radiograph shows local or diffuse patchy, poorly outlined densities, or irregular linear infiltrates; ABGs: hypoxemia and hypercarbia	Dyspnea, restlessness, hemoptysis, tachycardia, ineffective cough, crackles, decreased lung compliance
Tracheobronchial tear	Injury to tracheobronchial tree that can result in airway obstruction and tension pneumothorax Diagnostic findings: clinical findings are the basis of diagnosis: CT scan, endoscopic procedures or bronchoscopy confirms the tear	Fracture larynx: hoarseness, subcutaneous emphysema, palpable fracture Trachea injury: noisy breathing, depressed LOC, labored respiratory effort Bronchial injury: hemoptysis, subcutaneous emphysema, possible s/s of tension pneumothorax
Myocardial contusion	Injury to cardiac muscle that may result in dysrhythmias, muscle damage, cardiac rupture Diagnostic findings: no one diagnostic test is used, ECHO is helpful to evaluate abnormal wall motion; serial CKs may be used to evaluate myocardial damage	Chest discomfort, abnormal ECG changes: multiple PVCs, unexplained sinus tachycardia, atrial fibrillation, bundle branch block, and ST segment changes are the most common

PULM

Continued.

TABLE 2-16 Summary of Chest Injuries—cont'd

Injury	Clinical brief	Signs and symptoms
Diaphragm rupture	Tear in the diaphragm that may allow abdominal contents to herniate into thorax Diagnostic findings: chest radiograph with contrast confirms tear; NG tube may be observed curled in lower left chest; appearance of peritoneal lavage fluid in chest tube drainage confirms the diagnosis	Chest pain referred to shoulder, dyspnea, decreased breath sounds, bowel sounds auscultated in chest, possible rhonchi
Esophageal rupture	Perforation of the esophagus that allows gastric and esophageal contents to contaminate the mediastinum and pleura Diagnostic findings: chest radiograph visualizes mediastinal air on the left side, pleural effusion, pneumothorax; contrast studies and/or esophagoscopy confirms tear	Left pneumothorax or hemothorax without rib fracture; history of blow to lower sternum or epigastrium and pain or shock out of proportion to injury; particulate matter in chest tube

Patient-controlled analgesia (PCA)
Intercostal nerve block
Epidural analgesia
Detect/prevent clinical sequelae (Table 2-17)

▶ **Priority Nursing Diagnoses**
Impaired gas exchange
Altered tissue perfusion
Decreased cardiac output
Pain
Risk for altered protection (see p. 33)
Altered nutrition: less than body requirements
(see p. 41)
Risk for altered family process (see p. 29)

▶ **Nursing Diagnosis:** Impaired gas exchange related to ventilation-perfusion mismatch, decreased compliance, inadequate ventilation

OUTCOME CRITERIA
- Patient will be alert and oriented
- PaO_2 80-100 mm Hg
- pH   7.35-7.45
- $PaCO_2$ 35-45 mm Hg
- O_2 sat   ≥95%
- RR   12-20, eupnea
- $P(a/A)O_2$ 0.75-0.90
- Qs/Qt <5%
- Minute ventilation <10 L/min

PATIENT MONITORING
1. Continuously monitor ECG, since hypoxemia is a risk factor for dysrhythmias.
2. Continuously monitor oxygen saturation with pulse oximetry (SpO_2). Be alert for interventions and patient activities that may adversely affect oxygen saturation.
3. Continuously monitor end-tidal CO_2 with capnography (if available) to evaluate adequacy of ventilation (can also be used to select ventilator settings and calculate various oxygenation parameters).
4. Monitor pulmonary function by reviewing serial minute ventilation, calculating physiologic shunt (Qs/Qt), or calculating arterial-alveolar oxygen tension ratio $P(a/A)O_2$.
5. Monitor PA systolic (if available), since hypoxemia can increase sympathetic tone and increase pulmonary vasoconstriction. Monitor PVRI.

PULM

TABLE 2-17 Clinical Sequelae of Chest Trauma

Complication	Signs and symptoms
Hypoxemia	Restlessness, RR >30/min, HR >120 beats/min, labored breathing, increase in PAP
Pneumonia	Temperature >38.5° C (>101.3° F), purulent secretions
	Ineffective cough, diminished breath sounds
Tension pneumothorax	Severe dyspnea, tracheal deviation toward unaffected side, absence of breath sounds, distended neck veins, unequal chest symmetry (chest is larger on side of pneumothorax), cyanosis, hypotension
ARDS	Dyspnea, RR >30, labored breathing, tachycardia, decreased compliance (30-40 cm H_2O), PAWP <18 mm Hg, hypoxemia refractory to increase in FIO_2
Hemothorax shock	Decrease in sensorium; cool, clammy skin; HR >120 beats/min, SBP <90 mm Hg; urine output <0.5 ml/kg/hr
Pulmonary contusion Pulmonary edema	Tachypnea, cough, frothy sputum, crackles

6. Monitor the chest drainage system, which is used to drain air or fluid from the pleural space. Record drainage hourly; consult with physician if drainage >200 ml/hr. If drainage suddenly ceases, check the patient and system—a tension pneumothorax can develop. (See p. 569 for more information on chest drainage.)

7. If the patient is undergoing mechanical ventilation therapy, see p. 577 for more information.

PHYSICAL ASSESSMENT

1. Assess respiratory status and observe for respiratory distress and increased patient effort: RR >30; paradoxical motion of the ribcage and abdomen; and presence of intercostal and supraclavicular retraction. Auscultate lungs and note any adventitious sounds.

2. Assess for signs and symptoms of hypoxia: increased restlessness, increased complaints of dyspnea, and changes in LOC. Cyanosis is a late sign.

3. Assess the patient for development of clinical sequelae. (See Table 2-17.)

DIAGNOSTICS ASSESSMENT

1. Review ABGs for decreasing trend in PaO_2, despite increasing FIO_2, which may suggest ARDS; ARDS can develop with lung injury (e.g., flail chest, pulmonary contusion).

2. Review serial chest radiographs to evaluate patient progress or worsening lung condition and to verify the placement of CT and other invasive catheters.

3. Review Hgb and Hct levels, since oxygen-carrying capacity can be adversely affected with decreased Hgb.

PATIENT MANAGEMENT

1. Promote pulmonary hygiene with incentive spirometry, chest physiotherapy, postural drainage, C & DB therapy, and position changes q2h. Note sputum color and consistency. Patients with impaired breathing patterns who are immobilized and have an ineffective cough are at risk for atelectasis and secretion retention. Anticipate antibiotic therapy for pulmonary infections.

2. If the patient develops respiratory distress, be prepared for intubation and mechanical ventilation. Nonconventional modes of ventilation may be employed if ventilation and gas exchange do not improve. (See p. 577 for information on mechanical ventilation.)

3. Flail chest: Positive pressure ventilation with PEEP or pressure support ventilation may be required to splint the chest wall internally.

4. Open pneumothorax: Place a sterile dressing on the wound, taping only three sides; this type of dressing will allow air to escape but not reenter the pleural space. Continue to assess the patient for tension pneumothorax.

5. Pulmonary contusion: Methylprednisone (controversial) may be ordered to reduce inflammation.

6. Diaphragmatic and esophageal rupture: Anticipate NG insertion to decompress the stomach and reduce the risk of contaminating the thorax. Anticipate antibiotic therapy.

7. Prepare the patient for surgical repair of the injured structures.

▶ **Nursing Diagnoses:** Altered tissue perfusion related to **Decreased cardiac output** secondary to blood loss, development of tension pneumothorax, dysrhythmias

PULM

OUTCOME CRITERIA
- Patient will be alert and oriented
- Skin warm and dry
- Peripheral pulses strong
- HR   60-100 beats/min
- Absence of life-threatening dysrhythmias
- SBP   90-140 mm Hg
- MAP   70-105 mm Hg
- RR   12-20, eupnea
- Urine output 30 ml/hr or 0.5-1 ml/kg/hr
- O_2 sat   ≥95%
- Hgb   13-18 g/dl (males)
                  12-16 g/dl (females)
- CVP   2-6 mm Hg
- CI   2.5-4 L/min/m^2
- $\dot{D}o_2I$ 500-600 ml/min/m^2
- $\dot{V}o_2I$ 115-165 ml/min/m^2

PATIENT MONITORING
1. Measure hemodynamic pressure (as appropriate to patient's clinical condition). Obtain PA pressures and CVP hourly or more frequently if the patient's condition is unstable. Obtain CO/CI, and note trends or the patient's response to therapy.
2. Monitor arterial oxygen delivery ($\dot{D}o_2I$) and consumption ($\dot{V}o_2I$) to monitor indicators of tissue perfusion.
3. Obtain BP hourly or more frequently if the patient's condition is unstable, monitor MAP and pulse pressure, and note trends and patient response to therapy.
4. Monitor hourly urine output to evaluate effects of decreased CO and/or pharmacological intervention. Determine fluid volume balance q8h (1kg ~ 1000 ml of fluid).
5. Continuously monitor ECG for dysrhythmia development, which may further compromise cardiac output and tissue perfusion.
6. Continuously monitor oxygen saturation with pulse oximetry (Spo_2). Carefully monitor patient activities and nursing interventions that may adversely affect oxygen saturation.
7. Monitor the chest drainage system, which is used to drain air or fluid from the pleural space. Record drainage hourly; consult with the physician if drainage >200 ml/hr. If drainage suddenly ceases, check the patient and the system; a tension pneumothorax can develop. (See p. 569 for more information on chest drainage.)

8. If patient's lungs are being mechanically ventilated. (See p. 577 for more information on mechanical ventilation.)

PHYSICAL ASSESSMENT

1. Assess the patient's mentation, peripheral pulses, and skin, and note urine output at least hourly as indicators of tissue perfusion.
2. Obtain BP, HR, and RR q1h or more frequently if the patient's condition is unstable.
3. Check the patient for a deviated trachea; tracheal deviation, severe dyspnea, unilateral absence of breath sounds, and distended neck veins are highly suggestive of tension pneumothorax and must be treated immediately with CT insertion or needle decompression.
4. Assess the patient for development of clinical sequelae. (See Table 2-17.)

DIAGNOSTICS ASSESSMENT

1. Review ABGs (if available) for hypoxemia (PaO_2 <60 mm Hg) and acidosis (pH <7.35), since both conditions compromise CO and tissue perfusion.
2. Review Hgb and Hct levels to evaluate blood loss. Oxygen-carrying capacity can be adversely affected with blood loss.

PATIENT MANAGEMENT

1. Insert large-bore IV catheters to administer crystalloids and blood products as ordered to maintain intravascular volume and replace blood loss. Autotransfusion may be performed in patients with bleeding into the thorax. Measure PA pressures, CVP (if available), and BP to evaluate effectiveness of fluid resuscitation.
2. Pulmonary contusion: Limit IV fluids unless patient is in shock. Rapid fluid administration can increase hydrostatic pressure and cause pulmonary edema. Blood products and albumin may be given to replace blood loss and maintain oncotic pressure.
3. If tension pneumothorax is suspected, immediate treatment is required with needle decompression and CT insertion.
4. Be alert for dysrhythmia risk factors: anemia, hypovolemia, hypotension, hypokalemia, hyperkalemia, hypomagnesemia, acidosis, and decreased coronary perfusion pressure. Treat life-threatening dysrhythmias according to ACLS algorithms. (See Appendix A.)

▶ **Nursing Diagnosis:**   Pain related to injured body structures

OUTCOME CRITERION

• Patient communicates decreased pain.

PULM

PATIENT MONITORING
None
PHYSICAL ASSESSMENT
1. Use a visual analogue scale or rating scale to assess pain and evaluate effectiveness of analgesia. (See Figure 1-1.)
2. Assess respirations before administering medications. Do not administer CNS depressants if RR <12.

DIAGNOSTICS ASSESSMENT
None
PATIENT MANAGEMENT
1. Anticipate analgesia administration if the patient exhibits restlessness, increased HR, and increased BP and if hypoxemia is not the cause.
2. Administer medication as ordered, evaluating its effects on respiration and pain control.
3. Administer medication before initiating pulmonary hygiene; patients with chest trauma are reluctant to participate because of the pain.
4. Epidural analgesia, intercostal nerve blocks, or patient-controlled analgesia may be used to control pain.
5. Consult with the physician if the medication proves ineffective.
6. See Acute pain, p. 30.

PNEUMONIA

Clinical Brief

Pneumonia is an inflammation of the lung parenchyma caused by infectious agents or toxins via aspiration, inhalation, or translocation of organisms. Critically ill patients are at increased risk for nosocomial pneumonia because normal defense mechanisms are disrupted. Table 2-18 summarizes pathogens and risk factors for pneumonia.

Presenting signs and symptoms

The patient may have fever, chills, cough with purulent or rust-colored sputum, recent influenza, and shortness of breath.

Physical examination

Vital signs:
  HR: >100 beats/min
  RR: >24
  Temperature: >38.5° C (>101.3° F) rectally
Pulmonary: Tachypnea, crackles or bronchial breath sounds, nasal flaring or intercostal retractions may be present; dullness to percussion over the affected area may also be present

TABLE 2-18   Pathogens and Risk Factors Associated with Pneumonia

Type	Pathogen	Risk factors
Bacteria	*Streptococcus pneumoniae*	COPD, alcoholism, advanced age, multiple myeloma, recent influenza
	Staphylococcus aureus	Alcoholism, DM
	Haemophilus influenzae	COPD, alcoholism
	Pseudomonas aeruginosa	Mechanical ventilation
	Escherichia coli	Mechanical ventilation
	Klebsiella pneumonia	Advanced age, nosocomial infection
	Legionella pneumophila	Immunodeficiency
Viral	Cytomegalovirus	AIDS, lymphomas, organ transplantation
Fungal	*Candida species*	AIDS, immunosuppression
Protozoa	*Pneumocystis carinii*	AIDS, immunosuppression

PULM

Diagnostic findings
ROUTINE SPUTUM SPECIMEN
Characteristics: purulent or rust-colored. Gram stain is used to rapidly identify the pathogen. Specialized testing techniques are available for tuberculosis, fungi, and protozoa identification. Electron microscopes can be helpful to identify viruses. Cultures for precise identification take approximately 2 to 3 days.

BRONCHOALVEOLAR LAVAGE (BAL)
The established method for diagnosing opportunistic pneumonia in immunosuppressed patients.

CHEST RADIOGRAPH
Patchy, ill-defined, fluffy opacification, air bronchograms, or reticular shadows.

Acute Care Patient Management

Goals of treatment
Optimize oxygenation
  Oxygen therapy

Hydration with 3 L/day
Treat infectious process
Antibiotics
Detect/prevent clinical sequelae (Table 2-19)

▶ **Priority Nursing Diagnoses**
Impaired gas exchange
Hyperthermia
Altered protection (see p. 33)
Altered nutrition: less than body requirements
(see p. 41)
Risk for altered family process (see p. 29)

▶ **Nursing Diagnosis:** Impaired gas exchange related to ventilation-perfusion mismatch

OUTCOME CRITERIA
• Patient will be alert and oriented
• pH   7.35-7.45
• PaO_2 80-100 mm Hg
• $PaCO_2$ 35-45 mm Hg
• O_2 sat   ≥95%
• Lungs clear to auscultation
• RR   12-20, eupnea

PATIENT MONITORING
1. Continuously monitor oxygen saturation with pulse oximetry (SpO_2). Carefully monitor patient activities and nursing interventions that may adversely affect oxygen saturation.
2. Continuously monitor ECG, since hypoxemia is a risk factor for dysrhythmia development.
3. Monitor PA systolic pressure (if available), since hypoxemia can increase sympathetic tone and increase pulmonary vasoconstriction.

TABLE 2-19   Clinical Sequelae of Pneumonia

Complication	Signs and symptoms
Respiratory failure	Restlessness, increased RR, PaO_2 <50 mm Hg, $PaCO_2$ >50 mm Hg, pH <7.35
Septic shock	T >38° C or <36° C, SBP <90 mm Hg, HR >90 beats/min, RR >20 or $PaCO_2$ <32 mm Hg, PaO_2/FIO_2 <280, altered mental status, plasma lactate >2 mmol/L, urine output <0.5 ml/kg/hr, WBC >12,000 or <4000 or >10% neutrophils

PULM

PHYSICAL ASSESSMENT

1. Assess respiratory status: auscultate breath sounds; note rate, rhythm, depth, and use of accessory muscles. Observe for paradoxical breathing, increased restlessness, increased complaints of dyspnea, respiratory rate >30/min, and changes in LOC.
2. Assess for the presence of protective reflexes (e.g., gag and cough), since a loss of these reflexes increases the risk for aspiration.
3. Assess the patient for development of clinical sequelae. (See Table 2-19.)

DIAGNOSTICS ASSESSMENT

1. Review ABGs to evaluate oxygenation status and acid-base balance.
2. Review serial chest radiographs to evaluate improving or worsening condition.

PATIENT MANAGEMENT

1. Administer oxygen therapy as ordered and assist the patient to a position of comfort.
2. Reposition the patient to improve oxygenation and mobilize secretions. Evaluate the patient's response to position changes with ABGs to determine the best position for oxygenation.
3. Provide chest physiotherapy and postural drainage to mobilize secretions, followed by deep breathing and coughing or suctioning. Perform endotracheal suctioning when rhonchi are present in the intubated patient, nasopharyngeal suctioning in patients unable to expectorate secretions. Document the color and consistency of sputum.
4. If the patient's lungs are mechanically ventilated, see p. 577 for more information on mechanical ventilation.
5. Maintain endotracheal cuff pressure between 15-25 cm H_2O or maximal occlusive volume. However, even properly inflated cuffs do not prevent aspiration. Carefully monitor patients receiving tube feedings.
6. Reduce oxygen demand: pace patient activities, relieve anxiety and pain, and decrease fever.

▶ **Nursing Diagnosis:** Hyperthermia

OUTCOME CRITERION

• Temperature: 36.5° C (97.7° F) to 38.3° C (100.9° F)

PATIENT MONITORING

1. Monitor temperature q4h; obtain temperature 1 hour after antipyretics have been administered. If a hypothermia

blanket is being used, continuously monitor core temperature. (See p. 548 for more information on thermal regulation.)

2. Monitor BP, CO/CI, PA pressures, PVRI, SVRI, pulse pressure, and MAP, since hemodynamic changes occur in the presence of sepsis.

PHYSICAL ASSESSMENT

1. Assess for chills, rigors, diaphoresis.
2. Assess the patient for development of clinical sequelae. (See Table 2-19.)

DIAGNOSTICS ASSESSMENT

1. Review culture reports for identification of the infecting pathogen.
2. Review serial WBC count to monitor infective process.

PATIENT MANAGEMENT

1. Consult with the physician when temperature >38.5° C (>101.3° F). Obtain cultures before initiating antibiotics whenever possible.
2. Administer acetaminophen as ordered and monitor patient response. A hypothermia blanket may be required to decrease temperature. (See p. 548 for more information on thermal regulation.)
3. Prevent the patient from shivering by covering the patient with a light blanket or using pharmacological agents if necessary, since shivering can cause an increase in oxygen demand.

PULMONARY EMBOLUS

Clinical Brief

A pulmonary embolus is an occlusion in pulmonary vasculature that occurs from a fibrin or blood clot. Most commonly emboli are detached from the deep veins of the legs. Predisposing factors include Virchow's triad: acute injury to blood vessel walls, venous stasis, and hypercoagulable states. Air emboli usually result from air entering the circulatory system through intravascular catheters. Fat emboli occur with long-bone fractures.

Presenting signs and symptoms

The hemodynamic effects depend upon the size of the embolus, presence of cardiopulmonary disease, and the neuro hormonal response to the embolus. The patient may be apprehensive and exhibit dyspnea, pleuritic pain, hemoptysis, tachycardia, tachypnea, crackles, cough, and diaphoresis.

Physical examination

Appearance: Restless, anxious
Vital signs:
  BP: Normal or ↑ BP as a result of anxiety
  HR: Normal or ↑ HR >100 beats/min
  RR: ↑ rate
CV: Increased intensity of pulmonic S_2, S_4
Pulmonary: SOB, crackles (localized)
Massive PE: Cyanosis, altered LOC, sudden shock
DVT symptoms: Calf swelling, warmth, and tenderness

Diagnostic findings

HISTORY OF RISK FACTORS

Immobility, traumatic injury, pregnancy, use of oral contraceptives, atrial fibrillation, or mitral stenosis

ARTERIAL BLOOD GASES

Pao_2 ≤80 mm Hg, $Paco_2$ <35 mm Hg, and pH >7.45
Increased alveolar-arterial oxygen tension gradient

CHEST RADIOGRAPH

Initially normal; later findings include pleural effusions, wedge collapse, focal oligemic lung

ECG

Usually nonspecific; right-axis deviation, ST-segment depression in V_1-V_4, new right bundle branch block, and tachycardic rhythms all are suggestive

VENTILATION-PERFUSION LUNG SCAN

Results are suggestive of PE if a perfusion defect is found with normal ventilation.

PULMONARY ANGIOGRAPHY

Pulmonary angiography is the most definitive test for PE, showing an abrupt cutoff of a vessel or a filling defect. PA pressures may be elevated; PVR may be increased.

Acute Care Patient Management

Goals of treatment

Optimize tissue oxygenation
  Oxygen therapy
  Pulmonary embolectomy
  Thrombolytic therapy
  Analgesia
Prevent embolic phenomenon
  Sequential compression devices
  Antithromboemboli stockings
  Anticoagulation

PULM

Filter or ligation of vena cava
Detect/prevent clinical sequelae (Table 2-20)

▶ **Priority Nursing Diagnoses**
Impaired gas exchange
Altered tissue perfusion: cardiopulmonary
Risk for injury
Risk for altered protection (see p. 33)
Altered nutrition: less than body requirements
(see p. 41)
Risk for altered family process (see p. 29)

▶ **Nursing Diagnosis:** Impaired gas exchange related to ventilation-perfusion mismatch; hypoventilation secondary to pain

OUTCOME CRITERIA
- Patient will be alert and oriented
- PaO_2 80-100 mm Hg
- O_2 sat   ≥95%
- RR   12-20
- Eupnea
- Absence of adventitious breath sounds
- $P(a/A)O_2$ ratio >0.60

PATIENT MONITORING
1. Continuously monitor oxygen saturation with pulse oximetry (SpO_2). Carefully monitor patient activities and interventions that may adversely affect oxygen saturation.
2. Continuously monitor ECG for dysrhythmias or ischemic changes.
3. Calculate $P(a/A)O_2$ ratio to evaluate intrapulmonary shunt.

TABLE 2-20   Clinical Sequelae of Pulmonary Emboli

Complication	Signs and symptoms
Pulmonary infarction	Pleuritic pain, friction rub, hemoptysis, elevated temperature, cyanosis, shock, death
Pleural effusions	On affected side: decreased respiratory excursion and breath sounds, dullness on percussion
Right ventricular failure	Jugular venous distention; increased CVP, RAP, and RV pressure; Kussmaul's sign

PULM

PHYSICAL ASSESSMENT

1. Assess respiratory status: note rate and depth of respirations; observe for dyspnea and restlessness. Hypoxia may be manifested as increased restlessness or change in level of consciousness and respiratory rate >30/min. Auscultate breath sounds; crackles and pleuritic rub may be present.
2. Assess pain using a visual analogue scale. (See Figure 1-1.)
3. Assess the patient for development of clinical sequelae. (See Table 2-20.)

DIAGNOSTICS ASSESSMENT

1. Review ABGs for changes in SaO_2 and PaO_2 to evaluate improvement or deterioration in the patient's pulmonary status.

PATIENT MANAGEMENT

1. Place patient on bed rest initially and assist patient to assume a comfortable position.
2. Administer supplemental oxygen as ordered.
3. Place activities to decrease the patient's oxygen demand, allowing adequate time for patient recovery.
4. Turn, C & DB the patient q4h; note the color and character of sputum.
5. Administer analgesics as ordered to prevent splinting and improve chest excursion.

▶ **Nursing Diagnosis:** **Altered tissue perfusion: cardiopulmonary** related to embolic phenomenon

OUTCOME CRITERIA

- Patient will be alert and oriented
- RR   12-20
- Eupnea
- PaO_2 80-100 mm Hg
- O_2 sat   ≥95%
- Lungs clear to auscultation
- SBP   90-140 mm Hg
- HR   60-100 beats/min
- Peripheral pulses strong
- Skin pink, warm, and dry
- Absence of jugular venous distention (JVD)
- CI   2.5-4 L/min/m²
- PVRI   200-450 dynes/sec/cm⁻⁵/m²

PATIENT MONITORING

1. Continuously monitor oxygen saturation with pulse oximetry (SpO_2). Carefully monitor patient activities and interventions that may adversely affect oxygen saturation.

2. Continuously monitor ECG for dysrhythmias and ischemic changes. Tachycardia may reflect compensation to maintain CI.
3. Monitor CO/CI, PA pressure (if available), CVP, arterial BP and PVRI. Pulmonary embolism can cause an increase in RV workload or afterload and ultimately reduce CO.

PHYSICAL ASSESSMENT
1. Assess for thrombophlebitis: warmth, redness, tenderness, and swelling of lower extremity.
2. Assess the patient for manifestations of right ventricular failure: JVD, peripheral edema.
3. Assess respiratory status: auscultate breath sounds, note increased work of breathing (e.g., increased respiratory rate, use of accessory muscles, and dyspnea).
4. Be alert for emboli in other body systems. Assess level of consciousness and muscle strength to monitor for cerebral infarction; note any abdominal pain, nausea or vomiting, or decreased or absent bowel sounds to monitor for GI infarction; check for decreased urinary output and hematuria to monitor for renal infarction.
5. Assess the patient for development of clinical sequelae. (See Table 2-20.)

DIAGNOSTICS ASSESSMENT
1. Review serial ABGs to evaluate oxygenation status.
2. Review cardiac profile (if available) for evidence of myocardial infarction.
3. Review serial BUN and creatinine studies to evaluate renal function.

PATIENT MANAGEMENT
1. Assist the patient to a position that will promote chest excursion and ease of breathing.
2. Administer oxygen therapy as ordered.
3. Administer anticoagulants as ordered. An initial bolus of 5000 to 10,000 units of heparin may be required, followed by a continuous infusion at a rate of approximately 1000 U/hr. Monitor PTT results; therapeutic range is 1.5 to 2.5 times control.
4. Reduce risk factors: conduct range-of-motion exercises to extremities; avoid sharp flexion at knees and groin; apply antithromboembolism stockings and sequential compres-

sion devices on admission. Remove devices every shift to assess skin and prevent skin breakdown. Mobilize the patient as soon as possible.

5. See p. 618 for information on thrombolytic therapy.

▶ **Nursing Diagnosis: Risk for injury: bleeding** related to anticoagulant or thrombolytic agents

OUTCOME CRITERIA

- Absence of bleeding
- Hct   40%-54% (males)
             37%-47% (females)
- Hgb   14-18 g/dl (males)
             12-16 g/dl (females)
- PTT within therapeutic range
- SBP   90-140 mm Hg
- HR   60-100 beats/min

PATIENT MONITORING

None specific

PHYSICAL ASSESSMENT

1. Assess the patient for bleeding from puncture sites, wounds, gums, or any body orifice. Note any altered level of consciousness or abdominal pain that may indicate internal bleeding.

2. Test NG aspirate, emesis, urine, stool, and sputum for occult blood.

DIAGNOSTICS ASSESSMENT

1. Review serial Hgb and Hct levels for decreasing trend that may suggest bleeding.

2. Review serial PTT results. If results are greater than two times the control, consult with the physician.

3. Review serial platelet counts to monitor for thrombocytopenia.

PATIENT MANAGEMENT

1. Reposition the patient at least q2h to prevent high pressure areas. Handle the patient gently to prevent bruising.

2. An arterial line should be used to obtain specimens when at all possible. If venipuncture becomes necessary, apply direct pressure to the puncture site for 10 to 15 minutes and then apply a pressure dressing. When discontinuing intravenous or arterial catheters apply pressure for 20 to 30 minutes, then apply a pressure dressing to assure hemostasis. Reassess sites within

PULM

30 minutes for further bleeding or hematoma formation.

3. Antacids and/or H_2 antagonists may be ordered to prevent gastric bleeding. Monitor gastric pH.

4. Stool softeners should be administered to prevent straining and rectal bleeding.

5. Avoid aspirin or aspirin-containing products, which may contribute to bleeding.

Cardiovascular Disorders

ACUTE MYOCARDIAL INFARCTION (MI)

Clinical Brief

The death of myocardial tissue is a result of decreased blood supply to the myocardium. A myocardial infarction can go unnoticed (silent MI) or produce major hemodynamic consequences and death. It may result from arteriosclerosis, coronary artery spasm, or coronary thrombosis.

Risk factors

Risk factors mirror the risk factors for coronary artery disease: cigarette smoking, hyperlipidemia, hypertension, diabetes, obesity, and stress. Men, especially if over 50 years of age, are predisposed to MI, as are postmenopausal women. A positive family history of cardiovascular disease is also a predisposing factor.

Presenting signs and symptoms

Chest discomfort >20-30 min unrelieved by NTG, anxiety, feelings of impending doom, nausea/vomiting, dyspnea, weakness, diaphoresis, palpitations.

Physical examination

Appearance: Anxious, pale

Vital signs:

BP may be ↑ in response to pain, or ↓ secondary to hemodynamic compromise

HR may be ↑ in response to pain or ↓ secondary to ischemia and/or pharmacological therapy; may be irregular secondary to dysrhythmias

Cardiovascular: S_3, S_4, murmur, and/or rubs may be present

Pulmonary: SOB, tachypnea, crackles

RV Infarction

Cardiovascular: distended jugular veins, hypotension, Kussmaul's sign, heart block may be present

Pulmonary: clear lungs

Diagnostic findings

Cardiac enzymes: Characteristic changes are evident (Table 2-21).

Isoenzymes: CK-MB are cardiac specific, positive MB is diagnostic for MI; LDH_1 and LDH_2 are cardiac specific, an LDH "flip" ($LDH_1 > LDH_2$) is diagnostic for MI.

TABLE 2-21 Cardiac Enzymes

Enzyme	Onset	Peak	Return to normal
CK	2-5 hr	~24 hr	2-3 days
CK-MB	4-8 hr	16-24 hr	2-3 days
AST (SGOT)	6-8 hr	24-48 hr	4-8 days
LDH	6-12 hr	48-72 hr	7-10 days
LDH_1	6-12 hr	24-48 hr	Variable

ECG changes: usually occur from hours to within 7 days (Table 2-22).

Q-wave infarctions: pathological Q waves (≥0.04 sec or 25% of the height of the R wave), ST segment elevation with reciprocal ST depression in opposite leads; T-wave changes are initially positive, then become negative in leads facing the infarcted area.

Non-Q-wave infarction: ST depression and inverted T waves in leads facing the epicardial surface overlying the infarction; ST elevation and upright T waves in opposite leads.

Acute Care Patient Management
Goals of treatment
Salvage myocardium/limit infarction size
   Thrombolytic therapy
   Intraaortic balloon pump (IABP) counterpulsation
   Percutaneous transluminal coronary angioplasty (PTCA)
Improve myocardial oxygen supply
   Supplemental oxygen
   Heparin
   Calcium channel blocking agents
   Antiplatelet agents
Decrease myocardial oxygen demand
   Mechanical assist devices
   Bed rest
   NPO, liquid/soft diet
   β-Adrenergic blocking agents
Decrease preload
   Morphine sulfate
   Nitroglycerin
   Diuretic agents

TABLE 2-22   ECG Changes Associated with Myocardial Infarction

Type	Indicative changes	Reciprocal changes
Anterior	V_2-V_4	II, III, aV_F
Anteroseptal	V_1-V_4	
Anterolateral	I, aV_L, V_3-V_6	
Lateral	I, aV_L, V_5-V_6	II, III, aV_F
Inferior	II, III, aV_F	I, aV_L, V_1-V_4
Posterior		V_1-V_3

Note: Right ventricular infarction demonstrates ST segment elevation in V_{3R}, V_{4R}.

Decrease afterload
　　Morphine sulfate
　　Nitroglycerin
　　Calcium channel blocking agents
　　Angiotensin converting enzyme (ACE) inhibitors
Increase contractility
　　Dobutamine
Maintain electrophysiological stability
　　Lidocaine
　　β-Adrenergic blocking agents
　　Calcium channel blocking agents
　　Magnesium sulfate
Maintain hemodynamic stability
　　Volume loading to provide adequate filling pressure
Detect/prevent clinical sequelae
　　See Table 2-23

▶ **Priority Nursing Diagnoses**
Pain
Decreased cardiac output
Altered tissue perfusion
Risk for altered protection (see p. 33)
Risk for altered family process (see p. 29)

▶ **Nursing Diagnosis:**   Pain related to impaired myocardial oxygenation
OUTCOME CRITERIA
• Patient communicates pain relief
• Absence of ST, T-wave changes

CV

TABLE 2-23 Clinical Sequelae Associated with Myocardial Infarction

Complication	Signs and symptoms
Heart failure (HF)	Sustained elevated HR, cough, S_3, crackles
Pulmonary edema	Worsening HF, breathlessness, moist cough, frothy sputum, diaphoresis, cyanosis, ↓PaO_2, ↑RR, ↓BP, PAWP >25 mm Hg
Reinfarction/extension of infarction	Recurrence of chest pain, ST, T-wave changes, hemodynamic changes
Cardiogenic shock	↓ Mentation, ↑↓ HR, SBP <90 mm Hg, CI <2, urine output <20ml/hr, cool, clammy, mottled skin
Dysrhythmias/sudden death	Change in rate or rhythm, change in LOC, syncope, chest discomfort, ↓ BP
Pericarditis	Chest discomfort aggravated by supine position or on deep inspiration, intermittent friction rub may be present, fever
Papillary muscle rupture	Abrupt onset holosystolic murmur, sudden left ventricular failure, S_3, S_4, midsystolic ejection click, crackles
Ventricular aneurysm	Paradoxical pulse, ventricular ectopy, MAP <80 mm Hg, possible atrial fibrillation with BP changes, change in HR, outward bulging of precordium
Ventricular septal rupture	Sudden onset of palpable thrill, holosystolic murmur at LSB, sudden left ventricular failure, SOB, cough

PATIENT MONITORING

1. Continuous ECG monitoring to evaluate ST, T-wave changes, which may indicate ischemia, injury, or infarction (extension or new onset) and to detect the onset of dysrhythmias or conduction problems.

PHYSICAL ASSESSMENT

1. Assess pain to validate ischemic origin. (See Table 2-25.) Use a visual analogue scale (see Figure 1-1) to evaluate the severity of the pain.
2. Check VS frequently during pain episode and with administration of antianginal agents. Hypotension can occur with these agents.
3. Assess patient for development of clinical sequelae. (See Table 2-23.)

DIAGNOSTICS ASSESSMENT

1. Obtain 12-lead ECG and compare with previous ECGs, if available.
2. Review cardiac enzyme results, if ordered.

PATIENT MANAGEMENT

1. Stay with the patient, providing a calm, quiet environment.
2. Maintain O_2 therapy and assist the patient to a position of comfort.
3. Administer NTG: sublingual, 1 tablet q5min × 3; as an infusion, start at 5 µg/min; titrate to desired response or SBP >90 mm Hg. Increase dosage q5 to 10 min by 5 to 10 µg/min. If hypotension occurs, raise legs and stop infusion.
4. Administer morphine sulfate as ordered. Give IVP in 2 mg increments q5min to relieve chest discomfort. Dilute with 5 ml NS and administer over 4 to 5 minutes. Monitor respirations.
5. Administer β-Adrenergic blocking agents such as atenolol, metoprolol, or propranolol as ordered. These pharmacological agents decrease SNS tone, reduce cardiac demand, and have been shown to prevent myocardial reinfarction. Monitor drug's effect on HR and BP.
6. Administer a calcium channel blocking agent such as cardizem as ordered to reduce coronary vasospasm; these agents can also reduce afterload and control dysrhythmias. Monitor drug's effect on HR and BP.
7. Administer antiplatelet agents to prevent platelet adherence in coronary arteries.

CV

8. Administer an anticoagulant such as heparin as ordered. This agent may be given prophylactically or with thrombolytic therapy to prevent further clot formation. Monitor patient for overt and covert bleeding and check daily PTT for therapeutic anticoagulation (1.5 to 2.5 times normal).

9. IABP insertion may be required. (See p. 600 for information on IABP.)

10. Thrombolytic therapy may be required. (See p. 618 for information on thrombolytic therapy.)

▶ **Nursing Diagnosis:** Decreased cardiac output related to electrophysiological instability and impaired inotropic state

OUTCOME CRITERIA

- Patient will be alert and oriented
- Skin warm and dry
- Pulses strong, equal bilaterally
- Capillary refill <3 sec
- SBP   90-140 mm Hg
- MAP   70-105 mm Hg
- Pulse pressure 30-40 mm Hg
- HR   60-100 beats/min
- Absence of life-threatening dysrhythmias
- Urine output 30 ml/hr or 0.5-1 ml/kg/hr
- CVP   2-6 mm Hg
- PAS   15-30 mm Hg
- PAD   5-15 mm Hg
- PAWP   4-12 mm Hg
- CI   2.5-4 L/min/m^2
- SVRI   1700-2600 dynes/sec/cm^{-5}/m^2
- PVRI   200-450 dynes/sec/cm^{-5}/m^2
- Svo_2 60%-80%
- $\dot{D}o_2I$ 500-600 ml/min/m^2
- $\dot{V}o_2I$ 115-165 ml/min/m^2

PATIENT MONITORING

1. Monitor in the lead appropriate for ischemia or dysrhythmia identification. Place in lead II to monitor for SVT and axis deviation. Place in lead MCL$_1$ to differentiate between ventricular ectopy and aberrantly conducted beats, to determine types of BBB, or to verify RV pacemaker beats (paced QRS beat should be negative). (See Table 2-24 for site of infarction and related conduction problems.)

2. Analyze ECG rhythm strip at least q4h and note rate, rhythm, PR, QRS, and QT intervals (prolonged QT is

TABLE 2-24   Infarction and Related Conduction Problems

Site	ECG changes
Anterior MI	BBB as a result of septal involvement; check widened QRS
	RBBB = rSR′ in V_1, Rs in V_6
	LBBB = rS in V_1, large monophasic R wave in V_6
	Left anterior hemiblock: LAD >−45°; negative QRS in II, III, aV_F
	Second-degree AV block, Type II
	Complete heart block
Inferior MI	Bradycardia, second-degree AV block, Type I
	Complete heart block
Posterior MI	See Inferior MI
Right ventricular infarction	Second degree AV block

CV

associated with torsade de pointes). Note ST, T-wave changes, which may indicate ischemia, injury, or infarction. Note occurrence of PACs or PVCs, since premature beats are frequently the forerunner of more serious dysrhythmias. Mobitz type II heart block may progress to complete heart block. (See p. 500 for information on the dysrhythmia interpretation.)

3. Obtain PA pressures and CVP (RA) hourly (if available) or more frequently if titrating pharmacological agents. Obtain CO as patient condition indicates. Note trends in CI, PVRI, and SVRI, and patient response to therapy. Note LVSWI, RVSWI to evaluate contractility.
4. Monitor arterial oxygen delivery index ($\dot{D}o_2I$) and oxygen consumption index ($\dot{V}o_2I$) as indicators of tissue perfusion.
5. Obtain BP hourly; note trends in MAP and pulse pressure, and patient response to therapy.
6. Monitor hourly urine output to evaluate effects of decreased CO and/or pharmacological intervention. Determine fluid balance each shift. Compare serial weights for rapid changes (0.5 to 1 kg/day) suggesting fluid gain or loss.

7. Continuously monitor Svo$_2$ (if available) to evaluate oxygen supply and demand; a downward trend can indicate decreased supply or increased demand.

PHYSICAL ASSESSMENT

1. Obtain HR, RR, BP q15min during acute phase and when titrating vasoactive drugs. Obtain T q4h.
2. Assess patient's mentation, skin color and temperature, capillary refill, and peripheral pulses at least hourly to monitor adequacy of CO.
3. Assess patient for development of clinical sequelae. (See Table 2-23.)

DIAGNOSTICS ASSESSMENT

1. Review serial 12-lead ECGs to determine location and extension of MI.
2. Review serial electrolyte levels, since a disturbance in potassium or magnesium is a risk factor for dysrhythmia development.
3. Review serial ABGs for hypoxemia and acidosis, since these conditions increase the risk for dysrhythmias and decreased contractility.

PATIENT MANAGEMENT

1. Provide oxygen at 2 to 4 L/min to maintain or improve oxygenation.
2. Minimize oxygen demand: decrease anxiety, keep the patient NPO or provide a liquid diet in the acute phase, decrease pain.
3. Maintain patient on bed rest to decrease myocardial oxygen demand during the acute phase.
4. Initiate IV to ensure emergency vascular access.
5. Administer IV fluids as ordered to provide adequate filling pressures that maintain CO. A PAD ~15 to 20 mm Hg may be required.
6. Be alert for dysrhythmia risk factors: anemia, hypovolemia, hypokalemia, hypomagnesemia, acidosis, decreased coronary perfusion pressure, administration of digitalis and other antidysrhythmic agents, pain, or CVP/PA or pacemaker catheter misplacement. Treat life-threatening dysrhythmias according to ACLS algorithms. (See Appendix A.)
7. Lidocaine may be used prophylactically to prevent ventricular dysrhythmias. The patient may be given a bolus dose of 1 to 1.5 mg/kg, followed with infusion: 1 to 4 mg/min. Do not exceed 4 mg/min. Magnesium sulfate

may also be used prophylactically to prevent ventricular dysrhythmias. The recommended dose is 1 to 2 g in 50 to 100 ml of D_5W administered IV over 5 to 60 min; an infusion of 0.5 to 1 g/hr should follow for up to 24 hours.

8. If the patient is bradycardic, be prepared to administer atropine 0.5 mg IV if the patient manifests the following: SBP <90 mm Hg, decreased mentation, PVCs, chest discomfort, or dyspnea. Pacemaker insertion may be required.

9. If the patient is tachycardic, check BP and mentation. Drug therapy depends on the tachydysrhythmia. (See Appendix A.) Be prepared to countershock/defibrillate.

10. Administer nitroglycerin and calcium channel blocking agents as ordered to reduce preload and afterload. Monitor drug effects on BP and HR.

11. Administer furosemide as ordered to rid the body of excess fluid. Monitor urine output and electrolytes.

12. Dobutamine may be required to enhance contractility. Dopamine may be ordered to increase renal blood flow.

13. Invasive therapeutic modalities may be required: counterpulsation (IABP), percutaneous transluminal coronary angioplasty (PTCA), thrombolytic therapy; or revascularization surgery.

► **Nursing Diagnosis:**   Altered tissue perfusion related to inadequate cardiac output

OUTCOME CRITERIA
- Patient will be alert and oriented
- Skin warm and dry
- Pulses strong, equal bilaterally
- Capillary refill <3 sec
- Urine output 30 ml/hr or 0.5-1 ml/kg/hr
- HR   60-100 beats/min
- Absence of life-threatening dysrhythmias
- SBP   90-140 mm Hg
- Pulse pressure 30-40 mm Hg
- MAP   70-105 mm Hg
- CI   2.5-4 L/min/m²
- $\dot{D}o_2I$ 500-600 ml/min/m²
- $\dot{V}o_2I$ 115-165 ml/min/m²
- $S\bar{v}o_2$ 60%-80%
- O_2 sat   ≥95%

PATIENT MONITORING

1. Obtain PA pressures and CVP (RA) hourly (if available) or more frequently if titrating pharmacological agents. Obtain CO and monitor CI as patient condition indicates; note trends and the patient's response to therapy.
2. Monitor arterial oxygen delivery index (Do_2I) and oxygen consumption index (Vo_2I) as indicators of tissue perfusion.
3. Obtain BP hourly or more frequently if the patient's condition is unstable; note trends in MAP and pulse pressure, and patient response to therapy.
4. Monitor hourly urine output to evaluate effects of decreased CO and/or pharmacological intervention.
5. Continuously monitor oxygen status with pulse oximetry (Spo_2) or Svo_2 (if available) and monitor patient activities and nursing interventions that may adversely affect oxygenation.

PHYSICAL ASSESSMENT

1. Obtain HR, RR, BP q15min during acute phase and when titrating vasoactive drugs.
2. Assess mentation, skin temperature and color, capillary refill, and peripheral pulses as indicators of tissue perfusion.
3. Assess chest discomfort to validate ischemic origin (Table 2-25). Use a visual analogue to evaluate severity of pain. (See Figure 1-1.)
4. Assess the patient for development of clinical sequelae. (See Table 2-23.)

DIAGNOSTICS ASSESSMENT

1. Review serial ABGs for hypoxemia (<60 mm Hg) and acidosis (pH <7.35), which may further compromise tissue perfusion.
2. Review lactate levels, an indicator of anaerobic metabolism.
3. Review serial BUN and creatinine levels to evaluate renal function; BUN >20 and creatinine >1.5 suggest renal impairment, which may be a result of decreased renal perfusion.
4. Review echocardiography or cardiac catheterization results (if available) to assess ventricular function (ejection fraction and wall motion).

PATIENT MANAGEMENT

A progressive reduction in cardiac output leading to decreased tissue perfusion in the MI patient may be a result of heart failure (see p. 179), cardiogenic pulmonary edema (see p. 153), or cardiogenic shock (see p. 159).

ANGINA

Clinical Brief

Angina is a subjective experience of chest discomfort resulting from an imbalance in myocardial oxygen supply and demand. Etiological factors in angina are usually related to the atherosclerotic disease process, whereby the coronary arteries lose their ability to dilate and increase blood flow in the presence of increased oxygen consumption. Angina may be classified as (1) stable angina, which typically results from atherosclerotic vessel changes, (2) unstable angina, which usually results from accelerated or multivessel disease, and (3) Prinzmetal's angina, which usually results from coronary artery vasospasm. Prolonged myocardial ischemia may ultimately result in a myocardial infarction.

Risk factors mirror the risk factors for coronary artery disease: cigarette smoking, hyperlipidemia, hypertension, diabetes, obesity, and stress; angina occurs most frequently in men, especially those over 50 years of age, or in postmenopausal women. A positive family history of cardiovascular disease predisposes an individual to angina.

Presenting signs and symptoms

Stable angina: chest discomfort that is predictable to the patient; usually follows exertion, meals, or increased activity levels; is relieved by rest and/or nitroglycerin; and manifests as ST segment depression (subendocardial ischemia) on ECG during the episode of discomfort.

Unstable angina (crescendo or preinfarction angina): chest discomfort that is new onset or has changed in character and is now more severe, lasts longer, is more difficult to relieve and occurs with less exertion than previously.

Prinzmetal's angina (variant angina): chest discomfort that is nontypical; occurs with rest, not relieved with nitroglycerin or rest, manifests as ST segment elevation on ECG during the episode of discomfort.

Physical examination

Appearance: Anxious

Vital signs:

BP may be elevated or decreased

HR may be elevated secondary to pain

Cardiovascular: S_4 may be present

Pulmonary: Dyspnea, tachypnea may be present

Diagnostic findings

ECG changes: ST segment depression (classic and unstable) or ST segment elevation (Prinzmetal)

Acute Care Patient Management

Goals of treatment

Improve myocardial oxygen supply
    Supplemental oxygen
    Nitroglycerin
    Calcium channel blocking agents
    Possible PTCA or CABG

Decrease myocardial oxygen demand
    Bed rest
    Nitroglycerin
    β-Adrenergic blocking agents
    Calcium channel blocking agents

▶ **Priority Nursing Diagnoses**

Pain

Risk for altered family process (see p. 29)

Knowledge deficit (see p. 43)

▶ **Nursing Diagnosis:** Pain related to impaired myocardial oxygenation

OUTCOME CRITERIA

- Patient communicates pain relief.
- ST segment returns to baseline.

PATIENT MONITORING

1. Continuous ECG monitoring to evaluate ST, T-wave changes, which may indicate ischemia, injury, or infarction, and to detect dysrhythmia development.

PHYSICAL ASSESSMENT

1. Assess pain to validate ischemic origin (Table 2-25). Use a visual analogue scale (see Figure 1-1) to evaluate the severity of the pain.
2. Check VS frequently during anginal episode and with administration of antianginal agents. Hypotension can occur with these agents.

DIAGNOSTICS ASSESSMENT

1. Review 12-lead ECG for evidence of a critical lesion of the LAD (Wellen's Syndrome). See characteristics—p. 456.
2. Review serial 12-lead ECGs to evaluate patterns of ischemia, injury, and infarction.
3. Review cardiac enzyme laboratory results (if available) for characteristic changes of myocardial infarction.

TABLE 2-25 Differentiating Chest Pain

Type	Symptoms	Signs	Pain relief
Cardiac			
Ischemic	Substernal "crushing" chest pain; may radiate to LUE and/or jaw (common), or RUE and/or back (less common)	Anxiety; skin: pale/cyanotic, diaphoretic	Depends on specific ischemic condition
Stable angina	Predictable: follows exertion, meals, or increased activity	ECG: ST seg ↓	Rest, NTG, O$_2$
Unstable or crescendo or preinfarction angina	Less predictable: occurs with less exertion than before	ECG: ST seg ↓	Rest, NTG, O$_2$
Prinzmetal's or variant	Unpredictable: may occur at rest	ECG: ST seg ↑	Not relieved by NTG or rest
MI	May not differ from angina; SOB, crackles, S$_3$, S$_4$, nausea	ECG: new Q waves ST seg ↑ or ST seg ↓, T waves inverted, cardiac enzymes ↑	Thrombolytic therapy Rest, O$_2$, and NTG may not relieve pain; MSo$_4$ may or may not relieve pain

Continued.

CV

TABLE 2-25 Differentiating Chest Pain—cont'd

Type	Symptoms	Signs	Pain relief
Cardiac—cont'd			
Nonischemic			
Pericarditis	Severe, sharp, precordial pain that may radiate to LUE	Pt appears restless; friction rub, pulsus paradoxus, dyspnea, ↑ RR ECG: diffuse ST seg ↑, T-wave inversion	Leaning forward, shallow breathing, indomethacin, ibuprofen
Gastrointestinal			
Gastric reflux	"Burning" pain, midepigastric area; nonradiating	Anxiety Skin: diaphoretic/pale Hx peptic ulcer, hiatal hernia	Antacids, cimetidine/ranitidine, viscous lidocaine
Musculoskeletal			
Costochondritis	Chest pain that may/may not be discrete; ↑ when ribs/sternum palpated and on deep inspiration	Anxiety Skin: diaphoretic/pale Shallow respirations ↑ ESR, ↑ WBCs	Position changes, ibuprofen, indomethacin

Chest wall trauma	Chest pain that may/may not be discrete; ↑ on deep inspiration	Anxiety Skin: diaphoretic/pale May see bruises/lacerations/distortion/crepitus/subcutaneous emphysema Hx of trauma	Position changes, depends on cause
Pulmonary			
Pulmonary embolism	Severe, sharp chest pain that is usually diffuse; "breathlessness"	Anxiety Skin: pale/diaphoretic Dyspnea/tachypnea, hyperpnea ABG: ↓ O_2 sat, ↓ $Pa O_2$, ↓ $Pa CO_2$ May see hemoptysis	Analgesic support may provide some relief; narcotics are usually contraindicated or used with caution.
Pleurisy	Sudden onset Stabbing chest pain that may/may not be discrete; ↑ with deep inspiration	Anxiety Rapid, shallow respirations	ASA /ibuprofen; position changes; codeine may be used with caution

CV

4. Review results of cardiac catheterization (if available) for degree of coronary artery disease involvement.

PATIENT MANAGEMENT

1. Stay with the patient, providing a calm, quiet environment. Assess level of anxiety and other factors that increase myocardial oxygen demand, such as fever, dysrhythmias, anger, hypertension, and hypoxemia.

2. Provide oxygen at 2 to 4 L/min to maintain or improve oxygenation.

3. Initiate and maintain IV line(s) for emergent drug and fluid resuscitation.

4. Administer nitroglycerin as indicated to decrease pre-load, decrease myocardial oxygen demand, and increase myocardial oxygen supply: sublingual, 1 tablet q5min × 3; intravenous, start with an infusion of 5 μg/min; titrate to desired response or to maintain SBP >90 mm Hg. Increase dosage q5 to 10 min by 5 to 10 μg/min. If hypotension occurs, raise the patient's legs and stop infusion.

5. Administer morphine sulfate as ordered. Give IVP in 2 mg increments q5min to relieve chest discomfort. Dilute with 5 ml NS and administer over 4 to 5 minutes. Monitor the patient's respirations, because narcotics are respiratory depressants. Notify the physician if pain is not relieved despite pharmacological intervention or if pain has subsided but recurs.

6. Administer calcium channel blockers such as diltiazem or nifedipine as ordered to decrease myocardial oxygen demand, increase myocardial oxygen supply, and decrease coronary artery vasospasm. Monitor drug effects on HR and BP.

7. Administer β blockers such as propranolol as ordered to decrease myocardial oxygen demand. Monitor drug effects on HR and BP.

8. Administer ASA or other antiplatelet drug as ordered to decrease chance of thrombus formation. IV heparin may be ordered for patients with unstable angina who do not have contraindications to the drug.

9. Angioplasty or revascularization surgery may be indicated.

AORTIC DISSECTION

Clinical Brief

Aortic dissection involves a tear in the intimal layer of the aortic wall, causing blood to extravasate into the media and thus compromising blood flow to the brain, heart, and other organs.

Usually the causative factor is an underlying disease of the media. Dissection can be classified by the site(s) involved: (1) DeBakey type I—classified by a tear antegrade around the aortic arch and into the descending aorta, (2) DeBakey type II—classified by a tear of the ascending aorta, and (3) DeBakey type III—classified by a tear of the descending aorta distal to the origin of the subclavian artery.

Demographic risk factors include being male, black, and in the fifth to seventh decade of life. Medical risk factors include having hypertension, aortic valve disease, coarctation of the aorta, Marfan's syndrome, recent deceleration injury, cocaine use, and/or complications from invasive procedures such as angiography or intra-aortic balloon.

Presenting signs and symptoms

The patient experiences severe, "tearing" pain that may be localized in the anterior chest, abdomen, or lumbar area. The pain is usually nonprogressive and most intense at its onset.

Physical examination

Appearance: Anxiety, paleness

Vital signs:
↑ BP, diastolic BP may be greater than 150 mm Hg
↓ BP, if hypovolemic (aortic rupture) or cardiac tamponade develops

Neurological: May have intermittent episodes of lightheadedness, clouded mentation

Cardiovascular:
Systolic and diastolic murmurs may be present
Pulse deficits and BP differences between right and left limbs may be noted

Diagnostic findings

Chest radiographs: changes seen may include a widened mediastinum, enlarged ascending aorta, blurring of the aortic knob and/or a left-sided effusion.

Transesophageal echocardiography: identifies presence and location of tear; may also identify degree of aortic insufficiency present.

Aortography: confirms presence and location of tear.

Acute Care Patient Management

Goals of treatment

Reduce BP to prevent further dissection of aorta and relieve pain
Antihypertensive agents

Propranolol
Relief of stress/anxiety
Correct problem
Aortic resection

▶ **Priority Nursing Diagnoses**
Altered tissue perfusion
Pain
Risk for altered protection (see p. 33)
Risk for altered family process (see p. 29)

▶ **Nursing Diagnosis:** Altered tissue perfusion related to compromised arterial blood flow secondary to blood extravasation via aortic dissection

OUTCOME CRITERIA
- Patient will be alert and oriented
- Skin warm and dry
- SBP 100-120 mm Hg or as low as can possibly maintain systemic perfusion
- Urine output 30 ml/hr or 0.5-1 ml/kg/hr
- Pulses strong, equal bilaterally
- Capillary refill <3 sec
- Pupils equal and normoreactive
- Extremities strong, equal bilaterally

PATIENT MONITORING
1. Continuously monitor arterial BP during acute phase to evaluate the patient's response to therapy.
2. Monitor hourly urine output, since a drop in output may indicate renal artery dissection or a decrease in arterial blood flow.
3. Continuously monitor ECG for dysrhythmia formation or ST, T-wave changes suggesting coronary artery involvement or a decrease in arterial blood flow.

PHYSICAL ASSESSMENT
1. Assess neurological status to evaluate the course of dissection. Confusion or changes in sensation and motor strength may indicate compromised cerebral blood flow.
2. Assess cardiovascular status for signs and symptoms of heart failure (e.g., sustained tachycardia, S_3, crackles), which may indicate that the dissection involves the aortic valve.
3. Compare BP from both arms to determine differences. Assess pulses for differences in quality.

DIAGNOSTICS ASSESSMENT
1. Review serial BUN and creatinine levels to evaluate renal function.

2. Review cardiac enzymes, since a dissection involving coronary arteries may result in MI.
3. Review the ECG for patterns of ischemia, injury, and infarction.

PATIENT MANAGEMENT

1. Administer oxygen therapy as ordered.
2. Keep patient on bed rest to prevent further dissection.
3. Nitroprusside may be ordered to lower BP. Titrate the infusion to desired BP. Dose may range from 0.5 to 10 μg/kg/min. Do not administer more than 10 μg/kg/min, or the patient may exhibit signs and symptoms of cyanide toxicity: tinnitus, blurred vision, delirium, and muscle spasm.
4. A β-blocking agent such as propranolol may be ordered to reduce stress on the aortic wall.
5. Nifedipine may be given sublingually in an emergent situation to rapidly lower BP. Administer 10 to 20 mg as directed by the physician by expelling the contents of the capsule under the patient's tongue.
6. Anticipate surgical intervention. Surgery typically consists of resection of the torn portion of the aorta and replacement with a prosthetic graft. With severe aortic regurgitation, valve replacement may also be indicated.

▶ **Nursing Diagnosis:** Pain related to aortic dissection

OUTCOME CRITERION

• Patient communicates that pain is reduced or tolerable.

PATIENT MONITORING

1. Monitor vital signs for evidence of pain and anxiety (e.g., increased HR, SBP, and RR). Be sure to differentiate these signs of pain from signs of hypovolemic shock.

PHYSICAL ASSESSMENT

1. Note facial expression and evidence of guarding. Use a visual analogue to evaluate course of pain. (See Figure 1-1.) Increased severity may indicate increasing dissection. Note BP, since an increased BP can cause further dissection and increase pain.

DIAGNOSTICS ASSESSMENT

None specific

PATIENT MANAGEMENT

1. Administer antihypertensive agents to control BP.
2. Small amounts of morphine may be given as ordered, depending on patient status.

CV

3. Alleviate anxieties by providing realistic assurances and providing family support as indicated. Administer anti-anxiety agents as ordered.

CARDIAC TAMPONADE

Clinical Brief

Cardiac tamponade is the accumulation of excess fluid within the pericardial space, resulting in impaired cardiac filling, reduction in stroke volume, and epicardial coronary artery compression with resultant myocardial ischemia. Clinical signs of cardiac tamponade depend on the rapidity of fluid accumulation as well as fluid volume. The acute accumulation of 200 ml of blood within the pericardium as a result of blunt or penetrating trauma to the thorax will result in rapid evidence of decompensation, whereas an insidious effusion may not evidence decompensation until as much as 2000 ml of fluid have slowly accumulated.

Risk factors include recent cardiac trauma such as open trauma to the thorax (gunshot wounds and stabs), closed trauma to the thorax (impact of the chest on a steering wheel from a motor vehicle accident), cardiac surgery, cardiac catheterization, or pacemaker electrode perforation; nontraumatic factors include metastatic neoplasm, tuberculosis, acute viral or idiopathic pericarditis, renal failure, and hemopericardium from anticoagulant therapy.

Presenting signs and symptoms

Symptoms are highly variable and depend on the cause. However, decreased cardiac output and poor tissue perfusion are the net result.

Physical examination

Pulsus paradoxus >10 mm Hg (hallmark)

Narrowed pulse pressure (<30 mm Hg)

Hypotension

Neurological: anxiety, confusion, obtunded if decompensation is advanced

Cardiovascular:

    Jugular venous distention

    Kussmaul's sign (rise in venous pressure with inspiration) may be present

    Muffled, distant heart sounds

    Pericardial rub may be present

Skin: cool, pale, may be clammy

Diagnostic findings

Cardiac tamponade should be suspected if there is a rise in CVP and PAWP, fall in arterial pressure, and a decrease in heart tones.

OTHER

ECG: usually nonspecific; may note electrical alternans and/or diffuse low voltage of QRSs

CXR: in acute cases, is rarely diagnostic. Chronic effusions may result in a "water bottle" appearance of the cardiac silhouette

Echocardiography: usually reveals widespread compression of the heart as well as inferior and superior vena cava congestion; evidence of pericardial effusion

Hemodynamics: as cardiac tamponade progresses, RA pressure begins to approximate PAWP (pressure plateau), ↑ SVRI

Acute Care Patient Management

Goals of treatment

Maintain hemodynamic stability
    Supplemental oxygen
    Volume expanders
    β-Adrenergic agents: isoproterenol
Relieve cardiac compression
    Pericardiocentesis/pericardiectomy
    Possible thoracotomy

▶ **Priority Nursing Diagnoses**
Decreased cardiac output
Risk for altered protection (see p. 33)
Risk for altered family process (see p. 29)

▶ **Nursing Diagnosis:** Decreased cardiac output related to reduced ventricular filling secondary to increased intrapericardial pressure

OUTCOME CRITERIA

- Patient will be alert and oriented
- Skin warm and dry
- Pulses strong, equal bilaterally
- Capillary refill <3 sec
- HR   60-100 beats/min
- SBP   90-140 mm Hg
- Pulse pressure   30-40 mm Hg
- MAP   70-105 mm Hg
- CVP   2-6 mm Hg

- PAWP   4-12 mm Hg
- CO   4-8 L/min
- CI   2.5-4 L/min/m^2
- SVRI   1700-2600 dynes/sec/cm^{-5}/m^2
- Urine output 30 ml/hr or 1 ml/kg/hr

PATIENT MONITORING

1. Continuously monitor ECG for dysrhythmia formation, which may be a result of myocardial ischemia secondary to epicardial coronary artery compression. Electrical alternans, a waxing and waning of the R wave, may be evident.
2. Monitor the BP q5 to 15 min during the acute phase. Monitor for pulsus paradoxus via arterial tracing or during manual BP reading. A drop in SBP >10 mm Hg during the inspiratory phase of a normal respiratory cycle confirms the presence of pulsus paradoxus.
3. Monitor PA pressures and CVP (if available) for pressure plateau. Right atrial and wedge pressures will equalize as fluid accumulates in the pericardial space.
4. Monitor MAP, SVRI and pulse pressure to evaluate patient response to increasing intrapericardial pressure and/or therapy. As the pressure increases, MAP will fall, pulse pressure will narrow, and SVRI will increase.
5. Monitor urine output hourly; a drop in urine output may indicate decreased renal perfusion as a result of decreased stroke volume secondary to cardiac compression.

PHYSICAL ASSESSMENT

1. Assess cardiovascular status: determine jugular venous pressure and presence of Kussmaul's sign. Note skin temperature and color and capillary refill. Assess amplitude of femoral pulse during quiet breathing. Pulse amplitude that decreases or disappears may indicate pulsus paradoxus. Auscultate the anterior chest for muffled or distant heart sounds.
2. Assess LOC for changes that may indicate decreased cerebral perfusion.

DIAGNOSTICS ASSESSMENT

None specific

PATIENT MANAGEMENT

1. Provide supplemental oxygen as ordered.
2. Initiate two large-bore IVs for fluid administration to maintain filling pressure.

3. Pharmacological therapy may include isoproterenol to enhance myocardial contractility and decrease peripheral vascular resistance. This is a temporary measure to maintain CO and tissue perfusion until the tamponade can be relieved. Isoproterenol infusion can be initiated at 1 μg/min. Monitor for cardiac dysrhythmias and hypotension.

4. Pericardiocentesis may be performed. Monitor the patient for dysrhythmias, coronary artery laceration (chest discomfort suggestive of ischemia), or hemopneumothorax (dyspnea, decreased or absent ipsilateral breath sounds, contralateral tracheal shift).

5. Surgical intervention to identify and repair bleeding site and evacuate clots in the mediastinum, or resection of the pericardium may be required.

CARDIOGENIC PULMONARY EDEMA

Clinical Brief

Pulmonary edema is an abnormal accumulation of extravascular fluid in the lung parenchyma that interferes with adequate gas exchange. This is a life-threatening situation that needs immediate treatment. The most common cause of cardiogenic pulmonary edema is left ventricular failure. Risk factors include ischemic heart disease, cardiomyopathy, and valvular disease.

Presenting signs and symptoms

Signs and symptoms include shortness of breath, orthopnea, moist cough with pink frothy sputum, chest discomfort, and palpitations.

Physical examination

Appearance: Anxious
Vital signs:
    HR sustained tachycardia
    SBP <90 mm Hg
    RR >30/min
Cardiovascular:
    Alteration in rhythm with ectopy
    Murmur
    S_3 with possible S_4
Pulmonary:
    Respiratory distress
    Orthopnea
    Coarse bilateral crackles
    Frothy sputum

Diagnostic findings

ABGs: Acidosis (pH <7.35) with hypoxemia (Pao$_2$ <60)

CXR:

  Increased heart shadow

  Kerley B lines

  Increased distribution of fluid to upper lobes

  Intraalveolar fluid

PAWP: >25 mm Hg

Acute Care Patient Management

Goals of treatment

Reduce extravascular fluid in lung

  Diuretics: furosemide, bumetanide

Improve LV function

  Bed rest

  Diuretics: furosemide, bumetanide

  Inotropes: digoxin, dobutamine, amrinone, milrinone, dopamine

  Vasodilators: morphine sulfate, nitroglycerin, nitroprusside

Improve oxygenation/ventilation

  Bed rest

  Supplemental oxygen

  Diuretics: furosemide, bumetanide

  Endotracheal intubation and mechanical ventilation

▶ **Priority Nursing Diagnoses**

Impaired gas exchange

Decreased cardiac output

Risk for altered protection (see p. 33)

Risk for altered family process (see p. 29)

▶ **Nursing Diagnosis:**   Impaired gas exchange related to increased pulmonary congestion secondary to increased LVEDP

OUTCOME CRITERIA

- RR   12-20/min
- Eupnea
- Lungs clear to auscultation
- pH   7.35-7.45
- Pao$_2$ 80-100 mm Hg
- Paco$_2$ 35-45 mm Hg
- O$_2$ sat   ≥95%
- Svo$_2$ 60%-80%
- P(a/A)o$_2$ ratio 0.75-0.95

PATIENT MONITORING

1. Obtain PA pressures (if available) including PAWP, to evaluate course of pulmonary edema and/or patient response to therapy.

2. Continuously monitor oxygenation status with pulse oximetry (SpO_2) or SvO_2 monitoring. Note patient activities and nursing interventions that may adversely affect oxygen saturation.

3. Continuously monitor ECG for dysrhythmia development that may be related to hypoxemia or acid-base imbalance.

4. Calculate arterial-alveolar oxygen tension ratio ($P(a/A)O_2$) as an index of gas exchange efficiency.

5. Monitor fluid volume status, since excess fluid can further compromise myocardial functioning. Measure I & O hourly; determine fluid balance each shift. Compare serial weights. Rapid (0.5 to 1 kg/day) changes in weight suggest fluid gain or loss.

PHYSICAL ASSESSMENT

1. Measure HR, RR, BP q15min to evaluate patient response to therapy and detect cardiopulmonary deterioration.

2. Assess the patient for changes that may indicate respiratory compromise, necessitating intubation and mechanical ventilation: air hunger, acute onset of production of pink, frothy sputum, diaphoresis, and cyanosis.

DIAGNOSTICS ASSESSMENT

1. Review ABGs for hypoxemia (PaO_2 <60 mm Hg) and acidosis (pH <7.35), which may further compromise tissue perfusion.

2. Review lactate levels, an indicator of anaerobic metabolism.

3. Review serial chest radiographs for worsening or resolving pulmonary congestion.

PATIENT MANAGEMENT

1. Be prepared to provide assisted ventilation; PEEP will most likely be employed to improve gas exchange. (See p. 577 for information on mechanical ventilation.)

2. Minimize oxygen demand: decrease anxiety, keep the patient NPO in the acute phase, pace nursing interventions, and provide uninterrupted rest periods.

3. Position the patient to maximize chest excursion; evaluate patient response to position changes with SpO_2 or SvO_2 monitoring.

CV

4. Once the patient's condition is stabilized, promote pulmonary hygiene to reduce risk of pneumonia and atelectasis: C & DB the patient, encourage incentive spirometry, and reposition the patient frequently.
5. Low-dose morphine sulfate may be ordered to promote venous pooling, decrease anxiety, and decrease dyspnea.
6. Diuretic agents may be ordered to reduce circulating volume. Monitor urine output and electrolytes.

▶ **Nursing Diagnosis:** Decreased cardiac output related to impaired LV function

OUTCOME CRITERIA
- Patient will be alert and oriented
- Skin warm and dry
- Pulses strong, equal bilaterally
- Capillary refill <3 sec
- SBP   90-140 mm Hg
- MAP   70-105 mm Hg
- Pulse pressure 30-40 mm Hg
- HR   60-100 beats/min
- Absence of life-threatening dysrhythmias
- Urine output 30 ml/hr or 0.5-1 ml/kg/hr
- CVP   2-6 mm Hg
- PAS   15-30 mm Hg
- PAD   5-15 mm Hg
- PAWP   4-12 mm Hg
- SVRI   1700-2600 dynes/sec/cm^{-5}/m^2
- PVRI   200-450 dynes/sec/cm^{-5}/m^2
- CI   2.5-4 L/min/m^2
- Svo$_2$ 60%-80%

PATIENT MONITORING
1. Obtain PA pressures and CVP (RA) hourly (if available) or more frequently if titrating pharmacological agents. Obtain CO as patient condition indicates and monitor CI. Note trends or the patient's response to therapy.
2. Obtain BP hourly or more frequently if the patient's condition is unstable. Note trends in MAP and pulse pressure, and the patient's response to therapy.
3. Monitor hourly urine output to evaluate effects of decreased CO and/or pharmacological intervention.
4. Analyze ECG rhythm strip at least q4h and note rate, rhythm, PR, QRS, and QT intervals. Note ST and T-wave changes, which may indicate ischemia.

PHYSICAL ASSESSMENT

1. Obtain HR, RR, BP q15min during acute phase and when titrating vasoactive drugs.
2. Assess for changes in neurological function hourly and as clinically indicated; note orientation to person, place, and time, arousability to verbal and/or tactile stimuli, and bilateral motor and sensory responses.
3. Assess skin for warmth and uniform color. Assess briskness of capillary refill. Assess distal pulses bilaterally for strength, regularity, and symmetry.
4. Assess for chest discomfort, because myocardial ischemia may be the result of hypoxemia and decreased CO.
5. Assess heart and lung sounds q4h and as clinically indicated to evaluate the course of pulmonary edema.

DIAGNOSTICS ASSESSMENT

1. Review serial BUN and creatinine levels to evaluate renal function; BUN >20 and creatinine >1.5 suggest renal impairment, which may be a result of decreased renal perfusion.
2. Review echocardiography or cardiac catheterization results (if available) to assess ventricular function (ejection fraction and wall motion).

PATIENT MANAGEMENT

1. Mechanical ventilation with adjunctive PEEP therapy may be required. (See p. 577 for information on mechanical ventilation.)
2. Minimize oxygen demand: decrease anxiety, keep the patient NPO or provide liquid diet in the acute phase, decrease pain.
3. Initiate an IV line to ensure emergency vascular access. Multiple IV sites may be necessary to maintain multiple vasopressor drips. Verify drug compatibilities should IV sites need to be shared by more than one IV drug.
4. Administer pharmacological agents as ordered to reduce preload and afterload (e.g., diuretics such as furosemide or bumetanide). Administer furosemide IVP as ordered at the rate of 20 mg/min. Doses as high as 120 mg may be required. Administer bumetanide 0.5 to 1 mg IVP at the rate of 0.5 mg/min. Doses may be repeated as indicated q2h, not to exceed 10 mg in 24 hours. A common effect of furosemide and bumetanide administration is potassium depletion; therefore monitor serum

potassium before and after administration of furosemide and administer potassium supplements orally and/or intravenously as ordered. Serum potassium levels should range from 3.5 to 5. Signs and symptoms of hypokalemia (K^+ <3.5) include muscle weakness, tetany, and dysrhythmia formation.

5. Administer vasodilators as ordered to reduce preload and afterload. Administer morphine sulfate as ordered. Give IVP in 2 mg increments q5min to relieve symptoms. Dilute with 5 ml NS and administer over 4 to 5 min. Nitroglycerin may be administered emergently: sublingual, 1 tablet q5min × 3; IV, start with an infusion of 5 µg/min; titrate to desired response or to maintain SBP >90 mm Hg. Increase dosage q5 to 10 min by 5 to 10 µg/min. If hypotension occurs, raise the patient's legs and stop the infusion. Sodium nitroprusside may be administered continuously via intravenous drip emergently in patients whose SBP is >100 mm Hg. Do not administer more than 10 µg/kg/min, or patient may exhibit signs and symptoms of cyanide toxicity: tinnitus, blurred vision, delirium, and muscle spasm.

6. Titrate pharmacological agents as ordered to enhance contractility (e.g., digoxin, dopamine, dobutamine, milrinone, and amrinone). Monitor serum digoxin levels within the first 24 hours of administration for efficacy. Note for signs and symptoms of digitalis toxicity, which may include dysrhythmia formation, AV dissociation, PSVT, nausea, vomiting, diarrhea, and blurred or yellow vision. Monitor serum potassium levels closely, especially if digoxin is given concomitantly with furosemide or bumetanide. Signs and symptoms of digitalis toxicity will be exhibited earlier if the patient is hypokalemic. Dobutamine can be initiated at 0.5 mg/kg/min. Amrinone is typically administered via initial IV bolus, followed by a maintenance drip. An initial IV bolus should be given as 0.75 mg/kg over 2 to 3 min. Follow this with an infusion, titrating the dose at 5 to 10 µg/kg/min to the desired effects. Total 24-hour dose should not exceed 10 mg/kg. Milrinone is administered as a 50 µg/kg bolus over 10 min, followed by an infusion of 0.5 µg/kg/min. Dopamine administered at low dose (1 to 2 µg/kg/min) increases renal blood flow; at moderate doses (2 to 10 µg/kg/min), contractility is enhanced.

CARDIOGENIC SHOCK

Clinical Brief

Left ventricular dysfunction resulting from myocardial infarction is the most common cause of cardiogenic shock. The loss of viable myocardium and consequently impaired contractility adversely affect stroke volume. Other causes include ventricular septal defect, papillary muscle rupture, pulmonary embolism, endstage cardiomyopathies, and valvular disorders. The primary defect in this acute circulatory failure is severe left ventricular dysfunction.

Presenting signs and symptoms

Appearance: Restlessness progressing to unresponsiveness

Vital signs:

HR >100 beats/min

SBP <80 mm Hg

RR >20/min

Physical examination

Neurological: agitation, restlessness progressing to unresponsiveness

Cardiovascular: weak, thready pulses; rhythm may be irregular; S_3, S_4

Pulmonary: crackles, rapid respirations

Skin: cool, clammy skin, color pale, delayed capillary refill

Diagnostic findings

Clinical manifestations and hemodynamic findings are the basis for diagnosis.

CI <2 L/min/m²

PAWP >18 mm Hg

SVRI increasing trend

Pulse pressure narrowed

SI decreasing trend

LVSWI decreasing trend

Urine output <0.5 ml/kg/hr

Acute Care Patient Management

Goals of treatment

Optimize oxygen delivery

Supplemental oxygen

Intubation and mechanical ventilation

Morphine sulfate

Inotropes: dopamine, dobutamine, amrinone

CV

Vasopressors: norepinephrine, epinephrine, phenyl-
ephrine, methoxamine hydrochloride
Mechanical support: IABP, VAD
ECMO
PTCA, CABG
Reduce oxygen demand
Morphine sulfate
Diuretics: furosemide, bumetanide
Vasodilators: nitroglycerin
Mechanical support: IABP, VAD
Detect/prevent clinical sequelae
See Table 2-26
▶ **Priority Nursing Diagnoses**
Altered tissue perfusion
Impaired gas exchange
Altered protection (see p. 33)
Risk for altered family process (see p. 29)
Altered nutrition: less than body requirements
(see p. 41)
▶ **Nursing Diagnoses:** Altered tissue perfusion related
to Decreased cardiac output secondary to decreased con-
tractility
OUTCOME CRITERIA
• Patient will be alert and oriented
• Skin warm and dry

TABLE 2-26 Clinical Sequelae Associated with
Cardiogenic Shock

Complication	Signs and symptoms
Cardiopulmonary arrest	Nonpalpable pulse, absent respirations
Extension of MI	Cardiac pain, ST, T-changes involving more leads
Pulmonary edema	Dyspnea, cough, frothy sputum, cyanosis $\downarrow PaO_2$, $\uparrow RR$, $\downarrow BP$, PAWP >25 mm Hg
Renal failure	Urine output <0.5 ml/kg/hr, steady rise in creatinine
GI dysfunction/bleed	Blood in NG aspirate, emesis, stool; absent bowel sounds, distention

- Peripheral pulses strong
- HR   60-100 beats/min
- Absence of life-threatening dysrhythmias
- Coronary perfusion pressure 60-80 mm Hg
- Urine output 30 ml/hr or 0.5-1 ml/kg/hr
- SBP   90-140 mm Hg
- MAP   70-105 mm Hg
- CI   2.5-4 L/min/m²
- SVRI   1700-2600 dynes/sec/cm⁻⁵/m²
- PVRI   200-450 dynes/sec/cm⁻⁵/m²
- O_2 sat   ≥95%
- Svo_2 60%-80%
- $\dot{D}o_2I$ 500-600 ml/min/m²
- $\dot{V}o_2I$ 115-165 ml/min/m²

PATIENT MONITORING

1. Monitor BP continuously via arterial cannulation since cuff pressures are less accurate in shock states. Monitor MAP, an indicator that accurately reflects tissue perfusion. MAP <60 mm Hg adversely affects cerebral and renal perfusion.
2. Continuously monitor ECG to detect life-threatening dysrhythmias or HR >140 beats/min, which can adversely affect stroke volume. Monitor for ischemia (ST, T-wave changes) associated with decreased coronary perfusion.
3. Calculate coronary perfusion pressure; a decrease promotes further myocardial ischemia and necrosis.
4. Obtain CO/CI at least q8h or more frequently to evaluate patient response to changes in therapies.
5. Note trends in LVSWI/RVSWI to evaluate myocardial contractility. An increase reflects improved contractility.
6. Monitor trends in SVRI and PVRI. An increasing trend reflects increased afterload and increased myocardial oxygen consumption, which can further compromise myocardial function.
7. Monitor trends in $\dot{D}o_2I$ and $\dot{V}o_2I$ to evaluate effectiveness of therapies. Inadequate oxygen delivery or consumption produces tissue hypoxia.
8. Monitor PA pressures and CVP (if available) hourly or more frequently to evaluate patient response to treatment. Both parameters reflect the capacity of the vascular system to accept volume and can be used to monitor for fluid overload and pulmonary edema.

9. Continuously monitor Svo_2. A decreasing trend may indicate decreased CO and increased tissue oxygen extraction (inadequate perfusion).

10. Monitor hourly urine output to evaluate renal perfusion.

PHYSICAL ASSESSMENT

1. Obtain HR, RR, BP q15min to evaluate patient response to therapy and detect cardiopulmonary deterioration.

2. Assess mentation, skin temperature, and peripheral pulses and the presence of cardiac or abdominal pain to evaluate CO and state of vasoconstriction.

3. Assess the patient for development of clinical sequelae. (See Table 2-26.)

DIAGNOSTICS ASSESSMENT

1. Review ABGs for hypoxemia and acidosis, since these conditions can precipitate dysrhythmias or affect myocardial contractility. O_2 sat should be ≥95%.

2. Review serial ECGs to evaluate myocardial injury, ischemia, necrosis.

3. Review Hgb and Hct levels and note trends. Decreased RBCs can adversely affect oxygen-carrying capacity.

4. Review lactate levels, an indicator of anaerobic metabolism. Increased levels may signal decreasing oxygen delivery.

5. Review BUN, creatinine, and electrolytes and note trends to evaluate renal function.

PATIENT MANAGEMENT

1. Administer low dose morphine sulfate as ordered to promote venous pooling and decrease dyspnea, anxiety, and pain.

2. Administer inotropes such as dobutamine and dopamine to increase contractility, increase stroke volume, and raise cardiac output.

3. Administer vasodilators such as nitroglycerin (mainly venous effects) and nitroprusside (mainly arterial effects) to reduce preload and afterload, improve stroke volume, and reduce myocardial oxygen consumption. Monitor BP closely to avoid hypotension. Nitroglycerine may have more beneficial effects with myocardial ischemia or infarction than nitroprusside.

4. Administer colloids as ordered if the patient is hypovolemic (CVP <6 mm Hg; PAWP <18 mm Hg). Cardiac patients generally require a higher filling pressure

(preload). Monitor PAWP closely; >25 mm Hg is associated with pulmonary edema.

5. Administer diuretics (furosemide, bumetanide) as ordered to decrease circulating volume and decrease preload as necessary. Monitor CVP and PAWP for decreasing trends that would suggest hypovolemia. Monitor for hypokalemia secondary to diuresis and correct imbalance.

6. Correct an acidotic state, since acidosis blocks or diminishes responsiveness to drug therapy. Monitor potassium levels in addition to pH, since excessive sodium bicarbonate administration is associated with hypokalemia.

7. Provide oxygen therapy as ordered. Anticipate intubation and mechanical ventilation if the oxygenation status deteriorates or cardiopulmonary arrest ensues.

8. Treat dysrhythmias according to ACLS. (See Appendix A.)

9. Prepare the patient for IABP, VAD, or ECMO. (See Chapter 7 for specific therapy.)

10. PTCA and CABG may be performed to interrupt the progressive myocardial necrosis associated with myocardial infarction.

11. Other surgical interventions (e.g., VSD repair, aneurysm resection) may be required.

▶ **Nursing Diagnosis: Impaired gas exchange** related to increased LVEDP and pulmonary edema associated with severe LV dysfunction

OUTCOME CRITERIA
- Patient will be alert and oriented
- PaO_2 80-100 mm Hg
- pH   7.35-7.45
- $PaCO_2$ 35-45 mm Hg
- O_2 sat   ≥95%
- RR   12-20 min, eupnea
- Lungs clear to auscultation
- PAWP   4-12 mm Hg

PATIENT MONITORING

1. Continuously monitor oxygenation status with pulse oximetry. Be alert for effects of interventions and patient activities that may adversely affect oxygen saturation.

2. Continuously monitor ECG, since hypoxia is a risk factor for dysrhythmias, which can further aggravate ventricular dysfunction.

CV

3. Continuously monitor PA systolic pressure, since hypoxia can increase sympathetic tone and increase pulmonary vasoconstriction.
4. Note trends in PAD and PAWP; increasing values may indicate pulmonary congestion.
5. Monitor fluid volume status; measure hourly I & O and measure serial weights (1 kg weight gain reflects ~ 1000 ml fluid retention).

PHYSICAL ASSESSMENT
1. Obtain HR, RR, BP q15min to evaluate patient response to therapy and detect cardiopulmonary deterioration.
2. Assess the patient's respiratory status: RR >30/min suggests impending respiratory dysfunction. Note the use of accessory muscles and respiratory pattern. Note the presence of adventitious breath sounds suggesting worsening pulmonary congestion.
3. Assess for signs and symptoms of hypoxia: increased restlessness, increased complaints of dyspnea, changes in LOC. Cyanosis is a late sign.
4. Assess for excess fluid volume, which can further compromise myocardial function: note pulmonary congestion, increased jugular venous distention, ascites, peripheral edema, and positive hepatojugular reflex.
5. Assess the patient for development of clinical sequelae. (See Table 2-26.)

DIAGNOSTICS ASSESSMENT
1. Review ABGs for decreasing trends in PaO_2 (hypoxemia) or pH (acidosis). These conditions can adversely affect myocardial contractility and stroke volume. O_2 sat should be ≥95%.
2. Review serial chest radiographs to evaluate the patient's progress or a worsening lung condition.
3. Review Hgb and Hct levels and note trends. Decreased RBCs can adversely affect oxygen-carrying capacity.

PATIENT MANAGEMENT
1. Provide supplemental oxygen as ordered. If the patient develops respiratory distress, be prepared for intubation and mechanical ventilation. (See p. 577 for information on mechanical ventilation.)
2. Administer low-dose morphine sulfate as ordered to promote venous pooling and decrease dyspnea.
3. When the patient is hemodynamically stable, promote pulmonary hygiene with cough, deep breathing, and position changes q2h.

4. Minimize oxygen demand by decreasing anxiety, fever, and pain.
5. Administer diuretics as ordered to reduce circulating volume and decrease preload.
6. Position patient for maximum chest excursion and comfort.

CARDIOMYOPATHY

Clinical Brief

Cardiomyopathy is a dysfunction of cardiac muscle not associated with coronary artery disease (CAD), hypertension (HTN), or valvular, vascular, or pulmonary disease. Cardiomyopathies are classified into three groups:

- Dilated, or congestive, cardiomyopathy (DC) is characterized by ventricular dilation and impaired systolic function. Emboli may occur because of blood stasis in the dilated ventricles. This is the most common type of cardiomyopathy.
- Restrictive cardiomyopathy (RC) is characterized by a decreased diastolic compliance. The ventricular cavity is decreased, and clinical manifestations are similar to chronic constrictive pericarditis.
- Hypertrophic cardiomyopathy (HC) is characterized by inappropriate myocardial hypertrophy without ventricular dilation. Obstruction to left ventricular outflow may or may not be present. Ventricular compliance is decreased and diastolic filling is impaired.

Presenting signs and symptoms

Signs and symptoms of cardiomyopathy include manifestations of heart failure, dysrhythmias, or conduction disturbances. Sudden death may result from cardiomyopathy.

Physical examination

Vital signs:
    HR increased, irregular rhythm
    BP ↑ or ↓, depending on underlying disease or degree of heart failure
    RR may be ↑, depending on degree of heart failure
Cardiovascular:
    Murmurs
    S_3 and/or S_4
    Ectopy
    ↑JVP
Pulmonary:
    Crackles
    Dry cough

Diagnostic findings

ECG: Supraventricular and ventricular dysrhythmias, LV hypertrophy and/or strain or RV hypertrophy and/or strain, abnormal Q waves without infarction

CXR: Evidence of heart failure, enlarged cardiac silhouette, possibly pleural effusion

Echocardiogram:
 LV hypertrophy
 RV hypertrophy
 ↓EF
 ↓CO
 Possible area of hypokinesia

Hemodynamics:
 ↑PAWP
 ↑SVRI

Acute Care Patient Management

Goals of treatment

Maximize cardiac output
 Bed rest
 Inotropic drugs: digoxin, dobutamine, amrinone, milrinone*
 Antidysrhythmic agents
 β Blockers: propranolol
 Percutaneous laser myoplasty (HC)
 Surgery: heart transplant (DC)
           myotomy/myectomy (HC)
Decrease myocardial work
 Supplemental oxygen
 Diuretics: furosemide, bumetanide*
 Vasodilators: nitroglycerin, nitroprusside, captopril*
 β Blockers: propranolol
Detect/prevent clinical sequelae
 See Table 2-27

▶ **Priority Nursing Diagnoses**
Decreased cardiac output
Pain
Impaired gas exchange
Fluid volume excess
Risk for altered protection (see p. 33)

Note: Inotropic, diuretic, and vasodilator agents are contraindicated in the early stages of HC.

TABLE 2-27 Clinical Sequelae Associated with Cardiomyopathy

Complication	Signs and symptoms
Pulmonary edema	Worsening HF: breathlessness, moist cough, frothy sputum, ↑Pao$_2$, ↑RR, ↓BP
Cardiogenic shock	↓Mentation, ↑ or ↓ HR, SBP <90 mm Hg, CI <2 L/min/m², urine output <0.5 ml/kg/hr; cool, clammy, mottled skin
Dysrhythmias/sudden death	Change in rate and/or rhythm, change in LOC, syncope, chest discomfort
Thrombus with embolic event	Change in LOC, ECG changes indicative of ischemia, dysrhythmias, renal failure, GI ileus, abdominal pain, SOB, ↓Pao$_2$, crackles

Risk for altered family process (see p. 29)
Altered nutrition: less than body requirements (see p. 41)
▶ **Nursing Diagnosis:** Decreased cardiac output related to dysrhythmias and left ventricular dysfunction
OUTCOME CRITERIA
- Patient will be alert and oriented
- Skin warm and dry
- Pulses strong, equal bilaterally
- Capillary refill <3 sec
- SBP   90-140 mm Hg
- MAP   70-105 mm Hg
- Pulse pressure 30-40 mm Hg
- HR   60-100 beats/min
- Absence of life-threatening dysrhythmias
- Urine output 30 ml/hr or 0.5-1 ml/kg/hr
- CVP   2-6 mm Hg
- PAS   15-30 mm Hg

CV

- PAD $\quad$ 5-15 mm Hg
- PAWP $\quad$ 4-12 mm Hg
- SVRI $\quad$ 1700-2600 dynes/sec/cm^{-5}/m^2
- PVRI $\quad$ 200-450 dynes/sec/cm^{-5}/m^2
- CI $\quad$ 2.5-4 L/min/m^2

PATIENT MONITORING

1. Obtain PA pressures and CVP (RA) hourly (if available) or more frequently if titrating pharmacological agents. Obtain CO as patient condition indicates and monitor CI. Note trends or patient's response to therapy.
2. Obtain BP hourly or more frequently if the patient's condition is unstable. Note trends in MAP and pulse pressure, and patient's response to therapy.
3. Monitor hourly urine output to evaluate effects of decreased CO and/or pharmacological intervention.
4. Analyze ECG rhythm strip at least q4h and note rate, rhythm, PR, QRS, and QT intervals. Note ST, T-wave changes, which may indicate ischemia.

PHYSICAL ASSESSMENT

1. Obtain HR, RR, BP q15min during acute phase and when titrating vasoactive drugs.
2. Assess for changes in neurological function hourly and as clinically indicated; note orientation to person, place, and time, arousability to verbal and/or tactile stimuli, and bilateral motor and sensory responses.
3. Assess skin for warmth and uniform color. Assess briskness of capillary refill. Assess distal pulses bilaterally for strength, regularity, and symmetry.
4. Assess for chest discomfort, because myocardial ischemia may be the net result of poor perfusion secondary to decreased cardiac output.
5. Assess heart and lung sounds to evaluate course of heart failure.
6. Assess the patient for development of clinical sequelae. (See Table 2-27.)

DIAGNOSTICS ASSESSMENT

1. Review signal-averaged ECG, echocardiography, or cardiac catheterization results (if available) and note ventricular function (ejection fraction and wall motion).

PATIENT MANAGEMENT

1. Provide O$_2$ at 2 to 4 L/min to maintain or improve oxygenation.
2. Minimize oxygen demand: decrease anxiety, keep the patient NPO or provide a liquid diet in acute phase.

3. Maintain patient on bed rest to decrease myocardial oxygen demand during the acute phase.

4. Initiate and maintain IV line(s) for emergent drug and/or fluid resuscitation.

5. Administer pharmacological agents as ordered to reduce preload and afterload (e.g., diuretics such as furosemide or bumetanide). Administer furosemide IVP as ordered at the rate of 20 mg/min. Doses as high as 120 mg may be required. Administer bumetanide IVP at the rate of 0.5 mg/min. Doses may be repeated as indicted q2h not to exceed 10 mg in 24 hours. A common effect of furosemide and bumetanide administration is potassium depletion; therefore monitor serum potassium before and after administration of furosemide and administer potassium supplements orally and/or intravenously as ordered. Serum potassium levels should range from 3.5 to 5. Signs and symptoms of hypokalemia (K^+ <3.5) include muscle weakness, tetany, and dysrhythmia formation.

6. Administer vasodilators to reduce preload and afterload in patients with dilated cardiomyopathy. Vasodilators are contraindicated in hypertrophic cardiomyopathy. If nitroglycerin is ordered, start the infusion at 5 μg/min; titrate to desired response or to maintain SBP >90 mm Hg. Increase dosage q5 to 10 min by 5 to 10 μg/min. If hypotension occurs, raise the patient's legs and stop the infusion. If nitroprusside is ordered, titrate the infusion to maintain systolic BP at 100 to 120 mm Hg. Dose may range from 0.5 to 10 μg/kg/min. Do not administer more than 10 μg/kg/min or patient may exhibit signs and symptoms of cyanide toxicity: tinnitus, blurred vision, delirium, and muscle spasm.

7. Titrate pharmacological agents as ordered if necessary to enhance contractility (e.g., digoxin, dobutamine, milrinone, and amrinone). Monitor drug effects on hemodynamic states. Note CI, SVRI, PVRI, MAP, and pulse pressure. Patients may require digitalization. Monitor serum digoxin levels within the first 24 hours of administration for efficacy. Assess for signs and symptoms of digitalis toxicity: dysrhythmia formation, AV dissociation, PSVT, nausea, vomiting, diarrhea, blurred or yellow vision. Monitor serum potassium levels closely, especially if digoxin is given concomitantly with furosemide or bumetanide, since hypokalemia increases the risk for toxicity. Dobutamine may be required; initiate the infusion

CV

at 0.5 μg/kg/min. Amrinone may be required. It is typically administered via initial IV bolus, followed by a maintenance drip. An initial IV bolus should be given as 0.75 mg/kg over 2 to 3 min. Follow this with an infusion, titrating the dose at 5 to 10 mg/kg/min to the desired effects. Total 24-hour dose should not exceed 10 mg/kg. Milrinone is administered as a 50 mg/kg bolus over 10 min, followed by an infusion of 0.5 mg/kg/min.

8. Prophylactic heparin may be ordered to prevent thromboembolus formation secondary to venous pooling. Generally, 5000 U are given subcutaneously bid.

▶ **Nursing Diagnosis:** **Pain** related to decreased oxygen supply secondary to outflow tract obstruction (hypertrophic cardiomyopathy) or impaired systolic function (dilated cardiomyopathy)

OUTCOME CRITERIA
• Patient communicates pain relief
• Absence of ST, T-wave changes

PATIENT MONITORING
1. Continuously monitor ECG to evaluate ST, T-wave changes, which may indicate ischemia, injury, or infarction and to detect dysrhythmia development.

PHYSICAL ASSESSMENT
1. Assess pain to validate ischemic origin. (See Table 2-25.) Use a visual analogue scale to evaluate severity of pain. (See Figure 1-1.)
2. Check VS frequently during anginal episode and with administration of antianginal agents. Hypotension can occur with these agents.
3. Assess patient for development of clinical sequelae. (See Table 2-27.)

DIAGNOSTICS ASSESSMENT
1. Review serial 12-lead ECGs to evaluate effects of the ischemic episode.

PATIENT MANAGEMENT
1. Stay with the patient, providing a calm, quiet environment. Assess the level of anxiety and other factors that increase myocardial oxygen demand, such as fever, dysrhythmias, anger, hypertension, and hypoxemia.
2. Provide supplemental oxygen at 2 to 4 L/min to maintain or improve oxygenation.
3. Initiate and maintain IV line(s) for emergent drug and fluid resuscitation.

4. Administer NTG to patients with dilated cardiomyopathy as indicated to decrease afterload, decrease myocardial oxygen demand, and increase myocardial oxygen supply: sublingual, 1 tablet q5min × 3; IV, start with an infusion of 5 μg/min; titrate to desired response or to maintain SBP >90 mm Hg. Increase dosage q5 to 10 min by 5 to 10 μg/min. If hypotension occurs, raise the patient's legs and stop the infusion. Nitroglycerin may aggravate angina in patients with hypertrophic cardiomyopathy.

5. Administer morphine sulfate as ordered. Give IVP in 2 mg increments q5min to relieve chest discomfort. Dilute with 5 ml NS and administer over 4 to 5 min. Monitor respirations, because narcotics are respiratory depressants.

6. Notify the physician if pain is not relieved despite pharmacological intervention or if pain has subsided but recurs.

7. Administer β blockers such as propranolol as ordered to decrease myocardial oxygen demand. Monitor drug effects of HR and BP.

8. Avoid drugs that may increase outflow obstruction in patients with hypertrophic cardiomyopathy (e.g., digitalis, β-Adrenergic agents, and vasodilators).

▶ **Nursing Diagnosis:** **Impaired gas exchange** related to increased pulmonary congestion secondary to increased left ventricular end diastolic pressure associated with ventricular failure

OUTCOME CRITERIA
- PaO_2 80-100 mm Hg
- pH   7.35-7.45
- $PaCO_2$ 35-45 mm Hg
- O_2 sat   ≥95%
- RR   12-20/min, eupnea
- Lungs clear to auscultation

PATIENT MONITORING
1. Obtain PA pressures (if available), including PAWP; increasing PAWP may signal development of pulmonary edema. Increasing PA systolic pressure may signal hypoxia. Monitor PVRI.

2. Continuously monitor oxygenation status with pulse oximetry (SpO_2) or SvO_2 monitoring. Note patient activities and nursing interventions that may adversely affect oxygen saturation.

3. Continuously monitor ECG for dysrhythmia development that may be related to hypoxemia or acid-base imbalance.

CV

4. Calculate arterial-alveolar oxygen tension ratio ($P[a/A]O_2$ ratio) as an index of gas exchange efficiency.
5. Monitor fluid volume status, since excess fluid can further compromise myocardial functioning. Measure I & O hourly. Determine fluid balance each shift. Compare serial weights. Rapid (0.5 to 1 kg/day) changes in weight suggest fluid gain or loss.

PHYSICAL ASSESSMENT
1. Assess respiratory status frequently during the acute phase. RR >30/min, increasing complaints of dyspnea, increasing restlessness, and use of accessory muscles indicate respiratory distress and increased patient effort. Cyanosis is a late sign.
2. Assess lung sounds for adventitious sounds and to evaluate the course of pulmonary congestion.
3. Assess the patient for the development of clinical sequelae. (See Table 2-27.)

DIAGNOSTICS ASSESSMENT
1. Review serial ABGs for hypoxemia (PaO_2 <60 mm Hg) and acidosis (pH <7.35), which may further compromise tissue perfusion.
2. Review lactate levels, an indicator of anaerobic metabolism.
3. Review serial chest radiographs for pulmonary congestion.

PATIENT MANAGEMENT
1. Provide supplemental oxygen as ordered to maintain or improve oxygenation. If patient develops respiratory distress, be prepared for intubation and mechanical ventilation.
2. Minimize oxygen demand: decrease anxiety, keep the patient NPO or provide a liquid diet in the acute phase, decrease pain, limit patient activities, pace activities and nursing interventions, and provide uninterrupted rest periods.
3. Maintain the patient on bed rest to decrease myocardial oxygen demand during the acute phase.
4. Position the patient to maximize chest excursion; evaluate patient response to position changes with SpO_2 or SvO_2 monitoring.
5. Promote pulmonary hygiene to reduce the risk of pneumonia and atelectasis; C & DB the patient, encourage incentive spirometry, and reposition the patient frequently.
6. Low-dose morphine sulfate may be ordered to promote venous pooling and decrease dyspnea.
7. Diuretic agents may be ordered to reduce circulating volume. Monitor urine output and electrolytes.

▶ **Nursing Diagnosis:** Fluid volume excess related to fluid retention secondary to decreased renal perfusion

OUTCOME CRITERIA
- Absence of peripheral edema
- Lungs clear to auscultation
- PAWP   4-12 mm Hg or not to exceed 18 mm Hg
- PAS   15-30 mm Hg
- PAD   5-15 mm Hg
- CVP   2-6 mm Hg
- Urine output 30 ml/hr or 0.5-1 ml/kg/hr

PATIENT MONITORING
1. Obtain PA pressures and CVP readings (if available) hourly or more frequently, depending on patient condition. Both parameters reflect the capacity of the vascular system to accept volume and can be used to monitor for fluid overload.
2. Monitor fluid volume status; measure I & O hourly and determine fluid balance each shift. Compare serial weights. Rapid (0.5 to 1 kg/day) changes in weight suggest fluid gain or loss (NOTE: 1 kg ~ 1000 ml fluid).

PHYSICAL ASSESSMENT
1. Assess fluid volume status: note increase in JVP, peripheral edema, tachycardia, S_3, adventitious breath sounds.
2. Assess the patient for development of clinical sequelae. (See Table 2-27.)

DIAGNOSTICS ASSESSMENT
1. Review serial BUN and creatinine levels to evaluate renal function. BUN >20 and creatinine >1.5 suggest renal impairment.

PATIENT MANAGEMENT
1. Administer diuretic agents as ordered and monitor urine output and electrolytes.
2. Provide meticulous skin care and reposition the patient frequently.
3. Titrate pharmacological agents as ordered to improve cardiac output to kidneys.

ENDOCARDITIS

Clinical Brief

Endocarditis is an inflammation of the endocardium; it is usually limited to the membrane lining the valves. The cause of endocarditis may be viral, fungal, or, most commonly, bacterial; the most common agent is *Streptococcus viridans.* Vegetations (growths or lesions) may cause valvular dysfunction.

Risk factors include any high-risk individual (such as a patient with valvular disease or mitral valve prolapse) undergoing any type of invasive procedure, especially dental surgery; any chronically ill individual, especially one who is immunosuppressed; any individual with previously damaged or congenitally malformed valves or who has prosthetic valves; and illicit drug users.

Presenting signs and symptoms

Signs and symptoms may be nonspecific. Fever is the most common early manifestation.

Physical examination

Physical findings are nonspecific. A new murmur may be auscultated. Signs/symptoms of heart failure may be present.

Diagnostic findings

History and physical examination: High index of suspicion in individuals with fever of unknown origin, who are anemic, and who have the presence of a new murmur.

Blood cultures and sensitivity, aerobic and anaerobic, may isolate the offending organism.

CXR: findings consistent with heart failure:
Possible enlargement of heart shadow
Redistribution of fluid to upper lobes
Kerley B lines
Pleural effusion
Dilated aorta
Left atrial enlargement

Enchocardiogram: valve disease or vegetations may be seen

Acute Care Patient Management

Goals of treatment

Eliminate infection
Antibiotic therapy
Maintain valvular integrity or improve myocardial function
Surgical valve repair and/or replacement
Supplemental oxygen
Inotropic drugs: digoxin, dobutamine, amrinone, milrinone
Vasodilators: nitroglycerin
Reduce myocardial work
Bed rest
Vasodilators: nitroglycerin
Reduce circulating volume
Diuretics: furosemide, bumetanide
Vasodilators: nitroglycerin

▶ **Priority Nursing Diagnoses**
Decreased cardiac output
Altered tissue perfusion
Risk for altered protection (see p. 33)
Risk for altered family process (see p. 29)
Altered nutrition: less than body requirements
(see p. 41)

▶ **Nursing Diagnosis:** Decreased cardiac output secondary to valvular dysfunction from infective process

OUTCOME CRITERIA

- Patient will be alert and oriented
- Skin warm and dry
- Pulses strong, equal bilaterally
- Capillary refill <3 sec
- SBP   90-140 mm Hg
- MAP   70-105 mm Hg
- Pulse pressure 30-40 mm Hg
- HR   60-100 beats/min
- Absence of life-threatening dysrhythmias
- Urine output 30 ml/hr or 0.5-1 ml/kg/hr
- CVP   2-6 mm Hg
- PAS   15-30 mm Hg
- PAD   5-15 mm Hg
- PAWP   4-12 mm Hg
- CI   2.5-4 L/min/m²
- SVRI   1700-2600 dynes/sec/cm⁻⁵/m²
- PVRI   200-450 dynes/sec/cm⁻⁵/m²

PATIENT MONITORING

1. Monitor PA pressure and CVP (if available) hourly or more frequently if titrating pharmacological agents. Obtain CO as patient condition indicates and note CI. Note trends or patient's response to therapy.
2. Obtain BP hourly or more frequently if the patient's condition is unstable. Note trends in MAP and pulse pressure and patient response to therapy.
3. Monitor hourly urine output to evaluate effects of decreased CO and/or pharmacological intervention.
4. Analyze ECG rhythm strip at least q4h and note rate, rhythm, PR, QRS, and QT intervals. Note ST, T-wave changes, which may indicate ischemia.
5. Continuously monitor Svo_2 (if available) to evaluate oxygen supply and demand; a downward trend can indicate decreased supply or increased demand.

CV

PHYSICAL ASSESSMENT

1. Obtain HR, RR, BP q15min if the patient is exhibiting signs and symptoms of heart failure and vasoactive drugs are being administered. If the patient is stable and not in heart failure, vital signs may be obtained hourly or less frequently, depending on patient condition.
2. Assess for changes in neurological function hourly and as clinically indicated; note orientation to person, place, and time, arousability to verbal and/or tactile stimuli, and bilateral motor and sensory responses.
3. Assess skin for warmth and uniform color. Assess briskness of capillary refill. Assess distal pulses bilaterally for strength, regularity, and symmetry.
4. Assess for chest discomfort, because myocardial ischemia may be the net result of poor perfusion secondary to decreased cardiac output.
5. Assess heart and lung sounds q4h and as clinically indicated for signs of progressive valvular dysfunction. Note the degree of jugular venous distention, dyspnea, sustained tachycardia, and crackles.

DIAGNOSTICS ASSESSMENT

1. Review BUN and creatinine levels to evaluate renal function; BUN >20 and creatinine >1.5 suggest renal impairment, which may be a result of decreased renal perfusion.
2. Review echocardiography findings (if available) for valvular and ventricular function (ejection fraction and wall motion) and presence of vegetations.
3. Review WBC counts to evaluate course of infection.

PATIENT MANAGEMENT

1. Provide supplemental oxygen at 2 to 4 L/min to maintain or improve oxygenation.
2. Minimize oxygen demand: decrease anxiety, maintain the patient on bed rest if in acute heart failure, and keep NPO or on a clear liquid diet as tolerated during the acute phase.
3. Initiate and maintain IV line(s) for emergent drug and fluid resuscitation.
4. Administer IV antibiotics as ordered and obtain serum antibiotic peak and trough levels as ordered to determine efficacy.
5. Administer antipyretics as ordered and monitor patient's temperature.
6. Administer pharmacological agents as ordered if the patient is in acute heart failure to reduce preload and

afterload (diuretics such as furosemide or bumetanide). Administer furosemide IVP as ordered at the rate of 20 mg/min. Administer bumetanide IVP at the rate of 0.5 mg/min. Doses may be repeated as indicated q2h, not to exceed 10 mg in 24 hours. A common effect of furosemide and bumetanide administration is potassium depletion; therefore monitor serum potassium before and after administration of furosemide and administer potassium supplements orally and/or intravenously as ordered. Serum potassium levels should range from 3.5 to 5. Signs and symptoms of hypokalemia (K^+ <3.5) include muscle weakness, tetany, and dysrhythmia formation. Nitroglycerin may be administered to decrease preload. Start the infusion at 5 µg/min; titrate to desired response or to maintain SBP >90 mm Hg. Increase dosage q5 to 10 min by 5 to 10 µg/min. If hypotension occurs, raise the patient's legs and stop the infusion.

7. Titrate pharmacological agents as ordered to enhance contractility (e.g., digoxin, dopamine, dobutamine, and amrinone). Monitor drug effects on hemodynamic status (e.g., CI, SVRI, PVRI, pulse pressure, and MAP if a PA catheter is utilized). Patients may require digitalization. Monitor serum digoxin levels within the first 24 hours of administration for efficacy. Assess for signs and symptoms of digitalis toxicity: dysrhythmia formation, AV dissociation, PSVT, nausea, vomiting, diarrhea, blurred or yellow vision. Monitor serum potassium levels closely, especially if digoxin is given concomitantly with furosemide or bumetanide, since hypokalemia increases the risk for digitalis toxicity. Dobutamine may be required; initiate the infusion at 0.5 µg/kg/min Amrinone may be required. It is typically administered via an initial IV bolus, followed by a maintenance drip. The initial IV bolus should be given as 0.75 mg/kg over 2 to 3 min. Follow this with an infusion, titrating the dose at 5 to 10 µg/kg/min to the desired effects. Total 24-hour dose should not exceed 10 mg/kg. Milrinone is administered as a 50 µg/kg bolus over 10 min, followed by an infusion of 0.5 µg/kg/min. Dopamine at low doses (1 to 2 µg/kg/min) increases renal blood flow and enhances contractility at moderate doses (2 to 10 µg/kg/min).

8. Prepare the patient for anticipated surgical intervention to repair/replace affected valve(s). In stable patients, this

will usually occur 6 weeks after the completion of antibiotic therapy. In patients with acute heart failure, this surgery may be performed emergently.

▶ **Nursing Diagnosis:** Altered tissue perfusion secondary to embolic event

OUTCOME CRITERIA
- Patient will be alert and oriented
- Vision unchanged
- RR 12-20/min, regular and nonlabored
- Urine output 30 ml/hr or 0.5 ml/kg/hr and clear yellow
- Skin warm and dry
- No c/o pain to either flank, LUQ, or periphery

PATIENT MONITORING
1. Monitor hourly urine output for volume and clarity. Check for hematuria.

PHYSICAL ASSESSMENT
1. Assess neurological status: note any change in LOC or change in motor or sensory responses.
2. Assess for chest discomfort that may signal myocardial infarction.
3. Note skin color and temperature of extremities. Check pulses and capillary refill for development of peripheral emboli.
4. Assess respiratory status for increasing dyspnea, restlessness, tachypnea, pleuritic chest pain, and tachycardia suggesting a pulmonary embolus.
5. Investigate complaints of LUQ pain or flank pain, which may suggest decreased perfusion to the spleen or kidney.

DIAGNOSTICS ASSESSMENT
1. Review results of echocardiogram for presence of vegetations and extent of myocardial compromise.
2. Review ABGs to evaluate oxygenation and acid-base status.
3. Monitor serial BUN and creatinine levels to evaluate renal function; BUN >20 and creatinine >1.5 suggest renal impairment, which may be a result of decreased renal perfusion.
4. Review results of blood cultures to determine the infecting organism.

PATIENT MANAGEMENT
1. Administer antibiotics as ordered in a timely fashion.
2. Protect IV site, since antibiotic therapy may be required over several weeks. Observe the site for redness, tenderness, or infiltration.

3. Provide pulmonary hygiene to decrease the risk of atelectasis and pneumonia during the acute phase when the patient is maintained on bed rest. C & DB the patient, encourage incentive spirometry, and reposition the patient frequently.
4. Assist with ROM exercises while the patient is maintained on bed rest.

HEART FAILURE (HF)

Clinical Brief
HF is the inability of the heart to maintain adequate cardiac output to meet the metabolic and oxygen demands of the tissues despite adequate venous return. Conditions that produce abnormal cardiac muscle contraction and/or relaxation (cardiomyopathies), conditions that lead to pressure or volume overload (increased preload or increased afterload), and conditions or diseases that greatly increase demands on the heart (anemia, thyrotoxicosis) are associated with the development of HF.

Risk factors
Risk factor for HF include ischemic heart disease, valvular disease, cardiomyopathies, high cardiac output.

Presenting signs and symptoms

Left-sided heart failure	Right-sided heart failure
Cardiomegaly	RV heave
LV heave	JVD
S_3, S_4	Ascites
Crackles	Hepatomegaly
Dyspnea	Dependent edema
Orthopnea	RUQ pain
Nocturia and night cough	Anorexia and bloating

Both right- and left-sided heart failure
Fatigue

Increased RR, HR

Decreased pulses

Pulsus alternans

S_3

Cheyne-Stokes respirations (associated with advanced failure)

CV

Physical examination
See Presenting signs and symptoms.
Diagnostic findings
ECG: may have evidence of LV hypertrophy and/or strain
    pattern, evidence of RV hypertrophy and/or strain
    pattern
CXR:
    Heart shadow may be enlarged
    Redistribution of fluid to upper lobes
    Kerley B lines
    Pleural effusion
    Dilated aorta
    Left atrial enlargement
CXR findings may lag clinical presentation by 24 hours.

Acute Care Patient Management
Goals of treatment
Improve myocardial function
    Supplemental oxygen
    Inotropes: digoxin, dobutamine, amrinone, milrinone
Reduce myocardial work
    Bed rest
    Vasodilators: nitroglycerin, captopril, hydralazine,
        prazosin
Reduce circulating volume
    Diuretics: furosemide, bumetanide
    Vasodilators: nitroglycerin, captopril, hydralazine, pra-
        zosin, nitroprusside
Detect/prevent clinical sequelae
    See Table 2-28
▶ **Priority Nursing Diagnoses**
Decreased cardiac output
Impaired gas exchange
Fluid volume excess
Risk for altered protection (see p. 33)
Risk for altered family process (see p. 29)
▶ **Nursing Diagnosis:**   Decreased cardiac output related to
impaired inotropic state of the myocardium
    OUTCOME CRITERIA
    • Patient will be alert and oriented
    • Skin warm and dry
    • Pulses strong, equal bilaterally
    • Capillary refill <3 sec

TABLE 2-28 Clinical Sequelae Associated with Heart Failure

Complication	Signs and symptoms
Pulmonary edema	Worsening HF, breathlessness, ↑RR, ↓BP, moist cough, frothy sputum, diaphoresis, cyanosis, ↓Pao$_2$
Acute myocardial infarction	ECG and cardiac enzyme changes consistent with AMI, dysrhythmias, ↓BP, hemodynamic compromise
Cardiogenic shock	↓Mentation, ↑HR, SBP <90 mm Hg, CI <2, urine output <20 ml/hr, cool/clammy mottled skin
Embolic events	
Spleen	Sharp LUQ pain, splenomegaly, local tenderness, abdominal rigidity
Kidneys	Flank pain, hematuria
Small, peripheral vessels	Mottled, cool skin; peripheral pain
CNS	Change in LOC, focal signs, loss of vision
Lungs	↑RR, SOB, ↓Pao$_2$

- SBP   90-140 mm Hg
- MAP   70-105 mm Hg
- Pulse pressure 30-40 mm Hg
- HR   60-100 beats/min
- Absence of life-threatening dysrhythmias
- Urine output 30 ml/hr or 0.5-1 ml/kg/hr
- CVP   2-6 mm Hg
- PAS   15-30 mm Hg
- PAD   5-15 mm Hg
- PAWP   4-12 mm Hg
- SVRI   1700-2600 dynes/sec/cm^{-5}/m^2
- PVRI   200-450 dynes/sec/cm^{-5}/m^2
- CI   2.5-4 L/min/m^2

CV

PATIENT MONITORING

1. Obtain PA pressures and CVP (RA) hourly (if available) or more frequently if titrating pharmacological agents. Obtain CO as patient condition indicates and monitor CI. Note trends and the patient's response to therapy.
2. Obtain BP hourly or more frequently if the patient is unstable; note trends in MAP and pulse pressure and the patient's response to therapy.
3. Monitor hourly urine output to evaluate effects of decreased CO and/or pharmacological intervention.
4. Analyze ECG rhythm strip at least q4h and note rate, rhythm, PR, QRS, and QT intervals. Note ST, T-wave changes, which may indicate ischemia.

PHYSICAL ASSESSMENT

1. Obtain HR, RR, BP q15min during acute phase and when titrating vasoactive drugs.
2. Assess for changes in neurological function hourly and as clinically indicated; note orientation to person, place, and time, arousability to verbal and/or tactile stimuli, and bilateral motor and sensory responses.
3. Assess skin for warmth and uniform color. Assess briskness of capillary refill. Assess distal pulses bilaterally for strength, regularity, and symmetry.
4. Assess for chest discomfort, because myocardial ischemia may be the net result of poor perfusion secondary to decreased cardiac output.
5. Assess heart sounds q4h and as clinically indicated. S_3 is a hallmark of heart failure. Note degree of jugular vein distention and presence of peripheral edema.
6. Assess the patient for development of clinical sequelae. (See Table 2-28.)

DIAGNOSTICS ASSESSMENT

1. Review serial BUN and creatinine levels to evaluate renal function. BUN >20 and creatinine >1.5 suggest renal impairment that may be a result of decreased renal perfusion.
2. Review echocardiography or cardiac catheterization results (if available) to assess ventricular function (ejection fraction and wall motion).

PATIENT MANAGEMENT

1. Provide supplemental oxygen at 2 to 4 L/min to maintain or improve oxygenation.

2. Minimize oxygen demand; decrease anxiety, keep the patient NPO or provide a liquid diet in the acute phase, decrease pain.

3. Maintain the patient on bed rest to decrease myocardial oxygen demand during the acute phase.

4. Initiate and maintain IV line(s) for emergent drug and/or fluid resuscitation.

5. Administer pharmacological agents as ordered to reduce preload and afterload (e.g., diuretics such as furosemide or bumetanide). Administer furosemide IVP as ordered at the rate of 20 mg/min. Doses as high as 120 mg may be required. Furosemide may also be given as a continuous infusion. Administer bumetanide IVP at the rate of 0.5 mg/min. Doses may be repeated as indicated q2h not to exceed 10 mg in 24 hours. A common effect of furosemide and bumetanide administration is potassium depletion; therefore monitor serum potassium before and after administration of diuretics and administer potassium supplements orally and/or intravenously as ordered. Serum potassium levels should range from 3.5 to 5. Signs and symptoms of hypokalemia (K^+ <3.5) include muscle weakness, tetany, and dysrhythmia formation.

6. Administer vasodilators (e.g., captopril, hydralazine, prazosin, nitroprusside) to reduce preload and afterload. Nitroglycerin may be administered emergently: sublingual, 1 tablet q5min × 3; IV, start with an infusion of 5 μg/min; titrate to desired response or to maintain SBP >90 mm Hg. Increase dosage q5 to 10 min by 5 to 10 μg/min. If hypotension occurs, raise the patient's legs and stop the infusion.

7. Titrate pharmacological agents as ordered to enhance contractility (e.g., digoxin, dopamine, dobutamine, milrinone, and amrinone). Monitor drug effects on hemodynamic states. Note CI, SVRI, PVRI, MAP, and pulse pressure. Patients may require digitalization. Monitor serum digoxin levels for efficacy within the first 24 hours of administration. Assess for signs and symptoms of digitalis toxicity: dysrhythmia formation, AV dissociation, PSVT, nausea, vomiting, diarrhea, blurred or yellow vision. Monitor serum potassium levels closely, especially if digoxin is given concomitantly with furosemide or bumetanide, since hypokalemia increases the risk for digitalis toxicity.

Dobutamine may be required; initiate the infusion at 0.5 μg/kg/min. Amrinone or milrinone may be required. Amrinone is typically administered via initial IV bolus, followed by a maintenance drip. Initial IV bolus should be given as 0.75 mg/kg over 2 to 3 min. Follow this with an infusion, titrating the dose at 5 to 10 μg/kg/min to the desired effects. Total 24-hour dose should not exceed 10 mg/kg. Milrinone is administered as a 50 mg/kg bolus over 10 min, followed by an infusion of 0.5 μg/kg/min.

8. Prophylactic heparin may be ordered to prevent thromboembolus formation secondary to venous pooling. Generally, 5000 U are given subcutaneously bid.

▶ **Nursing Diagnosis:** Impaired gas exchange related to increased pulmonary congestion secondary to increased left ventricular end diastolic pressure (LVEDP)

OUTCOME CRITERIA
- PaO_2 80-100 mm Hg
- pH   7.35-7.45
- $PaCO_2$ 35-45 mm Hg
- O_2 sat   ≥95%
- SvO_2 60%-80%
- RR   12-20/min
- Lungs clear to auscultation
- PAWP   4-12 mm Hg
- $P(a/A)O_2$ ratio 0.75-0.90

PATIENT MONITORING
1. Obtain PA pressures (if available), including PAWP; increasing PAWP may signal development of pulmonary edema. Increasing PA systolic pressure may signal hypoxia. Monitor PVRI.

2. Continuously monitor oxygenation status with pulse oximetry (SpO_2) or SvO_2 monitoring. Note patient activities and nursing interventions that may adversely affect oxygen saturation.

3. Continuously monitor ECG for dysrhythmia development that may be related to hypoxemia or acid-base imbalance.

4. Calculate arterial-alveolar oxygen tension ratio ($P[a/A]O_2$ ratio) as an index of gas exchange efficiency.

5. Monitor fluid volume status, since excess fluid can further compromise myocardial functioning. Measure I & O hourly. Determine fluid balance each shift. Compare serial weights. Rapid (0.5 to 1 kg/day) changes in weight suggest fluid gain or loss.

PHYSICAL ASSESSMENT

1. Assess respiratory status frequently during the acute phase. RR >30, increasing complaints of dyspnea, increasing restlessness, and use of accessory muscles indicate respiratory distress and increased patient effort. Cyanosis is a late sign.
2. Assess lung sounds for adventitious sounds and to evaluate the course of pulmonary congestion.
3. Assess the patient for the development of clinical sequelae. (See Table 2-28.)

DIAGNOSTICS ASSESSMENT

1. Review serial ABGs for hypoxemia (PaO_2 <60 mm Hg) and acidosis (pH <7.35), which may further compromise tissue perfusion.
2. Review lactate levels, an indicator of anaerobic metabolism.
3. Review serial chest radiographs for pulmonary congestion.

PATIENT MANAGEMENT

1. Provide supplemental oxygen as ordered to maintain or improve oxygenation. If patient develops respiratory distress, be prepared for intubation and mechanical ventilation.
2. Minimize oxygen demand: decrease anxiety, keep the patient NPO or provide liquid diet in the acute phase, decrease pain, limit patient activities, pace activities and nursing interventions, and provide uninterrupted rest periods.
3. Maintain the patient on bed rest to decrease myocardial oxygen demand during the acute phase.
4. Position the patient to maximize chest excursion. Evaluate patient response to position changes with SpO_2 or SvO_2 monitoring.
5. Promote pulmonary hygiene to reduce risk of pneumonia and atelectasis; C & DB the patient, encourage incentive spirometry, and reposition the patient frequently.
6. Low-dose morphine sulfate may be ordered to promote venous pooling and decrease dyspnea.
7. Diuretic agents may be ordered to reduce circulating volume. Monitor urine output and electrolytes.

▶**Nursing Diagnosis:**   **Fluid volume excess** related to fluid retention secondary to decreased renal perfusion

OUTCOME CRITERIA

- Absence of peripheral edema
- Lungs will be clear to auscultation
- PAWP   4-12 mm Hg or not to exceed 18 mm Hg
- PAS   15-30 mm Hg

- PAD   5-15 mm Hg
- CVP   2-6 mm Hg
- Urine output 30 ml/hr or 0.5-1 ml/kg/hr

PATIENT MONITORING

1. Obtain PA pressures and CVP readings hourly or more frequently, depending on patient condition. Both parameters reflect the capacity of the vascular system to accept volume and can be used to monitor for fluid overload.
2. Monitor fluid volume status; measure I & O hourly and determine fluid balance each shift. Compare serial weights. Rapid (0.5 to 1 kg/day) changes in weight suggest fluid gain or loss (NOTE: 1 kg ~ 1000 ml fluid).

PHYSICAL ASSESSMENT

1. Assess fluid volume status: note increase in JVP, peripheral edema, tachycardia, S_3, adventitious breath sounds.
2. Assess the patient for development of clinical sequelae. (See Table 2-28.)

DIAGNOSTICS ASSESSMENT

1. Review serial BUN and creatinine levels to evaluate renal function. BUN >20 and creatinine >1.5 suggest renal impairment.

PATIENT MANAGEMENT

1. Administer diuretic agents as ordered and monitor urine output and electrolytes. Monitor for s/s hypovolemia, dehydration.
2. Provide meticulous skin care and reposition the patient frequently.
3. Titrate pharmacological agents (e.g., dopamine, dobutamine) as ordered to improve cardiac output to kidneys.

HYPERTENSIVE CRISIS

Clinical Brief

Hypertensive crisis is an emergent situation in which a marked elevation in diastolic BP can cause end organ damage. Severe hypertension (usually a diastolic reading above 120 mm Hg) can cause irreversible injury to the brain, heart, and kidneys and can rapidly lead to death. Hypertensive crisis can occur in patients with either essential hypertension, which has no known cause, or secondary hypertension, which can be a result of renal or endocrine disease. Emergencies include hypertension in association with encephalopathy, acute aortic dissection, pulmonary edema, pheochromocytoma crisis, intracranial bleeding, and eclampsia.

Presenting signs and symptoms
Signs and symptoms depend on the underlying disease and end-organ damage. Headache, nausea, dizziness, and visual disturbances may be present.
Physical examination
DBP >120 mm Hg. (See Presenting signs and symptoms.) Other findings may be the result of damage to end organs (Table 2-29).
Diagnostic findings
Diagnostic tests are used to evaluate the effects of ↑ BP on target organs or to determine the cause of secondary hypertension.

TABLE 2-29   Clinical Sequelae Associated with Hypertensive Crisis

Complication	Signs and symptoms
Heart failure	Sustained elevated HR, cough, S_3, crackles, PAWP >20 mm Hg
Pulmonary edema	Worsening heart failure, breathlessness, ↑ RR, ↑ HR, moist cough, frothy sputum, diaphoresis, cyanosis, PAWP >25 mm Hg
Acute myocardial infarction	Chest pain, ECG and cardiac enzyme changes indicative of ischemia/infarct, hemodynamic compromise
CVA	Change in LOC, change in focal neurological signs, pupil changes
Renal failure	Urine output <0.5 ml/kg/hr, edema
Aortic dissection	Severe pain to chest, abdomen, or lumbar area; pulse and BP differentials between RUE and LUE; murmur; initial ↑ BP followed by drop in BP and tachycardia
Hypertensive encephalopathy	Change in LOC, ↑ ICP, retinopathy with papilledema, seizures

CV

Acute Care Patient Management
Goals of treatment
Reduce BP
  Vasodilators: nitroprusside, diazoxide
  Sympatholytics: labetalol
  Calcium channel blocking agents: nicardipine
  Ganglionic blocking agents: trimethaphan
  Surgical intervention
Detect/prevent clinical sequelae
  See Table 2-29

▶ **Priority Nursing Diagnoses**
Risk for injury
Risk for altered protection (see p. 33)
Risk for altered family process (see p. 29)
Altered nutrition: less than body requirements
(see p. 41)

▶ **Nursing Diagnosis:** Risk for injury: end organ damage secondary to severe hypertension
OUTCOME CRITERIA
- Patient will be alert and oriented
- Skin warm and dry
- Pulses strong, equal bilaterally
- Capillary refill <3 sec
- MAP   70-120 mm Hg
- HR   60-100 beats/min
- Absence of life-threatening dysrhythmias
- Urine output 30 ml/hr or 0.5-1 ml/kg/hr
- BUN   <20 mg/dl, creatinine <1.5 mg/dl

PATIENT MONITORING
1. Monitor arterial BP continuously and note sudden increases or decreases in readings. A precipitous drop in blood pressure can cause reflex ischemia to the heart, brain, kidneys, and/or the GI tract. Note trends in MAP and the patient's response to therapy.
2. Monitor hourly urine output and note any presence of blood in the urine.
3. Continuously monitor the ECG for dysrhythmias or ST, T-wave changes associated with ischemia.

PHYSICAL ASSESSMENT
1. Assess the patient for development of clinical sequelae. (See Table 2-29.)

DIAGNOSTICS ASSESSMENT

1. Review BUN and creatinine to evaluate the effect of BP on kidneys. BUN >20 and creatinine >1.5 suggest renal impairment.
2. Review serial chest radiography for pulmonary congestion.
3. Review serial 12-lead ECGs for patterns of injury, ischemia, and infarction.

PATIENT MANAGEMENT

1. Provide oxygen at 2 to 4 L/min to maintain or improve oxygenation.
2. Minimize oxygen demand: decrease anxiety and keep the patient NPO or provide a liquid diet in the acute phase.
3. Maintain the patient on bed rest to decrease myocardial oxygen demand during the acute phase.
4. Vasodilators such as nitroprusside or diazoxide may be ordered. Nitroprusside can be initiated with an infusion at a rate 0.5 µg/kg/min, not to exceed 10 µg/kg/min. Diazoxide can be given as miniboluses or as an infusion. If hypotension occurs, raise the patient's legs and stop the infusion.
5. Labetalol may be given intravenously, usually 20 to 80 mg bolus every 10 to 15 min to rapidly lower BP. Mini-boluses or an infusion may be ordered.
6. A ganglionic blocking agent such as trimethaphan camsylate may be ordered to emergently lower BP. Begin continuous IV infusion and titrate to the desired BP response. The usual dosage range may be 0.5 to 5 mg/min. If hypotension occurs, raise the patient's legs and stop the infusion.
7. Prepare the patient and family for surgical intervention to correct the underlying cause, if this is indicated.

HYPOVOLEMIC SHOCK

Clinical Brief

Hemorrhage is a major cause of hypovolemic shock. However, plasma loss and interstitial fluid accumulation (third spacing) can also adversely reduce circulating volume and consequently decrease oxygen availability to cells. The primary defect is decreased preload.

Presenting signs and symptoms

Appearance: Anxiety progressing to coma

Vital signs:
>   BP normal to unobtainable
>   Palpable radial pulse reflects SBP of 80 mm Hg
>   Palpable femoral pulse reflects SBP of 70 mm Hg
>   Palpable carotid pulse reflects SBP of 60 mm Hg
>   HR normal to >140 beats/min
>   RR normal to >35/min

Physical examination

Cardiovascular: weak, thready pulse
Pulmonary: deep or shallow rapid respirations, lungs usually
>   clear

Skin:
>   Cool, clammy skin, pale color
>   Delayed/absent capillary refill
>   Lips cyanotic (late sign)

Diagnostic findings

Clinical findings are the basis for diagnosis. Other findings
include the following:
>   CI <2 L/min/m^2
>   Lactate >2 mmol/L
>   Svo$_2$ <60%
>   MAP <80 mm Hg
>   PAP declining trend
>   CVP declining trend
>   PAWP declining trend

Acute Care Patient Management

Goals of treatment

Reestablish intravascular volume
>   Blood, blood products
>   Autotransfusion
>   Colloids, crystalloids

Optimize oxygen delivery
>   Oxygen therapy, intubation, and mechanical
>   ventilation
>   Inotropes, vasopressors

Treat underlying problem
>   Surgery

Detect/prevent clinical sequelae
>   See Table 2-30

▶ **Priority Nursing Diagnoses**
Altered tissue perfusion
Altered protection (see p. 33)

TABLE 2-30   Clinical Sequelae Associated with Hypovolemic Shock

Complication	Signs and symptoms
Cardiopulmonary arrest	Nonpalpable pulse, absent respirations
ARDS	Dyspnea, tachypnea, labored breathing, tachycardia, PAWP <18 mm Hg, hypoxemia refractory to increases in FIO_2, decreased compliance
Acute tubular necrosis/renal failure	Urine output <0.5 ml/kg/hr, steady rise in creatinine
GI dysfunction/ bleeding	Blood in NG aspirate, emesis, stool; absent bowel sounds, abdominal pain, N/V, jaundice
DIC	Bleeding from puncture sites, mucous membranes; hematuria, ecchymoses; prolonged PT and PTT; decreased fibrinogen, platelets, factors V, VIII, XIII, II; increased FSP

Altered nutrition: less than body requirements
(see p. 41)
Risk for altered family process (see p. 29)
▶ **Nursing Diagnosis: Altered tissue perfusion** related to
blood loss and hypotension
OUTCOME CRITERIA
- Patient will be alert and oriented
- Skin warm and dry
- Peripheral pulses strong
- Urine output 30 ml/hr or 0.5-1 ml/kg/hr
- Hct   ~32%
- SBP   90-140 mm Hg
- MAP   70-105 mm Hg
- CI   2.5-4 L/min/m²
- O_2 sat   ≥95%
- $S\bar{v}O_2$ 60%-80%
- $\dot{D}O_2I$ 500-600 ml/min/m²
- $\dot{V}O_2I$ 115-165 ml/min/m²
- ERO_2 25%

PATIENT MONITORING

1. Monitor BP continuously via arterial cannulation since cuff pressures are less accurate in shock states. Monitor MAP, an indicator that accurately reflects tissue perfusion. MAP <60 adversely affects cerebral and renal perfusion.
2. Obtain CO/CI at least q8h or more frequently to evaluate patient response to changes in therapies.
3. Monitor trends in $\dot{D}o_2I$ and $\dot{V}o_2I$ to evaluate effectiveness of therapies. Inadequate oxygen delivery or consumption produces tissue hypoxia. Calculate ERo_2; a value >25% suggests increased oxygen consumption, decreased oxygen delivery, or both.
4. Monitor PA pressures and CVP (if available) hourly or more frequently to evaluate patient response to treatment. Both parameters reflect the capacity of the vascular system to accept volume and can be used to monitor for fluid overload and pulmonary edema.
5. Continuously monitor Svo_2. A decreasing trend may indicate decreased CO and increased tissue oxygen extraction.
6. Continuously monitor ECG to detect life-threatening dysrhythmias or HR >140 beats/min, which can adversely affect stroke volume.
7. Monitor hourly urine output to evaluate renal perfusion.
8. Measure blood loss (if possible) to quantify the loss and evaluate progression or improvement of the problem.

PHYSICAL ASSESSMENT

1. Obtain HR, RR, BP q15min to evaluate patient response to therapies and detect cardiopulmonary deterioration.
2. Assess mentation, skin temperature, and peripheral pulses to evaluate CO and state of vasoconstriction.
3. Assess the patient for development of clinical sequelae. (See Table 2-30.)

DIAGNOSTICS ASSESSMENT

1. Review Hgb and Hct levels and note trends. Decreased RBCs can adversely affect oxygen-carrying capacity.
2. Review lactate levels, an indicator of anaerobic metabolism. Increased levels may signal decreasing oxygen delivery or utilization.
3. Review ABGs for hypoxemia and acidosis, since these conditions can precipitate dysrhythmias and affect myocardial contractility. O_2 sat should be ≥95%.
4. Review BUN, creatinine, and electrolytes and note trends to evaluate renal function.

PATIENT MANAGEMENT

1. Use a large-bore (16- to 18-gauge) cannula for IVs to replace volume rapidly.
2. Administer blood and blood products as ordered to reestablish intravascular volume and improve oxygen-carrying capacity. (See p. 534 for information on blood administration.)
3. Colloids (albumin) and crystalloids (LR or NS) can be administered in addition to blood. Monitor CVP and PAWP to evaluate response to fluid resuscitation. A PAWP >25 mm Hg is associated with pulmonary edema.
4. Avoid dextran infusions for hypovolemia secondary to hemorrhage, since coagulation problems can occur and enhance the bleeding problem.
5. Pharmacological agents may be used if intravascular volume is replaced and CI, $\dot{D}o_2I$, and $\dot{V}o_2I$ are not improved. Correct acidotic state, since acidosis blocks or diminishes responsiveness to drug therapy. Inotropes (dopamine or dobutamine) may be used if HR <130 beats/min. Vasopressors (dopamine or norepinephrine) may be used to maintain a MAP adequate for cerebral and coronary perfusion.
6. Provide oxygen therapy as ordered. Anticipate intubation and mechanical ventilation if oxygenation status deteriorates or cardiopulmonary arrest ensues.
7. If the site of bleeding is known (e.g., GI bleeding) anticipate appropriate treatment.
8. A pneumatic antishock garment or military antishock trousers may be used in addition to other therapies, although controversy in their use still exists.
9. Prepare the patient for surgical intervention if required.

PERICARDITIS

Clinical Brief

Pericarditis is an inflammation of the pericardium, the sac that contains the heart. The inflammation may spread to the epicardium or pleurae. Atrial and ventricular dysrhythmias may result. Resulting fibrosis and/or pericardial fluid accumulation may limit the cardiac chamber's ability to fill, affecting cardiac output.

Risk factors include infections, vasculitis-connective tissue disease, myocardial infarction, uremia, neoplasms, and trauma;

iatrogenic (after cardiac surgery, drugs, cardiac resuscitation) and idiopathic pericarditis may also occur.

Presenting signs and symptoms

Chest pain is the most common manifestation. A pericardial friction rub is a clinical hallmark sign. Typically, the pain begins suddenly, is severe and sharp, and is aggravated by inspiration and deep breathing. Pain is usually anterior to the precordium, radiates to the left shoulder, and is generally relieved by sitting up and leaning forward.

Physical examination

Appearance:
    Restlessness
    Irritability
    Weakness
Vital signs:
    HR increased
    Temperature increased
    RR increased
Cardiovascular:
    Friction rub
    Pulsus paradoxus
Pulmonary: Dyspnea

Diagnostic findings

ECG: early phase—diffuse ST segment elevation with concave curvature representing injury caused by inflammation, present in all leads except aV$_L$ and V$_1$; several days later—ST segments return to normal; T-wave inversion may be apparent

Cardiac enzymes: normal, but are increased with underlying acute myocardial infarction

Echocardiogram: may indicate presence of pericardial effusion

Acute Care Patient Management

Goals of treatment

Treat underlying disease and relieve pain
    Antibiotic therapy
    Surgery
    Supplemental oxygen
    Antiinflammatory agents: indomethacin, ibuprofen, ASA, and prednisone
Detect/prevent clinical sequelae
    See Table 2-31

TABLE 2-31   Clinical Sequelae Associated with Pericarditis

Complication	Signs and symptoms
Cardiac tamponade	↓ SBP, narrowed pulse pressure, pulsus paradoxus, ↑ CVP, ↑ JVP, ↑ HR, ↑ RR, possible friction rub, muffled heart sounds, low-voltage ECG, electrical alternans, rapidly enlarging cardiac silhouette on CXR, peripheral cyanosis, anxiety, chest pain
	If PA line in place, RAP = PADP = PAWP (equalization of pressures in all chambers)

▶ **Priority Nursing Diagnoses**
Pain
Risk for altered protection (see p. 33)
Risk for altered family process (see p. 29)
▶ **Nursing Diagnosis:** Pain related to inflammation and aggravated by position and inspiration
OUTCOME CRITERIA
• Patient communicates pain relief
• Patient breathes with comfort
• O₂ sat   ≥95%
PATIENT MONITORING
1. Check temperature q4h to evaluate course of inflammatory process.
PHYSICAL ASSESSMENT
1. Assess pain to validate inflammation-type chest pain versus ischemic pain. (See Table 2-25.) Use a visual analogue scale to evaluate severity of pain. (See Figure 1-1.)
2. Auscultate the anterior chest to determine the quality of the friction rub.
3. Assess respiratory status, since the patient may hypoventilate as a result of pain. Note respiratory rate and depth and ease of breathing.
4. Assess the patient for development of clinical sequelae. (See Table 2-31.)

Diagnostics Assessment

1. Review ABGs to evaluate oxygenation and acid-base status.
2. Review results of echocardiogram, if available. Pleural and pericardial effusion can be identified with echocardiography.
3. Review serial ECGs for changes. ST segments generally return to baseline within 7 days, followed by T-wave inversion within 1 to 2 weeks from the onset of pain.

Patient Management

1. Administer pharmacological agents such as ibuprofen and indomethacin as ordered to reduce inflammation and pain. Other agents may be ordered for pain relief; note patient response to therapy.
2. Stay with the patient, providing a calm, quiet environment.
3. Assist the patient to maintain a position of comfort (leaning forward may help).
4. Ensure activity restrictions while the patient is symptomatic, febrile, or if a friction rub is present.
5. Promote pulmonary hygiene to prevent risk of atelectasis; C & DB the patient and encourage incentive spirometry.

SUDDEN CARDIAC DEATH

Clinical Brief

Sudden cardiac death is the unexpected collapse and cardiopulmonary arrest that occurs within minutes to 1 hour after the collapse in a previously well-appearing individual. Sudden cardiac death occurs as a primary manifestation of ischemic heart disease with victims usually suffering from multivessel coronary artery atherosclerosis.

Risk factors mirror the risk factors for coronary artery disease: cigarette smoking, hyperlipidemia, hypertension, diabetes, obesity, stress, and a positive family history of cardiovascular disease; men, especially those over 50 years of age, are susceptible, as are postmenopausal women. In addition, patients who (1) are known sudden cardiac death survivors, (2) have had an acute MI within the last 6 months and evidenced early dysrhythmias and/or who had demonstrated left ventricular ejection fractions <40%, and (3) had QT intervals that were prolonged and who had a history of syncopal episodes are particularly at risk for sudden cardiac death.

Presenting signs and symptoms

A previously normal-appearing adult will suddenly collapse with cardiopulmonary arrest, not associated with accidental or traumatic causes. There may be a brief period of chest discomfort just before the arrest; however, most commonly there are no prodromal symptoms.

Physical examination
Full cardiopulmonary arrest
Pulselessness
No respirations
Monitor may depict VT/VF

Diagnostic findings
Clinical findings are the basis for diagnosis of sudden cardiac death.

Acute Care Patient Management

Goals of treatment
Salvage the victim
    CPR and ACLS protocols
    Supplemental oxygen
Salvage myocardium at risk
    Supplemental oxygen
    Morphine sulfate
    Antidysrhythmic agents
    Implantable cardiac defibrillator (ICD)
Detect/prevent clinical sequelae
    See Table 2-32

▶ **Priority Nursing Diagnoses**
Decreased cardiac output
Risk for altered family process (see p. 29)

▶ **Nursing Diagnosis:** Decreased cardiac output related to electrophysiological instability.

OUTCOME CRITERIA
• Patient will be alert and oriented
• Skin warm and dry
• HR   60-100 beats/min
• Absence of lethal dysrhythmias
• SBP   90-140 mm Hg
• MAP   70-105 mm Hg
• Urine output 30 ml/hr or 0.5-1 ml/kg/hr
• CI   2.5-4 L/min/m^2

PATIENT MONITORING
1. Monitor in the lead appropriate for ischemia or dysrhythmia identification. Place in lead II to monitor for SVT and axis deviation. Place in lead MCI_1 to differentiate between ventricular ectopy and aberrantly conducted

TABLE 2-32 Clinical Sequelae Associated with Sudden Cardiac Death

Complication	Signs and symptoms
Cardiopulmonary (CP) arrest	Pulselessness, absence of respirations
Acute myocardial infarction	ECG and cardiac enzyme changes indicative of AMI (See Tables 2-21 and 2-22); dysrhythmias, ↓ BP
Dysrhythmias	Change in rate and rhythm, change in LOC, syncope, chest discomfort, ↓ SBP (<90 mm Hg)
Heart failure (HF)	Sustained elevated HR, cough, S_3, PAWP >20 mm Hg
Pulmonary edema	Worsening HF, breathlessness, moist cough, frothy sputum, diaphoresis, cyanosis ↓Pao_2, ↑ RR, ↓ SBP (<90 mm Hg)

beats, to determine types of BBB, or to verify RV pacemaker beats (paced QRS beat should be negative). Recurrence of dysrhythmias is most common within the first 72 hours.

2. Analyze ECG rhythm strip at least q4h and note rate, rhythm, PR, QRS, and QT intervals (prolonged QT is associated with torsade de pointes). Note ST, T-wave changes, which may indicate ischemia, injury, or infarction. Note occurrence of PACs or PVCs, since premature beats are frequently the forerunner of more serious dysrhythmias. Mobitz type II heart block may progress to complete heart block. (See p. 500 for information on dysrhythmia interpretation.)

3. Obtain PA pressures and CVP (RA) hourly (if available) or more frequently if titrating pharmacological agents. Obtain CO as patient condition indicates. Note trends in CI, PVRI, and SVRI and patient response to therapy. Note LVSWI, RVSWI to evaluate contractility.

4. Monitor arterial oxygen delivery ($\dot{D}o_2$) and oxygen consumption ($\dot{V}o_2$) as indicators of tissue perfusion.
5. Obtain BP hourly; note MAP and pulse pressure and patient response to therapy.
6. Monitor hourly urine output to evaluate effects of decreased CO and/or pharmacological intervention. Determine fluid volume balance each shift. Compare serial weights. A rapid (0.5 to 1 kg/day) change in weight suggests fluid gain or loss (1 kg ~ 1 L fluid).
7. Continuously monitor Svo_2 (if available) to evaluate oxygen supply and demand; a downward trend can indicate decreased supply or increased demand.

PHYSICAL ASSESSMENT
1. Obtain HR, RR, BP q15min during acute phase and when titrating vasoactive drugs. Obtain T q4h.
2. Assess patient's mentation, skin temperature and color, and peripheral pulses at least hourly to monitor adequacy of CO.
3. Be alert to the development of dysrhythmias (i.e., change in rate or rhythm, change in LOC, syncope, chest discomfort, hypotension, and/or pulselessness).
4. Assess patient for development of clinical sequelae. (See Table 2-32.)

DIAGNOSTICS ASSESSMENT
1. Review serial 12-lead ECGs and cardiac enzymes to determine whether MI has occurred.
2. Review signal averaged ECG, holter monitor, and echocardiogram (if available) to identify the high-risk patient for sudden death.
3. Review serial electrolyte levels, since a disturbance in potassium or magnesium is a risk factor for dysrhythmia development.
4. Review ABGs for hypoxemia and acidosis, since these conditions increase the risk for dysrhythmias and decreased contractility.

PATIENT MANAGEMENT
1. Provide supplemental oxygen to maintain or improve oxygenation. Patient may be intubated and mechanically ventilated.
2. Minimize oxygen demand: decrease anxiety, keep the patient NPO or provide a liquid diet in the acute phase, decrease pain.

3. Maintain patient on bed rest to decrease myocardial oxygen demand during the acute phase.

4. Initiate and maintain IV line(s) for emergent drug and fluid resuscitation.

5. Be alert for dysrhythmia risk factors: anemia, hypovolemia, hypokalemia, hypomagnesemia, acidosis, decreased coronary perfusion pressure, administration of digitalis and other antidysrhythmic agents, pain, or CVP/PA or pacemaker catheter misplacement. Treat life-threatening dysrhythmias according to ACLS algorithms. (See Appendix A.) Be prepared to countershock/defibrillate the patient.

6. Lidocaine may be used prophylactically to prevent ventricular dysrhythmias. Administer a bolus dose 1 to 1.5 mg/kg, follow with infusion: 1 to 4 mg/min. Do not exceed 4 mg/min. Magnesium sulfate may also be used prophylactically to prevent ventricular dysrhythmias. The recommended dose is 1 to 2 g in 50 to 100 ml of D_5W administered IV over 5 to 60 min; an infusion of 0.5 to 1 g/hr should follow for up to 24 hours.

7. Since most sudden cardiac death occurrences are secondary to a lethal dysrhythmia, 24-hour Holter monitoring and possible electrophysiological study (EPS) may be done to determine the effectiveness of a pharmacological regimen. Cardiac catheterization may be indicated to determine underlying disease.

8. Anticipate ICD insertion. (See p. 599 for information on ICD.)

VALVULAR DISORDERS

Clinical Brief

Valvular disorders may be congenital or acquired. Common causes of acquired valvular heart disease include rheumatic heart disease (which is declining in incidence), infective endocarditis, ischemia (which usually affects the mitral valve), traumatic damage (commonly caused by blunt chest trauma), and syphilitic disease (aortic valvular disease). When valve leaflets fail to close properly, blood leaks from one chamber back into another; this is called a *regurgitant valve*. When the valve orifice is restricted and is not allowed to open properly, forward blood flow is obstructed and the valve is described as *stenotic*. All valves can be diseased; however, the mitral and aortic valves are most commonly affected. Murmurs and related valvular disorders are listed in Table 2-33.

TABLE 2-33 Valvular Disorders

Type	Physical examination	Diagnostic study findings
Mitral stenosis	Diastolic heart murmur Dyspnea on exertion (DOE) Weakness Fatigue Predisposition to respiratory infections Orthopnea Paroxysmal nocturnal dyspnea Palpitations (from atrial fibrillation) Hemoptysis	ECG: Left atrial enlargement Prolonged, notched P waves (P mitrale) or atrial fibrillation Right ventricular hypertrophy Chest radiograph: Left atrial enlargement Pulmonary venous congestion Interstitial pulmonary edema Right ventricular enlargement Cardiac catheterizaton: ↑ Pressure across mitral valve ↑ Left atrial pressure ↑ PAWP ↓ CO Echocardiogram: ↓ Excursion of leaflets Diminished E-F slope

Continued.

CV

TABLE 2-33 Valvular Disorders—cont'd

Type	Physical examination	Diagnostic study findings
Mitral regurgitation	Murmur throughout systole Weakness Fatigue DOE Palpitations	ECG: Left atrial enlargement (P mitrale) Left ventricular hypertrophy Atrial fibrillation Chest radiograph: Left atrial enlargement Left ventricular enlargement Pulmonary vascular congestion Cardiac catheterization: Angiography used to identify and quantify regurgitation Echocardiogram: Left atrial enlargement Hyperdynamic left ventricle

Aortic stenosis

Systolic murmur
Syncope (especially on exertion)
Angina pectoris
Left ventricular failure
Fatigue
Dyspnea

ECG:
Left ventricular hypertrophy
Chest radiograph:
Poststenotic aortic dilation
Aortic valve calcification
Cardiac catheterization:
Pressure gradient in systole between left ventricle
    and aorta (across aortic valve)
↑ Diastolic ventricular pressure
Normal left atrial and pulmonary pressures
Echocardiogram:
Restricted movement of aortic valve
Increased echoes
Thickening of left ventricular wall

Aortic regurgitation

Diastolic and systolic murmurs
Water-hammer pulse
Palpitations
Syncope
DOE
Chest pain
Heart failure

ECG:
Left ventricular hypertrophy
Chest radiograph:
Left ventricular enlargement
Dilation of ascending aorta
Cardiac catheterization:
↑ Pulse pressure
Angiography used to identify and quantify
    regurgitation

CV

Presenting signs and symptoms

Symptoms reflect left ventricular or biventricular failure. (See Heart failure, p. 179.) Atrial dysrhythmias can also be present.

Diagnostic findings

See Table 2-33

Acute Care Patient Management

See Cardiac surgery, p. 591, and Heart failure, p. 179.

ACUTE PANCREATITIS

Clinical Brief

Acute pancreatitis is an inflammation of the pancreas that results in intraparenchymal enzyme activation, tissue destruction, and ischemic necrosis. Alcohol abuse and biliary tract disease account for 80% of the cases of acute pancreatitis. Other causes include trauma or surgery, pharmacological agents (sulfonamides, tetracycline, lipids, procainamide, enalapril, furosemide), hyperlipidemia, ERCP examination, and infection.

The events that trigger the sequence of enzymatic reactions that initiate acute pancreatitis remain unknown. One of the most popular theories is that it results from obstruction to outflow of pancreatic juice or from excessive stimulation of pancreatic exocrine secretion.

Acute pancreatitis ranges from glandular swelling to hemorrhagic necrosis. Systemic effects depend on the severity of the inflammatory process. Hypoxemia is common, as are metabolic alterations, including hypocalcemia, hyperglycemia, hypertriglyceridemia, and acidosis. Hypotension and shock can also occur.

Presenting signs and symptoms

The hallmark of acute pancreatitis is a steady, dull, or boring pain in the epigastrium or left upper abdominal quadrant. This pain often radiates to the lower thoracic vertebral region and is worse in the supine position. Nausea and vomiting generally accompany the pain. The patient may be in respiratory distress and complain of thirst.

Physical examination

Vital signs:

BP and HR may be elevated as a result of pain or reduced as a result of hypovolemia and peripheral vasodilatation

Temperature is elevated

RR tachypnea

Neurological: Restlessness

Pulmonary:
  Dyspnea
  Crackles may be present
Abdominal:
  Distended, ascites may be present
  Cullen's sign (bluish-brown discoloration
    periumbilically)
  Bowel sounds decreased or absent
  Upper left quadrant (interstitial) or epigastric tenderness
    with deep palpation; initially no abdominal wall rigidity
    or rebound tenderness
Skin:
  Grey-Turner's sign (bluish-brown discoloration of flanks)
  Jaundice may be present
  Decreased turgor

Diagnostic findings

Diagnostic findings are dependent on the clinical examination: acute noncolicky epigastric pain, history of risk factors, and laboratory findings (Table 2-34). According to Ranson's criteria, the number of signs present during the first 48 hours of admission is directly related to the patient's chances for significant morbidity and mortality.

TABLE 2-34 Laboratory Findings in Acute Pancreatitis

Serum amylase	>200 U/dl	
Serum lipase	>24 IU/dl	
Pancreatic isoamylase	>50%	
Ranson's Criteria:	Alcoholic	Nonalcoholic
Age	>55 years	>70 years
WBC	>16,000/mm³	>18,000/mm³
LDH	>300 IU/L	>400 IU/L
AST (SGOT)	>250 U/L	>250 IU/L
Blood glucose	>200 mg/dl	>220 mg/dl
Within 48 hours:		
Hematocrit drop	>10% points	>10% points
Base deficit	>4 mEq/L	>5 mEq/L
Serum calcium	<8 mg/dl	<8 mg/dl
Serum BUN rise	>5 mg/dl	>2 mg/dl
Arterial Pao$_2$	<60 mm Hg	<60 mm Hg
Fluid sequestration	>6 L	>4 L

Acute Care Patient Management
Goals of treatment
Restore fluid and electrolyte balance
    Crystalloids, colloids
    Electrolyte replacement
Maintain adequate oxygenation
    Supplemental oxygen
    Intubation/mechanical ventilation
Alleviate the pain
    Meperidine
Rest the pancreas
    NPO, NG intubation
    Antacids, parenteral nutrition
Treat the cause
    Appropriate therapy
Detect/prevent clinical sequelae
    See Table 2-35

▶ **Priority Nursing Diagnoses**
Fluid volume deficit
Impaired gas exchange
Pain
Altered nutrition: less than body requirements
(see p. 41)
Risk for altered protection (see p. 33)
Risk for altered family process (see p. 29)

▶ **Nursing Diagnosis:**   Fluid volume deficit related to fluid sequestration to retroperitoneum and interstitium, intraperitoneal bleed, vomiting, or NG suction
OUTCOME CRITERIA
- CVP   2-6 mm Hg
- PAS   15-30 mm Hg
- PAD   5-15 mm Hg
- SBP   90-140 mm Hg
- MAP   70-105 mm Hg
- Serum sodium 135-145 mEq/L
- Serum potassium 3.5-4.5 mEq/L
- Serum calcium 8.5-10.5 mg/dl
- HR   60-100 beats/min
- Hgb   12-16 g/dl (females); 13.5-17.5 g/dl (males)
- Hct   37%-47% (females); 40%-54% (males)
- Moist mucous membranes
- Elastic skin turgor
- Urine output 30 ml/hr or 0.5-1 ml/kg/hr

GI

TABLE 2-35 Clinical Sequelae Associated with
Acute Pancreatitis

Complication	Signs and symptoms
Shock	Tachycardia, hypotension, altered mentation, cool clammy skin
Respiratory insufficiency	Dyspnea, hypoxemia, tachypnea, crackles, use of accessory muscles
Acute tubular necrosis	Oliguria, increased BUN and creatinine levels, urine sodium >30 mEq/L; urine casts, red cells and protein
Sepsis	2 or more of the following: HR >90 beats/min, RR >20/min or $PaCO_2$ <32 mm Hg, T >38° C or <36° C, WBC >12,000 or <4000 or >10% neutrophils; infection
Coagulopathies	Thrombocytopenia, delayed thrombin time, decreased fibrinogen, elevated fibrin degradation products
Diabetes	Elevated serum glucose, glycosuria
Pancreatic abscess	Increasing temperature, elevated WBC count, abdominal distention, pain
Pancreatic cutaneous fistula	Drainage through skin tract
Pseudocysts	Seen on CT, ultrasound evaluation

PATIENT MONITORING
1. Obtain CVP, PA pressures (if available), and BP qlh or more frequently during rapid fluid resuscitation. Monitor MAP, an indicator of tissue perfusion. MAP <60 mm Hg adversely affects renal and cerebral perfusion.
2. Monitor fluid volume status: measure urine output hourly and other bodily drainage to determine fluid balance q8h. Compare serial weights for rapid (0.5 to 1 kg/day) changes that suggest fluid imbalances (1 kg ~ 1000 ml fluid).
3. Continuously monitor ECG for dysrhythmias secondary to electrolyte imbalance associated with NG suction.

PHYSICAL ASSESSMENT
1. Assess tissue perfusion: note level of mentation, skin color and temperature, peripheral pulses, and capillary refill.

2. Assess hydration status: note skin turgor on inner thigh or forehead, condition of buccal membranes, development of edema or crackles. Fever increases fluid loss.
3. Assess abdomen: measure abdominal girth once each shift to determine the degree of ascites.
4. Assess for signs and symptoms of electrolyte imbalance.
5. Assess the patient for development of clinical sequelae. (See Table 2-35.)

DIAGNOSTICS ASSESSMENT
1. Review serial serum electrolytes to evaluate degree of imbalance or the patient's response to therapy.
2. Review serial serum Hgb and Hct, since intraperitoneal bleeding may occur.
3. Review serum albumin and protein levels since these will be decreased with third spacing of fluid.

PATIENT MANAGEMENT
1. Administer crystalloids for fluid resuscitation as ordered. Albumin may be required in hypoproteinemic patients to pull fluid back into the intravascular space. Blood or blood products may be required in case of bleeding or coagulopathies.
2. Calcium, magnesium, or potassium supplements may be needed to restore serum levels. (See pp. 277-300 for information on electrolyte imbalances.)
3. Sympathomimetic agents, such as dopamine or isoproterenol hydrochloride, may be necessary if hypotension persists despite fluid resuscitation.
4. See Hypovolemic shock, p. 189.

▶ **Nursing Diagnosis:** Impaired gas exchange related to pulmonary complications: infiltrates, atelectasis, diaphragmatic elevation, pleural effusion secondary to toxic effects of pancreatic enzymes on pulmonary membranes

OUTCOME CRITERIA
- RR 12-20/min, eupnea
- Pao_2 80-100 mm Hg
- $Paco_2$ 35-45 mm Hg
- pH 7.35-7.45
- O_2 sat ≥95%
- Lungs clear to auscultation
- HR 60-100 beats/min

PATIENT MONITORING
1. Continuously monitor ECG for dysrhythmias and ischemic changes (ST, T-wave changes) secondary to hypoxemia.

GI

2. Continuously monitor oxygen saturation with pulse oximetry (SpO_2). Monitor interventions and patient activities that may adversely affect oxygen saturation.

3. Continuously monitor PA systolic pressure (if available), since hypoxia can increase sympathetic tone and increase pulmonary vasoconstriction.

PHYSICAL ASSESSMENT

1. Assess respiratory status: note respiratory rate and depth, and use of accessory muscles; auscultate breath sounds and note onset of adventitious sounds or decreased breath sounds. Signs of hypoxemia include restlessness, RR >30/min, and altered mental status. ARDS may develop.

2. Assess the patient for development of clinical sequelae. (See Table 2-35.)

DIAGNOSTICS ASSESSMENT

1. Review serial ABGs; note trends of PaO_2, since pulmonary complications are associated with pancreatitis, and abdominal pain and distention may compromise ventilation. A decreasing trend in PaO_2, despite increases in FIO_2 administration, is indicative of ARDS.

2. Review serial chest radiographs for development or resolution of pleural effusions (left side most common), infiltrates, and atelectasis.

3. Review serum ionized calcium and magnesium levels as well as triglycerides. Hypocalcemia and hypertriglyceridemia (>1000 mg/dl) are risk factors for ARDS in patients with pancreatitis.

4. Review serum amylase and lipase levels to evaluate pancreatic function.

PATIENT MANAGEMENT

1. Administer supplemental oxygen; anticipate intubation and mechanical ventilation. (See p. 577 for information on mechanical ventilation.)

2. Elevate HOB if at all possible to improve chest excursion.

3. Reposition patient q2h; C & DB the patient hourly to prevent atelectasis and encourage incentive spirometry.

4. Administer nonopiate-containing analgesics such as meperidine (Demerol) for pain, since opiates may cause spasms of the sphincter of Oddi and increased pancreatic pain.

5. Assist the patient in assuming a position of comfort; provide a calm environment and explore alternate means of pain control (e.g., distraction, imagery).

6. A peritoneal lavage may be performed to remove toxic substances and fluid and to decrease the pressure on the diaphragm.

▶ **Nursing Diagnosis:** Pain related to edema/distention of pancreas, peritoneal irritation, and interruption of blood supply

OUTCOME CRITERION
• Patient will communicate pain relief.

PATIENT MONITORING
1. Monitor pain using a visual analogue scale or any pain rating scale. (See Figure 1-1.)

PHYSICAL ASSESSMENT
1. Assess for anxiety and fear, which may increase the release of enzymes and increase pain.
2. Note changes in HR, BP, and RR that may suggest SNS stimulation, which may signal pain.
3. Observe for cues such as grimacing, grunting, sobbing, irritability, withdrawal, or hostility, which may signal pain.

DIAGNOSTICS ASSESSMENT
None specific

PATIENT MANAGEMENT
1. Keep the patient NPO to rest the GI tract and stop pancreatic enzyme excretion.
2. Anticipate NG intubation if ileus or significant abdominal distention is present. Connect the NG tube to suction to decompress the stomach and prevent gastric stimulation of the pancreatic enzymes.
3. Ensure bed rest and limit activities to decrease the metabolic rate and the production of pancreatic enzymes.
4. Assist the patient to assume a position of comfort; provide a restful environment and explore alternate means of pain relief (e.g., distraction, imagery).
5. Administer nonopiate-containing analgesics such as meperidine as ordered, since opiates intensify spasms at the sphincter of Oddi.
6. See Acute pain, p. 30.

▶ **Nursing Diagnosis:** Altered nutrition: less than body requirements related to nausea, vomiting, hypermetabolic state, and NPO status

OUTCOME CRITERIA
• Absence of nausea and vomiting
• Positive nitrogen balance
• Serum albumin 3.5-5 g/dl
• Transferrin >230 mg/dl

GI

PATIENT MONITORING

1. Monitor I & O and caloric intake when the patient is ingesting food and fluids.
2. Compare serial weights to determine whether the target weight is being achieved.

PHYSICAL ASSESSMENT

1. Assess GI status: auscultate bowel sounds and evaluate abdominal distention; assess for nausea, vomiting, and anorexia.
2. Assess the patient for development of clinical sequelae. (See Table 2-35.)

DIAGNOSTICS ASSESSMENT

1. Review serum glucose levels, since pancreatitis-associated hyperglycemia can be aggravated once enteral or parenteral nutrition is initiated.
2. Review nutritional panel (e.g., albumin, serum transferrin, total lymphocytes, and creatinine-height index) to evaluate nutritional status.
3. Review results of 24-hour urine urea nitrogen; increased levels indicate protein loss is taking place.

PATIENT MANAGEMENT

1. An NG tube will be required to reduce vomiting and abdominal distention.
2. Consult with a dietitian for a formal nutritional work-up.
3. Administer parenteral nutrition and supplements as ordered during the acute phase. Insulin may be required to control glucose levels. Lipids are generally avoided because they increase pancreatic exocrine secretion. See p. 639 for information on nutrition.
4. Administer pharmacologic agents as ordered to reduce gastric acidity and pancreatic juices.
5. Oral feedings may be instituted once pain has subsided and GI function returns. Provide small feedings high in carbohydrates and low in proteins and fat. Note patient tolerance (i.e., absence of vomiting, abdominal distention, and pain).
6. Administer antiemetic as ordered and before meals if necessary. Supplemental nourishment may be needed. Provide good mouth care to enhance appetite.
7. Decrease metabolic demands: allow rest periods between nursing activities, reduce anxiety, control fever and pain.

HEPATIC FAILURE

Clinical Brief

Hepatic failure can result from acute liver injury (fulminant hepatic failure) or chronic liver disease (e.g., cirrhosis). An alteration in hepatocyte functioning affects liver metabolism, detoxification processes, and protein synthesis. Fulminant hepatic failure (FHF) occurs when severe hepatic injury results in encephalopathy and severe coagulopathy within 8 weeks of onset of symptoms. Without liver transplantation this form of hepatic failure causes significant morbidity and mortality. The most commonly identified cause of FHF is viral hepatitis, with nonA nonB being the single most frequent cause. Drugs, such as acetaminophen, isoniazid, halothane, and phenytoin are the second most common cause. Other causes include infection (cytomegalovirus, adenovirus), metabolic disorders (Wilson's disease, acute fatty liver of pregnancy), and severe ischemic insult (shock).

Cirrhosis is induced by alcohol (most common), decreased bile flow, severe long-term right-sided heart failure or necrotic damage due to hepatotoxins, chemicals, infection, or metabolic disorders. It is generally categorized by presentation and causative agent (i.e., alcoholic, biliary, postnecrotic, or cardiac cirrhosis). Generally patients with cirrhosis are admitted to intensive care as a result of GI bleeding (varices), spontaneous bacterial peritonitis, hepatic encephalopathy, and/or hepatorenal syndrome (a form of oliguric renal failure observed in severe liver disease in the absence of other known causes of renal failure). Hepatorenal syndrome is almost always fatal.

Presenting signs and symptoms

Manifestations depend on the complications associated with the liver dysfunction. Patient behavior may range from agitation to frank coma. Evidence of GI bleeding, renal failure, or respiratory distress may also be present. The initial manifestation in FHF is frequently jaundice.

Physical examination

Vital signs:
   SBP <90 mm Hg (with shock)
   HR >120 beats/min (with shock)
   Temperature may be elevated
   RR tachypnea initially progressing to respiratory
      depression associated with encephalopathy

GI

Neurological:
   Mildly confused to coma
   Personality changes
   Asterixis
Pulmonary:
   Crackles
   Labored respirations
Gastrointestinal:
   Hematemesis, melena
   Ascites
   Hepatomegaly may be present
   Fetor hepaticus
   Diarrhea
Skin:
   Jaundice, spider nevi may be present
   Ecchymosis
   Pruritis
   Edema

Diagnostic findings
The following laboratory findings reflect hepatocellular dysfunction:
Serum bilirubin >1.2 mg/dl
Prolonged prothrombin time; 10 sec > normal suggests
   massive liver necrosis
AST >40 U/ml
ALT >40 U/ml
Other laboratory findings vary, depending on the severity of the disease and its impact on other bodily functions.

Acute Care Patient Management
Goals of treatment
Restore fluid volume and electrolyte balance
   Crystalloids, colloids
   Electrolyte therapy
   Shunting procedures
   Diuretic therapy
Maintain adequate oxygenation
   Supplemental oxygen or intubation/mechanical
      ventilation
   Blood products
Decrease circulating ammonia and toxins
   Bowel evacuations
   Neomycin

TABLE 2-36 Clinical Sequelae Associated with Hepatic Failure

Complication	Signs and symptoms
Hepatorenal syndrome	Oliguria, azotemia, BUN/Cr ratio >30:1, urine osmolality >400 mOsm, urinary Na <10 mmol/L
Gastrointestinal hemorrhage	Frank bleeding from the upper or lower GI tract
Hepatic encephalopathy	Alterations in mentation advancing to coma
DIC	Prolonged bleeding from all sites, skin bruising, intracerebral bleeding
Septic shock	SBP <90 mm Hg, HR >90 beats/min, RR >20/min or $Paco_2$ <32 mm Hg, Pao_2/Fio_2 <280, T >38° C or <36° C, WBC >12,000 or <4000 or >10% neutrophils; altered mental status, urine output <0.5 ml/kg/hr, plasma lactate >2 mmol/L
Hypoglycemia	Headache, impaired mentation, hunger, irritability, lethargy
Respiratory failure	Restlessness, Pao_2 <50 mm Hg, $Paco_2$ >50 mm Hg, pH <7.35
Bacterial peritonitis	Fever, abdominal pain, leukocytosis

GI

    Lactulose
    Protein-restricted diet
Maintain coagulation factors
    Blood products
    Vitamin K
Decrease intracranial pressure (FHF)
    Head/bed positioning
    Control Pao_2 and Pco_2 levels
    Mannitol
    Barbiturate coma (if necessary)
Detect/prevent clinical sequelae
    See Table 2-36

▶ **Priority Nursing Diagnoses**
Fluid volume deficit
Impaired gas exchange
Risk for injury

Risk for altered protection (see p. 33)
Risk for altered family process (see p. 29)
Risk for altered nutrition: less than body requirements
(see p. 41)

▶ **Nursing Diagnosis:**   Fluid volume deficit related to fluid sequestration secondary to hypoalbuminemia, bleeding secondary to abnormal clotting factors or variceal hemorrhage, and diuretic therapy

OUTCOME CRITERIA

- SBP   90-140 mm Hg
- MAP   70-105 mm Hg
- CVP   2-6 mm Hg
- PAS   15-30 mm Hg
- PAD   5-15 mm Hg
- PAWP   4-12 mm Hg
- Serum albumin 3.5-5 mg/dl
- Hgb   12-16 g/dl (females)
               13-17.5 g/dl (males)
- Hct   37%-47% (females)
               40%-54% (males)
- Platelet count >50,000/mm³
- Urine output 30 ml/hr or 0.5-1 ml/kg/hr
- Serum sodium 135-145 mEq/L
- Serum potassium 3.5-5 mEq/L
- Intake approximates output

PATIENT MONITORING

1. Obtain PA pressures, CVP, BP continuously until the patient's condition is stable, then hourly. Monitor pulse pressure, MAP, PAWP, and CI to evaluate effectiveness of fluid resuscitation. Increased abdominal pressure secondary to fluid sequestration on the inferior vena cava can decrease venous return and consequently affect CO.

2. Continuously monitor ECG for lethal dysrhythmias that may result from electrolyte and acid-base imbalances.

3. Monitor fluid volume status: measure intake and urine output hourly; determine fluid balance q8h; compare serial weights to determine rapid (0.5 to 1 kg/day) changes indicating fluid imbalances.

PHYSICAL ASSESSMENT

1. Assess hydration status: note skin turgor on inner thigh or forehead, condition of buccal membranes, development of edema or crackles.

2. Assess for signs of bleeding: bleeding from gums or puncture sites, bruising or petechiae; test urine, stool, and gastric aspirate for occult blood.
3. Measure abdominal girth once each shift to determine progression of ascites. Percuss and palpate abdomen, since dullness is representative of fluid accumulation.
4. Assess respiratory status: note rate and depth of respirations; ascites may impair ventilation. Auscultate lungs for adventitious sounds.
5. Assess the patient for development of clinical sequelae. (See Table 2-36.)

DIAGNOSTICS ASSESSMENT

1. Review serial serum ammonia, albumin, bilirubin, AST (SGOT), ALT (SGPT), LDH, platelet count, PT, and PTT results to evaluate hepatic function.
2. Review serial serum electrolytes. Hypokalemia and other electrolyte imbalances can precipitate hepatic encephalopathy.
3. Review serial serum Hgb and Hct for decreasing values suggesting blood loss.
4. Review urine electrolytes, BUN, and creatinine to evaluate renal function.

PATIENT MANAGEMENT

1. Administer intravenous crystalloids as ordered: dextrose solutions will be needed in acute fulminant hepatic failure, since the patient is at risk for hypoglycemia; colloids may be given to increase oncotic pressure and pull ascitic fluid into intravascular space. Blood and blood products may be required to replace RBCs and clotting factors. Carefully monitor the patient for fluid volume overload during fluid resuscitation.
2. Administer potassium as ordered. Validate adequate urine output before potassium administration.
3. Sodium restriction of 0.5 g/day and fluid restriction to 1000 ml/day may be ordered.
4. Vitamin K may be required to promote clotting process. Protect the patient from injury; pad side rails, keep the bed in low position, and minimize handling; avoid injections or invasive procedures if at all possible if results of clotting studies are abnormal.
5. Institute bleeding precautions: avoid razor blades and use soft-bristled toothbrushes. Minimize needlesticks.

GI

6. In patients with ascites, diuretic agents may be required. Rapid diuresis (>2000 ml/day) can precipitate renal failure. Carefully monitor the patient for hypovolemia, electrolyte imbalances, and increasing BUN/Cr.

7. A peritoneovenous (LaVeen or Denver) shunt may be implanted to return ascitic fluid to the superior vena cava in patients who are refractory to medical therapy. Monitor patient for adverse affects: hemodilution, wound infection, clotting of shunt, bleeding problems, and leakage of ascitic fluid from incision.

8. Paracentesis may be performed if abdominal distention is severe. Note amount, color, and character of fluid. Monitor the patient for shock and hepatorenal syndrome.

9. See Hypovolemic shock, p. 189.

▶ **Nursing Diagnosis:** Impaired gas exchange related to intrapulmonary and portopulmonary shunt, hyperventilation secondary to ascites, pulmonary edema secondary to circulating toxic substances, or respiratory depression secondary to encephalopathy

OUTCOME CRITERIA
- PaO_2 80-100 mm Hg
- $PaCO_2$ 35-45 mm Hg
- pH   7.35-7.45
- O_2 sat   ≥95%
- RR   12-20/min, eupnea
- Lungs clear to auscultation

PATIENT MONITORING

1. Continuously monitor oxygen saturation with pulse oximetry (SpO_2). Monitor interventions and patient activities that may adversely affect oxygen saturation.

2. Continuously monitor ECG for dysrhythmias: hypoxemia is a risk factor for dysrhythmias.

PHYSICAL ASSESSMENT

1. Assess respiratory status: note respiratory rate and depth; RR >30/min or <12/min suggests impending respiratory dysfunction. Auscultate breath sounds q2h or more frequently during fluid resuscitation; note development of crackles or other adventitious sounds suggesting pulmonary congestion. Note dyspnea and cough, which may suggest pulmonary edema. Cyanosis is a late sign.

2. Assess the patient for development of clinical sequelae. (See Table 2-36).

DIAGNOSTICS ASSESSMENT

1. Review ABGs for decreasing trend in SaO_2, PaO_2 (hypoxemia), or pH (acidosis).
2. Review serial chest radiographs to evaluate a worsening lung condition. Right-sided pleural effusions are common in chronic liver disease.

PATIENT MANAGEMENT

1. Administer supplemental oxygen as ordered to prevent hypoxemia. Anticipate intubation and mechanical ventilation. See p. 577 for information on mechanical ventilation.
2. Reposition and C & DB patient q2h to prevent atelectasis. If necessary, suction secretions gently, being careful to avoid trauma to the mucosa, which can increase the risk for bleeding.
3. Elevate HOB to promote adequate chest excursion. A paracentesis may be performed to remove excess fluid from the abdomen and ease the work of breathing.

▶ **Nursing Diagnosis:** **Risk for injury** related to brain exposure to toxic substances (hepatic encephalopathy)

OUTCOME CRITERIA

• Patient will be alert and oriented
• Serum ammonia 12-55 µmol/L
• Patient will not injure self

PATIENT MONITORING

1. Monitor LOC using Glasgow coma scale.

PHYSICAL ASSESSMENT

1. Assess the patient's LOC at least hourly. A decreased awareness of the environment is an early manifestation of encephalopathy. Note any personality changes, slurred or slow speech. In acute liver failure, the mental impairment progresses to coma rapidly and includes a period of agitation, whereas the encephalopathy in chronic liver disease progresses gradually to coma without a phase of agitation.
2. Assess patient for asterixis (flapping tremors of the wrist when extended), an early manifestation of encephalopathy.
3. Assess sleep pattern, since a reversal of day-night sleep pattern is an early indicator of encephalopathy.
4. Assess for other etiologies of encephalopathy (e.g., hypoglycemia, hypoxemia, hemorrhage, sepsis, sedatives/hypnotics, electrolyte imbalance, acid-base disturbance, hypotension).
5. Assess the patient for development of clinical sequelae. (See Table 2-36.)

GI

DIAGNOSTICS ASSESSMENT

1. Monitor serum ammonia levels in patients with cirrhosis, since ammonia is thought to be a factor contributing to encephalopathy.
2. Monitor serum glucose levels; hypoglycemia is a common finding in acute liver failure and may further impair cerebral functioning.
3. Monitor serum sodium and potassium levels since imbalances can contribute to hepatic encephalopathy.

PATIENT MANAGEMENT

1. Administer ammonia-reducing medications as ordered (e.g., lactulose 10-30 ml or neomycin 1 g). Magnesium sulfate and lactulose enemas can be prescribed to cleanse the bowel of ammonia and prevent absorption of protein-breakdown products. The goal of therapy is 3 to 4 soft stools per day. If diarrhea occurs, hypovolemia and electrolyte imbalances may ensue. Avoid lactulose use in patients with FHF as it may increase the formation of colonic gas, which could hinder subsequent liver transplantation.
2. Maintain a safe environment; restrain the patient only if necessary for safety.
3. Restrict dietary protein to 20 to 40 g/day until normal mentation returns. If the patient is receiving TPN or enteral feedings, see pp. 636, 639 for patient care management guidelines.
4. NG intubation may be required to decompress the stomach, reduce absorption of protein breakdown products, and reduce the risk of aspiration in an unconscious patient.
5. Avoid sedatives if at all possible or use with extreme caution, since respiratory depression and circulatory collapse can result.
6. Patients with FHF may develop cerebral edema and increased intracranial pressure and require mannitol 20%; 0.5 to 1 g/kg hourly if adequate renal function. If renal failure is present, ultrafiltration may be required. Calculate serum osmolality; the goal is an osmolality <310 mOsm/L but in high normal range. Keep head/neck in neutral position, elevate HOB, and be alert to factors that may increase ICP (e.g., hypoxemia, fluid overload). See p. 511 for information on increased ICP.

PERITONITIS
Clinical Brief
Acute peritonitis is an inflammation of the peritoneal cavity caused by chemical irritation or an infective organism. Avenues by which organisms or chemicals may reach the peritoneum include perforation, suppuration, or ischemia of the GI or biliary tract; the female genital tract; penetrating abdominal injury; and the blood supply. Patients at risk for developing primary peritonitis include those with cirrhosis, nephrosis, ascites, tuberculosis, and immunosuppression. Patients at risk for developing secondary peritonitis include those with abdominal surgery, perforated ulcer or colon, ruptured appendix or viscus, bowel obstruction, gangrenous bowel, ischemic bowel disease, and peritoneal dialysis. The inflammatory response causes vascular dilatation and an increase in vascular permeability. These changes bring the necessary cells for removal of contaminants but also lead to fluid shifts from the extracellular compartment into the peritoneum, producing hypovolemia.

Presenting signs and symptoms
Signs and symptoms include a patient assuming a knees-flexed position, complaining of severe localized (parietal) or generalized (visceral) abdominal pain, nausea, vomiting, anorexia, and diarrhea.

Physical examination
Vital signs:
  HR tachycardia
  BP hypotension
  RR increased and shallow
  Temperature elevated
Neurological: Normal to decreased mentation
Skin: Pale, flushed, or diaphoretic
Cardiovascular: Pulse thready, weak, or may be bounding in presence of fever
Pulmonary: Breath sounds may be diminished secondary to shallow breathing
Abdominal:
  Rebound tenderness with guarding
  May have referred pain to the shoulder
  Rigid, distended abdomen
  Bowel sounds decreased to absent

GI

Diagnostic findings

Diagnostic findings are based on clinical manifestations of fever, abdominal pain, and rebound tenderness along with a history of precipitating factors. Cultures of peritoneal fluid will yield positive results.

In addition, the following may be found:

WBC >10 × 10³/μl
Serum protein <6 g/dl
Serum amylase >160 SU/dl

Acute Care Patient Management

Goals of treatment

Restore fluid and electrolyte balance
    Crystalloid, colloid, blood, and blood products
    Electrolyte replacement
Eradicate infection
    Antibiotic therapy
Control pain
    Analgesics
Rest GI tract
    NPO, NG intubation
Correct the underlying problem
    Surgery
Detect/prevent clinical sequelae
    See Table 2-37

▶ **Priority Nursing Diagnoses**
Fluid volume deficit
Pain
Ineffective breathing pattern
Risk for altered protection (see p. 33)
Risk for altered family process (see p. 29)
Risk for altered nutrition: less than body requirements (see p. 41)

▶ **Nursing Diagnosis:** Fluid volume deficit related to intravascular fluid shift to the peritoneal space and inability to ingest oral fluids

OUTCOME CRITERIA

- CVP   2-6 mm Hg
- SBP   90-140 mm Hg
- MAP   70-105 mm Hg
- PAS   15-30 mm Hg
- PAD   5-15 mm Hg

TABLE 2-37   Clinical Sequelae Associated with Peritonitis

Complication	Signs and symptoms
Septic shock	SBP <90 mm Hg, HR >90 beats/min, RR >20/min or $PaCO_2$ <32 mm Hg, PaO_2/FIO_2 <280, T >38° C or <36° C, WBC >12,000 or <4000 or >10% neutrophils; altered mental status, urine output <0.5 ml/kg/hr, plasma lactate >2 mmol/L
Paralytic ileus	Absent bowel sounds, abdominal distention
Respiratory failure	Restlessness, RR >30/min, labored breathing, PaO_2 <50 mm Hg, $PaCO_2$ >50 mm Hg, pH <7.35
Renal failure	Urinary output <30 ml/hr after fluid replacement, increasing BUN and creatinine
Liver failure	Jaundice, elevated AST (SGOT)
Dysrhythmias	Irregular rhythm, decreased mentation

- HR   60-100 beats/min
- Urine output 30 ml/hr or 0.5-1 ml/kg/hr

PATIENT MONITORING

1. Obtain PA pressures and CVP (if available) and monitor MAP hourly or more frequently if the patient's hemodynamic status is unstable. Note the patient's response to therapy. A MAP <60 mm Hg adversely affects cerebral and renal perfusion.
2. Monitor fluid volume status: measure urine output hourly, and NG and other bodily drainage. Determine fluid balance q8h. Urine output <0.5 ml/kg/hr may indicate renal insufficiency. Compare serial weights (1 kg ~ 1000 ml fluid) to evaluate for rapid (0.5 to 1 kg/day) changes, suggesting fluid imbalance.
3. Continuously monitor ECG for dysrhythmias resulting from electrolyte disturbances.

PHYSICAL ASSESSMENT

1. Assess tissue perfusion: note level of consciousness, skin color and temperature, pulses, and capillary refill.

GI

2. Assess hydration status: note skin turgor on inner thigh or forehead, condition of buccal membranes, development of edema or crackles.
3. Assess abdomen: note resolution of rigidity, rebound tenderness, and distention; auscultate bowel sounds.
4. Assess the patient for development of clinical sequelae. (See Table 2-37.)

DIAGNOSTICS ASSESSMENT

1. Review serum sodium and potassium levels, which may become depleted with nasogastric suctioning, or fluid shifts.
2. Review serial WBC count to evaluate the course of infection.

PATIENT MANAGEMENT

1. Administer crystalloid or colloid solutions to improve intravascular volume. CVP and PA pressures reflect the capacity of the vascular system to accept volume and can be used to monitor fluid volume status.
2. Replace potassium as ordered; validate adequate urine output before administration.
3. Keep the patient NPO if the patient is nauseated and vomiting. NG intubation with suction may be required to decompress the stomach and prevent aspiration. When vomiting and ileus resolve, provide the patient with oral fluids as tolerated.
4. Parenteral nutritional support may be required to provide nutrients while the patient is NPO.
5. Administer antibiotics as prescribed. Most patients will require surgery to treat the cause of peritonitis.

▶ **Nursing Diagnosis:** Pain related to inflammation of the peritoneal cavity

OUTCOME CRITERION

• Patient will communicate pain relief.

PATIENT MONITORING

1. Monitor the patient's level and location of pain using a visual analogue scale or rating scale. (See Figure 1-1.)

PHYSICAL ASSESSMENT

1. Observe for nonverbal cues of pain intolerance.
2. Assess abdomen for increasing girth or rigidity.
3. Obtain BP, HR; elevated values may reflect the presence of pain.

DIAGNOSTICS ASSESSMENT

None specific

Patient Management

1. Administer pain medication as ordered and evaluate its effectiveness. Assess respiratory status before administering analgesics that depress the central nervous system.
2. Administer antibiotics as ordered to eradicate the infecting organism.
3. Provide a relaxed environment to alleviate anxiety.
4. Place the patient in a position of comfort. Elevating the HOB will help to localize the infection and enhance chest excursion.
5. Instruct the patient to request pain medication before the pain is out of control.
6. Explore alternate methods of pain relief with patient (e.g., distraction, imagery).
7. See Acute pain, p. 30.

▶ **Nursing Diagnosis:** Ineffective breathing pattern related to abdominal distention and pain

Outcome Criteria

- RR   12-20/min, eupnea
- Pao_2 80-100 mm Hg
- $Paco_2$ 35-45 mm Hg
- pH   7.35-7.45
- Lungs clear to auscultation

Patient Monitoring

1. Continuously monitor oxygen saturation with pulse oximetry (Spo_2). Monitor interventions and patient activities that can adversely affect oxygen saturation.
2. Monitor PA systolic pressure (if available), since hypoxia can increase sympathetic tone and pulmonary vasoconstriction.

Physical Assessment

1. Assess respiratory status: note rate and depth of respirations. Rate >30, labored breathing, and restlessness suggest respiratory distress. Auscultate lungs; the onset of crackles may suggest fluid volume overload. Diminished lung sounds may be associated with shallow breathing, atelectasis, or pleural effusion.

Diagnostics Assessment

1. Review serial ABGs to identify decreasing trends in Pao_2 (hypoxemia), pH (acidosis), and Sao_2.
2. Review serial chest radiographs to identify improvement or worsening of the condition.

GI

PATIENT MANAGEMENT

1. Administer supplemental oxygen as ordered. See p. 577 for information on mechanical ventilation.
2. Elevate HOB to enhance chest excursion. C & DB the patient hourly to prevent atelectasis. Encourage slow, deep inspirations, since patients have a tendency to take short, shallow breaths.
3. Ensure NG tube patency to prevent gastric secretion accumulation, which might increase the risk for aspiration or increase abdominal distention and interfere with diaphragmatic motion.
4. Administer pain medication to promote pain-free respirations and deep breathing. Note the respiratory rate before and after pain-medication administration. Narcotics should not be given if respiratory rate <12/min.

UPPER GASTROINTESTINAL BLEEDING

Clinical Brief

Upper GI bleeding is characterized by the sudden onset of severe bleeding from an intestinal source proximal to the ligament of Treitz. Most upper GI bleeds are a direct result of peptic ulceration, erosive gastritis (resulting from alcohol or aspirin ingestion or stress), or esophageal varices (alcoholic cirrhosis, liver disease, and schistosomiasis). Mallory-Weiss tears can cause gastroesophageal bleeding as a result of severe wretching and vomiting. Hospitalized critically ill patients are also at risk for GI bleeding.

Mortality is highest among the elderly and in patients who have sustained multiple-organ hypoperfusion secondary to reduced blood volume.

Presenting signs and symptoms

Signs and symptoms depend on the amount and rapidity of blood loss; however, melena and hematemesis are usually present. Pain may be present with peptic ulcer disease, whereas the patient will be pain free if esophageal varices are the source of bleeding. Patients may have signs and symptoms of hypovolemic shock: cool clammy skin, pallor, apprehension to unresponsiveness, weak thready pulse, and hypotension.

Physical examination

Vital signs:

BP <90 mm Hg recumbent (>30% volume loss) or orthostatic BP (15%-30% volume loss)

HR >100 beats/min

RR tachypnea
Temperature may be elevated
Other: Obvious blood: hematemesis, melena, bloody stool
  with a fetid odor, coffee ground gastric aspirate
Neurological: Syncope, light-headed, altered mentation,
  apprehension
Skin:
  Pale, diaphoretic
  Cool, clammy skin
  Jaundice, petechiae, or hematomas may be present with
    liver disease
Cardiovascular:
  Weak, thready pulse
  Capillary refill >3 sec (shock)
Abdominal:
  May be tender with guarding
  Bowel sounds hyperactive or absent

Diagnostic findings

BUN >20 mg/dl (newly elevated)
Emesis and/or stool positive for occult blood
Decreasing trend to Hgb and Hct
Endoscopy and angiography may be used to diagnose the
  site of bleeding

Acute Care Patient Management

Goals of treatment

Optimize tissue oxygenation
  Supplemental oxygenation
  Intubation/mechanical ventilation
  Blood transfusion therapy
Stabilize the hemodynamic status
  Crystalloids, colloids, blood administration
Arrest/prevent bleeding and locate the source
  Gastric lavage
  Vasopressin therapy
  Esophageal tamponade (varices)
  Sclerotherapy (varices)
  Electrocoagulation
  Transjugular intrahepatic portosystemic shunt (varices)
  Surgical intervention
  H_2 receptor antagonists
  Antacids
  Cytoprotection

GI

Detect/prevent clinical sequelae
  See Table 2-38
▶ **Priority Nursing Diagnoses**
Fluid volume deficit
Altered tissue perfusion
Risk for aspiration
Risk for altered nutrition: less than body requirements
(see p. 41)
Risk for altered protection (see p. 33)
Risk for altered family process (see p. 29)
▶ **Nursing Diagnosis:** Fluid volume deficit related to
blood loss from hemorrhage
OUTCOME CRITERIA
• Patient will be alert and oriented
• Skin, pink, warm, and dry
• CVP   2-6 mm Hg
• PAS   15-30 mm Hg
• PAD   5-15 mm Hg

TABLE 2-38 Clinical Sequelae Associated with
Gastrointestinal Bleeding

Complication	Signs and symptoms
General	
Hypovolemic shock	SBP <90 mm Hg, HR >120 beats/min, cool, clammy skin
Aspiration pneumonia	↑ temperature, decreased breath sounds, ↓ PaO_2 and SaO_2
Myocardial, cerebral ischemia	ST, T-wave changes, chest pain, decreased LOC
DIC	Abnormal clotting factors, uncontrolled bleeding from all orifices
Peptic ulcer disease	
Perforation of stomach or intestine	Profound shock, sudden change in the character of the pain to include back pain and boardlike abdominal pain, rebound tenderness, absent bowel sounds
Gastric outlet obstruction	Protracted vomiting, visual peristaltic waves
Peritonitis	Elevated temperature, abdominal pain, ↑ WBCs

- SBP   90-140 mm Hg
- MAP   70-105 mm Hg
- HR   60-100 beats/min
- Urine output 30 ml/hr or 0.5-1 ml/kg/hr
- Hgb   12-16 g/dl (females)
               13.5-17.5 g/dl (males)
- Hct   37%-47% (females)
               40%-54% (males)

PATIENT MONITORING

1. Obtain PA pressures (if available), CVP, and BP q15min during acute episodes to evaluate fluid needs and patient response to therapy. Monitor MAP, an indicator of tissue perfusion. MAP <60 mm Hg adversely affects cerebral and renal perfusion. Orthostatic vital signs, a narrowed pulse pressure, and delayed capillary refill time indicate a loss of 15% to 30% of circulating blood volume.
2. Monitor fluid volume status: measure intake and urine output hourly to evaluate renal perfusion; measure blood loss if possible; determine fluid balance q8h. Compare serial weights to evaluate rapid (0.5 to 1 kg/day) changes suggesting fluid volume imbalance.
3. Continuously monitor ECG for dysrhythmias and myocardial ischemia (ST, T-wave changes) associated with reduced oxygen-carrying capacity associated with blood loss.

PHYSICAL ASSESSMENT

1. Assess patient for increased restlessness, apprehension, or altered consciousness, which may indicate decreased cerebral perfusion.
2. Assess hydration status: note skin turgor on inner thigh or forehead, condition of buccal membranes, development of edema or crackles.
3. Be alert for recurrence of bleeding.
4. Assess the patient for development of clinical sequelae. (See Table 2-38.)

DIAGNOSTICS ASSESSMENT

1. Review Hgb and Hct levels to determine the effectiveness of treatment or worsening of the patient's condition. The Hct should rise 2 to 3 points for each unit of PRBCs given.
2. Review clotting factors and serum calcium levels if multiple transfusions have been given.
3. Review serial BUN levels; elevated BUN (with a normal creatinine) can provide information about the degree of blood loss.

GI

4. Review serial ABGs to evaluate oxygenation and acid-base status. Hypoxia can lead to lactic acidosis.
5. Review the results of endoscopic evaluation or arteriogram if available.

PATIENT MANAGEMENT

1. Maintain a patent airway; administer supplemental oxygen as ordered; intubation and mechanical ventilation may be required. See p. 577 for information on mechanical ventilation.
2. Administer NS, LR, or colloids as ordered to restore intravascular volume. Intravenous fluids should contain multivitamins, magnesium, and thiamine with dextrose in patients with alcohol abuse. Carefully monitor patient response: note CVP, PA pressures, and BP.
3. Type and crossmatch for anticipated blood products. Transfuse the patient with blood or blood products to improve tissue oxygenation and correct coagulation deficiencies. Observe for transfusion reaction. (See Blood administration, p. 534.)
4. Evacuate the stomach contents with a large bore orogastric tube (34 to 36 Fr) and initiate lavages with room temperature tap water to clear blood clots from the stomach. Keep HOB elevated to reduce the risk of aspiration. Remove NG tube after irrigation.
5. Continue to monitor the patient closely once stabilized; rebleeding can occur even up to 1 week after the initial bleeding. Test all gastric secretions and stools for occult blood.
6. Vitamin K and/or fresh-frozen plasma may be ordered to correct coagulation deficiencies.
7. Administer H_2 receptor antagonists (ranitidine, cimetidine, famotidine) as ordered to decrease gastric acid secretion; cytoprotection may be provided with sucralfate to prevent mucosal lesion development; omeprazole may be ordered to decrease gastric acid secretion; antacids should be used cautiously as they may stimulate secretion of hydrochloric acid and increase rates of pneumonia. Gastric pH should be kept >3.5 or the value established by physician.
8. Explain all procedures and tests to the patient to help alleviate anxiety and decrease tissue oxygen demands.
9. Anticipate endoscopy and hemostatic therapy. Anticipate GI surgery (e.g., pyloroplasty, vagotomy, gastrectomy) if medical therapy unsuccessful.

MANAGEMENT OF ESOPHAGEAL VARICES

1. Administer fluids conservatively and monitor CVP (keep <8 mm Hg), since rapid volume expansion can increase portal and variceal pressures, causing further rupture and bleeding.

2. Administer vasopressin as ordered to control esophageal bleeding. Intraarterial or intravenous vasopressin is thought to constrict hepatic artery and splanchnic arterioles, thus decreasing portal venous pressure. Generally vasopressin is administered as a bolus 20 U over 20 min, followed by an infusion of 40 U/250 ml D_5W at a rate of 0.1 to 0.9 U/min. Subcutaneous infiltration can cause necrosis; therefore avoid peripheral veins if at all possible. Vasopressin can be given up to 24 hours after the bleeding has stopped. Observe for hypertension and myocardial and/or bowel ischemia. NTG may be given along with vasopressin to reduce the ischemic effects. Titrate the dose to desired effect; keep SBP >90 mm Hg.

3. Anticipate endoscopic sclerotherapy to obliterate the varices. (See Endoscopy, p. 461.)

4. Anticipate balloon tamponade to temporarily control esophageal bleeding if vasopressin and sclerotherapy are unsuccessful. (See Sengstaken-Blakemore tube, p. 626.)

5. Anticipate portosystemic shunting (transjugular intrahepatic portosystemic shunt [TIPS] or surgery) if medical treatment is unsuccessful. (See TIPS, p. 645.)

▶ **Nursing Diagnosis:** **Risk for aspiration** related to vomiting, esophageal tamponade, ileus, increased intragastric pressure, and altered mentation

OUTCOME CRITERIA

- Lungs clear to auscultation
- Pao_2 80-100 mm Hg
- O_2 sat   ≥95%
- Afebrile
- Absence of vomiting

PATIENT MONITORING

1. Monitor temperature q4h; elevation may indicate aspiration pneumonia.

2. Continuously monitor oxygen saturation with pulse oximetry (Spo_2). Monitor interventions and patient activities that may adversely affect oxygen saturation.

PHYSICAL ASSESSMENT

1. Assess LOC; patient may not be able to protect the airway if mentation is altered.

GI

2. Assess respiratory status: auscultate lungs for excessive secretions or absence of breath sounds that may indicate pneumonia.
3. Assess abdomen: auscultate bowel sounds; absence of intestinal peristalsis can cause increased intragastric pressure and vomiting.
4. If present, assess placement of nasoenteric tube.

DIAGNOSTICS ASSESSMENT
1. Review serial chest radiographs to evaluate placement of nasoenteric tubes and assess lung fields.
2. Review serial ABGs, since aspiration can decrease gas exchange.

PATIENT MANAGEMENT
1. Elevate HOB if the patient is hemodynamically stable; a right side-lying position may enhance gastric emptying if the patient can tolerate this position.
2. If present, maintain patency of the NG tube to promote adequate decompression of the stomach.
3. Secure all tubes to prevent dislodgement and excessive movement that can cause gastric irritation.
4. Restrain or sedate patient if necessary to prevent tubes from being inadvertently pulled out. Administer sedation cautiously in patients with underlying liver dysfunction.
5. Maintain esophageal tamponade with Sengstaken-Blakemore type tubes. (See p. 626.)

Endocrine Disorders

ADRENAL CRISIS

Clinical Brief

Adrenal crisis or acute adrenal insufficiency (AI) is a life-threatening state of acute suppression or absolute lack of secretion of glucocorticoids and/or mineralocorticoids. Lack of glucocorticoids is particularly serious due to their role in the body's defense mechanisms and response to stress. Adrenocortical insufficiency is classified as either primary (e.g., destruction of adrenal gland [Addison's disease]) or secondary (e.g., inadequate ACTH secretion as a result of an interruption in the hypothalamic-pituitary-adrenal axis).

Autoimmune destruction of the adrenal gland is the most common cause of adrenal insufficiency, but metastatic disease, infections (particularly tuberculosis), adrenal hemorrhage, sepsis, and autoimmune deficiency syndrome can also cause the disorder. Secondary adrenal insufficiency is usually associated with prolonged exogenous glucocorticoid (steroid) administration. Abrupt withdrawal or insufficient amounts of the exogenous steroid during stress can precipitate an adrenal crisis. Other causes include pituitary tumors, infarction, irradiation, hypophysectomy, or infection.

Presenting signs and symptoms

GI symptoms will be manifested: anorexia, nausea, vomiting, weight loss, and diarrhea. The patient may be anxious and complain of muscle weakness and fatigue or manifest the signs of shock.

Physical examination

Vital signs:

BP low or orthostatic hypotension (primary AI)

HR tachycardia (primary AI)

RR increased

Skin:

Pale

Hyperpigmentation (primary AI)

Dehydrated, decreased turgor

Neurological: Confusion, lassitude, progressing to unresponsiveness
Gastrointestinal: Nausea, vomiting, abdominal pain
Diagnostic findings
There should be a high index of suspicion if unexplained
hypotension (or hypotension unresponsive to vasopressors or
inotropes), hypoglycemia, hyperkalemia, and hyponatremia
are present. A lack of a response to IV cosyntropin confirms
AI. (A normal response is an increase in the corticol level of
at least 7 µg/dl over the basal level and a serum cortisol level
to at least 20 µg/dl).

Acute Care Patient Management

Goals of treatment
Replace glucocorticoids or mineralocorticoids
   Hydrocortisone
   Desoxycorticosterone
Restore fluid, glucose, and electrolyte balance
   Crystalloids
   Electrolyte therapy
Reduce stress
   Stress-free environment
Detect/prevent clinical sequelae
   See Table 2-39

▶ **Priority Nursing Diagnoses**
Fluid volume deficit
Altered protection
Risk for altered nutrition: less than body requirements
(see p. 41)
Risk for altered family process (see p. 29)

▶ **Nursing Diagnosis:** Fluid volume deficit related to
increased sodium and water excretion secondary to insufficient mineralocorticoids

OUTCOME CRITERIA
- Patient will be alert and oriented
- CVP   2-6 mm Hg
- PAS   15-30 mm Hg
- PAD   5-15 mm Hg
- CI   2.5-4 L/min/m²
- SBP   90-140 mm Hg
- MAP   70-105 mm Hg
- HR   60-100 beats/min
- Serum sodium 135-145 mEq/L

- Urine output 30 ml/hr or 0.5-1 ml/kg/hr
- Intake approximates output
- Elastic skin turgor
- Moist mucous membranes

PATIENT MONITORING

1. Obtain CVP, PA pressures (if available), and BP hourly or more frequently to evaluate hypovolemia and patient response to therapy. Monitor CI and MAP; MAP <60 mm Hg adversely affects cerebral and renal perfusion.
2. Monitor fluid volume status: measure urine output hourly; determine fluid balance q8h; compare serial weights for a rapid decrease (0.5 to 1 kg/day), suggesting fluid loss.
3. Continuously monitor ECG for dysrhythmias secondary to electrolyte imbalance.

PHYSICAL ASSESSMENT

1. Assess hydration status: thirst, skin turgor on inner thigh or forehead, buccal membranes, pulse pressure.
2. Assess indicators of tissue perfusion: note level of consciousness, skin color and temperature, peripheral pulses, and capillary refill.
3. Assess the patient for development of clinical sequelae (Table 2-39).

DIAGNOSTICS ASSESSMENT

1. Review serial serum sodium and potassium levels to evaluate the patient's response to therapy.
2. Review serial serum glucose levels; symptoms usually appear when level is <50 mg/dl.

PATIENT MANAGEMENT

1. Administer D_5NS rapidly to restore volume and provide a glucose source, since the patient may be hypoglycemic. Carefully monitor CVP, PA pressures, BP, and CI to determine fluid needs and signs of fluid volume overload.

ENDO

TABLE 2-39 Clinical Sequelae Associated with Acute Adrenal Crisis

Complication	Signs and symptoms
Shock	CI <2.5 L/min/m², SBP <90 mm Hg, HR >120 beats/min, change in mental status, cool clammy skin, oliguria
Electrolyte imbalances	Life threatening dysrhythmias

2. Administer glucocorticoids (hydrocortisone) as ordered, usually 100 mg IV q6h initially, then tapering the dosage as patient condition allows to an oral maintenance dose of 20 mg AM and 10 mg PM. If a diagnosis is not established, dexamethasone 1 to 4 mg IV may be required while giving the cosyntropin stimulation test. Long-term replacement therapy may include glucocorticoid preparations such as prednisone, methylprednisolone, or hydrocortisone.

3. Colloids may be required if fluids and steroid administration do not improve intravascular volume. Sympathomimetic agents will not be effective without glucocorticoid replacement.

4. Fludrocortisone may be required in patients with primary AI to help maintain sodium and potassium balance and control postural hypotension.

5. If the patient is able to take oral fluids, encourage fluids high in sodium to combat excessive sodium excretion.

▶ **Nursing Diagnosis:** Altered protection related to decreased immune response, decreased mentation and weakness secondary to insufficient adrenocorticoids, and electrolyte imbalance

OUTCOME CRITERIA
- Serum glucose 80-120 mg/dl
- Serum sodium 135-145 mEq/L
- Patient will be alert and oriented
- Absence of aspiration
- Patient will not injure self

PATIENT MONITORING
None specific

PHYSICAL ASSESSMENT
1. Assess level of consciousness since fluid and electrolyte imbalance can alter mentation, which increases the risk of patient injury.

2. Assess respiratory status, since a patient with altered mentation may be unable to protect the airway and is at risk for aspiration and respiratory distress. Note rate and depth of respirations; auscultate lungs for decreased or adventitious breath sounds.

3. Assess response to activity and monitor for fatigue since muscle strength may be affected.

4. Assess level of anxiety, since added stressors may further compromise patient condition.

DIAGNOSTICS ASSESSMENT
1. Review serum glucose levels. Signs and symptoms generally manifest at glucose levels <50 mg/dl.
2. Review sodium levels. Neurological signs generally manifest at sodium levels <125 mEq/L and become more severe at levels <115 mEq/L.

PATIENT MANAGEMENT
1. Protect the patient from stimuli or stressors; maintain a quiet, dimly lit room; control room temperature to avoid extremes; screen visitors to those who promote patient relaxation.
2. Explain all procedures and ICU routine so that the patient is not necessarily surprised.
3. Maintain bed rest and limit activities until the patient's condition stabilizes.
4. Maintain a patent airway and supply supplemental oxygen as ordered, especially with activity.
5. Increase activity gradually. Terminate activity if there are signs and symptoms of intolerance.
6. Keep the patient NPO until nausea and vomiting resolve and patient mentation improves.
7. Maintain sterile technique when performing invasive procedures to prevent infection.

DIABETES INSIPIDUS (DI)

Clinical Brief
Diabetes insipidus is a disorder characterized by impaired renal conservation of water resulting from a deficiency in ADH secretion or renal resistance to ADH. Excessive water loss, hyperosmolality, and hypernatremia result. DI is classified as either central, nephrogenic, or psychogenic. DI may be transitory or permanent, depending on the cause; however, profound diuresis regardless of the cause will occur. Central DI (decreased ADH production or release) may be idiopathic or result from pituitary surgery or conditions that disturb the hypothalamus (eg., head trauma, infection, cancerous brain tumors, or anoxic brain death). Nephrogenic DI occurs if the renal receptors are insensitive or resistant to circulating ADH. Causes include diseased kidneys or drug therapies (lithium carbonate, demeclocycline). Psychogenic DI occurs with compulsive water consumption. Patients can excrete from 4 to 24 L/day. As long as patients are able to

ENDO

respond to the thirst mechanism, serum osmolality will remain normal and dehydration will be prevented.

Presenting signs and symptoms

The alert patient will complain of polydipsia, polyuria, and fatigue as a result of lack of sleep from nocturia. Unresponsive patients will have profound dehydration or hypovolemic shock.

Physical examination

Vital signs:

    BP postural hypotension

    HR tachycardia

    RR eupnea

    Temperature normothermic

Cardiovascular:

    Cool, clammy skin

    Capillary refill >3 sec

    Pulse weak, thready

Skin: Decreased turgor; dry, sticky mucous membranes

Diagnostic findings

Water deprivation test demonstrates the following:

Serum osmolality >300 mOsm/kg

Serum sodium >145 mEq/L

Urine osmolality <200 mOsm/L

In addition:

Decreased serum ADH (nl = 1-5 pg/ml)

Urine specific gravity <1.005

Acute Care Patient Management

Goals of treatment

Restore fluid balance

    Hypotonic fluid replacement

    Vasopressin

    Treatment of the cause

Detect/prevent clinical sequelae

    See Table 2-40

▶ **Priority Nursing Diagnoses**

Fluid volume deficit

Risk for altered protection (see p. 33)

Risk for altered family process (see p. 29)

Risk for altered nutrition: less than body requirements (see p. 41)

▶ **Nursing Diagnosis:** Fluid volume deficit related to excessive diuresis of dilute urine secondary to inadequate ADH secretion/response

TABLE 2-40   Clinical Sequelae Associated with DI

Complication	Signs and symptoms
Circulatory collapse	Tachycardia, decreasing trend in BP, decreasing trend in urine output, diminished pulse, decreased sensorium, cool clammy skin, restlessness

OUTCOME CRITERIA
- Patient will be alert and oriented
- Moist buccal membranes
- Elastic skin turgor
- CVP   2-6 mm Hg
- PAS   15-30 mm Hg
- PAD   5-15 mm Hg
- SBP   90-140 mm Hg
- MAP   70-105 mm Hg
- Intake approximates output
- Urine osmolality 300-1400 mOsm/L
- Serum osmolality 275-295 mOsm/L
- Urine specific gravity 1.010-1.030
- Serum sodium 135-145 mEq/L

PATIENT MONITORING
1. Monitor CVP and PA pressures (if available) hourly or more frequently to evaluate volume status. Hypovolemic shock can occur.
2. Monitor MAP; MAP <60 mm Hg adversely affects cerebral and renal perfusion.
3. Monitor urine output hourly and determine fluid balance each shift. Urine output can exceed 1 L/hr. Compare daily weights; dramatic weight loss can occur if fluid replacement is inadequate. Neurosurgical patients (neurohypophysis destruction) may develop polyuria immediately after surgery, which lasts for approximately 24 to 48 hours, followed by oliguria for approximately 3 to 4 days before developing permanent polyuria and polydipsia.

PHYSICAL ASSESSMENT
1. Obtain VS hourly or more often if the patient's condition is unstable; hypovolemic shock can occur. Signs and

symptoms include restlessness, cool, clammy skin, tachycardia, SBP <90 mm Hg.

2. Assess hydration status to evaluate the patient's response to therapy. Note skin turgor on inner thigh or forehead, condition of buccal membranes, resolution of postural hypotension.

3. Assess LOC; changes in sensorium can be caused by decreased perfusion or dehydration.

4. Assess the patient for development of clinical sequelae. (See Table 2-40.)

DIAGNOSTICS ASSESSMENT

1. Monitor serum sodium, potassium, and osmolality as well as urine specific gravity and osmolality to evaluate water deficiency and the patient's response to therapy. Serum osmolality can be calculated:

2Na + K + BUN/3 + Glucose/18.

PATIENT MANAGEMENT

1. Administer hypotonic fluids as ordered to reduce serum hyperosmolality and prevent circulatory collapse. Fluids are usually titrated to hourly urine output. Monitor the patient for fluid volume overload. NS may be used if signs of circulatory collapse are present.

2. Recognize risk factors that may potentiate osmolality problems such as the administration of TPN or enteral feedings.

3. Aqueous vasopressin (Pitressin) will be required in patients who are unable to synthesize ADH; DDAVP 2 to 4 μg subq or IV, 10 to 40 μg intranasally may be used. Observe for abdominal cramps, hypertension, and coronary insufficiency with vasopressin administration.

4. In patients with nephrogenic DI, thiazide diuretics may be used to deplete Na$^+$ and cause increased renal water reabsorption. Nephrogenic DI does not respond to hormonal replacement.

5. Carbamazepine, clofibrate, or chlorpropamide may be helpful to produce and release endogenous vasopressin in patients with insufficient amounts of circulating ADH.

6. Restrict salt and protein intake for patients with nephrogenic DI.

7. Encourage iced fluids when the patient is able to take oral fluids.

8. Provide oral hygiene and meticulous skin care to preserve skin integrity. Vasopressin therapy may cause diarrhea, a risk factor for skin breakdown.
9. For hypernatremia, see p. 296-300.

DIABETIC KETOACIDOSIS (DKA)

Clinical Brief

Diabetic ketoacidosis, a common complication of insulin-dependent diabetes mellitus, is characterized by hyperglycemia, uncontrolled lipolysis (decomposition of fat), ketogenesis (production of ketones), negative nitrogen balance, fluid loss, electrolyte imbalance, and acid-base imbalance. As a result of a relative or absolute insulin deficiency, uptake of glucose by muscle cells is decreased, production of glucose by the liver is increased, and the metabolism of free fatty acids into ketones is increased. Despite the hyperglycemia, cells are unable to use the glucose as their energy source, requiring the conversion of fatty acids and protein into ketone bodies for energy.

Osmotic diuresis occurs; leading to cellular dehydration, hypotension, electrolyte loss, and severe metabolic acidosis. In 50% of the DKA episodes, insufficient insulin, an increase in the ingestion or production of glucose, or infection are precipitating factors. Other risk factors include pharmacotherapy with some medications (e.g., steroids, phenytoin sodium [Dilantin], thiazide diuretics) and stressful events (e.g., surgery, myocardial infarction, illnesses, psychological stress).

Presenting signs and symptoms

Neurological response may range from alert to comatose. Respirations are deep and rapid (Kussmaul) with a "fruity" acetone breath. The patient may be dehydrated and complain of extreme thirst, polyuria, and weakness. Nausea, vomiting, severe abdominal pain, and bloating are often present and can be mistaken for manifestations of an acute condition of the abdomen. Headache, muscle twitching, or tremors may also be present.

Physical examination

Vital signs:
    BP orthostatic hypotension
    HR tachycardia
    RR tachypnea to Kussmaul breathing
    Temperature may be elevated (infection) or decreased

ENDO

Skin:
  Dry, flushed
  Decreased turgor
  Dry buccal membranes
Pulmonary:
  Lungs clear
  Pleuritic pain, friction rubs (dehydration)
Abdominal:
  Tender, guarding
  Decreased bowel sounds
  Rigid, absent BS, rebound tenderness (severe DKA)
Musculoskeletal:
  Weakness
  Decreased deep tendon reflexes

Diagnostic findings
Serum glucose >300 mg/dl but not >800 mg/dl
Urine ketones strongly positive
Serum ketones >3 mOsm/L
Blood pH <7.30 (<7.1 common)
Serum bicarbonate <15 mEq/L
Serum osmolality increased but usually <330 mOsm/L
Anion gap >20 mmol/L
Serum potassium initially may be normal or high but will decrease with therapy.

Acute Care Patient Management

Goals of treatment
Provide cellular nutrition
  Insulin therapy
Restore fluid and electrolyte balance
  Crystalloids
  Colloids
  Electrolyte therapy
Determine and treat the cause
  Appropriate treatment
Detect/prevent clinical sequelae
  See Table 2-41

▶ **Priority Nursing Diagnoses**
Fluid volume deficit
Risk for injury
Risk for altered nutrition: less than body requirements (see p. 41)
Risk for altered family process (see p. 29)

TABLE 2-41 Clinical Sequelae Associated with DKA

Complication	Signs and symptoms
Circulatory collapse	SBP <90 mm Hg, HR >120 beats/min, change in mental status, cool clammy skin, diminished pulses
Renal failure	Oliguria, increasing BUN and creatinine
Electrolyte imbalances	Life-threatening dysrhythmias, ileus
Cerebral edema	Lethargy, drowsiness, headache during successful therapy

▶ **Nursing Diagnosis:** Fluid volume deficit related to osmotic diuresis secondary to hyperglycemia and lack of adequate oral intake

OUTCOME CRITERIA
- CVP   2-6 mm Hg
- PAS   15-30 mm Hg
- PAD   5-15 mm Hg
- SBP   90-140 mm Hg
- MAP   70-105 mm Hg
- HR   60-100 beats/min
- RR   12-20/min
- Urine output 30 ml/hr or 0.5-1 ml/kg/hr
- Serum glucose 150-250 mg/dl
- Serum osmolality 275-295 mOsm/kg
- Serum sodium 135-145 mEq/L
- Serum potassium 3.5-5.5 mEq/L
- Elastic skin turgor
- Moist buccal membranes

PATIENT MONITORING
1. Obtain PA pressures (if available), and CVP hourly or more frequently if the patient's condition is unstable or during fluid resuscitation. Both parameters reflect the capacity of the vascular system to accept volume and can be used to monitor fluid volume status. Increasing values suggest fluid overload; decreasing values suggest hypovolemia.
2. Monitor MAP; a MAP <60 mm Hg can adversely affect cerebral and renal perfusion.
3. Continuously monitor ECG to detect life-threatening dysrhythmias that may be caused by hypokalemia.

ENDO

4. Perform bedside glucose monitoring with finger-stick to evaluate the patient's response to therapy.

5. Accurately monitor fluid volume status: measure urine output hourly, determine fluid balance q8h, and compare serial weights. Average water deficit is 6 L.

6. Calculate serum osmolality and monitor trends.

PHYSICAL ASSESSMENT

1. Obtain VS: BP, MAP, HR, and RR, hourly or more frequently if the patient's condition is unstable or during fluid resuscitation to evaluate the patient's response to therapy. Kussmaul breathing is associated with a pH <7.2.

2. Assess hydration status: note skin turgor on inner thigh or forehead, condition of buccal membranes, development of edema or crackles.

3. Assess LOC carefully during fluid resuscitation, since brain edema may result from overly aggressive volume replacement.

4. Assess respiratory status to determine the rate and depth of respirations or adventitious breath sounds. Potassium imbalance can cause respiratory arrest; rapid fluid resuscitation may cause fluid overload.

5. Assess GI status: nausea, abdominal distention, and absence of bowel sounds may indicate ileus.

6. Assess the patient for development of clinical sequelae. (See Table 2-41.)

DIAGNOSTICS ASSESSMENT

1. Review serial serum glucose levels (in addition to bedside monitoring) to evaluate patient response to insulin therapy.

2. Review serum electrolytes (e.g., Na^+, K^+, and Mg^+), since imbalances are associated with osmotic diuresis. Potassium in particular should be evaluated every 1 to 2 hours. Seizures may be associated with hyponatremia; ileus and dysrhythmias may result with potassium imbalances.

3. Review indicators of renal function: creatinine and BUN.

4. Review ABGs to evaluate oxygenation status and resolution or worsening of metabolic acidosis.

5. Review culture reports to identify presence of infecting organism.

PATIENT MANAGEMENT

1. Administer crystalloids as ordered to correct dehydration. NS boluses of up to 1000 ml/hr may be required until

urine output, VS, and clinical assessment reflect an adequate hydration state. Half-strength solutions may follow once the patient's condition is stabilized or manifestations of heart failure develop.
2. Offer small, frequent sips of water or ice chips if the patient is permitted to take fluids by mouth.
3. Provide frequent oral hygiene, since dehydration causes drying of the mucous membranes.
4. Provide insulin therapy as ordered.

▶ **Nursing Diagnosis:** **Risk for injury** related to acidosis, electrolyte imbalances, and impaired glucose utilization secondary to lack of insulin

OUTCOME CRITERIA
• Patient will be alert and oriented
• Serum glucose 150-250 mg/dl
• Absence of serum/urine ketones
• pH 7.35-7.45
• Serum bicarbonate 22-26 mEq/L
• Patient will not injure self

PATIENT MONITORING
None specific

PHYSICAL ASSESSMENT
1. Assess LOC, which may range from confusion to frank coma. Too rapid a reduction in serum glucose (>100 mg/dl/hr) may also impair cerebral function. If patient experiences headache, lethargy, or drowsiness during successful therapy, suspect cerebral edema.
2. Assess the patient for development of clinical sequelae. (See Table 2-41.)

DIAGNOSTICS ASSESSMENT
1. Review serial serum glucose levels (in addition to bedside monitoring) to evaluate the patient's response to insulin therapy.
2. Review ABGs to evaluate oxygenation status and resolution or worsening of metabolic acidosis.

PATIENT MANAGEMENT
1. Administer regular insulin as ordered. Generally, 10 U is given initially as an IV bolus, followed with a continuous insulin infusion, 100 U/100 ml NS, infused at 5 to 10 U/hr (0.1 to 0.2 U/kg/hr). Glucose should drop 40 to 80 mg/dl/hr. Too rapid a fall in serum glucose levels can cause cerebral edema. If the serum glucose level does not decrease in 2 hours, doubling the

ENDO

dose of insulin infusion may be necessary. If cerebral edema occurs, anticipate mannitol administration.

2. Dextrose should be combined with half normal saline when the glucose level is 250 to 300 mg/dl to prevent hypoglycemia and cerebral edema.

3. Subcutaneous administration of regular insulin can be started when serum glucose is <250 mg/dl, pH is >7.2, or CO_2 is 15 to 18 mEq/L, and the patient is able to take fluids orally. Generally, an insulin infusion will be discontinued 1 to 2 hours after the patient receives subcutaneous insulin.

4. Anticipate potassium supplementation (KCl, KPO_4, K acetate) to replace potassium loss as a result of urinary excretion, correction of metabolic acidosis, or secondary to cellular uptake with insulin therapy. Validate urine output before administering potassium. If hypokalemia is refractory to therapy, consider Mg^+ replacement.

5. Na bicarbonate is considered only if the serum pH is <7.

6. NG intubation may be required to reduce the risk of vomiting and aspiration in the patient with altered mentation. Keep the patient NPO until the patient is alert, vomiting has ceased, and bowel sounds have returned.

7. Intubation and mechanical ventilation may be required if the patient is unable to protect the airway or adequately ventilate and oxygenate.

8. Cough and deep breathe the conscious patient to prevent pulmonary stasis and atelectasis. Reposition the unconscious patient every 1 to 2 hours and suction secretions as needed.

9. Provide meticulous skin care to prevent impaired skin integrity; inspect bony prominences. Maintain body alignment in the unconscious patient.

10. Frequently orient the patient to the surroundings. Keep the bed in low position and side rails up.

HYPERGLYCEMIC HYPEROSMOLAR NONKETOTIC COMA (HHNC)

Clinical Brief

HHNC is a condition of extreme hyperglycemia, dehydration, and minimal or absence of ketosis or acidosis. It occurs most often in the older population, either as a first symptom in a patient with undiagnosed type II diabetes or from an acute illness or infection in a patient with previously mild type II diabetes. Enteral or parenteral nutrition or certain medications have also been linked to the development HHNC. Certain drugs such as corticosteriods, thiazide diuretics, furosemide, cimetidine, phenytoin sodium, diazoxide, and propranolol hydrochloride may precipitate HHNC. Regardless of the cause, the body does not have sufficient insulin to prevent hyperglycemia, yet has enough insulin present to prevent lipolysis.

It is most clearly distinguished from diabetic ketoacidosis (DKA) by the lack of or mild ketoacidosis and higher serum glucose levels, which can reach 2000 mg/dl or more.

Presenting signs and symptoms

Signs and symptoms include severe dehydration with mild or no nausea and vomiting. HHNC will resemble DKA in many ways (with the exception of the profound dehydration): polyuria, polyphagia, weakness, and confusion (Table 2-42). Neurological signs are more predominant and frequently increased lethargy is the chief complaint. Up to half of the patients present comatose. Focal neurological signs such as hemisensory deficits, hemiparesis, aphasia, and seizures may mimic a cerebrovascular accident.

Physical examination

Vital signs:

HR tachycardia

BP low systolic, orthostatic hypotension

RR rapid and shallow (not Kussmaul), absence of fruity breath

Temperature normothermic or hyperthermic, depending on underlying process

TABLE 2-42 Comparison of Clinical Signs of DKA and HHNC

Parameter	DKA	HHNC
Respirations	Kussmaul	Regular
Serum glucose	300-800 mg/dl	>800 mg/dl
Serum osmolality	295-330 mOsm/L	>350 mOsm/L
Serum bicarbonate	<15 mEq/L	22-26 mEq/L
Blood pH	<7.3	Normal to mild acidosis
Serum ketones	>3 mOsm/L	Absent
Urine ketones	Strongly positive	Negative or slight
Serum sodium	Mean 132 mEq/L	Mean 145 mEq/L
BUN	Mean 41 mg/dl	Mean 65 mg/dl

ENDO

Neurological:
  Altered mental status
  Focal neurological signs may be present
  +4 reflexes
Skin:
  Pale, dry, with decreased turgor
  Dry buccal membranes
  Tongue dry, furrowed
Cardiovascular:
  Pulse weak and thready
  Capillary refill >3 sec

Diagnostic findings
Serum glucose >800 mg/dl, averaging 1200 mg/dl
Serum sodium >147 mEq/L
Serum potassium initially may be normal or high
pH normal to mild acidosis <7.3
Serum bicarbonate 22-26 mEq/L
Serum osmolality >350 mOsm/kg
Urine acetone negative or slight
Urine specific gravity >1.022

Acute Care Patient Management
Goals of treatment
Restore fluid and electrolyte balance
  Crystalloids
  Electrolyte therapy
Improve glucose/insulin ratio
  Insulin therapy
Determine and treat the cause
  Appropriate therapy
Detect/prevent clinical sequelae
  See Table 2-43

▶ **Priority Nursing Diagnoses**
Fluid volume deficit
Risk for injury
Risk for altered nutrition: less than body requirements
(see p. 41)
Risk for altered protection (see p. 33)
Risk for altered family process (see p. 29)
▶ **Nursing Diagnosis:** Fluid volume deficit related to
osmotic diuresis, inability to take oral fluids, nausea, and
vomiting
OUTCOME CRITERIA
• CVP   2-6 mm Hg

TABLE 2-43   Clinical Sequelae Associated with HHNC

Complication	Signs and symptoms
Neurological deficits	Focal changes, generalized seizures, hemiparesis, sensory deficits
Hypovolemic shock	SBP <90 mm Hg, HR >120 beats/min, weak thready pulse, progressive deterioration in LOC, cool/clammy skin
Renal failure	Decreased urinary output, increasing BUN and creatinine
Embolic phenomenon	Calf pain, SOB, neurological deficits

- PAS   15-30 mm Hg
- PAD   5-15 mm Hg
- SBP   90-140 mm Hg
- MAP   70-105 mm Hg
- Absence of nausea/vomiting
- Moist buccal membranes
- Elastic skin turgor
- Serum osmolality 275-295 mOsm/kg
- Serum potassium 3.5-5.5 mEq/L
- Urine output 30 ml/hr or 0.5-1 ml/kg/hr

PATIENT MONITORING

1. Obtain CVP, PA pressures (if available), and BP readings q15min during fluid resuscitation and evaluate the patient's response to therapy. Monitor MAP; MAP <60 mm Hg adversely affects cerebral and renal perfusion.
2. Monitor fluid volume status: measure urine output hourly, determine fluid balance q8h, compare serial weights for rapid (0.5-1 kg/day) changes that suggest fluid imbalance.
3. Continuously monitor ECG, since dysrhythmias may be precipitated by electrolyte imbalance associated with diuresis.

PHYSICAL ASSESSMENT

1. Monitor HR, RR, and BP q15min during fluid resuscitation and note the patient's response to therapy.
2. Assess the patient's hydration status: note skin turgor on inner thigh or forehead, condition of buccal membranes, development of edema or crackles. Calculate osmolality.
3. Assess tissue perfusion: note level of consciousness, peripheral pulses, skin temperature and moisture. Hypovolemia may lead to shock.

ENDO

4. Assess for gastric distention and absent bowel sounds, which would suggest ileus.
5. Assess the patient for development of clinical sequelae. (See Table 2-43.)

DIAGNOSTICS ASSESSMENT

1. Review serial ABGs to evaluate hypoxemia and acidosis, which may be present with shock.
2. Review serial electrolyte levels (e.g., Na^+, K^+, and Mg^+) to evaluate the need for replacement or patient response to therapy.
3. Review serial serum osmolality and evaluate patient's response to therapy.
4. Review serial Hgb and Hct levels; increased levels are associated with profound diuresis and increase blood viscosity.

PATIENT MANAGEMENT

1. Fluid resuscitation with NS at 1 L/hr may be required if the patient is hypotensive and tachycardic. Fluid requirements may exceed 10 L; 1/2 NS may be used if hypernatremia is present or the patient manifests signs and symptoms of heart failure. D_5W is administered when serum glucose reaches 250 to 300 mg/dl.
2. Administer insulin as ordered, usually 0.1 to 0.2 U/kg/hr.
3. Plasma expanders may be required if isotonic solutions do not improve intravascular volume.
4. Administer potassium supplements as ordered to prevent adverse effects on the myocardium, gastrointestinal, and respiratory muscles; validate adequate urine output before potassium administration. If hypokalemia is refractory to therapy, consider magnesium replacement.
5. Keep the patient NPO while nauseated and vomiting; NG intubation may be required if ileus develops or the patient is at risk for aspiration.
6. Prophylactic low-dose heparin therapy may be ordered to prevent clotting associated with increased blood viscosity secondary to profound diuresis.
7. Antibiotic therapy will be ordered if the patient has an underlying infection.
8. See electrolyte imbalances, pp. 277-300.

▶ **Nursing Diagnosis:** **Risk for injury** related to altered level of consciousness secondary to insulin insufficiency, cerebral edema, or cellular dehydration

OUTCOME CRITERIA
- Patient will be alert and oriented
- Patient will not injure self
- Absence of seizure activity
- Serum sodium 135-145 mEq/L
- Serum glucose <250 mg/dl
- Serum osmolality 275-295 mOsm/kg

PATIENT MONITORING
1. Monitor bedside serum glucose levels at least hourly.

PHYSICAL ASSESSMENT
1. Assess neurological status q15 to 30 min during fluid resuscitation when risk of cerebral edema is especially high. LOC will improve as osmolality decreases.
2. Assess the patient for development of clinical sequelae. (See Table 2-43.)

DIAGNOSTICS ASSESSMENT
1. Evaluate serum glucose and serum osmolality to determine effectiveness of therapy.
2. Carefully monitor hourly potassium levels; as hyperglycemia and fluid volume deficit are corrected, potassium will shift intracellularly, resulting in hypokalemia.

PATIENT MANAGEMENT
1. Administer insulin as ordered. Generally, a bolus of regular insulin 0.1 to 0.2 U/kg is given IV, followed by an insulin infusion at 0.1 to 0.2 U/kg/hr until the serum glucose reaches 250 mg/dl. Lowering serum glucose too rapidly (>100 mg/dl/hr) may result in hypoglycemia.
2. Institute seizure precautions: pad side rails, reduce environmental stimuli, place bed in low position, have emergency equipment (oral airway, suction) available.
3. Keep HOB elevated if BP has stabilized, and NG tube patent to decrease the risk of aspiration.

ENDO

HYPOGLYCEMIA (HYPERINSULINISM, INSULIN SHOCK, INSULIN COMA)

Clinical Brief

Hypoglycemia is a condition characterized by a serum glucose level less than 50 mg/dl caused by glucose production inadequate to meet glucose utilization demands. It is characterized either as postprandial or fasting. Postprandial primarily occurs after surgical modification of the upper gastrointestinal tract. Fasting hypoglycemia is most commonly caused by excessive administration of insulin or oral hypoglycemics, too much exercise, or too little food. Alcohol or salicylate ingestion, use of β-adrenergic blocking agents, and tapering of steroids can be contributing factors. Onset is rapid and the symptoms are varied. Iatrogenically induced hypoglycemia can result if serum glucose is rapidly reduced in the treatment of DKA. Repeated or prolonged periods of hypoglycemia can lead to permanent neurological damage (especially in children) or death. Elderly patients who have other disease conditions that cause them to be debilitated and patients with "hypoglycemia unawareness" (low blood sugar episodes without early-stage symptoms) are at risk for developing severe hypoglycemia.

Presenting signs and symptoms

Mild hypoglycemia is associated with adrenergic symptoms: pallor, diaphoresis, tachycardia, palpitations, hunger, widened pulse pressure, and shakiness. Patients who are taking β-adrenergic blocking agents may not exhibit these symptoms. Patients are totally alert during mild hypoglycemic episodes.

Moderate hypoglycemia is characterized by neuroglycopenic signs: headache, inability to concentrate, confusion, irrational behavior, slurred speech, blurred vision, paresthesias, fatigue, or somnolence. Severe hypoglycemia includes neuroglycopenic signs or loss of consciousness and seizures. Signs and symptoms will be particularly prominent if the serum glucose falls rapidly.

Physical examination

Vital signs:
    HR tachycardia
    BP hypertension initially, progressing to shock; widened pulse pressure
    RR shallow and rapid initially, progressing to bradypnea
    Temperature normal
Neurological:
    Visual disturbances
    Dilated pupils
    Numbness of tongue and lips
    Change in level of consciousness
    Seizures
    Paresthesias or paralysis
Skin: Pallor, diaphoresis, cool to touch

Diagnostic findings
Serum glucose <50 mg/dl
Serum ketones negative

Acute Care Patient Management

Goals of treatment
Restore serum glucose level
  10%-50% dextrose IV
  IV therapy with 5%-10% glucose solution
▶ **Priority Nursing Diagnoses**
Risk for injury
Risk for altered protection (see p. 33)
Risk for altered nutrition: less than body requirements
(see p. 41)
Risk for altered family process (see p. 29)
▶ **Nursing Diagnosis: Risk for injury** related to CNS dysfunction secondary to lack of glucose energy source

OUTCOME CRITERIA
- Patient will not injure self
- Patient will be alert and oriented
- Absence of seizures
- Serum glucose between 80-120 mg/dl

PATIENT MONITORING
1. Bedside glucose monitoring with finger-stick for quick evaluation of glucose level. May be performed hourly during initial treatment. Glucose should be raised to 100 mg/dl.

PHYSICAL ASSESSMENT
1. Observe for adrenergic symptoms: tachycardia, hypertension. Note onset of palpitations, shakiness, pallor, or diaphoresis. These symptoms may indicate recurrence of a hypoglycemic episode.
2. Assess for changes in LOC, speech, vision, and behavior, which may signal neuroglycopenia.

DIAGNOSTICS ASSESSMENT
1. Review daily serum glucose levels to monitor the patient's response to nutritional and glucose support.
2. If the patient remains unconscious with a serum glucose of 200 mg/dl, suspect neurological residual.

PATIENT MANAGEMENT
1. If the patient is symptomatic but conscious, administer a rapidly absorbed, glucose-containing food or liquid (e.g.,

ENDO

4 oz of orange juice or apple juice, sugar cubes, honey, hard candy, or syrup). At least 10 g of carbohydrate are required to raise the blood sugar. Repeat q5 to 10 min until symptoms begin to subside. Recheck glucose level in 20 to 30 minutes. IV therapy of D_5W may be ordered for continued glucose support.

2. If the patient is unconscious, administer dextrose 10% to 50% solution intravenously as ordered. IV therapy of D_5W or $D_{10}W$ may be ordered for continued glucose support. Hydrocortisone or glucagon may be added to each liter of fluid. Supplement IV dextrose with oral carbohydrates when patient awakens.

3. If long-acting oral hypoglycemic agents (e.g., sulfonylureas) have been implicated as the cause of the hypoglycemic episode, the patient is at risk for recurrences.

4. Institute seizure precautions: pad side rails, place the bed in low position; have emergency equipment available, such as oral airway and suction.

5. Alcoholic patients may require thiamine, since it promotes carbohydrate metabolism to prevent Wernicke-Korsakoff syndrome.

6. Maintain a safe environment.

MYXEDEMA COMA
Clinical Brief
Myxedema coma is a life-threatening condition in which patients with underlying thyroid dysfunction exhibit exaggerated manifestations of hypothyroidism. Precipitating factors may include (but are not limited to) infection, trauma, surgery, heart failure, stroke, or CNS depressants. Hypothyroidism depresses metabolic rate, thus seriously affecting all body systems. The clinical signs of myxedema coma and thyroid storm are compared in Table 2-44.
Presenting signs and symptoms
The predominant features are hypothermia, hypoventilation, and decreased mental function. Profound fatigue, activity intolerance, and hyporeflexia may precede its onset. Signs and symptoms of cardiac or respiratory failure may also be present.
Physical examination
Vital signs:
BP hypotension or hypertension
HR bradycardia

TABLE 2-44 Comparison of Clinical Signs of Thyroid Storm and Myxedema Coma

	Thyroid storm	Myxedema coma
Blood pressure	Increased	Decreased
Heart rate	Tachycardia	Bradycardia
Respiratory rate	Tachypnea	Bradypnea
Temperature	>39° C	<35° C
Fluid balance	Dehydrated	Overload
Serum glucose	Hyperglycemia	Hypoglycemia
Cardiac index	Increased	Decreased
SVRI	Decreased	Increased
Serum sodium	Hypo or hyper	Hyponatremia
Serum T_4	>12.5 mcg/dl	<5 mcg/dl
Serum T_3	>230 ng/100ml	<110 ng/100ml
Resin T_3 uptake	>35%	<25%

RR bradypnea
Temperature hypothermic <35° C (95° F)
Skin: Coarse and dry, possibly carotene color, edema
Neurological:
   Obtunded, coma or seizures
   Delayed reflexes
Gastrointestinal: Decreased bowel sounds

Diagnostic findings
Diagnosis is based on a high index of suspicion, and treatment should not be withheld until laboratory results confirm the diagnosis. Thyroid studies indicating primary hypothyroidism include the following:
Low free thyroxine index and elevated TSH level
Other: Hyponatremia and hypoglycemia may be present;
   ECG demonstrates low voltage, prolonged QT interval,
   flattened or inverted T wave
Cortisol level is usually low

Acute Care Patient Management
Goals of treatment
Increase thyroid hormone levels
   Thyroid replacement
Improve ventilation/oxygenation
   Supplemental oxygen
   Intubation/mechanical ventilation

Restore normothermia
  Warming methods
Restore hemodynamic stability
  Crystalloids
  Vasopressor agents
Detect/prevent clinical sequelae
  See Table 2-45

▶ **Priority Nursing Diagnoses**
Hypothermia
Impaired gas exchange
Decreased cardiac output
Risk for injury
Altered protection (see p. 33)
Risk for altered family process (see p. 29)

▶ **Nursing Diagnosis:** Hypothermia related to decreased metabolism secondary to hypothyroidism

OUTCOME CRITERION
• T 36.5° C (97.7° F) to 37.8° C (100° F)

PATIENT MONITORING
1. Continuously monitor core temperature (if possible) to evaluate the patient's response to therapy.
2. Assess the patient for development of clinical sequelae (Table 2-45).

PHYSICAL ASSESSMENT
1. Assess neurological status: note LOC.

DIAGNOSTICS ASSESSMENT
None specific

TABLE 2-45   Clinical Sequelae Associated with Myxedema Coma

Complication	Signs and symptoms
Respiratory failure	PaO_2 <50 mm Hg, $PaCO_2$ >50 mmHg pH <7.35
Cardiac failure	PAWP >20 mm Hg, increased JVP, crackles, S_3, decreased heart sounds, murmur
Bowel obstruction	Distended abdomen, vomiting, hypoactive/absent bowel sounds
Acute adrenal insufficiency	Hyponatremia, decreased cortisol, hypoglycemia

PATIENT MANAGEMENT

1. Administer thyroid hormone as ordered and carefully monitor cardiac patients for myocardial ischemia, chest pain, and ECG changes:

   Thyroxine: a loading dose is 300 to 500 µg IV, followed by a daily dose of 75 to 100 µg IV.

   Liothyronine sodium for a more rapid onset. Usual dose is 25 µg IV q6h.

   Triiodothyronine: 12.5 to 25 µg q6h. Combination therapy may be ordered: Thyroxine 200 to 300 µg + 25 µg triiodothyronine q12h initially, then reducing thyroxine dose to 100 µg on day 2, and 50 µg per day thereafter.

   Corticosteroids may also be administered.

2. Institute passive rewarming methods; a thermal blanket may be necessary to increase body temperature. Use cautiously; rewarming may cause vasodilation and hypotension. (See p. 548 for information about thermal regulation.)

▶ **Nursing Diagnosis:** Impaired gas exchange related to respiratory muscle weakness and blunted central respiratory response to hypoxemia and hypercapnia

OUTCOME CRITERIA

- Patient alert and oriented
- RR   12-20/min, eupnea
- PaO_2 80-100 mm Hg
- $PaCO_2$ 35-45 mm Hg
- pH   7.35-7.45
- O_2 sat   ≥95%

PATIENT MONITORING

1. Continuously monitor oxygen saturation with pulse oximetry (SpO_2). Monitor patient activities and interventions that can adversely affect oxygen saturation.

2. Continuously monitor ECG for dysrhythmias that may be related to hypoxemia or acid-base imbalance.

PHYSICAL ASSESSMENT

1. Assess respiratory status: note respiratory rate, rhythm, and depth. Patients are generally intubated and their lungs are mechanically ventilated.

2. Assess the patient for development of clinical sequelae. (See Table 2-45.)

DIAGNOSTICS ASSESSMENT

1. Review serial ABGs to evaluate oxygenation and acid-base balance.

ENDO

PATIENT MANAGEMENT

1. Administer supplemental oxygen as ordered (for patient management of mechanical ventilation, see p. 577.)
2. Administer thyroid medication as prescribed.
3. Reposition the patient to improve oxygenation and mobilize secretions. Evaluate the patient's response to position changes with SpO_2 or ABGs to determine the best position for oxygenation.
4. As the patient stabilizes hemodynamically, provide pulmonary hygiene to prevent complications.
5. Avoid administering CNS depressants, since they are slowly metabolized by the hypothyroid patient.

▶ **Nursing Diagnosis:**   Decreased cardiac output related to bradycardia and decreased stroke volume

OUTCOME CRITERIA

- Patient will be alert and oriented
- SBP   90-140 mm Hg
- MAP   70-105 mm Hg
- HR   60-100 beats/min
- Urine output 30 ml/hr or 0.5-1 ml/kg/hr
- Peripheral pulses palpable
- PAS   15-30 mm Hg
- PAD   5-15 mm Hg
- CI   2.5-4 L/min/m²

PATIENT MONITORING

1. Continuously monitor ECG for dysrhythmias or profound bradycardia that can adversely affect CO. A prolonged QT interval is associated with torsade de pointes.
2. Continuously monitor PA pressures, CVP (if available), and BP. Obtain CI and PAWP to evaluate cardiac function and the patient's response to therapy. Monitor MAP; a MAP <60 mm Hg adversely affects cerebral and renal perfusion.
3. Monitor fluid volume status: measure urine output hourly, determine fluid balance q8h; compare serial weights; a rapid (0.5 to 1 kg/day) change suggests fluid imbalance.

PHYSICAL ASSESSMENT

1. Assess cardiovascular status: note quality of peripheral pulses and capillary refill. Observe for increase in JVP and pulsus paradoxus, which may indicate pericardial effusion. Auscultate heart sounds, heart rate, and breath sounds for development of heart failure. Observe for

tachycardia and myocardial ischemia as thyroid hormone is being replaced.

2. Assess the patient for development of clinical sequelae. (See Table 2-45.)

DIAGNOSTICS ASSESSMENT

1. Review thyroid studies as available. TSH levels should decline within 24 hr of therapy and should normalize after 7 days of therapy.

PATIENT MANAGEMENT

1. Administer IV fluids as ordered to maintain SBP >90 mm Hg; carefully monitor for fluid overload and development of heart failure.

2. Vasopressor agents may be used if hypotension is refractory to volume administration and if thyroid replacement has not had time to act. Carefully monitor the patient for lethal dysrhythmias.

▶ **Nursing Diagnoses:**   **Risk for injury** related to altered level of consciousness and **Fluid volume deficit** secondary to impaired free water clearance

OUTCOME CRITERIA

- Patient will be alert and oriented
- Absence of seizures
- Patient will not injure self
- Intake approximates output
- Serum sodium 135-145 mEq/L
- Serum osmolality 275-295 mOsm/L
- Urine specific gravity 1.010-1.030

PATIENT MONITORING

1. Monitor fluid volume status: measure intake and output hourly, determine fluid balance q8h. Compare serial weights; a rapid (0.5 to 1 kg/day) change indicates fluid imbalance. Weight gain without edema may be observed.

2. Monitor LOC with Glasgow coma scale. Deterioration in LOC may be associated with water intoxication.

PHYSICAL ASSESSMENT

1. Assess for complaints of headache, fatigue, or weakness.

2. Assess hydration status: note skin turgor on inner thigh or forehead, observe buccal membranes, and assess thirst.

3. Assess the patient's lungs for adventitious sounds; assess heart sounds for development of S_3 (a hallmark of heart failure).

ENDO

4. Assess the patient for development of clinical sequelae. (See Table 2-45.)

DIAGNOSTICS ASSESSMENT

1. Review serum sodium, serum osmolality, and urine specific gravity. Hyponatremia may be contributing to the obtunded state.

PATIENT MANAGEMENT

1. If the sodium level is <120 mEq/L, isotonic saline may be administered and free water restricted. (See p. 296 for management of hyponatremia.)
2. Carefully administer fluids and diuretics. Explain fluid restriction to patient.
3. Institute seizure precautions.
4. Hydrocortisone 100 mg IV q6 to 8h may be ordered until adrenal function normalizes.
5. Maintain safe environment. Reorient the confused patient with each interaction.

SYNDROME OF INAPPROPRIATE ANTIDIURETIC HORMONE (SIADH)

Clinical Brief

SIADH is a condition that results from failure in the negative feedback mechanisms that regulate inhibition and secretion of ADH. It produces excess antidiuretic hormone (ADH), resulting in hyponatremia and hypo-osmolality of serum. The kidneys respond by reabsorbing water in the tubules and excreting sodium; thus the patient becomes severely water intoxicated. SIADH is most commonly caused by ectopic production of ADH by malignant tumors. It can be the result of CNS disorders, such as Guillain-Barré syndrome, meningitis, brain tumors, and head trauma. Pulmonary-related conditions, such as pneumonia, and positive-pressure ventilation can cause SIADH. Pharmacological agents such as general anesthetics, thiazide diuretics, oral hypoglycemics, chemotherapeutic agents, and analgesics, are also associated with SIADH release.

Presenting signs and symptoms

Signs and symptoms depend on the degree and rate of onset of hyponatremia. The patient may complain of a headache, muscle cramps, and lethargy or have seizures or coma. If alert, the patient usually complains of nausea, vomiting, and anorexia with related muscle weakness and loss. Weight gain may result from increased water retention, although the patient does not appear edematous.

Physical examination
Vital signs:
   BP ↑ or may be normal
   HR tachycardia
   Temperature ↓ or may be normal
Neurological:
   Alert to unresponsiveness
   Seizures
Cardiovascular: Bounding pulses
Pulmonary: Crackles may be present
Gastrointestinal:
   Cramps
   Decreased bowel sounds
   Vomiting
Musculoskeletal:
   Weakness
   Cramps
   Absent deep tendon reflexes

DIAGNOSTIC FINDINGS
A water load test confirms the diagnosis:
Serum sodium <120 mEq/L, normalizes with water restriction
Serum osmolality <250 mOsm/kg
Serum potassium <3.8 mEq/L
Serum calcium <8.5 mg/dl
Serum aldosterone level <5 ng/dl
Serum ADH >5 pg/ml
Urine osmolality >900 mOsm/kg, 50-150 mOsm/L
Urine sodium >200 mEq/24 hr, 20 mEq/L

Acute Care Patient Management

Goals of treatment
Restore fluid and electrolyte balance
   Fluid restriction <1000 ml/day
   Diuretic therapy
   Potassium supplementation
Control ADH excretion
   Lithium
   Demeclocycline
   Phenytoin
   Surgery
Prevent seizures
   Hypertonic saline
   Phenytoin

ENDO

Treat the cause
  Appropriate therapy
▶ **Priority Nursing Diagnoses**
Fluid volume excess
Risk for injury
Risk for altered protection (see p. 33)
Risk for altered nutrition: less than body requirements
(see p. 41)
Risk for altered family process (see p. 29)
▶ **Nursing Diagnosis:**   Fluid volume excess related to excessive amounts of ADH secretion
OUTCOME CRITERIA
• Intake approximates output
• Serum potassium 3.5-5.0 mEq/L
• Serum sodium 135-145 mEq/L
• Serum chloride 95-105 mEq/L
• Serum osmolality 275-295 mOsm/kg
• Urine specific gravity 1.003-1.035
• CVP   2-6 mm Hg
• PAWP   4-12 mm Hg

PATIENT MONITORING
1. Monitor PA pressures and CVP hourly (if available) or
   more frequently to evaluate the patient's response to
   treatment. Both parameters reflect the capacity of the
   vascular system to accept volume and can be used to
   monitor fluid volume status.
2. Monitor hourly intake and urine output and determine
   fluid balance q8h. Compare serial weights and note rapid
   (0.5 to 1 kg/day) changes in weight suggesting fluid
   imbalance.
3. Continuously monitor ECG for dysrhythmias resulting
   from electrolyte imbalance.

PATIENT ASSESSMENT
1. Obtain VS q1h or more frequently until the patient's
   condition is stable.
2. Evaluate hydration status q4h. Note skin turgor on inner
   thigh or forehead, condition of buccal membranes,
   development of edema or crackles.

DIAGNOSTICS ASSESSMENT
1. Review serum sodium and potassium, serum osmolality,
   urine specific gravity, and urine osmolality to evaluate the
   patient's response to therapy.

PATIENT MANAGEMENT

1. Restrict fluid as ordered, generally <500 ml/day in severe cases and 800 to 1000 ml/day in moderate cases. Water intake should not exceed urine output and insensible loss until sodium is normal and patient is asymptomatic. Encourage fluids high in sodium.
2. Administer potassium supplements as ordered; assess renal function and ensure adequate urine output before administering potassium.
3. As adjuncts to water restriction, demeclocycline may be ordered to inhibit the renal response to ADH in patients with lung malignancies; lithium carbonate may be used to alter psychogenic behavior.
4. Avoid hypotonic enemas to treat constipation, since water intoxication can be potentiated.

▶ **Nursing Diagnosis:** **Risk for injury** related to low serum sodium

OUTCOME CRITERIA

- Patient will be alert and oriented
- Patient will not injure self
- Absence of seizures
- Serum sodium 135-145 mEq/L

PATIENT MONITORING

1. Obtain PA pressures and CVP (if available) hourly or more frequently during hypertonic saline infusions to monitor for development of fluid overload.

PATIENT ASSESSMENT

1. Assess LOC hourly to evaluate effects of water intoxication. Patients may become symptomatic (e.g., confusion, seizures, coma) at sodium levels <125 mEq/L.

DIAGNOSTICS ASSESSMENT

1. Review serial serum sodium levels to evaluate the patient's response to therapy.

PATIENT MANAGEMENT

1. If the patient's sodium level <105 mEq/L, hypertonic saline (3% NaCl) may be used to slowly raise serum sodium to 125 mEq/L (serum sodium should be increased no faster than 1 to 2 mEq/L/hour). Too rapid an increase in serum sodium may further impair neurological function. Closely monitor for fluid overload and heart failure during hypertonic infusion: dyspnea, increased respiratory rate, crackles, moist

ENDO

cough, bounding pulses. Furosemide or other diuretic agents may be administered with hypertonic saline infusions to increase urinary excretion of free water.

2. Maintain airway.
3. Institute seizure precautions.
4. Reorient the confused patient to place, person, and time with each interaction.

THYROID STORM

Clinical Brief

Thyroid storm is a life-threatening condition in which patients with underlying thyroid dysfunction exhibit exaggerated signs and symptoms of hyperthyroidism. Thyroid storm is precipated by stressors such as infection, trauma, DKA, surgery, heart failure, or stroke. The condition can result from discontinuation of thyroid medication or as a result of untreated or inadequate treatment of hyperthyroidism. The excess thyroid hormones increase metabolism and affect the sympathetic nervous system, thus increasing oxygen consumption and heat production and altering fluid and electrolyte levels. The clinical signs of thyroid storm and myxedema coma are compared in Table 2-44.

Presenting signs and symptoms

Signs and symptoms include sudden onset of fever (>39° C), tremors, flushing, profuse palm sweating, tachydysrhythmias, and extreme restlessness. The patient may be unresponsive. GI symptoms may be present: nausea, vomiting, diarrhea, and weight loss. Fatigue and muscle weakness and atrophy are common. Older patients may manifest principally cardiac symptoms (e.g., heart failure, angina, dysrhythmias).

Physical examination

Vital signs:

BP systolic hypertension or hypotension (if shock)

HR tachycardia disproportionate to the degree of fever

RR >20/min

Temperature >39° C (102.2° F), can be up to 41° C (105.9° F)

Neurological: Agitated, tremulous, delirious to coma

Cardiovascular: Bounding pulses, systolic murmur, widening pulse pressure; ↑ JVP, S_3, weak thready pulses (depending on the degree of CV compromise)

Pulmonary: Tachypnea, crackles may be present
Gastrointestinal: ↑ Bowel sounds

Diagnostic findings

Diagnosis is based on a high index of suspicion (fever, tachycardia out of proportion to the fever, and central nervous system dysfunction), and treatment should not be withheld until laboratory results confirm hyperthyroidism. Studies indicating hyperthyroidism include the following:

↑ T_4
↑ T_3 resin uptake
↓ TSH

ECG may reveal atrial fibrillation, SVT

Acute Care Patient Management

Goals of treatment

Reduce oversecretion of thyroid hormone
    Antithyroid agents
    β-Adrenergic blocking agents
    Glucocorticoids
    Surgery
    Treatment of precipitating factor
Restore hemodynamic stability
    Supplemental oxygen
    Crystalloids
    Vasopressor agents
    Inotropic agents
    Diuretic agents
Restore normothermia
    Cooling methods
    Acetaminophen
Support nutrition
    Supplemental feedings
    TPN
Detect/prevent clinical sequelae
    See Table 2-46

► **Priority Nursing Diagnoses**

Hyperthermia
Decreased cardiac output
Ineffective breathing pattern
Altered nutrition: less than body requirements
Altered protection (see p. 33)
Risk for altered family process (see p. 29)

ENDO

TABLE 2-46 Clinical Sequelae Associated with Thyroid Storm

Complication	Signs and symptoms
Shock	SBP <90 mm Hg, HR >120 beats/min, altered mental state, cool clammy skin, ↓ urine output
Respiratory failure	PaO_2 <50 mm Hg, $PaCO_2$ >50 mm Hg, paradoxical breathing, restlessness, RR >30/min
Cardiac failure/pulmonary edema	Tachycardia, S_3, hypotension, ↑ JVP, crackles, tachypnea, dyspnea, frothy sputum

▶ **Nursing Diagnosis:** Hyperthermia related to increased metabolism

OUTCOME CRITERIA
- T 36.5° C (97.7° F) to 37.8° C (100° F)
- SBP   90-140 mm Hg

PATIENT MONITORING
1. Continuously monitor core temperature (if possible) to evaluate the patient's response to therapy.
2. Continuously monitor BP, since fever increases peripheral vasodilation, which can lead to hypotension.

PHYSICAL ASSESSMENT
1. Assess the patient for diaphoresis and shivering; shivering increases metabolic demand.
2. Assess the patient for development of clinical sequelae. (See Table 2-46.)

DIAGNOSTICS ASSESSMENT
1. Review culture reports for possible infection.

PATIENT MANAGEMENT
1. Administer acetaminophen as ordered and evaluate the patient's response.
2. Avoid aspirin administration, since salicylates increase circulating thyroid hormones.
3. Administer antithyroid pharmacological agents as prescribed: *Propylthiouracil (PTU):* Blocks thyroid hormone synthesis and inhibits conversion of T_4 to T_3; loading dose of 600 to 1000 mg, then 150 to 200 mg tid-qid.

Iodide: Inhibits the release of thyroid hormone and should be given at least 1 hr after PTU has been administered; SSKI—10 gtt q12h or Lugol's solution—4 gtt q12h or sodium iodide—500 to 1000 mg q12h may be ordered.

Methimazole: Inhibits thyroid hormone synthesis; loading dose of 60 to 100 mg, then 10 to 20 mg tid.

Dexamethasone: May be used to suppress conversion of T_4 and T_3 and to replace rapidly metabolized cortisol; 2 mg q6h.

Colestipol: May be used in extreme cases; 10 g q8h.

4. Institute cooling methods; a hypothermia blanket may be necessary to reduce body temperature. (See p. 548.)
5. Provide comfort measures, checking the patient for diaphoresis and changing patient's gown and bed linens as necessary.
6. Peritoneal dialysis and plasmapheresis have been reported to reduce thyroid hormone levels in extreme cases.

▶ **Nursing Diagnoses:** **Decreased cardiac output** related to increased cardiac work secondary to increased adrenergic activity; and **Fluid volume deficit** secondary to increased metabolism and diaphoresis

OUTCOME CRITERIA
- Patient will be alert and oriented
- Peripheral pulses palpable
- Lungs clear to auscultation
- Urine output 30 ml/hr or 0.5-1 ml/kg/hr
- SBP   90-140 mm Hg
- MAP   70-105 mm Hg
- HR   60-100 beats/min
- Absence of life-threatening dysrhythmias
- PAS   15-30 mm Hg
- PAD   5-15 mm Hg
- PAWP   4-12 mm Hg
- CI   2.5-4 L/min/m²
- SVRI   1700-2600 dynes/sec/cm⁵/m²
- LVSWI   45-60 g-m/m²

PATIENT MONITORING
1. Continuously monitor ECG for dysrhythmias or HR >140 beats/min that can adversely affect CO and monitor for ST segment changes indicative of myocardial ischemia.

2. Continuously monitor oxygen saturation with pulse oximetry (SpO_2). Be alert for patient activities or interventions that adversely affect oxygen saturation.
3. Continuously monitor PA pressures, CVP (if available), and BP. Obtain CI and PAWP to evaluate cardiac function and patient response to therapy. Monitor MAP; a MAP <60 mm Hg adversely affects cerebral and renal perfusion.
4. Monitor fluid volume status: measure urine output hourly, determine fluid balance q8h. Compare serial weights; a rapid (0.5 to 1 kg/day) change suggests fluid imbalance.

PHYSICAL ASSESSMENT

1. Assess cardiovascular status: note extra heart sounds (S_3 is a hallmark of heart failure), ↑ JVP, crackles, and prolonged capillary refill suggesting heart failure, which can progress to pulmonary edema (increasing dyspnea, frothy sputum). Assess the patient for myocardial ischemic pain.
2. Assess hydration status (e.g., thirst, mucous membranes, skin turgor), since dehydration can further decrease circulating volume and compromise CO.
3. Assess the patient for development of clinical sequelae. (See Table 2-46.)

DIAGNOSTICS ASSESSMENT

1. Review thyroid studies as available.
2. Review serial serum electrolytes, serum glucose, and serum calcium levels to evaluate the patient's response to therapy.
3. Review serial ABGs for hypoxemia and acid-base imbalance, which can adversely affect cardiac function.
4. Review serial chest radiographs for cardiac enlargement and pulmonary congestion.

PATIENT MANAGEMENT

1. Administer dextrose-containing IV fluids as ordered to correct fluid and glucose deficits. Carefully assess the patient for heart failure or pulmonary edema. Dopamine may be used to support BP.
2. Provide supplemental oxygen as ordered to help meet increased metabolic demands. Once patient is hemodynamically stable, provide pulmonary hygiene to reduce pulmonary complications.
3. Administer β-adrenergic blocking agents such as propranolol to control tachycardia and hypertension (also inhibits conversion of T_4 to T_3; 1 mg IV q5″ to achieve a HR ~90

to 100 beats/min, and 20 to 40 mg po q6h. Monitor HR for bradycardia and PA pressures (if available) to evaluate left ventricular function. A short-acting β-adrenergic blocking agent such as esmolol may also be tried.

4. If the patient is in heart failure, typical pharmacological agents include digitalis, furosemide, potassium supplements, and afterload-reduction agents. (See Heart failure, p. 179.)

5. Reduce oxygen demands: decrease anxiety, reduce fever, decrease pain, and limit visitors if necessary. Schedule uninterrupted rest periods. Approach the patient in a calm manner, explain procedures or provide information to decrease misperceptions. Keep the room cool and dimly lit and reduce external stimuli as much as possible.

6. Anticipate aggressive treatment of precipitating factor.

▶ **Nursing Diagnosis:** Ineffective breathing pattern related to intercostal muscle weakness

OUTCOME CRITERIA
- Patient will be alert and oriented
- RR   12-20/min, eupnea
- Pao_2 80-100 mm Hg
- $Paco_2$ 35-45 mm Hg
- pH   7.35-7.45
- O_2 sat   ≥95%

PATIENT MONITORING
1. Continuously monitor oxygen saturation with pulse oximetry (Spo_2). Monitor patient activities and interventions that can adversely affect oxygen saturation.

2. Continuously monitor ECG for dysrhythmias that may be related to hypoxemia or acid-base imbalance.

PHYSICAL ASSESSMENT
1. Assess respiratory status: note respiratory rate, rhythm, depth, and use of accessory muscles. Observe for paradoxical breathing pattern and increased restlessness, increased complaints of dyspnea, and changes in level of consciousness. Cyanosis is a late sign of respiratory distress.

2. Assess patient for development of clinical sequelae. (See Table 2-46.)

DIAGNOSTICS ASSESSMENT
1. Review serial ABGs to evaluate oxygenation and acid-base balance.

2. Review serial chest radiographs for pulmonary congestion.

ENDO

PATIENT MANAGEMENT

1. Administer supplemental oxygen as ordered. (For patient management of mechanical ventilation, see p. 577.)
2. Reposition the patient to improve oxygenation and mobilize secretions. Evaluate the patient's response to position changes with SpO_2 or ABGs to determine the best position for oxygenation.
3. As the patient's hemodynamics stabilize, provide pulmonary hygiene to prevent complications.
4. Decrease oxygen demands (e.g., reduce fever, alleviate anxiety, limit visitors if necessary, schedule uninterrupted rest periods).
5. Administer antithyroid medications as prescribed.

▶ **Nursing Diagnosis:**   Altered nutrition: less than body requirements related to increased metabolism

OUTCOME CRITERION

• Stabilized weight

PATIENT MONITORING

1. Conduct calorie counts to provide information about the adequacy of intake required to meet metabolic needs.
2. Compare serial weights; rapid (0.5 to 1 kg/day) changes indicate fluid imbalance and not an imbalance between nutritional needs and intake.

PHYSICAL ASSESSMENT

1. Assess GI status: absent or hyperactive bowel sounds, vomiting, diarrhea, or abdominal pain may interfere with nutritional absorption.
2. Assess the patient for development of clinical sequelae. (See Table 2-46.)

DIAGNOSTICS ASSESSMENT

1. Review serial serum glucose levels for hyperglycemia, since excessive circulating thyroid hormones increase glycogenolysis and decrease insulin levels.

PATIENT MANAGEMENT

1. Consult with a nutritionist to maximize intake of calories and protein to reverse the negative nitrogen balance.
2. Assist the patient with small, frequent feedings. TPN may be required. (See p. 639 for information on parenteral nutrition.)
3. Insulin therapy may be required to control hyperglycemia.
4. Avoid caffeine products, which may increase peristalsis.

ACUTE RENAL FAILURE

Clinical Brief

Acute renal failure is a clinical syndrome characterized by a sudden, rapid deterioration in kidney function, which results in the retention of nitrogenous waste (urea nitrogen and creatinine) and fluid, electrolyte, and acid-base imbalances. Causes of acute renal failure can be divided into three categories.

Prerenal: Factors that decrease renal perfusion (e.g., shock, intravascular volume depletion, occlusion or damage to the renal arteries, pharmacologic agents)

Intrarenal: Factors that damage the renal parenchyma (e.g., nephrotoxic agents [antibiotics, contrast media, pesticides, myoglobin], inflammation, trauma, and any prerenal process that results in renal ischemia); acute tubular necrosis (ATN) is a type of intrarenal failure

Postrenal: Factors that result from obstruction of urine flow from the kidneys to the external environment (e.g., prostatic hypertrophy, kidney stones, or bladder tumor)

Acute tubular necrosis (ATN) is the most common cause of acute renal failure. Acute renal failure and ATN often present with oliguria (less than 700 ml of urine in 24 hours). Patient mortality is significantly reduced if oliguric renal failure can be converted to nonoliguric failure.

Presenting signs and symptoms

The acute onset of renal failure is often accompanied by oliguria (but may be nonoliguric), and azotemia (accumulation of nitrogen waste products).

Physical examination

Vital signs:

 BP increased or decreased

 HR increased

 RR increased

 Temperature normal or increased

Neurological: Irritability, restlessness, change in LOC

Cardiovascular: S_3, S_4, JVD may be present

Pulmonary: Deep and rapid respirations, crackles

Gastrointestinal: Nausea, vomiting, anorexia

RENAL

Diagnostic findings

Diagnostic findings vary with category (Table 2-47).

NOTE: Diuretic administration will affect urine analysis.

Acute Care Patient Management

Goals of treatment

Optimize renal perfusion and urine output
Correction of suspected cause
Fluid challenge
Low-dose dopamine
Diuretic agents
Antihypertensive agents
Vasodilator agents
Avoidance of nephrotoxic agents
Normalize fluid status
Fluid challenge in prerenal patients
Fluid restriction in oliguric patients
Diuretic agents
Renal replacement therapy

TABLE 2-47   Categories of Acute Renal Failure and Related Laboratory Values

	Prerenal	Intrarenal (ATN)	Postrenal
Urine			
Volume	Low	Low or high	Low or high
Sodium	<20 mEq/L	>20 mEq/L	>40 mEq/L
Osmolality	>350 mOsm	<300 mOsm (fixed)	<350 mOsm (varies)
Specific gravity	>1.020	<1.010	
Creatinine	~Normal	Low	Low
FEna	≤1%	>1%	
Sediment	Normal	Normal	Cells, casts, protein
Plasma			
Urea (BUN)	High	High	High
Creatinine	~Normal	High	High
BUN: creatinine	20:1 or more	10:1 to 15:1	10:1

Remove nitrogen waste products
   Restriction of protein intake
   Increase in caloric intake
   Renal replacement therapy
Maintain electrolyte balance
   Restriction of sodium
   Restriction of potassium
   Phosphate-binding antacids
   For hyperkalemia:
      Kayexalate (with sorbitol)
      Glucose with insulin
      Sodium bicarbonate
Treat hypercatabolism
   Renal replacement therapy
   Nutrition: high calorie, low protein, high essential amino acids
Detect/prevent clinical sequelae
   See Table 2-48

TABLE 2-48 Clinical Sequelae Associated with Acute Renal Failure

Complication	Signs and symptoms
Hyperkalemia	Peaked T waves, prolonged PR interval, prolonged QRS duration, dysrhythmias; twitching, cramps, hyperactive reflexes
Pericarditis	Chest discomfort aggravated by supine position or deep inspiration, intermittent friction rub and/or fever may be present
Metabolic acidosis	pH <7.35 with $\downarrow HCO_3$ and normal or $Paco_2$; Kussmaul respirations (hyperventilation); headache, fatigue, altered mental status
Anemia	Decreasing hematocrit, active bleeding; pale, weak, tired; SOB
GI bleed	Occult or visible blood in stools or gastric contents, decreasing hematocrit
Infection	Elevated temperature (may be subtle); lungs, urinary tract, or wounds may be sources
Uremia	Lethargy progressing to coma, seizures, asterixis, heart failure, volume disturbances, pericarditis, N/V, anorexia, diarrhea, GI bleeding

RENAL

▶ **Priority Nursing Diagnoses**
Fluid volume excess
Fluid volume deficit
Risk for injury (see pp. 277-300)
Altered nutrition: less than body requirements
(see p. 41)
Altered protection (see p. 33)
Risk for altered family process (see p. 29)

▶ **Nursing Diagnosis:** Fluid volume excess related to decreased renal excretion (oliguria)

OUTCOME CRITERIA
- Patient at target body weight
- Intake approximates output
- MAP   70-105 mm Hg
- SBP   90-140 mm Hg
- Absence of edema
- Lungs clear to auscultation
- Patient alert and oriented
- Absence of heart failure
- CVP   2-6 mm Hg
- Electrolytes WNL
- Creatinine 0.6-1.2 mg/dl
- BUN   <100 mg/dl
- Urine specific gravity 1.003-1.030

PATIENT MONITORING
1. Monitor fluid volume status: measure urine output hourly, determine fluid balance q8h and include other bodily drainage. Compare serial weights for rapid changes; an increase of 1 to 2 pounds/day indicates fluid retention. The oliguria phase (urine output <400 ml/day) in ATN usually lasts 10 to 16 days, followed by a diuretic phase.
2. Obtain CVP, PA pressures (if available), and BP hourly or more frequently to evaluate the extent of fluid volume excess and the patient's response to therapy. Monitor MAP, an indicator of tissue perfusion; a decrease in MAP further insults the kidney.
3. Continuously monitor ECG for dysrhythmias secondary to electrolyte imbalance.

PHYSICAL ASSESSMENT
1. Assess fluid volume status; note any onset of S_3 and crackles, presence of edema, cough, or frothy sputum, increased work of breathing, decreased peripheral perfu-

sion, and increased JVP to determine development of heart failure or pulmonary edema.

2. Assess the patient for development of clinical sequelae. (See Table 2-48.)

DIAGNOSTICS ASSESSMENT

1. Review BUN, creatinine, and BUN/creatinine ratio. Serum creatinine reflects GFR. Estimating GFR is not accurate in acute renal failure and is assumed to be <10. Uremic symptoms may manifest if BUN is >70 to 100 mg/dl or GFR is <10 to 15 ml/min. A rise in BUN without a corresponding rise in creatinine may indicate bleeding.

2. Review urine sodium, urine osmolality, and urine specific gravity to evaluate renal function.

3. Review serial chest radiographs to evaluate pulmonary congestion.

4. Review serial ABGs to evaluate extent of acid-base imbalances.

5. Review serial electrolytes: hyperkalemia, hyponatremia, hypocalcemia, hyperphosphatemia, and hypermagnesemia are common in acute renal failure.

PATIENT MANAGEMENT

1. Restrict fluids to ~600 ml/day plus insensible losses in oliguric patients and restrict sodium intake to reduce fluid volume. Restrict protein intake to limit nitrogen accumulation. Increase caloric intake to minimize protein catabolism.

2. Concentrate medications when possible to minimize fluid intake.

3. Administer diuretics (furosemide, bumetanide) as ordered to produce diuresis. Closely monitor for signs of peripheral vascular collapse, hypovolemia, hypotension, hypokalemia, and hyponatremia during rapid diuresis. If possible, obtain a urine specimen for laboratory analysis before administering diuretics.

4. Administer dopamine in low doses (1 to 5 μg/kg/min) to increase renal perfusion by vasodilating renal vasculature. Monitor urine output.

5. If the patient is hypertensive, administer vasodilators or antihypertensive agents as ordered. Carefully monitor BP before administration; generally SBP should be >90 mm Hg.

6. Raise HOB if the patient is SOB without being hypotensive.

RENAL

7. Provide meticulous skin care to prevent skin breakdown and infection.

8. Anticipate hemodialysis or other form of continuous renal replacement therapy to remove excess fluid and/or solutes. See p. 647 for information on renal replacement therapy.

9. Avoid administration of nephrotoxic agents or administer at reduced dosage or frequency to prevent additional renal damage.

▶ **Nursing Diagnosis:** **Fluid volume deficit** related to volume depletion (diuretic phase)

OUTCOME CRITERIA
- MAP   70-105 mm Hg
- Urine output 30 ml/hr or 0.5-1 ml/kg/hr
- Intake approximates output
- Elastic skin turgor
- Moist mucous membranes
- HR   60-100 beats/min
- Electrolytes WNL

PATIENT MONITORING
1. Monitor I & O hourly to assess the fluid balance trend, reflective of renal function, Diuretic phase (>400 ml/day) of ATN may last 2 to 3 days or up to 12 days.

2. Compare daily weights to assess fluid volume status.

3. Obtain CVP, PA pressures (if available), HR, and BP hourly or more frequently as patient condition dictates. Monitor MAP, an indicator of tissue perfusion; a MAP <70 mm Hg further insults the kidney. Be alert for tachycardia and postural hypotension, which may indicate volume depletion.

PHYSICAL ASSESSMENT
1. Assess hydration state: note skin turgor on inner thigh or forehead, condition of buccal membranes. Flat neck veins, complaints of thirst, and decreased sensorium may signal volume depletion.

2. Assess the patient for development of clinical sequelae. (See Table 2-48.)

DIAGNOSTICS ASSESSMENT
1. Review urine sodium, osmolality, and specific gravity to assess volume status.

2. Review serial electrolytes, since severe imbalances can occur.

PATIENT MANAGEMENT

1. Administer aggressive fluid and electrolyte replacements as ordered to increase volume and maintain normal electrolyte and acid-base balance. Carefully monitor for increase in urine output and early signs of fluid volume excess when administering fluid challenges.
2. Avoid administration of nephrotoxic agents or administer at reduced dosage or frequency to prevent additional renal damage.
3. Avoid rapidly placing the patient in an upright position, because postural hypotension may result.
4. Provide meticulous skin care to avoid skin breakdown and oral care to soothe dry mucous membranes.
5. Check for occult blood in stools and NG aspirate, since GI bleeding can occur in patients with renal failure, contributing to signs and symptoms of volume deficit.
6. Restrict protein intake to reduce nitrogen waste product accumulation. Increase caloric intake to minimize protein catabolism.

ELECTROLYTE IMBALANCE: CALCIUM

Clinical Brief

Calcium imbalances occur as a result of changes in calcium ion concentrations in extracellular fluid. Because approximately half of the calcium is bound to albumin, evaluation of calcium levels must be done in conjunction with albumin levels. A falsely low calcium level is seen in the presence of low albumin levels. Changes in pH alter the amount of calcium bound to albumin, requiring that assessment of serum calcium levels ideally be done when the pH is normal.

Hypocalcemia frequently results from respiratory alkalosis associated with hyperventilation, receiving large amounts of stored blood, acute pancreatitis, decreased intake, or decreased absorption (from vitamin D deficiency, decreased parathyroid hormone release, hyperphosphatemia, chronic renal failure, or malabsorption). *Hypercalcemia* commonly occurs with malignancy (primarily cancer of the lung, breast, and hematologic tissues) and hyperparathyroidism. However, immobility and resumption of kidney function following renal transplantation can also cause hypercalcemia.

Presenting signs and symptoms

Signs and symptoms depend on the severity of the imbalance. (See Physical examination.)

RENAL

Physical examination

	Hypocalcemia	Hypercalcemia
Appearance:	Tired	Tired, lethargic, bone pain
Cardiovascular:	ECG: Prolonged QT interval Palpitations Decreased CO Dysrhythmias	ECG: Shortened QT interval Dysrhythmias, especially heart block; cardiac arrest
Pulmonary:	Stridor, bronchospasm, laryngospasm	
Neurological:	Cramping of hands, feet, circumoral paresthesia, hyperreflexia, tetany, carpal and pedal spasm, numbness, tingling, twitching, seizures, altered mental status	Hyporeflexia, altered mental status, headache
Gastrointestinal:	Abdominal cramps	Anorexia, thirst, nausea, vomiting, constipation

Diagnostic findings

Hypocalcemia is defined as an ionized serum calcium level of less than 4.5 mg/dl (total calcium of less than 9 mg/dl); *hypercalcemia* is an ionized calcium of greater than 5.5 mg/dl (total calcium greater than 11 mg/dl).

Acute Care Patient Management
Goals of treatment

	Hypocalcemia	Hypercalcemia
Maintain normal serum calcium level	Correct underlying problem High-calcium diet Vitamin D Oral calcium supplements 10% calcium gluconate Phosphate-binding antacids	Correct underlying problem Low-calcium diet Normal saline and diuretics Corticosteroids Calcitonin Mithramycin Etidronate Phosphates

Hypocalcemia

▶ **Priority Nursing Diagnosis:**   Risk for injury related to calcium imbalance: hypocalcemia

OUTCOME CRITERIA

- Serum calcium 4.5-5.5 mg/dl (total 9-11 mg/dl)
- Normal reflex activity
- Normal peripheral sensation and movement
- Patient alert and oriented
- HR   60-100 beats/min
- PR interval 0.12-0.20
- QT interval <½ of R-R interval
- Absence of life-threatening dysrhythmias
- MAP   70-105 mm Hg
- Absence of injury
- Absence of seizure activity
- RR   12-20/min
- Nonlabored respirations
- Absence of laryngeal stridor
- Absence of Trousseau's sign
- Absence of Chvostek's sign

PATIENT MONITORING

1. Continuously monitor ECG for dysrhythmias. Measure serial QT intervals; torsade de pointes is associated with prolonged QT intervals.
2. Monitor BP, since decreased myocardial contractility and hypotension are cardiovascular manifestations associated with hypocalcemia.

PHYSICAL ASSESSMENT

1. Assess for presence of cramps in hands, feet, and legs, and assess for circumoral paresthesia.
2. Assess respiratory rate and depth, work of breathing, and breath sounds at least q4h. Airway obstruction and respiratory arrest can occur. Monitor for stridor, bronchospasm, and laryngospasm.
3. Assess for signs of tetany; numbness and tingling in the fingers, around the mouth, and over the face, which may be followed by spasms of the face and extremities.
4. Assess for Trousseau's sign by inflating a blood pressure cuff above SBP for 2 to 5 minutes and assessing for carpopedal spasm of the hand. A positive test, which results when carpopedal spasm is present, is associated with hypocalcemia.
5. Assess for Chvostek's sign by tapping the facial nerve anterior to the ear and observing for lip and cheek

RENAL

spasms. Spasms indicate a positive test result and are associated with hypocalcemia.

6. Be alert for seizures, since hypocalcemia causes CNS irritability.

7. Assess patients taking digitalis for signs of digitalis toxicity; increasing calcium may cause digitalis toxicity.

DIAGNOSTICS ASSESSMENT

1. Review albumin levels, since hypoalbuminemia is the most common cause of hypocalcemia.

2. Review serial serum calcium levels in conjunction with pH and albumin levels, since alkalosis and hypoalbuminemia decrease calcium ionization. To correct for calcium in the presence of hypoalbuminemia, the following formula can be used: Corrected Ca = total calcium + 0.8 (4 – albumin). In addition, drugs can cause hypocalcemia: aminoglycosides, aluminum-containing antacids, corticosteroids, and loop diuretics.

PATIENT MANAGEMENT

1. Initiate seizure precautions by padding side rails, minimizing stimulation, assisting the patient with all activities, and keeping airway management equipment available. If seizures do occur, protect the patient and be prepared to correct hypocalcemia and administer antiseizure medications if ordered.

2. Have a tracheostomy tray available; be prepared to administer humidified air or oxygen, administer bronchodilators and/or assist with a tracheostomy if bronchospasm and laryngospasm occur.

3. If respiratory arrest occurs, institute emergency respiratory and cardiac support.

4. Administer vitamin D and oral calcium supplements 1 hour after meals and at bedtime to maximize calcium absorption and utilization.

5. Phosphate-binding antacids may be used to reduce phosphate absorption and cause an inverse increase in calcium. Administer antacids before meals.

6. For symptomatic hypocalcemia, administer undiluted 100 to 200 mg elemental calcium over 5 to 10 minutes. Calcium gluconate contains 90 mg of elemental calcium in 10 ml of a 10% solution; calcium chloride contains 272 mg of elemental calcium in 10 ml of a 10% solution. Administer through a central line if one is available since calcium is very irritating to the veins and will cause

tissue damage if it extravasates. Too rapid IV administration of calcium can lead to cardiac arrest. Monitor patients receiving digitalis closely for fatal dysrhythmias.

7. Encourage foods high in calcium (e.g., milk products, meats, and leafy green vegetables).
8. Assist with self-care activities, since the patient may develop poor coordination.
9. Evaluate the patient for hypomagnesemia since magnesium deficiency is often associated with hypocalcemia and impairs the restoration of normal calcium levels.

Hypercalcemia

▶ **Priority Nursing Diagnosis:** Risk for injury related to calcium imbalance: hypercalcemia

OUTCOME CRITERIA

- Serum calcium 4.5-5.5 mg/dl (total 9-11 mg/dl)
- Normal reflex activity
- Normal peripheral sensation and movement
- Patient alert and oriented
- HR   60-100 beats/min
- PR interval 0.12-0.20
- QT interval <½ of R-R interval
- Absence of life-threatening dysrhythmias
- MAP   70-105 mm Hg
- Absence of injury

PATIENT MONITORING

1. Continuously monitor ECG for dysrhythmias. Measure the QT interval.
2. Monitor fluid volume status: measure I & O hourly; hypercalcemia impairs the kidneys to concentrate urine and diuretic therapy will cause urine output to increase. Patients may receive an intake of up to 10 L of fluid a day.

PHYSICAL ASSESSMENT

1. Assess mentation and observe for behavior changes. Patients may be confused or develop psychotic behavior.
2. Assess patients receiving digitalis for signs of digitalis toxicity, since the inotropic effect of digitalis is enhanced by calcium. Digitalis dosage may need to be reduced.
3. Assess GI function: note abdominal distention and absent bowel sounds, anorexia, or N/V, which may suggest paralytic ileus.

DIAGNOSTICS ASSESSMENT

1. Review serial calcium levels to evaluate patient response to therapy.

RENAL

PATIENT MANAGEMENT

1. Anticipate the administration of normal saline to expand ECF volume along with diuretics to increase urinary excretion of calcium. Monitor for signs of fluid volume imbalances. Thiazide diuretics are avoided because they inhibit calcium excretion.

2. Etidronate may be administered intravenously for hypercalcemia associated with malignancy. Generally 7.5 mg/kg is given qd for 3 days.

3. Calcitonin may be required if serum calcium is >15 mg/dl or in patients who cannot tolerate sodium. Administer 3 to 4 U/kg subcutaneously q12 to 24h.

4. Corticosteroids may be initiated if hypercalcemia is associated with some types of granulomatous disorders.

5. Mithramycin may be given in hypercalcemia associated with malignancy. Administer over 4 hours to reduce nausea. Dilute medication to minimize irritation to the veins. Be alert for thrombocytopenia, hepatotoxicity, and nephrotoxicity.

6. Phosphates administered intravenously may be given as a last resort to lower calcium; fatal hypotension and widespread metastatic calcification may occur.

7. If the patient develops heart block, check BP, HR, pulse pressure; be prepared to administer atropine, calcium, and to assist with pacemaker insertion. Be prepared to initiate immediate emergency measures for cardiac arrest.

8. Encourage a diet low in calcium and protein.

9. Encourage mobility as soon as possible, since immobility results in the release of bone calcium; assist with ambulation, since muscle weakness may be present.

10. To prevent the formation of kidney stones, encourage a high fluid intake (avoiding milk products, which are high in calcium), distributed throughout the entire 24-hour period, to a level that maintains urine output of 2500 ml/day. Encourage prune or cranberry juice to maintain acidic urine, since calcium solubility is increased in acidic urine.

11. If the patient develops bone pain or pain from a kidney stone, initiate comfort measures (e.g., positioning, darkened room). Administer pain medications.

ELECTROLYTE IMBALANCE: MAGNESIUM

Clinical Brief

Magnesium imbalances occur as a result of changes in magnesium ion concentrations in extracellular fluid. *Hypomagnesemia* occurs as a result of malabsorption, starvation, hyperalimentation without magnesium, alcoholism, excessive diuretics, GI losses, pancreatitis, pregnancy toxemia, hypocalcemia, and hyperaldosteronism. *Hypermagnesemia* is associated with renal insufficiency, acidosis, adrenal insufficiency, hyperparathyroidism, and increased magnesium intake.

Magnesium is essential for the production of energy (all cellular enzymatic reactions require ATP) and the maintenance of normal intracellular electrolyte composition. Magnesium is critical for the activation of the NA^+/K^+. ATPase pump, which moves potassium into the cell and sodium out of the cell against the concentration gradient. Magnesium is also needed for protein synthesis within the cell and neuromuscular transmission.

Abnormalities in magnesium are often mistaken for potassium imbalances. Magnesium deficiency often makes hypokalemia refractory to treatment. Most significantly, magnesium has a profound effect on cardiac activity, and magnesium deficiency may cause hypertension and coronary artery vaospasm. Magnesium deficiency may contribute to sudden death from nonocclusive ischemic heart disease and increase the risk of myocardial infarction.

Presenting signs and symptoms

See Physical examination

Physical examination

	Hypomagnesemia	Hypermagnesemia
Appearance:	Weak, dizzy, cramping	Lethargic, flushed
VS:	↑ HR, ↑ BP	↓ RR, ↓ HR, ↓ BP
Cardiovascular:	ECG: flat or inverted T waves, prolonged PR or QT interval, dysrhythmias	ECG: peaked T waves, wide QRS; prolonged QT interval, bradycardia, cardiac arrest
Pulmonary:	Stridor, bronchospasm, laryngospasm	Shallow respirations, apnea

RENAL

Text continued on p. 284.

	Hypomagnesemia	Hypermagnesemia
Neurological:	Confusion, altered mental status, tremors, tetany, hyperreflexia, seizures	Altered mental status, hyporeflexia, seizures, muscle paralysis, coma
Gastrointestinal:	Anorexia, nausea	

Diagnostic findings

Hypomagnesemia is defined as a serum magnesium level less than 1.5 mEq/L. *Hypermagnesemia* is a serum magnesium level greater than 2.5 mEq/L. Reduced body stores of magnesium, referred to as magnesium deficiency, may be present with normal magnesium levels.

Acute Care Patient Management

Goals of treatment

	Hypomagnesemia	Hypermagnesemia
Normalize serum magnesium levels	High-magnesium diet Magnesium sulfate	Low-magnesium diet Diuretics Calcium gluconate

Hypomagnesemia

▶ **Priority Nursing Diagnosis:** Risk for injury related to magnesium imbalance: hypomagnesemia

OUTCOME CRITERIA
- Serum magnesium 1.5-2.5 mEq/L
- Normal reflex activity
- Normal peripheral sensation and movement
- HR   60-100 beats/min
- PR interval 0.12-0.20
- QT interval <½ of R-R interval
- T wave rounded
- Absence of life-threatening dysrhythmias
- MAP   70-105 mm Hg
- RR   12-20/min
- Nonlabored respirations
- Absence of laryngeal stridor
- Absence of injury
- Absence of seizure activity

PATIENT MONITORING

1. Continuously monitor ECG for changes in rate and rhythm. Measure PR and QT intervals. Torsade de pointes is associated with prolonged QT intervals. Dysrhythmias may occur: premature ventricular contractions, ventricular tachycardia, and ventricular fibrillation.

PHYSICAL ASSESSMENT

1. Assess mentation, changes in behavior, and ability to swallow.
2. Assess respiratory rate and depth, work of breathing, and breath sounds at least q4h. Monitor for stridor, bronchospasm, and laryngospasm, which can occur during acute hypomagnesemia.
3. Assess for signs of hypocalcemia, which often accompanies hypomagnesemia: muscle weakness, muscle pain, numbness and tingling, positive Trousseau's sign, and positive Chvostek's sign.
4. Assess patients taking digitalis for signs of digitalis toxicity, since hypomagnesemia predisposes the patient to toxicity. Digitalis dosage may need to be adjusted.
5. Be alert for seizures.

DIAGNOSTICS ASSESSMENT

1. Review magnesium levels when available, although serum levels do not reflect total body magnesium stores and thus are poor indicators of magnesium deficiency. Urinary excretion of magnesium or a magnesium load test may be done to further assess magnesium levels.
2. Review potassium levels, since magnesium imbalances are often mistaken for potassium imbalances.
3. Review calcium levels, since hypocalcemia often accompanies hypomagnesemia.

PATIENT MANAGEMENT

1. Encourage foods high in magnesium, such as seafood, green vegetables, bananas, grapefruits, oranges, nuts, and legumes. Diet can correct mild hypomagnesemia.
2. For symptomatic hypomagnesemia, administer intravenous magnesium as ordered. A rapid infusion may result in cardiac or respiratory arrest; 10% magnesium sulfate (1 g/10ml) should be administered no faster than 1.5 ml/min.
   a. Assess renal function before administering magnesium, since magnesium is removed from the body through the kidneys.

RENAL

b. Obtain BP, HR, and respirations every 15 minutes during infusion of large doses of magnesium, since vasodilation, bradycardia, and respiratory depression may occur.

c. Before and during the administration of magnesium, monitor for hypermagnesemia by assessing the patellar (knee-jerk) reflex. If the reflex is absent, stop the magnesium infusion and notify the physician. Hyporeflexia will precede respiratory depression.

d. If hypotension or respiratory depression occurs during magnesium infusion, stop the magnesium infusion, notify the physician, and be prepared to administer calcium and to support cardiac and respiratory functioning.

3. Seizures may result from hypomagnesemia. Initiate seizure precautions by padding side rails, minimizing stimulation, assisting the patient with all activities, and keeping airway management equipment available. If seizures do occur, protect the patient and be prepared to correct hypomagnesemia and administer antiseizure medications if ordered.

4. Have tracheostomy tray available. Be prepared to administer humidified air or oxygen, administer bronchodilators, and/or assist with a tracheostomy if bronchospasm and laryngospasm occur.

5. If dysrhythmia occurs, be prepared to begin treatment to increase the serum magnesium level. Be aware that antidysrhythmic agents and defibrillation are often ineffective in the presence of hypomagnesemia.

6. If respiratory arrest occurs, institute emergency respiratory and cardiac support.

7. Correct the magnesium level before correcting the potassium level, since hypokalemia is difficult to treat in the presence of hypomagnesemia.

8. Because patients with hypomagnesemia often experience muscle weakness, teach the patient methods for conserving energy; provide for rest periods and assist with self-care activities and ambulation.

Hypermagnesemia

▶ **Priority Nursing Diagnosis:** Risk for injury related to magnesium imbalance: hypermagnesemia

OUTCOME CRITERIA

- Serum magnesium 1.5-2.5 mEq/L
- Normal reflex activity

- Normal peripheral sensation and movement
- HR   60-100 beats/min
- PR interval 0.12-0.20
- QT interval <½ of R-R interval
- T wave rounded
- Absence of life-threatening dysrhythmias
- MAP   70-105 mm Hg
- RR   12-20/min
- Nonlabored respirations
- Absence of laryngeal stridor
- Absence of injury

PATIENT MONITORING

1. Continuously monitor the ECG for bradycardia and heart block. Measure PR and QT intervals.
2. Monitor BP for hypotension.

PHYSICAL ASSESSMENT

1. Assess LOC and note lethargy or drowsiness.
2. Assess the respiratory rate and pattern; note shallow respirations or periods of apnea.
3. Monitor patellar (knee-jerk) reflex, since absence of the reflex indicates severe hypermagnesemia that may proceed to respiratory or cardiac arrest.

DIAGNOSTICS ASSESSMENT

1. Review magnesium levels when available.
2. Review potassium levels, since magnesium imbalances are often mistaken for potassium imbalances.
3. Review calcium levels, since hypercalcemia often accompanies hypermagnesemia.

PATIENT MANAGEMENT

1. Restrict food high in magnesium, including seafood, green vegetables, bananas, grapefruits, oranges, nuts, and legumes.
2. Administer normal saline and diuretics as ordered to increase renal excretion of magnesium (if patient has urine output). If the patient is anuric, dialysis may be used.
3. If the patient is symptomatic (e.g., hypotension, shallow respirations, and/or decreased LOC), administer calcium gluconate (5 to 10 ml of 10% solution) as ordered.
4. If dysrhythmia occurs, be prepared to begin treatment to decrease the serum magnesium level and to administer antidysrhythmic agents as ordered.
5. If respiratory or cardiac arrest occurs, institute emergency respiratory and cardiac support.

RENAL

ELECTROLYTE IMBALANCE: PHOSPHORUS
Clinical Brief
Phosphorus imbalances occur as a result of changes in phosphorus ion concentrations in extracellular fluid. Phosphorus concentration in the extracellular fluid is in an inverse relationship with calcium concentration. *Hypophosphatemia* is associated with hyperparathyroidism, excessive diuresis, chronic alcohol abuse, carbohydrate load, hyperalimentation without phosphorus supplementation, respiratory alkalosis secondary to mechanical ventilation, malabsorption syndromes, and chronic use of antacids. *Hyperphosphatemia* occurs with hypoparathyroidism, acute and chronic renal failure, rhabdomyolysis, cytotoxic agents, metabolic acidosis, and excessive phosphate intake.

Presenting signs and symptoms
See Physical examination
Physical examination

	Hypophosphatemia	Hyperphosphatemia
Neuromuscular:	Malaise, muscle pain, muscle weakness, paresthesia, neuroirritability, confusion, tremors, seizures, coma	Fatigue, s/s of tetany
Gastrointestinal:	Anorexia	

Diagnostic findings
Hypophosphatemia is defined as a serum phosphorus level less than 3 mg/dl or 1.8 mEq/L. *Hyperphosphatemia* is a serum phosphorus level greater than 4.5 mg/dl or 2.6 mEq/L.

Acute Care Patient Management
Goals of treatment

	Hypophosphatemia	Hyperphosphatemia
Maintain normal serum phosphorus level	High-phosphorus diet Low-calcium diet Correct hypercalcemia Phosphorus	Low-phosphorus diet High-calcium diet Correct hypocalcemia Phosphate-binding antacids (aluminum hydroxide, aluminum carbonate)

Hypophosphatemia

▶ **Priority Nursing Diagnosis:** Risk for injury related to phosphorus imbalance: hypophosphatemia

OUTCOME CRITERIA

- Serum phosphorus 3-4.5 mg/dl (1.8-2.6 mEq/L)
- Serum calcium 4.5-5.5 mg/dl (total 9-11 mg/dl)
- Normal peripheral sensation and movement
- Absence of injury
- Hgb   12-16 g/dl (females)
              13.5-17.5 g/dl (males)
- Hct   37-47% (females)
              40-54% (males)

PATIENT MONITORING

None specific

PHYSICAL ASSESSMENT

1. Assess peripheral sensation and strength. Muscle weakness, muscle pain, numbness, and tingling often occur in patients with hypophosphatemia.
2. Assess neurological status for changes in mentation, confusion, or decreased LOC.
3. Be alert for development of hemolytic anemia: pallor, dyspnea, weakness, tachycardia, dysrhythmias.

DIAGNOSTICS ASSESSMENT

1. Review serum phosphorus levels in conjunction with calcium levels, since hypophosphatemia is usually associated with hypercalcemia.

PATIENT MANAGEMENT

1. Because patients with hypophosphatemia often experience muscle weakness, teach the patient methods for conserving energy and provide for rest periods.
2. Assist with self-care activities and ambulation.
3. Encourage a diet high in phosphorus by encouraging intake of hard cheeses, meats, fish, nuts, eggs, dried fruits and vegetables, and legumes.
4. When administering oral phosphorus supplements, mix them with ice water to increase palatability. Monitor for diarrhea.
5. Administer intravenous phosphate slowly to avoid rapidly decreasing calcium levels. The usual rate of administration is 20 mM over 4-6 hours. Observe for signs and symptoms of hypocalcemia, including tetany, fatigue, palpitations, hypotension, numbness and tingling, positive Trousseau's sign, and positive Chvostek's sign.

RENAL

6. If hemolytic anemia occurs, be prepared to administer oxygen, fluids, and blood products.

Hyperphosphatemia

▶ **Priority Nursing Diagnosis:** Risk for injury related to phosphorus imbalance: hyperphosphatemia

OUTCOME CRITERIA

- Serum phosphorus 3-4.5 mg/dl (1.8-2.6 mEq/L)
- Serum calcium 4.5-5.5 mg/dl (total 9-11 mg/dl)
- Normal peripheral sensation and movement
- Absence of injury
- Absence of seizure activity

PATIENT MONITORING

None specific

PHYSICAL ASSESSMENT

1. Assess BP to detect hypotension resulting from the hypocalcemia that often accompanies hyperphosphatemia.
2. Observe for signs and symptoms of hypocalcemia, including tetany, fatigue, palpitations, hypotension, numbness and tingling, positive Trousseau's sign, and positive Chvostek's sign, since hypocalcemia often accompanies hyperphosphatemia.
3. Be alert for the development of tremors and seizures.

DIAGNOSTICS ASSESSMENT

1. Review serial serum phosphorus levels in conjunction with calcium levels, since hyperphosphatemia is usually associated with hypocalcemia.

PATIENT MANAGEMENT

1. Restrict food high in phosphorus such as hard cheeses, meats, fish, nuts, eggs, dried fruits and vegetables, and legumes.
2. Because seizures may result from hyperphosphatemia, initiate seizure precautions by padding side rails, minimizing stimulation, assisting the patient with all activities, and keeping airway management equipment available. If seizures do occur, protect the patient and be prepared to correct hyperphosphatemia and hypocalcemia and administer antiseizure medications if ordered.
3. If ordered, administer phosphate-binding antacids (aluminum hydroxide, aluminum carbonate) before meals to reduce absorption of phosphorus.
4. In extreme situations, calcium administration may be required.

ELECTROLYTE IMBALANCE: POTASSIUM

Clinical Brief

Potassium imbalances occur as a result of changes in the concentration of potassium ions in the extracellular fluid. *Hypokalemia* is most frequently caused by losses of GI secretions, diuretic usage, decreased potassium intake, alkalemia, aldosterone excess, and is often associated with magnesium deficiency. *Hyperkalemia* occurs with decreased urine output, increased catabolism, increased potassium intake, acidemia, and hypoaldosteronism.

Presenting signs and symptoms

Signs and symptoms depend on the severity of the imbalance. See Physical examination.

Physical examination

Appearance: Weak, tired

Hypokalemia	Hyperkalemia
Cardiovascular:	
ECG: flat T waves, U waves, ST depression, prolonged QT interval, wide QRS, prolonged PR interval, dysrhythmias	ECG: tall, peaked T waves; prolonged PR interval; flat or absent P waves; prolonged QRS duration; dysrhythmias
Pulmonary: SOB may progress to respiratory arrest	SOB may progress to respiratory arrest
Neuromuscular: hypoactive reflexes, numbness, cramps, weakness, paralysis	Hyperactive reflexes, numbness, tingling, paralysis
Gastrointestinal: GI irritability, distention, ileus	Nausea, cramps, diarrhea

Diagnostic findings

Hypokalemia is defined as serum potassium <3.5 mEq/L; *hyperkalemia* is a serum potassium >5.5 mEq/L.

Acute Care Patient Management

Goals of treatment

	Hypokalemia	Hyperkalemia
Normalize serum potassium level	Treat underlying cause	Treat underlying cause
	High-potassium diet	Low-potassium diet
		Continued.

RENAL

Hypokalemia	Hyperkalemia
Correct alkalosis	Kayexalate with sorbitol
Oral potassium supplements	Hypertonic glucose and insulin
Intravenous potassium	Sodium bicarbonate (if not fluid over-loaded)
	Calcium gluconate
	Correct hypomag-nesemia

Hypokalemia

▶ **Priority Nursing Diagnosis:** Risk for injury related to hypokalemia

OUTCOME CRITERIA
- Serum potassium level 3.5-5.5 mEq/L
- Rounded P and T waves
- PR interval 0.12-0.20 seconds
- QRS duration 0.04-0.10 seconds
- Absence of dysrhythmias
- MAP   70-105 mm Hg
- RR   12-20/min
- Nonlabored respirations
- Deep, symmetrical chest expansion
- Normal reflex activity
- Normal peripheral sensation and movement
- Active bowel sounds
- Absence of injury

PATIENT MONITORING
1. Monitor ECG for changes in complex configuration, waveform, and duration. Flat or inverted T waves, U waves, ST segment depression, prolonged QT interval, wide QRS, and prolonged PR interval may be present. Dysrhythmias such as PVCs, heart blocks, VT, VF, and torsade de pointes may occur.
2. Monitor changes in intake or output that might affect potassium balance. Hypokalemia may occur with osmotic diuresis, renal insufficiency, and GI losses.

PHYSICAL ASSESSMENT
1. Observe for signs of alkalosis (pH >7.45, decreased respiratory rate, tingling, dizziness), since alkalosis shifts potassium into the cells, resulting in hypokalemia.

2. Assess patients on digitalis for signs of digitalis toxicity, since hypokalemia increases sensitivity to digitalis.

3. Assess muscle strength and monitor deep tendon reflex activity, since hypokalemia is associated with muscle weakness and hyporeflexia that may progress to tetany and respiratory arrest.

4. Assess abdomen size, shape, and bowel sounds q4h, since hypokalemia is associated with paralytic ileus.

DIAGNOSTICS ASSESSMENT

1. Review serial potassium levels to evaluate response to therapy and prior to administering diuretics. NOTE: Furosemide, dopamine, catecholamines, and antibiotics such as carbenicillin and gentamicin can cause hypokalemia.

2. Review magnesium levels, since abnormalities in magnesium are often mistaken for potassium imbalances. Hypokalemia that is refractory to treatment is often due to hypomagnesemia.

PATIENT MANAGEMENT

1. Ensure adequate urine output before administering potassium.

2. When administering oral potassium supplements, administer with food or immediately after meals to minimize GI irritation and diarrhea.

3. Ensure patency of the intravenous line before and during potassium administration, since potassium is irritating and potentially damaging to tissues. Dilute intravenous potassium to minimize irritation to the veins. A central line is preferable for potassium infusion. Administer intravenous potassium at a rate not to exceed 20 mEq/100 ml/hr; continuous cardiac monitoring should be employed. Rapid potassium infusions can result in cardiac arrest; potassium should never be given as a bolus. Check the potassium level and be alert for overcorrection of hypokalemia.

4. Evaluate for hypomagnesemia since magnesium deficiency is often associated with hypokalemia and impairs restoration of normal potassium levels.

5. Withhold oral intake and notify the physician if bowel sounds are severely diminished or absent. Otherwise, encourage foods rich in potassium such as apricots, bananas, cantaloupes, dates, raisins, avocados, beans, meats, potatoes, and orange juice.

6. If cardiac dysrhythmias or respiratory distress occurs, institute immediate treatment for hypokalemia while supporting cardiac and respiratory functioning.

RENAL

Hyperkalemia

▶ **Priority Nursing Diagnosis:**   Risk for injury related to hyperkalemia

OUTCOME CRITERIA

- Serum potassium level 3.5-5.5 mEq/L
- Rounded P and T waves
- PR interval 0.12-0.20 seconds
- QRS duration 0.04-0.10 seconds
- Absence of dysrhythmias
- MAP   70-105 mm Hg
- RR   12-20/min
- Nonlabored respirations
- Deep, symmetrical chest expansion
- Normal reflex activity
- Normal peripheral sensation and movement
- Active bowel sounds
- Absence of injury

PATIENT MONITORING

1. Monitor ECG for changes in complex configuration, waveform, and duration; tall peaked T waves and a shortened QT interval occur with potassium >6.5 mEq/L; the PR interval increases and QRS widens with potassium >8.0 mEq/L. Cardiac and renal patients are especially at risk for lethal effects of increased potassium on the electrical conduction system of the heart. Dysrhythmias such as bradycardia, heart blocks, extrasystoles, junctional rhythm, idioventricular rhythm, ventricular tachycardia or fibrillation, sine wave, and asystole can occur.

2. Note changes in I & O that might affect potassium balance. A decrease in renal function, as with acute renal failure, is a risk factor for hyperkalemia.

PHYSICAL ASSESSMENT

1. Observe for signs of acidosis (pH <7.35, increased respiratory rate and depth, confusion, drowsiness, headache), since acidosis shifts potassium out of the cells, resulting in hyperkalemia.

2. Assess muscle strength and monitor deep tendon reflex activity, since hyperkalemia is associated with muscle weakness and hyperreflexia. Numbness, tingling, muscle flaccidity, or paralysis may develop. Respiratory arrest may also occur.

DIAGNOSTICS ASSESSMENT

1. Review serial potassium levels and note the patient's response to therapy. Potassium-sparing diuretics

(spironolactone, triamterene and amiloride), penicillin G, succinylcholine, angiotensin-converting enzyme inhibitors, β-adrenergic blocking agents, salt substitutes as well as hemolyzed blood samples can cause hyperkalemia.

2. Review magnesium levels, since abnormalities in magnesium are often mistaken for potassium imbalances.

3. Review serial ABGs, since metabolic acidosis is associated with hyperkalemia.

PATIENT MANAGEMENT

1. Administer kayexalate with sorbitol orally (15 g l to 4 ×/day) or rectally (30 to 50 g) as ordered to treat mild hyperkalemia (potassium of 5.5 to 6.5 mEq/L). If administered rectally, encourage retention for 30 to 60 minutes for maximum effect. Kayexalate increases potassium excretion in the GI tract and each gram will remove 1 mEq of potassium. If kayexalate is used for several days, monitor for hypocalcemia, hypomagnesemia, and fluid overload (as a result of hypernatremia).

2. Anticipate furosemide and NS infusion to rid the body of excess potassium.

3. Hypertonic glucose (25 g of 50% dextrose) and insulin (10 U regular) for potassium of 6.5 to 7.5 mEq/L may be ordered to temporarily shift potassium into the cells.

4. A bolus of sodium bicarbonate (44 mEq) followed by an infusion (88 to 132 mEq $NaHCO_3$ per liter D_5NS) may be ordered to temporarily shift potassium into the cells. Carefully assess for signs of hypernatremia and fluid volume overload.

5. To antagonize the cardiac suppressoin associated with hyperkalemia, calcium gluconate may be ordered for severe hyperkalemia (potassium of >7.5 mEq/L). If not contraindicated, administer calcium gluconate slowly over 2 to 3 minutes while observing for ECG changes. Stop the infusion if bradycardia occurs.

6. While administering medications to treat hyperkalemia, monitor for correction of hyperkalemia and signs of hypokalemia that might result from overcorrection. Observe closely for returning signs of hyperkalemia 30 minutes after calcium administration and 2 to 3 hours after sodium bicarbonate or insulin with glucose treatment.

7. After emergency treatment of hyperkalemia, consult with the physician regarding follow-up treatment to permanently remove potassium.

RENAL

8. Restrict foods rich in potassium such as apricots, bananas, coffee, cocoa, tea, dried fruits, cantaloupes, avocados, beans, meats, potatoes, and orange juice.

ELECTROLYTE IMBALANCE: SODIUM

Clinical Brief

Sodium imbalances occur as a result of changes in soidum ion concentrations in extracellular fluid. *Hyponatremia* is a deficiency of sodium relative to water and can occur from (1) excess water, as with excessive water intake or syndrome of inappropriate antidiuretic hormone release (SIADH); (2) sodium depletion, as with GI losses, diaphoresis, diuretics, renal excretion of sodium, and adrenal insufficiency; and (3) combined water and sodium retention, as with heart failure, cirrhosis, or nephrotic syndrome. *Hypernatremia* is an excess of sodium relative to water and can occur from water depletion, as with diuretics, decreased intake, GI losses, hyperglycemia, diabetes insipidus; and sodium excess, as with large sodium intake (rare).

Sodium concentration is largely responsible for determining plasma osmolality. Symptoms associated with sodium imbalances are largely determined by the patient's volume status.

Presenting signs and symptoms

Signs and symptoms include complaints associated with dehydration or fluid retention. Patients with *hyponatremia* can have dehydration (circulatory insufficiency) or overhydration (fluid overload, pulmonary edema). Patients with *hypernatremia* usually have an ECF volume deficit (dehydration).

Physical examination

Dehydration (hyponatremia or hypernatremia)

Appearance: Fatigued, lethargic, loss of skin turgor, dry mucous membranes; with hypernatremia, flushed skin

Vital signs:

HR tachycardia

BP ↓ or orthostatic BP

Temperature elevated

Cardiovascular: Weak peripheral pulses, flat neck veins

Neurological: Confused, decreased mentation; irritability, twitching, and seizures (associated with sodium imbalances)

Genitourinary: Decreased urine output

Gastrointestinal: Abdominal cramps and nausea (hyponatremia)

Overhydration (hyponatremia or hypernatremia)
Appearance: Malaise, edema, flushed skin (hypernatremia)
Vital signs:
BP, increased
Cardiovascular: ↑ CO—bounding pulses, hypertension *or*
↓ CO— weak pulses, S_3, JVD
Pulmonary: Crackles, dyspnea
Neurological: Headache, confusion; irritability, twitching,
and seizures (associated with sodium imbalances)
Gastrointestinal: Abdominal cramps and nausea (hyponatremia)
Diagnostic findings
Hyponatremia is defined as a serum sodium of <135 mEq/L;
hypernatremia is a serum sodium of >145 mEq/L.

Acute Care Patient Management
Goals of treatment

	Hyponatremia	Hypernatremia
Maintain normal serum sodium and osmolality level	Correct underlying problem High sodium intake 3% saline 0.45 NS or 0.9 NS	Correct underlying problem Low sodium intake
Normalize fluid status and serum osmolality	Correct underlying problem If volume deficit: Fluids If volume excess: Restrict fluids Diuretics	Correct underlying problem If volume deficit: Fluids without salt If volume excess: Restrict fluids Diuretics

▶ **Priority Nursing Diagnoses**
Fluid volume deficit
Fluid volume excess
Risk for injury: neurological dysfunction
▶ **Nursing Diagnosis:** Fluid volume deficit related to
hypernatremia (hypertonic dehydration) or hyponatremia
(hypotonic dehydration) associated with decreased fluid
intake, GI losses, diaphoresis, diuretics, diabetes insipidus,
increased renal excretion of sodium, or adrenal insufficiency
OUTCOME CRITERIA
• Patient will be alert and oriented
• Serum sodium 135-145 mEq/L

RENAL

- Serum osmolality 275-295 mOsm/L
- MAP   70-105 mm Hg
- SBP   90-140 mm Hg
- Urine output 30 ml/hr or 0.5-1 ml/kg/hr
- CVP   2-6 mm Hg

PATIENT MONITORING

1. Monitor fluid volume status: obtain hourly I & O; include gastric and diarrheal fluid and diaphoresis in output when calculating fluid balance. Compare serial weights; a rapid decrease in weight (0.5 to 1 kg/day) suggests fluid volume loss.
2. Monitor BP, HR, and PA pressures (if available) to evaluate fluid volume status. An orthostatic BP suggests hypovolemia. Monitor MAP; a MAP <70 mm Hg adversely affects renal and cerebral perfusion.

PHYSICAL ASSESSMENT

1. Assess hydration state: note poor skin turgor on inner thigh or forehead, dry buccal membranes, flat neck veins, complaints of thirst, and decreased sensorium, which may signal volume depletion.
2. Assess for the development of hypovolemic shock: decreased weight, O > I, decreased mentation, SBP <90 mm Hg, urine output <0.5 ml/kg/hr, weak pulses, cool and clammy skin.

DIAGNOSTICS ASSESSMENT

1. Review serial serum sodium, serum osmolality, urine osmolality, and specific gravity to assess fluid volume status. Sodium <135 mEq/L, specific gravity <1.010, and serum osmolality <285 suggest overhydration; sodium >145 mEq/L, specific gravity >1.020 and serum osmolality >295 suggest dehydration.

PATIENT MANAGEMENT

1. Adjust oral intake of sodium as indicated by the serum sodium level. For a patient with *hyponatremia,* encourage fluids high in sodium, such as chicken or beef broths and canned tomato juice. For a patient with *hypernatremia,* encourage fluids low in sodium, such as distilled water, coffee, tea, and orange juice. Assist the patient with hypernatremia to avoid foods high in sodium.
2. Administer fluids and electrolytes as ordered. LR or 0.9 NS may be ordered for patients with hypovolemic hyponatremia. Patients should be carefully monitored for possible fluid overload as ECF volume is replaced.

3. Keep the patient supine until volume has been replaced. Assist the patient with position changes or ambulation, since orthostatic changes may occur while the patient is volume depleted.

► **Nursing Diagnosis:** Fluid volume excess related to hypernatremia or hyponatremia (excess fluid intake, heart failure, cirrhosis, or nephrotic syndrome)

OUTCOME CRITERIA
- Patient will be alert and oriented
- Serum sodium 135-145 mEq/L
- Serum osmolality 275-295 mOsm/L
- MAP   70-105 mm Hg
- SBP   90-140 mm Hg
- Lungs clear to auscultation
- CVP   2-6 mm Hg
- Intake approximates output

PATIENT MONITORING
1. Monitor fluid volume status: obtain hourly I & O; calculate fluid balance q8h. Compare serial weights; a rapid increase in weight (0.5 to 1 kg/day) suggests fluid volume retention.
2. Monitor BP, HR, and PA pressures (if available) to evaluate fluid volume status.

PHYSICAL ASSESSMENT
1. Assess fluid volume status; note the onset of S_3 and crackles, presence of edema, cough, or frothy sputum, increased work of breathing, decreased peripheral perfusion, and increased JVP to determine development of heart failure or pulmonary edema.
2. Assess for headache, blurred vision, and altered mentation and note pupil size and reaction, speech, motor strength, and tremors to determine development of cerebral edema. Neurological dysfunction is a major concern with hypernatremia.

DIAGNOSTICS ASSESSMENT
1. Review serial serum sodium, serum osmolality, urine osmolality, and specific gravity to assess fluid volume status. Sodium <135 mEq/L, specific gravity <1.010, and serum osmolality <285 suggest overhydration; sodium >145 mEq/L, specific gravity >1.020 and serum osmolality >295 suggest dehydration.

RENAL

PATIENT MANAGMENT

1. If *hypervolemic with hyponatremia,* anticipate salt and fluid restrictions. Concentrate medications when possible to minimize fluid intake.
2. If *hypervolemic with hypernatremia,* anticipate hypotonic fluids.
3. Administer diuretics as ordered to rid the body of excess fluid. Be alert for rapid diuresis and signs of volume depletion; check VS and potassium level.

▶ **Nursing Diagnosis:** Risk for injury: neurological dysfunction related to hypernatremia or hyponatremia

OUTCOME CRITERIA

- Patient will be alert and oriented
- Absence of neurological deficits
- Serum sodium 135-145 mEq/L

PATIENT MONITORING

None specific

PHYSICAL ASSESSMENT

1. Assess neurological status: note any change in mental status, presence of neuromuscular irritability, headache, blurred vision, focal neurological deficits, or seizure activity. Note pupil size and reaction, speech, motor strength, and presence of tremors to determine development of cerebral edema. Neurological dysfunction is a major concern with hypernatremia.

DIAGNOSTICS ASSESSMENT

1. Review serial serum sodium levels. Neurological signs generally manifest at sodium levels <125 mEq/L and become more severe at levels <115 mEq/L.

PATIENT MANAGEMENT

1. Primary problems (e.g., DI, SIADH, or AI) should be treated.
2. If the patient is *hyponatremic,* volume depleted, and asymptomatic, NS may be administered. If symptomatic hyponatremic develops, hypertonic saline (3% NaCl) in conjunction with diuretics may be administered. Generally sodium levels should be corrected no faster than 1 mEq/L/hr to 120 mEq/L or until symptoms subside.
3. If patient is *hypernatremic,* anticipate hypotonic solutions to gradually lower serum sodium. Rapid lowering of sodium can result in cerebral edema; carefully monitor neurological status.

ACQUIRED IMMUNODEFICIENCY SYNDROME (AIDS)

Clinical Brief

AIDS is caused by a retrovirus, human immunovirus (HIV), which infects and destroys T-helper lymphocytes (CD4 cells) and impairs the immune system. The blood-borne infection is transmitted in three ways: sexually, through transfer of infected blood, and from mother to infant. HIV disease has a wide clinical spectrum that ranges from no symptoms to complications associated with profound immunosuppression (AIDS).

Staging of HIV infection is done through CD4 counts. AIDS is defined as a CD4 count less than 200 cells/mm^3 plus an AIDS defining diagnosis. Patients with HIV infection admitted to ICU usually have pulmonary or central nervous system infections and sepsis.

Presenting signs and symptoms

Signs and symptoms vary, depending on the stage of illness and the presence of an opportunistic infection.

Physical examination

Skin: Purplish lesions (Kaposi's sarcoma)

Neurological: Irritability, depression, personality changes to coma; weakness to paralysis; seizures (CNS involvement)

Pulmonary: Dyspnea, dry, nonproductive cough (*Pneumocystis carinii*)

Gastrointestinal: Watery diarrhea

Diagnostic findings

Positive result to Western blot test

Polymerase chain reaction (PCR)

Acute Care Patient Management

Goals of treatment

Minimize further immune system damage

    Antiviral agents: zidovudine, dideoxyinosine (ddI), dideoxycytidine (ddC)

Treat opportunistic infections

    Pneumocystis carinii

        Antiprotozoal agents:

        Sulfamethoxazole

MULTI

    Pentamidine isethionate
    Dapsone, and trimethoprim
    Corticosteroids
  Kaposi's sarcoma
    Interferon alfa-2A
    Vinblastine, vincristine
  Toxoplasmosis
    Pyrimethamine, sulfadiazine, folinic acid
    Clindamycin, Leucovorin
  Herpes
    Acyclovir, vidarabine, foscarnet
  Cytomegalovirus
    Ganciclovir
    Foscarnet
    Acyclovir
  Cryptococcus
    Amphotericin B
    Flucytosine, fluconazole
    Ketoconazole
  Candida
    Fluconazole
    Amphotericin B
    Ketoconazole
  Mycobacterium tuberculosis
    Isoniazid, ethambutol, rifampin, pyrazinamid
Detect/prevent clinical sequelae
  See Table 2-49

▶ **Priority Nursing Diagnoses**
Impaired gas exchange
Altered protection
Fluid volume deficit
Altered nutrition: less than body requirements
(see p. 41)
Risk for altered family process (see p. 29)

▶ **Nursing Diagnosis:** Impaired gas exchange related to infectious processes impairing oxygen diffusion and decreasing lung compliance
OUTCOME CRITERIA
- Patient will be alert and oriented
- Pao_2 80-100 mm Hg
- pH   7.35-7.45
- $Paco_2$ 35-45 mm Hg
- O_2 sat   ≥95%
- RR   12-20, eupnea

TABLE 2-49 Clinical Sequelae Associated with HIV

Complication	Signs and symptoms
Respiratory failure	Restlessness, tachypneic, PaO_2 <50 mm Hg, $PaCO_2$ >50 mm Hg, pH <7.35
Septic shock	SBP <90 mm Hg, HR >90 beats/min, RR >20/min or $PaCO_2$ <32 mm Hg, PaO_2/FIO_2 <280, T >38° C or <36° C, WBC >12,000 or <4000 or >10% neutrophils; altered mental status, urine output <0.5 ml/kg/hr, plasma lactate >2 mmol/L
DIC	Bleeding from any orifice and mucous membranes; cool, clammy skin; abnormal clotting studies, D-dimer >2; FDP 1:40
AIDS dementia complex	Forgetfulness, personality changes, clumsiness, ataxia, weak or paralyzed extremities, aphasia
Meningitis	Nuchal rigidity, headache, fever, lethargy, confusion, seizures
Lymphoma (CNS)	Symptoms depend on tumor site, paresthesia, visual loss, ataxia, paresis, seizures
CMV retinitis	Progressive visual loss
Peripheral nervous system disease	Ascending paralysis, burning pain in feet, absent achilles tendon reflex, hypersensitivity, decreased sensation, muscle weakness

- Lungs clear to auscultation
- Minute ventilation <10 L/min
- Vital capacity 15 ml/kg
- Lung compliance 60-100 ml/cm H_2O

PATIENT MONITORING

1. Continuously monitor oxygenation status with pulse oximetry (SpO_2). Be alert for effects of interventions and patient activities, which may adversely affect oxygen saturation.
2. Monitor serial lung compliance values to assess progression of lung stiffness.

MULTI

3. Monitor pulmonary function by assessing minute ventilation and vital capacity measurements. A vital capacity of >15 ml/kg is generally needed for spontaneous breathing.

PHYSICAL ASSESSMENT

1. Assess respiratory status: RR >30/min suggests respiratory distress. Note the use of accessory muscles and the respiratory pattern. Note the presence of breath sounds and adventitious sounds suggesting worsening pulmonary congestion.
2. Assess for signs and symptoms of hypoxemia: increased restlessness, increased complaints of dyspnea, changes in LOC. Cyanosis is a late sign.
3. Assess the patient for development of clinical sequelae. (See Table 2-49.)

DIAGNOSTICS ASSESSMENT

1. Review ABGs for decreasing trends in PaO_2 (hypoxemia) or pH (acidosis). O_2 sat should be ≥95%.
2. Review serial chest radiographs to evaluate patient progress or worsening lung condition.
3. Review culture reports for identification of the infecting organism.

PATIENT MANAGEMENT

1. Provide supplemental oxygen as ordered. If the patient develops respiratory distress, be prepared for intubation and mechanical ventilation. (See p. 577 for information on mechanical ventilation.)
2. Promote pulmonary hygiene with chest physiotherapy and postural drainage if necessary. C & DB the patient and reposition the patient at least q2h. Encourage incentive spirometry to decrease risk of atelectasis. Suction secretions prn and note the color and consistency of sputum. Position the patient for maximum chest excursion.
3. Minimize oxygen demand by decreasing anxiety, fever, and pain.
4. Administer chemotherapeutic agents as ordered. Be alert for further decreases in WBC, RBC, platelets, and fluid and electrolyte imbalance. Orthostatic hypotension can occur with parenteral pentamidine administration.
5. Steroids may be administered to decrease the interstitial inflammatory response.

▶ **Nursing Diagnosis:** Altered protection related to immune dysfunction, chemotherapeutic agents, and central nervous system involvement

OUTCOME CRITERIA
- Absence of injury
- Absence of aspiration
- Absence of additional infections
- T 36.5° C (97.7° F)-37.8° C (100° F)
- Urine output 30 ml/hr or 0.5-1 ml/kg/hr
- BUN 10-20 mg/dl
- Creatinine 0.6-1.2 mg/dl
- WBCs 5-10 × 10³/µl
- RBCs 4.2-6.2 × 10⁶/µl
- Platelets >150 × 10³/µl

PATIENT MONITORING
1. Monitor urine output hourly and note a decreasing trend, which may suggest renal insufficiency.
2. Monitor temperature to evaluate patient's condition and response to therapy.

PHYSICAL ASSESSMENT
1. Assess for fever, chills, and night sweats. Be alert to signs of sepsis and septic shock.
2. Assess neurological status: a decreased sensorium decreases protective reflexes and increases the risk for aspiration. Changes in LOC, cognition, or personality, the onset of numbness/tingling, weakness of extremities, uncoordination, paralysis, or visual loss may indicate CNS infection or side effects of chemotherapeutic agents. Nuchal rigidity may indicate meningitis.
3. Assess for signs and symptoms of infection: redness, tenderness, drainage at IV sites; cloudy urine; purulent sputum; white patches on oral mucosa.
4. Assess for bleeding: test urine and stool; note gingival bleeding or oozing of blood from IV sites; note any petechiae.
5. Inspect skin for new lesions, rashes, or breaks in skin.
6. Assess the patient for clinical sequelae. (See Table 2-49.)

DIAGNOSTICS ASSESSMENT
1. Review CD4 counts to evaluate immune status.
2. Review serial WBC counts and cultures to evaluate course of infection.
3. Review serial Hgb, Hct, and platelets to evaluate anemia and extent of thrombocytopenia.
4. Review serial BUN and creatinine levels to evaluate renal function.

MULTI

PATIENT MANAGEMENT

1. Provide oral hygiene before and after meals to treat stomatitis associated with chemotherapy. Apply lip balm to prevent cracks and crustations.
2. Provide meticulous body hygiene, especially after diarrheal episodes to prevent spread of organisms from stool. Use of A & D ointment or zinc oxide may prevent skin excoriation around the anorectal area.
3. Turn and reposition the patient at least q2h and provide ROM and skin care to improve circulation and prevent skin breakdown. A therapeutic bed may be required.
4. Encourage fluids to maintain hydration and minimize nephrotoxic effects of drugs.
5. Keep HOB elevated or the patient in a side-lying position to prevent aspiration if the level of consciousness is decreased and/or the patient is receiving enteral feedings. Keep suction equipment available.
6. Ensure a safe environment: bed in low position, call bell in reach, soft restraints if indicated.
7. Institute seizure precautions as necessary.
8. Institute bleeding precautions if the patient is thrombocytopenic.
9. Assist the patient with activities to prevent falls.
10. Hematest body fluids for occult blood. Spontaneous bleeding (e.g., hemoptysis, hematuria) may indicate DIC.
11. Orient the patient as needed.

▶ **Nursing Diagnosis:** Fluid volume deficit related to severe diarrhea, vomiting, poor oral intake, intestinal malabsorption, and night sweats

OUTCOME CRITERIA

- Moist mucous membranes
- Elastic skin turgor
- T 36.5° C (97.7° F) to 37.8° C (100° F)
- Intake approximates output
- Urine specific gravity 1.001-1.035
- Serum osmolality 275-295 mOsm/kg
- SBP   90-140 mm Hg
- MAP   70-105 mm Hg

PATIENT MONITORING

1. Continuously monitor CVP and PA pressures (if available) to evaluate trends. Decreasing trends suggest hypovolemia.
2. Monitor MAP; a value <60 mm Hg adversely affects renal and cerebral perfusion.

3. Monitor fluid status: calculate hourly I & O to determine fluid balance. Compare daily weights; a loss of 0.25 to 0.5 kg/day reflects excess fluid loss. Include an accurate stool count, since patients may exceed 10 L of fluid per day with watery diarrhea.
4. Measure urine specific gravity to evaluate hydration status. Increased values reflect dehydration or hypovolemia.

PHYSICAL ASSESSMENT

1. Obtain BP and HR q1h to evaluate the patient's fluid volume status: HR >120 and SBP <90 mm Hg suggest hypovolemia; orthostatic hypotension reflects hypovolemia.
2. Evaluate mucous membranes by checking the area where the cheek and gum meet; dry, sticky membranes are associated with hypovolemia. Test skin turgor on the sternum or the inner aspects of thighs for best assessment.
3. Assess the patient for clinical sequelae. (See Table 2-49.)

DIAGNOSTICS ASSESSMENT

1. Review stool cultures for identification of any infectious agent.
2. Review serial electrolytes, since diarrhea and vomiting can result in a severe electrolyte imbalance.
3. Review serial serum osmolality to evaluate hydration status; increased values are associated with dehydration/hypovolemia.

PATIENT MANAGEMENT

1. Administer fluids as ordered, carefully monitoring for fluid overload.
2. Administer antidiarrheal agents as ordered to help control diarrhea.
3. Administer antiemetic agents as ordered to help control vomiting and increase the patient's ability to take oral food and fluids. Anticipate administration of nutritional supplementation either parenterally or enterally. Consult with a nutritionist to assess the patient's needs.
4. Administer antipyretics as ordered to control temperature.
5. Provide small portions of food more frequently. Include high-caloric, high-protein snacks. Avoid spicy or greasy foods. Cold entrees may be more palatable.
6. Low-fiber, lactulose-free, or pectin-containing formulas may help reduce diarrheal episodes.

MULTI

ANAPHYLACTIC SHOCK

Clinical Brief

Drugs, blood, and blood products can cause anaphylactic reactions. In addition, insect bites and vaccines can also produce this respiratory and circulatory emergency. A stimulus triggers a release of biochemical mediators, which causes a change in vascular permeability, leading to fluid accumulation in the interstitial spaces and a decreased circulating volume. Increased bronchial reactivity produces bronchial edema and bronchoconstriction, causing alveolar hypoventilation and respiratory distress.

Presenting signs and symptoms

Signs and symptoms include itching, chest tightness, difficulty breathing, and a feeling of impending doom.

Appearance: restless, anxious

Vital signs:

> BP normal to hypotensive
>
> HR >100 beats/min
>
> RR tachypnea

Physical examination

Neurological: Anxious progressing to unresponsive

Cardiovascular: Tachycardia with ectopic beats

Pulmonary: Stridor, wheezes, crackles

Skin: Erythema, urticaria, flushing, angioedema

Diagnostic findings

Clinical manifestations are the basis for diagnosis.

Acute Care Patient Management

Goals of treatment

Remove cause if possible

Maintain airway

> Oxygen, intubation/mechanical ventilation
>
> Aminophylline
>
> Epinephrine
>
> Diphenhydramine
>
> Inhaled Beta$_2$ adrenergic agonists

Optimize oxygen delivery

> Colloids (albumin)
>
> Epinephrine
>
> Vasopressors: dopamine, norepinephrine

▶ **Priority Nursing Diagnoses**

Impaired gas exchange

Altered tissue perfusion
Altered protection (see p. 33)
Risk for altered family process (see p. 29)

▶ **Nursing Diagnosis:** Impaired gas exchange related to bronchoconstriction, pulmonary edema, or obstructed airway

OUTCOME CRITERIA
- Patient will be alert and oriented
- PaO_2 80-100 mm Hg
- pH   7.35-7.45
- $PaCO_2$ 35-45 mm Hg
- O_2 sat   ≥95%
- Lungs clear to auscultation
- RR   12-20/min, eupnea

PATIENT MONITORING
1. Continuously monitor oxygenation status via pulse oximetry (SpO_2).

PHYSICAL ASSESSMENT
1. Obtain VS q15min during the acute phase.
2. Assess for hoarseness, stridor, and upper airway obstruction. Late phase reactions may occur 6 to 12 hours after the initial event.
3. Assess lung sounds and respiratory rate and depth to evaluate the degree of respiratory distress. Decreased air movement indicates severe respiratory distress.
4. Assess for signs and symptoms of hypoxemia: increased restlessness, increased complaints of dyspnea, changes in LOC. Cyanosis is a late sign.

DIAGNOSTICS ASSESSMENT
1. Review ABGs to evaluate hypoxemia and acid-base status. Hypoxemia and acidosis are risk factors for dysrhythmias. O_2 sat should be ≥95%.

PATIENT MANAGEMENT
1. Establish/maintain an airway and provide supplemental oxygen. Endotracheal intubation or tracheostomy may be required.
2. Racemic epinephrine may be prescribed via nebulizer (0.3 ml racemic epinephrine in 3 ml NS) for laryngeal edema.
3. Epinephrine 1 to 5 ml of 1:10,000 solution (0.1 to 0.5 mg) may be prescribed to reverse bronchoconstriction and hypotension. May be administered via ET tube if unable to establish IV access.
4. Corticosteroids may be administered to decrease or control edema.

MULTI

5. Aminophylline infusion may be ordered to relieve bronchoconstriction. Assess lungs for air movement and resolution of wheezes.

6. Metaproterenol 0.2 to 0.3 ml (5% solution) in 2.5 ml NS may be administered via nebulizer, or ipratropium bromide (36 μg inhaled) may be used for persistent bronchospasm.

7. Diphenhydramine (benadryl) may be used to reduce the effects of histamine. Usual dose is 25 to 50 mg IV.

8. Position the patient for maximum chest excursion.

9. Administer CPR and follow the ACLS protocol should cardiopulmonary arrest occur.

▶ **Nursing Diagnosis:** Altered tissue perfusion related to decreased circulating volume associated with permeability changes and loss of vasomotor tone

OUTCOME CRITERIA
- Patient will be alert and oriented
- Skin warm and dry
- Peripheral pulses strong
- Urine output 30 ml/hr or 0.5-1 ml/kg/hr
- Absence of edema
- SBP   90-140 mm Hg
- MAP   70-105 mm Hg
- O_2 sat   ≥95%

PATIENT MONITORING

1. Monitor BP continuously via arterial cannulation, if possible. Monitor MAP, an indicator that accurately reflects tissue perfusion. MAP <60 mm Hg adversely affects cerebral and renal perfusion.

2. Continuously monitor ECG to detect life-threatening dysrhythmias or HR >140 beats/min, which can adversely affect stroke volume.

3. Continuously monitor oxygenation status via pulse oximetry (SpO_2).

4. Monitor hourly urine output to evaluate renal perfusion.

5. Monitor PA pressures and CVP (if available) hourly or more frequently to evaluate the patient's response to treatment. Both parameters reflect the capacity of the vascular system to accept volume and can be used to monitor for fluid overload and pulmonary edema.

PHYSICAL ASSESSMENT

1. Obtain HR, RR, BP q15min to evaluate patient response to therapies and detect cardiopulmonary deterioration.

2. Assess mentation, skin temperature, and peripheral pulses to evaluate CO and state of vasoconstriction.
3. Assess periorbital area, lips, hands, feet, and genitalia to evaluate interstitial fluid accumulation.

DIAGNOSTICS ASSESSMENT
1. Review lactate levels, an indicator of anaerobic metabolism. Increased levels may signal decreasing oxygen delivery.
2. Review ABGs for hypoxemia and acidosis, since these conditions can precipitate dysrhythmias and affect myocardial contractility.
3. Review BUN, creatinine, and electrolytes and note trends to evaluate renal function.

PATIENT MANAGEMENT
1. Administer colloids (albumin) or crystalloids (LR) as ordered to restore intravascular volume.
2. An infusion of epinephrine (2 to 4 µg/min) or norepinephrine (4 to 8 µg/min) may be required.
3. Dopamine may also be tried to improve blood pressure.
4. Provide oxygen therapy as ordered. Anticipate intubation and mechanical ventilation if the oxygenation status deteriorates or cardiopulmonary arrest ensues. See p. 577 for information on mechanical ventilation.

BURNS

Clinical Brief
Thermal, electrical, or chemical media are common causes of burns. The severity of the burn is determined by the percentage or extent of the burn wound size and the depth of the burn wound. In addition to burn depth and percentage, the patient's age, medical history, and cause and location of the burn are investigated. Burn depth is described as superficial, partial-thickness, deep partial-thickness, or full thickness. Thermal burns can also be classified into concentric zones of injury. Hyperemia is the outermost zone and is the least damaged; stasis is the middle zone in which tissue perfusion is compromised; the innermost zone is coagulation, where cellular death occurs. In full thickness burns, the zone of coagulation involves the entire thickness of the dermis.

Presenting signs and symptoms
Superficial: skin is red, blanches, and is painful (e.g., sunburn).
Partial-thickness: pink or mottled, red, blisters; wound is painful.

Deep partial-thickness: pale, mottled, pearly white; dry, painful.

Full thickness: involves all layers of the skin and subcutaneous tissue; the wound varies from waxy white or charred to red or brown and leathery; the area is insensitive to pain, although surrounding areas may be painful. Injury may involve muscles, tendons, or bones.

Inhalation injury: chest tightness, hoarseness, dyspnea, tachypnea.

Physical examination

Skin: area of body burned (Figure 2-2, Table 2-50) depth of burn

Burns of head/neck/face/chest/mouth/nose/pharynx correlate with inhalation injury

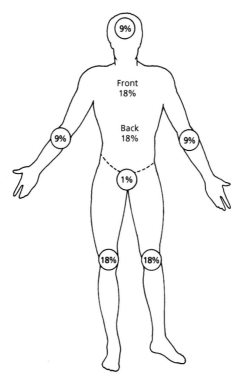

Figure 2-2   Rule of nines.

TABLE 2-50   Berkow Formula for Calculating
% BSA Burns

Area	Years					
	0-1	2-4	5-9	10-14	15	>15
Head	19	17	13	11	9	7
Neck	2	2	2	2	2	2
Ant. trunk	13	13	13	13	13	13
Post. trunk	13	13	13	13	13	13
R buttock	2.5	2.5	2.5	2.5	2.5	2.5
L buttock	2.5	2.5	2.5	2.5	2.5	2.5
Genitalia	1	1	1	1	1	1
R U arm	4	4	4	4	4	4
L U arm	4	4	4	4	4	4
R L arm	3	3	3	3	3	3
L L arm	3	3	3	3	3	3
R hand	2.5	2.5	2.5	2.5	2.5	2.5
L hand	2.5	2.5	2.5	2.5	2.5	2.5
R thigh	5.5	6.5	8	8.5	9	9.5
L thigh	5.5	6.5	8	8.5	9	9.5
R leg	5	5	5.5	6	6.5	7
L leg	5	5	5.5	6	6.5	7
R foot	3.5	3.5	3.5	3.5	3.5	3.5
L foot	3.5	3.5	3.5	3.5	3.5	3.5

Hallmark of smoke inhalation: hypercapnea, hypoxemia,
widened alveolar-arterial oxygen gradient, and increased
carboxyhemoglobin levels. Stridor, crackles, and carbonaceous sputum may be present. Charred eyebrows, eye-
lashes, nasal hair, and facial hair may also be present.

Diagnostic findings
Other findings may include the following:
SBP <90 mm Hg and HR >120 beats/min if shock is present

Acute Care Patient Management
Goals of treatment
Maintain airway and oxygenation
    Supplemental oxygen
    Intubation/mechanical ventilation
Restore intravascular volume
    Crystalloids, colloids

MULTI

TABLE 2-51 Clinical Sequelae Associated with Burns

Complication	Signs and symptoms
Burn shock (hypovolemic)	SBP <90 mm Hg, HR >100 beats/min, urine output <5 ml/kg/hr, cool, clammy skin
Renal failure	Urine output <5 ml/kg/hr, steady rise in BUN, creatinine
Respiratory distress	Carbon flecks in sputum, carbon monoxide levels >15%, RR >30/min, PaO_2 <60 mm Hg, stridor, noisy respirations, restlessness, change in LOC
Loss of limb	Pulselessness, pain, paresthesia, paralysis
Burn wound sepsis	Purulent exudate; focal black, grey, or dark brown discoloration; hemorrhagic discoloration and vascular thrombosis of underlying fat; erythema or edema of unburned skin at the wound margins; unexpected rapid eschar separation; greater than 100,000 organism-per-gram tissue
Curling's ulcer	Blood in emesis, NG aspirate, or stool; decreasing trend in Hgb and Hct
Septic shock	SBP <90 mm Hg, HR >90 beats/min, RR >20/min or $PaCO_2$ <32 mm Hg, PaO_2/FIO_2 <280, T >38° C or <36° C, WBC >12,000 or <4000 or >10% neutrophils; altered mental status, urine output <0.5 ml/kg/hr, plasma lactate >2 mmol/L

Control pain
  Morphine sulfate
Maximize wound closure
  Topical antimicrobials, wound management
Detect/prevent clinical sequelae
  See Table 2-51
▶ **Priority Nursing Diagnoses**
Impaired gas exchange
Fluid volume deficit
Altered tissue perfusion
Pain
Risk for infection

Altered nutrition: less than body requirements
(see p. 41)
Altered protection (see p. 33)
Risk for altered family process (see p. 29)

▶ **Nursing Diagnosis:** Impaired gas exchange related to inhalation injury: carbon monoxide poisoning, chemical pneumonitis, and upper airway obstruction

OUTCOME CRITERIA
- Patient will be alert and oriented
- Pao_2 80-100 mm Hg
- $Paco_2$ 35-45 mm Hg
- pH   7.35-7.45
- O_2 sat   ≥95%
- Lungs clear to auscultation
- RR   12-20/min, eupnea

PATIENT MONITORING
1. Continuously monitor oxygenation status with pulse oximetry (Spo_2). Be alert for effects of interventions and patient activities that may adversely affect oxygen saturation.
2. Calculate $P(a/A)o_2$ ratio to estimate intrapulmonary shunting and evaluate degree of lung dysfunction. The higher the ratio, the better the lung function.

PHYSICAL ASSESSMENT
1. Obtain BP, HR, RR q15min during the acute phase. Patients with carbon monoxide poisoning are tachycardic and tachypneic.
2. Assess for headache, confusion, n/v, and dyspnea. Note skin and mucous membranes—cherry red color reflects carbon monoxide poisoning. As the carbon monoxide level increases, the patient will become less responsive.
3. Assess the rate and depth of respirations; note stridor or noisy respirations that may indicate respiratory distress. Laryngeal edema can develop over 72 hours after the burn event. In patients with burns of the chest, carefully assess chest excursion, since burns to this area may result in hypoventilation and decreased compliance.
4. Note the presence of carbonaceous sputum, an indicator of inhalation injury.
5. Assess for signs and symptoms of hypoxia: increased rest-lessness, increased complaints of dyspnea, changes in LOC.
6. Assess the patient for development of clinical sequelae. (See Table 2-51.)

MULTI

DIAGNOSTICS ASSESSMENT

1. Review carboxyhemoglobin levels for carbon monoxide reflecting smoke inhalation (normal is <5% saturation of Hgb in nonsmokers; <10% in smokers).
2. Review ABGs for decreasing trends in PaO_2 (hypoxemia) or pH (acidosis). O_2 sat should be ≥95%.
3. Review serial chest radiographs to evaluate the patient's progress or a worsening lung condition.
4. Review Hgb and Hct levels and note trends. Decreased RBCs can adversely affect oxygen-carrying capacity.

PATIENT MANAGEMENT

1. Maintain oral airway and administer supplemental oxygen as ordered. FIO_2 of 1 is used to treat carbon monoxide poisoning. Anticipate intubation and mechanical ventilation with PEEP for respiratory failure. See p. 577 for information on mechanical ventilation.
2. Anticipate escharotomies to chest, if full thickness burns present, to improve compliance and ventilation.
3. Promote pulmonary hygiene: position the patient for maximum chest excursion, cough and deep breathe to mobilize secretions, and encourage incentive spirometry to prevent atelectasis; chest physiotherapy and suction may be required.
4. Bronchodilators may be used to treat bronchospasm.

▶ **Nursing Diagnosis:** Fluid volume deficit related to plasma loss, increased capillary permeability with interstitial fluid accumulation, and increased insensible water loss

OUTCOME CRITERIA

- Patient will be alert and oriented
- HR   60-100 beats/min
- SBP   90-140 mm Hg
- Urine output 30-50 ml/hr or 0.5-1 ml/kg/hr
- Urine specific gravity 1.005-1.030
- Lungs clear to auscultation
- Serum sodium 135-145 mEq/L
- Serum potassium 3.5-5.5 mEq/L

PATIENT MONITORING

1. Monitor fluid volume status: massive fluid shifts will occur within the first 72 hours of a burn event. Measure hourly I & O to determine fluid balance. Compare daily weights (1 kg ~ 1000 ml of fluid); a 15% to 20% weight gain within the first 72 hours can be anticipated. The

diuresis phase begins approximately 48 to 72 hours after the burn event.

2. Monitor MAP; a value <60 mm Hg adversely affects renal and cerebral perfusion.

3. If a pulmonary artery catheter has been inserted, monitor PAWP to evaluate fluid status. CO/CI will be increased due to a hypermetabolic state.

4. If a CVP line is indicated, frequently monitor pressure during fluid resuscitation to evaluate the patient's response to therapy. CVP can be estimated; see p. 17.

5. Continuously monitor the ECG for dysrhythmias.

PHYSICAL ASSESSMENT

1. Obtain VS q15min during the acute phase to detect cardiopulmonary deterioration.

2. Assess fluid volume status: Dry mucous membranes, decreased pulse pressure, tachycardia, furrowed tongue, absent JVD, and complaints of thirst suggest hypovolemia. Bounding pulses, cough, dyspnea, and crackles suggest volume overload.

3. Assess the patient for development of clinical sequelae. (See Table 2-51.)

DIAGNOSTICS ASSESSMENT

1. Review serum electrolyte levels closely during the fluid resuscitation period; either hyperkalemia or hypokalemia can occur; hyponatremia is not uncommon. Electrolyte imbalances can occur as a result of loss of fluids via burns, shifts into interstitial spaces, drainage, or fluid resuscitation.

2. Review serial Hgb, Hct, osmolality, and urine specific gravity and note trends. An increase in values may indicate hypovolemia.

PATIENT MANAGEMENT

1. Fluid administration is usually instituted for burns >20%. Administer LR as ordered. The American Burn Association (ABA) recommends 2 to 4 ml/kg/%BSA burned. Give the first half during the first 8 hours from the time of the burn injury and the second half during the next 16 hours. Colloids may be administered during the second 24 hours to maintain intravascular volume. As diuresis occurs, infusion rates may be decreased. Dextrose in water solutions may be used to maintain serum sodium within normal limits in the second 24

MULTI

hours. Hyperglycemia may occur with dextrose in water solutions.

2. Blood or blood products may be administered as needed. See p. 534 for information on blood transfusion.
3. Administer potassium as ordered to replace potassium lost through the urine.

▶ **Nursing Diagnosis:** Altered tissue perfusion related to hypovolemia, circumferential burns of extremities, and presence of myoglobin

OUTCOME CRITERIA
• Patient will be alert and oriented
• Peripheral pulses strong
• Bowel sounds present
• Absence of GI bleeding
• Gastric pH 5-7
• Urine output 30-50 ml/hr or 0.5-1 ml/kg/hr
• SBP   90-140 mm Hg
• MAP   70-105 mm Hg
• CVP   2-6 mm Hg

PATIENT MONITORING
1. Monitor MAP, an indicator of tissue perfusion. A MAP <60 mm Hg adversely affects cerebral and renal perfusion.
2. If a CVP line is indicated, continuously monitor pressure as an index of fluid volume status. CVP can be estimated. See p. 17.
3. Measure hourly I & O and urine specific gravity to evaluate adequacy of hydration; if urine output falls below 30 ml/hr, suspect renal ischemia secondary to hypovolemia or damage to tubules by myoglobin.
4. Monitor the color of the urine; if it is a port-wine color, suspect myoglobinuria.

PHYSICAL ASSESSMENT
1. Assess for systemic hypoperfusion: absent/decreased peripheral pulses, cool pale skin, capillary refill <3 sec.
2. Assess neurovascular status q15-30min the first 24 to 48 hours: pulselessness, pallor, pain, paresthesia, and paralysis can signal nerve ischemia. Damaged sensory nerve fibers may be misinterpreted as improvement in neurovascular status, when in fact a loss of a limb may be the outcome.
3. Assess GI status: test gastric pH, auscultate bowel sounds, and test stool for occult blood. Decreased perfusion to the GI system contributes to Curling's ulcer.
4. Assess the patient for development of clinical sequelae. (See Table 2-51.)

THE CRITICALLY ILL PATIENT

DIAGNOSTICS ASSESSMENT
1. Check the urinalysis for myoglobin level (myoglobin can cause tubular destruction and ATN).
2. Check urine specific gravity to determine hydration status and renal function.
3. Review serial BUN, creatinine, and potassium results for a steady rise in values, which may indicate renal failure.
4. Review Hgb and Hct levels for decreasing trends, which may suggest blood loss secondary to Curling's ulcer.

PATIENT MANAGEMENT
1. Administer fluids as ordered to optimize oxygen delivery and tissue perfusion.
2. Anticipate administration of mannitol, an osmotic diuretic, to flush kidneys and maintain a urine output >100 ml/hr if the patient has myoglobinuria.
3. Anticipate NG intubation for abdominal distension secondary to reflex paralytic ileus, and/or antacid administration.
4. Maintain gastric pH at 5 to 7 with antacids and H_2 antagonists as ordered to help prevent Curling's ulcer.
5. Elevate edematous extremities to increase venous return and to decrease edema, which may adversely affect tissue perfusion. Be prepared for an escharotomy or fasciotomy to improve circulation if circumferential burns are present.
6. Maintain a warmer than normal room temperature and keep wounds covered to prevent hypothermia and vaso-constriction.

▶ **Nursing Diagnosis:** Pain related to burned tissues and wound debridement

OUTCOME CRITERION
• Patient will communicate pain relief.

PATIENT MONITORING
1. Use a visual analogue scale (see Figure 1-1) to evaluate pain and the patient's response to therapy. An increase in intensity of pain may indicate ischemia. A decrease in pain may be misinterpreted as an improvement, when in fact sensory nerve fibers may be damaged.

PHYSICAL ASSESSMENT
1. Note changes in HR, BP, and RR that may suggest SNS stimulation, which may signal pain.
2. Observe for cues such as grimacing, grunting, sobbing, irritability, withdrawal, or hostility, which may signal pain.

MULTI

DIAGNOSTICS ASSESSMENT
None specific
PATIENT MANAGEMENT
1. Administer an analgesic as ordered (usually IV morphine sulfate) before debridement and at frequent intervals for controlled pain management. Pain increases catecholamine release and the metabolic rate, which puts an added burden on an already hypermetabolic state.
2. Plan diversional activities appropriate for the patient's developmental level and the severity of burn incurred (e.g., music, television).
3. Promote relaxation through controlled breathing and guided imagery.
4. Reposition the patient frequently to promote comfort and avoid deformities.
5. Keep partial-thickness burn wounds covered, since any stimulus to these wounds can cause pain.
6. If the open method of wound treatment is used, keeping the room warm (85° F, 29° C) and preventing drafts may help to decrease pain.
7. See Acute Pain, p. 30.

▶ **Nursing Diagnoses:** Risk for infection secondary to Impaired skin integrity related to severe burns
OUTCOME CRITERIA
- T 36.5° C (97.7° F) to 37.8° C (100° F)
- Negative wound biopsy
- Healing by secondary intention or skin grafting without purulent drainage

PATIENT MONITORING
None specific
PHYSICAL ASSESSMENT
1. Obtain temperature q4h to monitor inflammatory response.
2. Assess the wound daily and note color, drainage, odor, and the presence of epithelial buds. Rapid eschar separation, disappearance of well-defined burn margins, discoloration, and purulent exudates are indicative of infection. In skin grafts, bright red blood drainage and pooling of fluid will inhibit successful grafting. Check for adherence and closure of interstices. Check the donor site for infection development.

3. Assess the patient for development of clinical sequelae. (See Table 2-49.)

DIAGNOSTICS ASSESSMENT

1. Review wound biopsy reports for identification of the infecting organism (>100,000 organisms per gram tissue = burn wound sepsis).
2. Review serial WBC counts; silver sulfadiazine may decrease WBCs; an increase may be associated with sepsis, although the leukocytosis may be caused by the inflammatory process.

PATIENT MANAGEMENT

1. Handwashing is the most effective weapon against transmission of infection.
2. Patients should be assigned their own equipment including stethoscopes, thermometers, etc.
3. Avoid placing IV lines through burned skin. Remove invasive lines as early as possible.
4. Verify tetanus prophylaxis.
5. Regulate environmental temperature to 85° F to 90° F (29° C to 32° C) to avoid excess heat loss when wounds are open.
6. Wound management depends on institutional protocol:
   - Premedicate the patient.
   - Generally wound cleansing and debridement are performed daily.
   - Strict aseptic technique is used. Hair may need to be clipped around burn wounds to prevent infection.
   - Open treatment involves exposure of the wounds; isolation technique is required.
   - Closed treatment involves covering wounds with dressings; treatment includes washing of the wound and applying dressings with a topical agent per protocol.
   - Observe for impaired circulation caused by the dressings.
7. Anticipate a wound excision and skin grafting to speed healing, prevent contractures, and shorten convalescence.
8. Administer antibiotics as ordered when an invasive burn wound infection has been identified.
9. Anticipate nutritional support that supplies adequate protein, carbohydrate, and fat calories, zinc, vitamins, and minerals to promote tissue healing. Energy requirements may be as high as 5000 kcal/day. High-nitrogen diets by the enteral route may offer immunological benefits.

MULTI

DISSEMINATED INTRAVASCULAR COAGULATION (DIC)

Clinical Brief

DIC is a coagulation disorder characterized by inappropriate concurrent thrombus formation and hemorrhage secondary to overstimulation of the clotting cascade. It is a secondary complication of many underlying conditions (e.g., shock, sepsis, crush injuries, obstetrical complications, burns, and ARDS).

Presenting signs and symptoms

Signs and symptoms include abdominal, back, or joint pain; bleeding from multiple orifices and mucous membranes; and a feeling of impending doom.

Physical examination

Depends on the underlying condition:

Vital signs:

    HR >100 beats/min

    BP <90 mm Hg

    RR >20/min

Neurological: Restless, anxious, altered LOC, seizures, unresponsive

Skin: Mottled, cold fingers and toes; ecchymoses, petechiae, gingival bleeding

Cardiovascular: Tachycardia, murmurs may be noted

Pulmonary: Dyspnea, tachypnea, hemoptysis

Gastrointestinal: Hematemesis, melena, abdominal tenderness

Renal: Urine output <0.5 ml/kg/hr, hematuria

Other: Bleeding from any orifice

Diagnostic findings

Clinical manifestations are the basis for diagnosis. Sudden onset of bleeding (petechia, purpura, ecchymosis, oozing from puncture sites) and thrombosis (gangrene, acral cyanosis, skin necrosis, DVT). Other findings include the following:

Platelets <100×10^3/μl

PT >15 sec

PTT >40 sec

Fibrinogen <150 mg/dl

Fibrin split products >8 μg/ml

Fibrin degradation products >1:40

D-dimers >2

Antithrombin III decreased

Blood smear shows schistocytes and burr cells
Positive protamine sulfate test results

Acute Care Patient Management
Goals of treatment
Treat primary problem
  Surgery, antibiotics
Optimize oxygen delivery
  Crystalloids
  Supplemental oxygen/mechanical ventilation
  RBCs
  Positive inotropes: dopamine, dobutamine
Reverse clotting mechanism
  Heparin (controversial)
  Aminocaproic acid and heparin
Replace coagulation components
  Platelets, FFP, cryoprecipitate
Correct hemostatic deficiency
  Folic acid, vitamin K
Detect/prevent clinical sequelae
  See Table 2-52
▶ **Priority Nursing Diagnoses**
Altered tissue perfusion
Altered protection (see p. 33)
Altered nutrition: less than body requirements
(see p. 41)

TABLE 2-52 Clinical Sequelae Associated with DIC

Complication	Signs and symptoms
ARDS	Dyspnea, hypoxemia refractory to increases in FIO_2, cyanosis, PaO_2/FIO_2 <175, PAWP <18 mm Hg
Intracerebral bleeding	Change in sensorium, headache, seizures, extremity weakness/paralysis
GI dysfunction	Absent bowel sounds, abdominal pain, diarrhea, upper and lower GI bleeding
Renal failure	Urine output <0.5 ml/kg/hr, steady rise in creatinine
Shock	SBP <90 mm Hg, HR >100 beats/min, patient anxious to unresponsive, cold clammy skin, urine output <0.5 ml/kg/hr

MULTI

Risk for altered family process (see p. 29)

▶ **Nursing Diagnosis:** Altered tissue perfusion (peripheral, renal, cerebral, GI, and pulmonary) related to concurrent thrombus formation and bleeding

OUTCOME CRITERIA

- Patient will be alert and oriented
- Absence of neurological deficits
- Skin warm and dry
- Peripheral pulses strong
- Absence of acral cyanosis (mottled, cool toes and fingers)
- Absence of chest pain
- Absence of hemoptysis
- RR   12-20/min, eupnea
- Absence of hematemesis, melena
- Active bowel sounds
- Urine output 30 ml/hr or 0.5-1 ml/kg/hr
- Absence of hematuria
- Absence of pain, tenderness, redness, and venous distention in calves
- Platelets >50,000/μl
- Fibrinogen >100 mg/dl
- SBP   90-140 mm Hg
- MAP   70-105 mm Hg
- CI   2.5-4 L/min/m²
- O_2 sat   ≥95%
- SvO_2 60%-80%
- Hct   37%-47% (females)
              40%-54% (males)

PATIENT MONITORING

1. Monitor BP continuously via arterial cannulation, since cuff pressures can cause further injury and bleeding. Monitor MAP, an indicator that accurately reflects tissue perfusion. MAP <60 mm Hg adversely affects cerebral and renal perfusion.

2. Monitor PA pressures and CVP hourly or more frequently to evaluate patient response to treatment. Both parameters reflect the capacity of the vascular system to accept volume and can be used to monitor for fluid overload and pulmonary edema.

3. Obtain CO/CI at least q8h or more frequently to evaluate the patient's progress or deterioration.

4. Calculate $\dot{D}o_2I$ and $\dot{V}o_2I$ to evaluate oxygen transport; inadequate oxygen delivery and consumption produce tissue hypoxia.

5. Continuously monitor Svo$_2$ (if available). A decreasing trend may indicate decreased oxygen delivery and/or increased tissue oxygen extraction.
6. Continuously monitor oxygen status with pulse oximetry. Be alert for effects of interventions and patient activities, which may adversely affect oxygen saturation.
7. Continuously monitor ECG to detect life-threatening dysrhythmias and ST, T-wave changes.
8. Monitor fluid balance: record hourly I & O; include blood loss in determining fluid balance.

PHYSICAL ASSESSMENT
1. Obtain HR, RR, BP q15min to evaluate the patient's response to therapies and detect cardiopulmonary deterioration.
2. Assess peripheral pulses, capillary refill, and the color and temperature of extremities to evaluate thrombotic-ischemic changes.
3. Assess skin, mucous membranes, and all orifices for bleeding. Test emesis, urine, stool, NG aspirate, and drainage from tubes, drains, etc. for blood. Assess invasive line sites for oozing of blood.
4. Assess for the presence of headache or any change in LOC that might suggest impaired cerebral perfusion or intracranial bleeding; check extremities for strength and movement to identify neurological involvement.
5. Assess the patient for development of clinical sequelae. (See Table 2-52.)

DIAGNOSTICS ASSESSMENT
1. Review coagulation studies: INR, PTT, TT, fibrinogen level, platelet count, fibrin degradation products, and factors II, V, VII, and VIII to evaluate resolution or worsening of DIC.
2. Review Hgb and Hct levels and note trends. Decreased RBCs can adversely affect oxygen-carrying capacity.
3. Review ABGs for hypoxemia and acidosis, which can signal pulmonary involvement and impaired gas exchange.

PATIENT MANAGEMENT
1. Administer blood and blood products as ordered to replace coagulation components. (See p. 534 for information on blood transfusion.)
2. Administer crystalloids (LR or NS) as ordered to optimize oxygen delivery. Monitor CVP and PAWP to evaluate response to fluid resuscitation.

3. Avoid dextran infusions for hypovolemia secondary to hemorrhage, since coagulation problems can occur and enhance the bleeding problem.
4. Heparin may be ordered in select cases. Observe the patient for increased bleeding.
5. Dopamine or dobutamine may be used to enhance contractility; dopamine may be used to improve renal and splanchic blood flow.
6. Provide oxygen therapy as ordered.
7. Do not disturb established clots; use cold compresses or pressure to stop bleeding. Use an arterial line to minimize the number of peripheral sticks, thus minimizing thrombosis.
8. Avoid trauma and excessive manipulation of the patient to prevent further bleeding. Use gentle oral care, keep the patient's lips moist, avoid tape on the skin, use an electric razor, and use suction at the lowest pressure possible.
9. Avoid aspirin products, which could potentiate bleeding.
10. Administer pharmacological agents such as folic acid and vitamin K as ordered to correct hemostatic deficiency.

SEPTIC SHOCK

Clinical Brief

Sepsis is a systemic inflammatory response to the presence of infection. It involves a continuum of severity with cellular and immunologic components that is triggered by a pathogen and can lead to organ system dysfunction and shock. Septic shock is a result of an overwhelming mediator response that induces pathologic changes in the host. Septic shock is defined as sepsis-induced hypotension that persists despite adequate fluid resuscitation along with hypoperfusion and abnormalities or organ dysfunction.

Presenting signs and symptoms

Signs and symptoms are associated with systemic inflammatory response syndrome, infection, and hypotension

Septic shock

Sepsis + hypotension and hypoperfusion

SBP <90 mm Hg

Lactic acidosis, oliguria, altered mental status, Pao_2/Fio_2 <280

Sepsis

SIRS + infection

SIRS

Manifested by two or more of the following:

T >38° C or <36° C

HR >90 beats/min

RR >20/min or $PaCO_2$ <32 mm Hg

WBC >12,000/cu mm or <4000/cu mm or >10% immature neutrophils

Physical examination

Neurological: Unresponsive, difficult to arouse

Cardiovascular: Weak, thready pulses

Pulmonary: Crackles, wheezes, respiratory distress

Skin:

   Cool, clammy skin

   Color pale

Other: Evidence of multiple organ failure

Diagnostic findings

Clinical manifestations are the basis for diagnosis.

Acute Care Patient Management

Goals of treatment

Optimize oxygen delivery

   Colloids, crystalloids

    Vasopressors: dopamine, norepinephrine, phenylephrine

    Inotropes: dobutamine

    Intubation/mechanical ventilation

    Blood products

Treat underlying problem

   Antibiotics

   Surgery

Detect/prevent clinical sequelae

   See Table 2-53

▶ **Priority Nursing Diagnoses**

Altered tissue perfusion

Impaired gas exchange

Ineffective thermoregulation

Altered protection (see p. 33)

Altered nutrition: less than body requirements (see p. 41)

Risk for altered family process (see p. 29)

▶ **Nursing Diagnosis:** Altered tissue perfusion related to maldistribution of blood flow and depressed myocardial function

MULTI

TABLE 2–53 Clinical Sequelae Associated with Septic Shock

Complication	Signs and symptoms
Cardiopulmonary arrest	Nonpalpable pulse, absent respirations
Multiple organ dysfunction (MOD)	
ARDS	Hypoxemia refractory to increases in FIO_2, decreased compliance PaO_2/FIO_2 <175, PAWP <18 mm Hg
Renal dysfunction	Urine output <0.5 ml/kg/hr, steady rise in creatinine
GI bleed/dysfunction	Blood in NG aspirate, emesis, stool; absent bowel sounds, distention
Hepatic dysfunction	Jaundice, bilirubin >2 mg/dL, Rise in LFTs, decreased albumin
DIC	Bleeding from puncture sites and mucous membranes, hematuria, ecchymoses, prolonged PT and PTT; decreased fibrinogen, platelets, factors V, VIII, XIII, II; increased FSP; FDP 1:40; D-dimers >2

OUTCOME CRITERIA
- Patient will be alert and oriented
- Skin warm and dry
- Peripheral pulses strong
- Urine output 30 ml/hr or 0/5-1 ml/kg/hr
- SBP   90-140 mm Hg
- MAP   70-105 mm Hg
- CI   ~4.5 L/min/m²
- O_2 sat   ≥95%
- SvO_2 60%-80%
- $\dot{D}O_2I$ >600 ml/min/m²
- $\dot{V}O_2I$ >165 ml/min/m²
- ERO_2 25%

PATIENT MONITORING
1. Monitor BP continuously via arterial cannulation, since cuff pressures are less accurate in shock states. Monitor

MAP, an indicator that accurately reflects tissue perfusion. MAP <60 mm Hg adversely affects cerebral and renal perfusion.

2. Monitor PA pressures and CVP hourly or more frequently to evaluate the patient's response to treatment. Both parameters reflect the capacity of the vascular system to accept volume and can be used to monitor for fluid overload and pulmonary edema.

3. Obtain CO/CI at least q4h or more frequently to evaluate the patient's response to changes in therapies.

4. Calculate $\dot{D}o_2I$ and $\dot{V}o_2I$ to evaluate effectiveness of therapies. Supranormal levels of $\dot{D}o_2$ may be necessary to optimize $\dot{V}o_2$. Calculate ERo_2; a value >25% suggests increased oxygen consumption, decreased oxygen delivery, or both.

5. Continuously monitor Svo_2. A decreasing trend may indicate decreased CO and increased tissue oxygen extraction (inadequate perfusion). Calculating $Ca\text{-}vo_2$ (arteriovenous oxygen content difference) also provides information regarding oxygen uptake at the tissue level.

6. Monitor hourly urine output to evaluate renal perfusion.

PHYSICAL ASSESSMENT

1. Obtain HR, RR, BP q15min to evaluate patient response to therapy and detect cardiopulmonary deterioration.

2. Assess mentation, skin temperature, and peripheral pulses and the presence of cardiac or abdominal pain to evaluate CO and the state of vasoconstriction.

3. Assess the patient for development of clinical sequelae. (See Table 2-53.)

DIAGNOSTICS ASSESSMENT

1. Review ABGs for hypoxemia and acidosis, since these conditions can precipitate dysrhythmias or affect myocardial contractility. Hypoxemia refractory to increasing Fio_2 may signal ARDS.

2. Review WBC counts for leukocytosis as the body attempts to fight infection or for leukopenia as the bone marrow becomes exhausted.

3. Review culture reports for identification of the infecting pathogen.

4. Review Hgb and Hct levels and note trends. Decreased RBCs can adversely affect oxygen-carrying capacity.

5. Review lactate levels, an indicator of anaerobic metabolism. Increased levels signify that cells are not consuming

MULTI

the oxygen they need. However, lactate levels may be less useful in severe septic shock.

6. Review BUN, creatinine, and electrolytes and note trends to evaluate renal function.

PATIENT MANAGEMENT

1. Administer colloids (albumin) and crystalloids (LR or NS) to increase preload as ordered. Monitor CVP and PAWP to evaluate the patient's response to fluid resuscitation.

2. To increase oxygen transport, inotropes such as dobutamine may be required to increase myocardial contractility, stroke volume, cardiac output, and blood pressure. Blood may also be given to increase Hgb and improve oxygen-carrying capacity.

3. Administer vasopressors such as dopamine, norepinephrine, or phenylephrine as ordered to oppose vasodilation.

4. Correct an acidotic state since acidosis blocks or diminishes responsiveness to drug therapy.

5. Provide oxygen therapy as ordered. Anticipate intubation and mechanical ventilation before severe respiratory distress or cardiopulmonary arrest ensues.

6. Neuromuscular blockade with sedation/pain control may be instituted to reduce oxygen consumption and improve ventilation.

7. Administer antibiotics as ordered. Antibiotic therapy may not be effective in the first 48 to 72 hours; thus interventions to support BP and oxygenation are required.

8. Treat dysrhythmias according to ACLS.

9. Prepare the patient for surgical intervention if required (e.g., abscess drainage).

▶ **Nursing Diagnosis:** Impaired gas exchange related to increased pulmonary vascular resistance, pulmonary interstitial edema, and pulmonary microthrombi

OUTCOME CRITERIA

- Patient will be alert and oriented
- pH   7.35-7.45
- PaO_2 80-100 mm Hg
- $PaCO_2$ 35-45 mm Hg
- O_2 sat   ≥95%
- RR   12-20/min, eupnea
- Lungs clear to auscultation

PATIENT MONITORING

1. Continuously monitor oxygenation status with pulse oximetry (SpO_2). Be alert for effects of interventions and

patient activities, which may adversely affect oxygen saturation.

2. Continuously monitor PA systolic pressure (if available), since hypoxia can increase sympathetic tone and increase pulmonary vasoconstriction.

PHYSICAL ASSESSMENT

1. Obtain HR, RR, BP q15mm to evaluate patient response to therapy and detect cardiopulmonary deterioration.

2. Assess respiratory status: RR >30 beats/min suggests respiratory distress. Note the use of accessory muscles and respiratory pattern. Note the presence of breath sounds and adventitious sounds, suggesting worsening pulmonary congestion.

3. Assess for signs and symptoms of hypoxemia: increased restlessness, increased complaints of dyspnea, changes in LOC. Cyanosis is a late sign.

4. Assess the patient for development of clinical sequelae. (See Table 2-53.)

DIAGNOSTICS ASSESSMENT

1. Review ABGs for PaO_2 refractory to increases in FIO_2 that may suggest ARDS. O_2 sat should be ≥95%.

2. Review serial chest radiographs to evaluate patient progress or worsening lung condition.

3. Review Hgb and Hct levels and note trends. Decreased RBCs can adversely affect oxygen-carrying capacity.

PATIENT MANAGEMENT

1. Provide supplemental oxygen as ordered. Intubation and mechanical ventilation should be considered before severe respiratory distress develops.

2. When hemodynamically stable, promote pulmonary hygiene: C & DB and reposition the patient q2h to mobilize secretions and prevent atelectasis.

3. Minimize oxygen demand by decreasing anxiety, fever, shivering, and pain.

4. Position patient for maximum chest excursion and comfort.

▶ **Nursing Diagnosis:** Ineffective thermoregulation related to infecting pathogen

OUTCOME CRITERIA

• T 36.5° C (97.7° F) to 37.8° C (100° F)
• Absence of shivering

PATIENT MONITORING

1. Continuously monitor core temperature for any changes.

MULTI

PHYSICAL ASSESSMENT

1. Obtain HR and BP and evaluate trends to detect hemodynamic compromise.
2. Assess skin temperature and presence of diaphoresis. Note any chills or shivering, which increases oxygen demand.
3. Assess the patient for the development of clinical sequelae. (See Table 2-53.)

DIAGNOSTICS ASSESSMENT

1. Review culture reports for identification of infecting pathogen.
2. Review WBC counts; an increase suggests the body's attempt to fight the infection; a decrease suggests bone marrow exhaustion.

PATIENT MANAGEMENT

1. Regulate environmental temperature to help maintain patient temperature between 36.5° C (97.7° F) to 38° C (100.4° F).
2. Apply extra bed linens or blankets during hypothermia and shivering episodes.
3. Remove extra linens during hyperthermia episodes.
4. Tepid sponge baths or a cooling blanket may be needed during hyperthermia episodes.
5. Administer antipyretics as ordered to reduce fever.
6. Administer antibiotics as ordered to eradicate infection.
7. See p. 548 for information on thermal regulation.

REFERENCES

1. ACCP/SCCM Consensus Conference Committee: Definitions for sepsis and organ failure and guidelines for the use of innovative therapies in sepsis, *Chest* 101(6):1644-1655, 1992.
2. Acute Pain Management Guideline Panel: Acute pain management: operative or medical procedure and trauma, *Clinical practice guidelines AHCPR PUB* no. 92-0032, Rockville, MD, February 1992, Agency for Health Care Policy and Research, Public Health Service, U.S. Department of Health and Human Services.
3. Agency for Health Care Policy and Research: Diagnosing and managing unstable angina, *Clinical practice guidelines AHCPR PUB* no. 94-0602, Rockville, MD, 1994, U.S. Department of Health and Human Services.
4. Al-Ghamdi SMG, Cameron EC, Sutton RAL: Magnesium deficiency: pathophysiologic and clinical overview, *Am J Kidney Dis* 24(5):737-752, 1994.
5. American College of Surgeons: Thoracic trauma. In *Advanced trauma life support course for physician's manual,* Chicago, 1993, American College of Surgeons Committee on Trauma.

6. American Heart Association: Adjuncts for airway control, ventilation, and oxygenation. In Cummins RO, ed: *Advanced cardiac life support,* Dallas, 1994, American Heart Association.

7. Armstrong SL: Cerebral vasospasm: early detection and intervention, *Crit Care Nurse* 14(4):33-37, 1994.

8. Astiz M, Galeka-Santiago A, Rackow E: Intravascular volume and fluid therapy for severe sepsis, *New Horizons* 1(1):127-136, 1993.

9. Axelrod L, Levitsky LL: Hypoglycemia. In Kahrn CR, Weir GC, eds: *Joslin's diabetes mellitus,* ed 13, Philadelphia, 1994, Lea & Febiger.

10. Baer CL, Lancaster LE: Acute renal failure, *Crit Care Nurs Q* 14(4):1-21, 1992.

11. Barker E: *Neuroscience nursing,* St Louis, 1994, Mosby.

12. Batcheller J: Disorders of antidiuretic hormone secretion, *AACN Clin Issues Crit Care Nurs* 3(2):370-378, 1992.

13. Batcheller J: Syndrome of inappropriate antidiuretic hormone secretion, *Crit Care Nurs Clin North Am* 6(4):687-692, 1994.

14. Bell TN: Diabetes insipidus, *Crit Care Nurs Clin North Am* 6(4):675-685, 1994.

15. Blissitt PA: Ticlopidine hydrochloride, *J Neurosci Nurs* 24(5):296-300, 1992.

16. Bone R: Sepsis and its complications, the clinical problem, *Crit Care Med* 22(7):S8-S11, 1994.

17. Brewer TG: Treatment of acute gastroesophageal variceal hemorrhage, *Med Clin North Am* 77(5):993-1014, 1993.

18. Bridges J, Strong A: Angiotensin converting enzyme inhibition: pharmacologic management to minimize postinfarction heart failure, *Crit Care Nurs Q* 16(2):17-26, 1993.

19. Brodrick RL: Preventing complications in acute pancreatitis, *DCCN* 10(5):262-270, 1991.

20. Brown K: Critical interventions in septic shock, *AJN* 94(10):20-25, 1994.

21. Brown K: Septic shock: how to stop the deadly cascade, *AJN* 94(9):20-26, 1994.

22. Burroughs AK: Variceal hemorrhage. In Misiewicz JJ, Pounder RE, Venables CW, eds: *Diseases of the gut and pancreas,* ed 2, Boston, 1994, Blackwell Scientific Publications.

23. Calleja GA, Barkin JS: Acute pancreatitis, *Med Clin North Am* 77(5):1037-1056, 1993.

24. Carson MM et al: Managing pain during mediastinal chest tube removal, *Heart Lung* 23(6):500-505, 1994.

25. Christoph SB: Pain assessment: the problem of pain in the critically ill patient, *Crit Care Nurs Clin North Am* 3(1):11-16, 1991.

26. Civetta J, Taylor R, Kirby R: *Critical care,* ed 2, Philadelphia, 1992, J.B. Lippincott.

27. Cook HA: Aneurysmal subarachnoid hemorrhage: neurosurgical frontiers and nursing challenges, *AACN Clin Issues Crit Care Nurs* 2(4):665-674, 1991.

28. Covington H: Nursing care of patients with alcoholic liver disease, *Crit Care Nurse* 13(3):47-57, 1993.

29. Cullen L: Interventions related to fluid and electrolyte balance, *Nurs Clin North Am* 27(2):569-597, 1992.

30. Dantzker D: Adequacy of tissue oxygenation, *Crit Care Med* 21(2):S40-S43, 1993.

31. Dark D, Pingleton S: Nutrition and nutritional support in critically ill patients, *J Intensive Care Med* 8(1):16-33, 1993.

32. Davis M, Lucatorto M: Mannitol revisited, *J Neurosci Nurs* 26(3):170-174, 1994.

33. Doody SB, Smith C, Webb J: Nonpharmacologic interventions for pain management, *Crit Care Nurs Clin North Am* 3(1):69-76, 1991.

34. Dougherty C: Longitudinal recovery following sudden cardiac arrest and internal cardioverter defibrillator implantation: survivors and their families, *Am J Crit Care* 3(2):145-154, 1994.

35. Douglas S: Acute tubular necrosis: diagnosis, treatment, and nursing implications, *AACN Clin Issues Crit Care Nurs,* 1992.

36. Dronfield MW: Upper gastrointestinal bleeding. In Misiewicz JJ, Pounder RE, Venables CW, eds: *Diseases of the gut and pancreas,* ed 2, Boston, 1994, Blackwell Scientific Publications.

37. Emergency Cardiac Care Committee and Subcommittees, American Heart Association: Guidelines for cardiopulmonary resuscitation and emergency cardiac care, *JAMA* 268(16):2216-2230, 1992.

38. Enfanto P et al: Percutaneous laser myoplasty: nursing care implications, *Crit Care Nurse* 14(3):94-101, 1994.

39. Epstein CD: Adrenocortical insufficiency in the critically ill patient, *AACN Clin Issues Crit Care Nurs* 3(3):705-713, 1992.

40. Epstein D: Changing interpretations of angina pectoris associated with transient myocardial ischemia, *J Cardiovasc Nurs* 7(1):1-13, 1992.

41. Fedullo PF: Pulmonary embolism. In Tierney DF, ed: *Current pulmonology,* vol 14, St Louis, 1993, Mosby.

42. Feld H: New treatment strategies for cardiogenic shock in acute MI, *J Crit Illn* 7(8):1277-1294, 1992.

43. Funk M, Pooley-Richards R: Predicting hospital mortality in patients with acute myocardial infarction, *Am J Crit Care* 3(3):168-176, 1994.

44. Gianino S, St. John, R: Nutritional assessment of the patient in the intensive care unit, *Crit Care Nurs Clin North Am* 5(1):1-15, 1993.

45. Gillum R: Trends in acute myocardial infarction and coronary heart disease death in the United States, *J Am Coll Cardiol* 23(6):1273-1277, 1994.

46. Grimes DE, Grimes RM: *AIDS and HIV infection,* St Louis, 1994, Mosby.

47. Guidelines Committee, American College of Critical Care Medicine, Society of Critical Care Medicine and the Transfer Guidelines Task Force, American Association of Critical-Care Nurses: Guidelines for the transfer of critically ill patients, *Am J Crit Care* 2(3):189-195, 1993.

48. Gujol MC: A survey of pain assessment and management practices among critical care nurses, *Am J Crit Care* 3(2):123-128, 1994.

49. Gupta PK, Fleischer DE: Nonvariceal upper gastrointestinal bleeding, *Med Clin North Am* 77(5):973-992, 1993.

50. Guzzetta C, Dossey B: *Cardiovascular nursing,* St Louis, 1992, Mosby.

51. Hanson J: Modifiable risk factors for coronary heart disease in women, *Am J Crit Care* 3(3):177-184, 1994.

52. Haupt M: Anaphylaxis and anaphylactic shock. In Parrillo JE, Bone RC, eds: *Critical care medicine principles of diagnosis and management,* St Louis, 1995, Mosby.

53. Hennekens C et al: The benefits of aspirin in acute myocardial infarction: still a well-kept secret in the United States, *Arch Intern Med* 154(1):37-39, 1994.

54. Hickey JV: *Neurological and neurosurgical nursing,* ed 3, Philadelphia, 1992, J.B. Lippincott.

55. Hutchinson GH: Disease of the peritoneum. In Misiewicz JJ, Pounder RE, Venables CW, eds: *Diseases of the gut and pancreas,* ed 2, Boston, 1994, Blackwell Scientific Publications.

56. Jacobson IM: Fulminant hepatic failure. In Barie PS, Shires GT, eds: *Surgical intensive care,* Boston, 1993, Little, Brown & Co.

57. Jones RL: From diabetic ketoacidosis to hyperglycemic hyperosmolar nonketotic syndrome, *Crit Care Nurs Clin North Am* 6(4):703-720, 1994.

58. Kadakia SC: Biliary tract emergencies: acute cholecystitis, acute cholangitis, and acute pancreatitis, *Med Clin North Am* 77(5):1015-1036, 1993.

59. Kaplan N: Management of hypertensive emergencies, *Lancet* 344(8933):1335-1338, 1994.

60. Keller K, Lemberg L: Q and non-Q wave myocardial infarctions, *Am J Crit Care* 3(2):158-161, 1994.

61. Keller K, Lemberg L: The importance of magnesium in cardiovascular disease, *Am J Crit Care* 2(4):348-350, 1993.

62. Kernicki J: Differentiating chest pain: advanced assessment techniques, *Dimens Crit Care Nurs* 12(2):66-76, 1993.

63. Kerr ME, Brucia J: Hyperventilation in the head-injured patient: an effective treatment modality? *Heart Lung* 22(6):516-522, 1993.

64. Kinney M et al: *AACN's clinical reference for critical-care nursing,* ed 3, St Louis, 1993, Mosby.

65. Kirby RR, Taylor RW, Civetta JM: *Handbook of critical care,* Philadelphia, 1994, J.B. Lippincott.

66. Larsen G et al: Recurrent cardiac events in survivors of ventricular fibrillation or tachycardia, *JAMA* 1(17):1335-1339, 1994.

67. Leach RM, Treacher DF: Oxygen transport: the relation between oxygen delivery and consumption, *Thorax* 47:971-978, 1992.

68. Lee LM, Bumowski J: Adrenocortical insufficiency: a medical emergency, *AACN Clin Issues Crit Care Nurs* 3(2):319-330, 1992.

69. Leor J et al: Cardiogenic shock complicating acute myocardial infarction in patients without heart failure on admission: incidence, risk factors and outcome, *Am J Med* 94(3):265-273, 1993.

70. Libman H: Pathogenesis, natural history and classification of HIV infection, *Crit Care Clin* 9(1):13-30, 1993.

71. Long C, Greeneich D: Family satisfaction techniques—meeting family expectations, *Dimens Crit Care Nurs* 13(2):104-111, 1994.

72. Loriaux DL, McDonald WJ: Adrenal insufficiency. In DeGroot LJ et al, eds: *Endocrinology,* ed 3, Philadelphia, 1995, W.B. Saunders.

73. Mancini D et al: Prognostic value of an abnormal signal-averaged electrocardiogram in patients with nonischemic congestive cardiomyopathy, *Circulation* 98(4):1083-1092, 1993.

74. Martin S, Danziger L: Continuous infusion of loop diuretics in the critically ill: a review of the literature, *Crit Care Med* 22(8):1323-1329, 1994.

75. McCauley M: Pulmonary artery balloon counterpulsation as a treatment for right ventricular failure, *J Cardiovasc Nurs* 8(2):61-68, 1994.

76. McLean R: Magnesium and its therapeutic uses: a review, *Am J Med* 96(2):63-75, 1994.

77. McMahon MJ: Acute pancreatitis. In Misiewicz JJ, Pounder RE, Venables CW, eds: *Diseases of the gut and pancreas,* ed 2, Boston, 1994, Blackwell Scientific Publications.

78. McMorrow ME: The elderly and thyrotoxicosis, *AACN Clin Issues Crit Care Nurs* 3(1):114-119, 1992.

79. McQuaid KR, Isenberg JI: Medical therapy of peptic ulcer disease, *Surg Clin North Am* 72(2):285-316, 1992.

80. Miller TA, Reed RL, Moody FG: Gastrointestinal hemorrhage. In Baire PS, Shires GT, eds: *Surgical intensive care,* Boston, 1993, Little, Brown & Co.

81. Moore K, Trifiletti E: Stroke: the first critical days, *RN* 57(2):22-27, 1994.

82. Moser D, Woo J: Recurrent ventricular tachycardia, *Crit Care Nurs Clin North Am* 6(1):15-26, 1994.

83. Mudge C, Carlson L: Hepatorenal syndrome, *AACN Clin Issues Crit Care Nurs* 3(3):614-632, 1992.

84. Mulcahy K: Hypoglycemic emergencies, *AACN Clin Issues Crit Care Nurs* 3(2):361-369, 1992.

85. Murray M, Plevak D: Analgesia in the critically ill patient, *New Horizons* 2(1): 56-63, 1994.

86. Natanson C, Hoffman WD, Parrillo JE: Septic shock and multiple organ failure. In Parrillo JE, Bone RC, eds: *Critical care medicine principles of diagnosis and management,* St Louis, 1995, Mosby.

87. Nathens AB, Rotstein OD: Therapeutic options in peritonitis, *Surg Clin North Am* 74(3):677-692, 1994.

88. Nayduch D, Lee A, Butler D: High-dose methylprednisolone after acute spinal cord injury, *Crit Care Nurse* 14(4):69-78, 1994.

89. Neagley SR: The pulmonary system. In Grif Alspach J, ed: *AACN core curriculum for critical care nursing,* ed 4, Philadelphia, 1991, W.B. Saunders.

90. Nolan S: Current trends in the management of acute spinal cord injury, *Crit Care Nurs Q* 17(1):64-78, 1994.

91. Om A et al: Management of cocaine-induced cardiovascular complications, *Am Heart J* 125(2):469-475, 1993.

92. Packer M: Treatment of chronic heart failure, *Lancet* 340(8811):92-95, 1992.

93. Parrillo JE, Bone RC, eds: *Critical care medicine: principles of diagnosis and management,* St Louis, 1995, Mosby.

94. Pasquale MD, Cipolle MD, Cerra FB: Oxygen transport: does increasing supply improve outcome? *Respir Care* 38(7):800-828, 1993.

95. Peitzman AB, Arnold SA, Boone DC: *Trauma manual,* Pittsburgh, 1994, University of Pittsburgh Medical Center Publication.

96. Peterson WL, Laine L: Gastrointestinal bleeding. In Sleisenger MH, Fordtran JS, eds: *Gastrointestinal disease: pathophysiology/diagnosis/management,* ed 5, Philadelphia, 1993, W.B. Saunders.

97. Pires L, Huang S: Nonsustained ventricular tachycardia: identification and management of high-risk patients, *Am Heart J* 126(1):189-200, 1993.

98. Pontoppidan H, Geffin B, Lowenstein E: Acute respiratory failure in the adult, *N Engl J Med* 287:690-698, 743-792, 799-806, 1972.

99. Porembka D: Cardiovascular abnormalities in sepsis, *New Horizons* 1(2):324-341, 1993.

100. Quenzer R, Allen S: Infections in the critically ill. In Bongard FS, Sue DY, eds: *Current critical care diagnosis and treatment,* Norwalk, CT, 1994, Appleton & Lange.

101. Ranson JC: Risk factors in acute pancreatitis, *Hosp Pract* 20(4):69-73, 1985.

102. Rattner DW, Warshaw AL: Acute pancreatitis. In Barie PS, Shires GT, eds: *Surgical intensive care,* Boston, 1993, Little, Brown & Co.

103. Reischtein J: Liver failure: case study of a complex problem, *Crit Care Nurse* 13(5):36-44, 1993.

104. Riegler JL, Lake JR: Fulminant hepatic failure, *Med Clin North Am* 77(5):1057-1083, 1993.

105. Rinaldo JE: The adult respiratory distress syndrome. In Tierney DF, ed: *Current pulmonology,* Philadelphia, 1994, Mosby.

106. Runyon BA: Ascites and spontaneous bacterial peritonitis. In Sleisenger MH, Fordtran JS, eds: *Gastrointestinal disease: pathophysiology/diagnosis/management,* ed 5, Philadelphia, 1993, W.B. Saunders.

107. Runyon BA: Surgical peritonitis and other disease of the peritoneum, mesentery, omentum, and diaphragm. In Sleisenger MH, Fordtran JS, eds: *Gastrointestinal disease: pathophysiology/diagnosis/management,* ed 5, Philadelphia, 1993, W.B. Saunders.

108. Ruppel G: *Manual of pulmonary function tests,* ed 6, St Louis, 1994, Mosby.

109. Russell JA, Phang PT: The oxygen delivery/consumption controversy, *Am J Respir Crit Care Med* 149:533-537, 1994.

110. Russell S: Hypovolemic shock, *Nursing 94* 24(4):34-51, 1994.

111. Ryder M: Peripherally inserted central venous catheters, *Nurs Clin North Am* 28(4):937-971, 1993.

112. St. George CL: Spasticity: mechanisms and nursing care, *Nurs Clin North Am* 28(4):819-827, 1993.

113. Sauve DO, Kessler CA: Hyperglycemic emergencies, *AACN Clin Issues Crit Care Nurs* 3(2):350-360, 1992.

114. Schneider K, Ladewig N: Subarachnoid hemorrhage. In Urban N, ed: *Guidelines for critical care nursing,* St Louis, 1995, Mosby.

115. Shah P: Acute aortic dissection: Part 1—clues that signal impending disaster, Part 2—choosing among management options, *J Crit Illn* 7(7):1047-1072, 1075-1078, 1992.

116. Sheridan R, Tompkins R, Burke J: Management of burn wounds with prompt excision and immediate closure, *J Intensive Care Med* 90:6-19, 1994.

117. Shoemaker W et al: Hemodynamic and oxygen transport monitoring to titrate therapy in septic shock, *New Horizons* 1(1):145-159, 1993.

118. Sinski A: Surfactant replacement in adults and children with ARDS—an effective therapy? *Crit Care Nurse* 14(6):54-59, 1994.

119. Siperstein MD: Diabetic ketoacidosis and hyperosmolar coma, *Endocrinol Metab Clin North Am* 21(2):415-432, 1992.

120. Smallridge RC: Metabolic and anatomic thyroid emergencies: a review, *Crit Care Med* 20(2):276-291, 1992.

121. Snider S: Use of muscle relaxants in the ICU: nursing implications, *Crit Care Nurse* 13(6):55-60, 1993.

122. Soergel KH: Acute pancreatitis. In Sleisenger MH, Fordtran JS, eds: *Gastrointestinal disease: pathophysiology/diagnosis/management,* ed 5, Philadelphia, 1993, W.B. Saunders.

123. Sonnenblick E: Intravenous milrinone: a new inotropic vasodilator, *Resident and Staff Physician* 39(9):49-55, 1993.

124. Spittle L: Diagnoses in opposition: thyroid storm and myxedema coma, *AACN Clin Issues Crit Care Nurs* 3(2):300-308, 1992.

125. Stark JL: Acute tubular necrosis: differences between oliguria and nonoliguria, *Crit Care Nurs Q* 14(4):22-27, 1992.

126. Stein JH: Acute renal failure: lessons from pathophysiology, *West J Med* 156:176-182, 1992.

127. Stewart-Amidei C: Hypervolemic hemodilution: a new approach to subarachnoid hemorrhage, *Heart Lung* 18(6):590-598, 1989.

128. Stewart J et al: Cardiomyoplasty: treatment of the failing heart using the skeletal muscle wrap, *J Cardiovasc Nurs* 7(2):23-31, 1993.

129. Stiesmeyer J: Unstable angina associated with critical proximal left anterior descending coronary artery stenosis, *Am J Crit Care* 2(3):248-253, 1993.

130. Sue DY: Respiratory failure. In Bongard FS, Sue DY, eds: *Current critical care diagnosis and treatment*, Norwalk, CT, 1994, Appleton & Lange.

131. Task force of the stroke council of the AHA: Guidelines for the management of aneurysmal subarachnoid hemorrhage, *Circulation* 90(5):2592-2605, 1994.

132. Task force of the stroke council of the AHA: Guidelines for the management of patients with acute ischemic stroke, *Circulation* 90(3):1588-1601, 1994.

133. Ten Cafe H et al: Disseminated intravascular coagulation: pathophysiology, diagnosis and treatment, *New Horizons* 1(2):312-323, 1993.

134. Terry J: The major electrolytes: sodium, potassium, chloride, *J IV Nurs* 17(5):240-247, 1994.

135. Thelan L et al: *Critical care nursing*, ed 2, St Louis, 1994, Mosby.

136. Tisdale L, Drew B: ST segment monitoring for myocardial ischemia, *AACN Clin Issues Crit Care Nurs* 4(1):34-43, 1993.

137. Toto KH, Yucha CB: Magnesium: homeostasis, imbalances, and therapeutic uses, *Crit Care Nurs Clin North Am* 6(4):767-784, 1994.

138. Uber L, Uber W: Hypertensive crisis in the 1990s, *Crit Care Nurs Q* 16(2):27-34, 1993.

139. Urban N et al: *Guidelines for critical care nursing*, St Louis, 1995, Mosby.

140. Uszenski H et al: Hypertrophic cardiomyopathy: medical, surgical, and nursing management, *J Cardiovasc Nurs* 7(2):13-22, 1993.

141. Vaca K et al: Cardiac surgery in the octogenarian: nursing implications, *Heart Lung* 23(5):413-422, 1994.

142. Vincent JL, Preiser JC: Inotropic agents, *New Horizons* 1(1):127-136, 1993.

143. Whalen D, Izzi G: Pharmacologic treatment of acute heart failure resulting from left ventricular systolic or diastolic dysfunction, *Crit Care Nurs Clin North Am* 5(2):261-269, 1993.

144. Whang R, Whang DD, Ryan MP: Refractory potassium repletion: a consequence of magnesium deficiency, *Arch Intern Med* 152(1):40-45, 1992.

145. Whitney F: Drug therapy for acute stroke, *J Neurosci Nurs* 26(2):111-117, 1994.

146. Willich S et al: Sudden cardiac death: support for a role of triggering in causation, *Circulation* 87(5):1442-1450, 1993.

147. Woeber KA: Thyrotoxicosis and the heart, *N Engl J Med* 327:94-98, 1992.

148. Workman ML: Magnesium and phosphorus: the neglected electrolytes, *AACN Clin Issues Crit Care Nurs* 3(3):655-663, 1992.

149. Worthley LIG: *Synopsis of intensive care medicine,* London, 1994, Churchill Livingstone.

150. Yucha CB, Toto KH: Calcium and phosphorus derangements, *Crit Care Nurs Clin North Am* 6(4):747-766, 1994.

151. Zehender J et al: Right ventricular infarction as an independent predictor of prognosis after acute inferior myocardial infarction, *N Engl J Med* 328(14):981-988, 1993.

Management of Behavioral Manifestations in the Critically Ill Patient

A patient may experience a myriad of fears and concerns when admitted to the technologically sophisticated world of critical care. The patient enters a complex setting where staff members converge with a variety of procedures and supportive devices in an attempt to monitor, strengthen, or stabilize the physiological condition. The patient is immediately separated from significant others and surrounded by strangers who move about the critical care environment with familiarity and professional expertise. Although the patient may feel secure knowing that skilled and knowledgeable health care personnel are attending to the physiological crisis, feelings of anxiety, anger, depression, hopelessness, and powerlessness may also be experienced during the critical illness.

Anxiety occurs as a reaction to a threat to the person; the threat encompasses potential physiological loss, lifestyle changes, potential death, invasive procedures, or concerns about the unknown. The critically ill patient's biological integrity has been temporarily or permanently compromised, and the patient responds by becoming anxious.

As the patient's illness, injury, or disease begins to stabilize, anger may be manifested. Anger may be expressed verbally or turned inward in the form of blame or depression. The critically ill patient who has always enjoyed good health experiences tremendous stress when confronted with an illness that leads to limitations, disability, or disfigurement.

Depression can also result when feelings associated with a major loss have broken through an individual's defense. The patient's normal performance is decreased, leading to a perceived negative view of self, experiences, and the future. Depression is also a manifestation of felt hopelessness.

Hopelessness is associated with the patient's feeling of personal deficit and is an attempt to ward off feelings of despair. The critically ill patient may feel that a particular physiological alteration is irreversible and that there are no alternatives available. Generally the patient is unable to cope and unable to mobilize energy on his or her own behalf.

Powerlessness is a perceived lack of control. The patient feels unable to control the outcomes of the illness. In this instance, the critically ill patient feels physiological, cognitive, environmental, and decisional powerlessness.

Regardless of the specific behavioral manifestations, critical care nurses can reduce the patient's feelings of anxiety, direct anger to the appropriate source, and assist the patient in recognizing a positive view of self, experiences, and the future. The nurse can also provide a realistic sense of hope and foster physiological, cognitive, environmental, and decisional control.

ANXIETY

Clinical Brief

Anxiety is a state of apprehension or tension within a person that occurs when an interpersonal need for security and/or freedom from tension is not met. Anxiety's origin is nonspecific or unknown to the individual.

Risk factors

Lack of control over events
Threats to self-control
Threat of illness or disease
Threat of hospital environment
Separation from others
Role changes
Sensorimotor loss
Financial problems
Threat of death
Divorce
Unemployment
Forced retirement
Threat of invasive procedures or supportive devices
Situational or maturational crisis
Loss of status
Unfamiliar environmental settings

Inability to comprehend the consequences of illness
Obstruction of goals
Dependence
Lack of knowledge
Loss of decision-making power

Presenting signs and symptoms

Regulatory	Cognitive
Palpitations	Apprehension
Nausea	Nervousness
Increased respiratory rate	Fear
Increased heart rate	Agitation
Diaphoresis	Irritability
Muscle tension	Withdrawal
Vertigo	Anger
Elevated blood pressure	Regression
Hand tremors	Inability to concentrate
Increased palmar sweating	Forgetfulness
Increased gastrointestinal activity	Lack of initiative or motivation
Insomnia	Escape behavior
Urinary frequency and urgency	Helplessness
Dilated pupils	Loss of control
Flushing	Thinking of past versus present
Faintness	Crying
Dry mouth	Loss of self-confidence
Paresthesia	Worry
Vomiting	Tension
Dilation of bronchioles	Overexcitement
Weakness	Reduced perceptual field
	Excessive verbalization

▶ **Nursing Diagnosis:**   Anxiety
OUTCOME CRITERIA
- The patient recognizes the anxiety and communicates anxious feelings.
- The patient's agitation eases in response to specific therapeutic relaxation interventions.
- The patient, family, or significant other exhibits a reduction in anxiety.
- The patient experiences an increase in physiological comfort.
- The patient initiates measures to decrease the onset of anxiety.

- The patient uses appropriate coping mechanisms in controlling anxiety.

INTERVENTIONS

1. Establish a reassuring interpersonal relationship with the patient.
2. Provide information about threatening or stressful situations, including invasive procedures and the sensations that might be expected.
3. Use simple terms and repetition to provide information regarding the current illness, the purpose of interventions, and changes in care.
4. Encourage patients to acknowledge and communicate their fears; clarify the patient's reaction to anxiety.
5. Minimize anxiety-provoking stimuli in the environment and encourage the use of progressive muscle relaxation, biofeedback, hypnosis, autogenic relaxation, meditation, or imagery.
6. Use therapeutic touch to relax the patient before and during perceived stressful situations.
7. Help the patient establish goals, knowing that small accomplishments can promote feelings of independence and self-esteem and allow the patient a degree of control.
8. Give the patient positive feedback when alternative coping strategies are used to counteract feelings of anxiety.
9. Discuss the ICU transfer plans with the patient to keep the patient aware of his or her progress and impending discharge. (See p. 45.)
10. Administer antianxiety agents and monitor the patient's response, noting potential side effects.

ANGER

Clinical Brief

Anger is an emotional defense that occurs in an attempt to protect the individual's integrity and does not involve a destructive element. Anger is a relatively automatic response that occurs when the individual is threatened, and can be internalized or externalized.

Risk factors

Anger expression inhibited: internalization

    Perceived threat involving:

        Blocked goal

        Failure of individuals to live up to the patient's expectations

        Disappointment

        Blow to self-concept

        Illness perceived to be life-threatening

        Physical dependence

        Altered social integrity

    Agent of harm located:

        Authoritative figure (health care giver) perceived to be
          threatening

        Family

        Self

Anger directly expressed: externalization

    Perceived threat involving:

        Obstructed goal

        Role changes

        Financial dependence

    Agent of harm located:

        Environment

        Critical care team

Presenting signs and symptoms

Regulatory	Cognitive
Increased blood pressure	Clenched muscles or fists
Increased pulse rate	Turned away body
Increased respirations	Avoidance of eye contact
Muscle tension	Tardiness
Perspiration	Silence
Flushed skin	Sarcasm
Nausea	Insulting remarks
Dry mouth	Verbal abuse
	Argumentativeness
	Demanding attitude

▶ **Nursing Diagnosis:**   Individual coping, ineffective: anger
OUTCOME CRITERIA
- The patient is able to identify situations contributing to
  expressions of anger.
- The patient monitors behavior leading to internalization
  or externalization of anger.

INTERVENTIONS
1. Establish a reassuring interpersonal relationship and encourage the patient to acknowledge and express feelings of anger.
2. Assist the patient in identifying situations contributing to
   the expression of anger.

3. Explore with the patient reasons behind angry feelings and ways in which the patient's behavior can change.
4. Teach the patient to evaluate feelings that lead to either internalization or externalization of anger.
5. Encourage the family to accept the patient's behavior without judgment.
6. Encourage the patient to participate in decision-making and self-care.
7. Provide diversional activities as ways to reduce stress.
8. Teach the patient to use progressive relaxation technique, meditation, or guided imagery to reduce feelings of anger and hostility.
9. Assist the patient in identifying positive aspects of the illness or injury and assist the patient in using alternative coping strategies.

DEPRESSION

Clinical Brief

Depression is any decrease in normal performance, such as slowing of psychomotor activity or reduction of intellectual functioning. It covers a wide range of changes in the affective state, ranging in severity from normal, everyday moods of sadness or despondency to psychotic episodes with risk of suicide.

Risk factors

DISEASES
    Acute life-threatening illnesses
    Chronic and/or end stage diseases
DRUGS
    Sedatives
    Tranquilizers
    Antihypertensive medications
    Corticosteroids
ELECTROLYTE IMBALANCES
    Bicarbonate excess
    Hypercalcemia
    Hypomagnesemia
    Hyperkalemia
    Hypokalemia
    Hyponatremia
LOSS
    Financial loss
    Loss of control

Separation/loss from significant others
Loss of bodily function
Feeling of powerlessness or guilt
Role or lifestyle changes

Presenting signs and symptoms

Regulatory	Cognitive
Constipation	Agitation
Diarrhea	Anger
Headaches	Anxiety
Indigestion	Avoidance
Insomnia	Boredom
Menstrual changes	Careless appearance
Muscle aches	Confusion
Nausea	Crying
Tachycardia	Denial
Ulcers	Dependence
Weight loss or gain	Emptiness
Anorexia	Fatigue
	Fearfulness
	Feeling of worthlessness
	Guilt
	Hopelessness
	Indecisiveness
	Indifference
	Irritability
	Loss of interest
	Loss of feeling
	Low self-esteem
	Poor communication skills
	Sadness
	Self-criticism
	Sleep disturbance
	Slow thinking
	Social withdrawal
	Submissiveness
	Tension
	Tiredness

▶ **Nursing Diagnosis:** Individual coping, ineffective: depression
OUTCOME CRITERIA
• The patient will be able to communicate when feeling depressed.

- The patient initiates measures to decrease feelings of depression.
- The patient uses appropriate coping mechanisms in controlling depression.

INTERVENTIONS

1. Assist the patient in identifying situations contributing to feelings of depression.
2. Encourage the patient to discuss the illness, treatment, or prognosis.
3. Assist the patient in achieving a positive view of self by facilitating accurate perception of the illness, disease, or injury.
4. Assist the patient in establishing realistic goals, knowing that small accomplishments can enhance positive feelings of the future.
5. Encourage the patient to participate in self care and to assume decision-making control in the care.
6. Assist the patient in facilitating realistic appraisal of role changes.
7. Provide the patient with personal space in the technical environment.
8. Give the patient positive feedback when the patient accomplishes specific tasks.
9. Administer antidepressive agents and monitor the patient's response, noting any potential side effects.

HOPELESSNESS

Clinical Brief

Hopelessness is an emotional state displaying the sense of impossibility, the feeling that life is too much to handle. It is a subjective state in which an individual sees limited or no alternatives or personal choices available and is unable to mobilize energy in own behalf.

Risk factors

Threats to internal resources:
    Autonomy
    Self-esteem
    Independence
    Strength
    Integrity
    Biological security
Threats to perceptions of external resources:
    Environment

Staff
Family
Abandonment
Failing or deteriorating condition
Long-term stress

Presenting signs and symptoms

Regulatory	Cognitive
Weight loss	Reduced activity
Appetite loss	Lack of initiative
Weakness	Decreased response to stimuli
Sleep disorder	Decreased affect
	Passivity
	Interference with learning
	Muteness
	Closing eyes
	Saddened expression
	Noncompliance with treatment regimen

▶ **Nursing Diagnosis:** Hopelessness
OUTCOME CRITERIA
- The patient will regain adequate self-care.
- The patient will assess situations causing feelings of hopelessness.
- The patient will identify feelings of hopelessness and goals for self.
- The patient will maintain relationships with significant others.

INTERVENTIONS
1. Provide an atmosphere of realistic hope.
2. Inform the patient of progress with the illness, disease, or injury.
3. Teach the patient how to identify feelings of hopelessness and encourage the patient to accept help from others.
4. Encourage the patient to express feelings about self and illness by active listening and asking open-ended questions.
5. Evaluate whether physical discomfort is causing the patient's feeling of hopelessness.
6. Create the environment to facilitate the patient's active participation in self-care.
7. Encourage physical activities that give the patient a feeling of progress and hope.
8. Provide the patient with positive feedback for successful attempts at becoming involved in self-care.

9. Assist the patient in identifying and using alternative coping mechanisms.

POWERLESSNESS

Clinical Brief

Powerlessness is the perceived lack of control over current and future physiological, psychological, and environmental situations.

Risk factors

Sensorimotor loss
Inability to communicate
Inability to perform roles
Lack of knowledge
Lack of privacy
Social isolation
Inability to control personal care
Separation from significant others
Loss of control to others
Lack of decision-making control
Fear of pain

Presenting signs and symptoms

Regulatory	Cognitive
Tiredness	Apathy
Fatigue	Withdrawal
Dizziness	Resignation
Headache	Empty feeling
Nausea	Feeling of lack of control
	Fatalism
	Malleability
	Lack of knowledge of illness
	Anxiety
	Uneasiness
	Acting out of behavior
	Restlessness
	Sleeplessness
	Aimlessness
	Lack of decision-making
	Aggression
	Anger
	Expression of doubt about role performance
	Dependence on others
	Passivity

▶ **Nursing Diagnosis:** Powerlessness

OUTCOME CRITERIA

- The patient identifies situations causing feelings of powerlessness.
- The patient exhibits control over the illness and care.
- The patient experiences an increase in physiological control.
- The patient engages in problem-solving and decision-making behaviors.
- The patient seeks information about the illness, treatment, and prognosis.
- The patient establishes realistic goals that foster an increased sense of control.

INTERVENTIONS

1. Provide consistent health care members to provide care and information regarding the illness, treatment, and prognosis.
2. Encourage the patient to express feelings about self and illness, and situations in which powerlessness is felt.
3. Accept the patient's feelings of anger caused by a loss of control and provide the opportunity for control (e.g., in establishing privacy, informing the patient about sensory changes associated with invasive procedures).
4. Encourage the use of progressive relaxation, meditation, and guided imagery techniques to achieve a sense of acceptance or uncontrol (letting go).
5. Encourage the patient to ask questions, seek information, and participate in making decisions pertaining to self-care.
6. Teach the patient how to accept the illness and potential changes in lifestyle.
7. Listen to the patient's discussion regarding possible role changes and financial concerns and assist the patient in redefining the illness situation to identify positive aspects.
8. Teach the patient how to document progress through maintaining a journal.

REFERENCES

1. Averill J: *Anger and aggression: an essay on emotion,* New York, 1982, Springer-Verlag.
2. Biaggio MK: Therapeutic management of anger, *Clin Psychol Rev* 7:663-675, 1987.

3. Carpenito LJ: Anxiety. *Nursing diagnosis application to clinical practice,* New York, 1983, J.B. Lippincott.

4. Carpenito LJ: Powerlessness. *Nursing diagnosis application to clinical practice,* New York, 1983, J.B. Lippincott.

5. Field N: Physical causes of depression, *J Psychosoc Nurs Ment Health Serv* 23:7-11, 1985.

6. Kendell PC, Watson D: *Anxiety and depression distinctive and overlapping features,* New York, 1989, Academic Press, Inc.

7. Light RW et al: Prevalence of depression and anxiety in patients in COPD, *Chest* 87:35-38, 1985.

8. McFarland GK, McFarlane EA: Anxiety. *Nursing diagnosis and interventions: planning for patient care,* ed 2, St Louis, 1993, Mosby.

9. McFarland GK, McFarlane EA: Hopelessness. *Nursing diagnosis and interventions: planning for patient care,* ed 2, St Louis, 1993, Mosby.

10. Moch SD: Towards a personal control/uncontrol balance, *J Adv Nurs* 13:119-123, 1988.

11. North American Nursing Diagnosis Association: *Classification of nursing diagnosis: proceedings of the ninth national conference,* St Louis, 1990, Mosby.

12. Noyes R, Roth M, Burrows GD: *Handbook of anxiety,* New York, 1988, Elsevier Publishing.

13. Roberts SL: Anger. *Nursing diagnosis and the critically ill patient,* Norwalk, CT, 1987, Appleton & Lange.

14. Roberts SL: Anger and hostility. *Behavioral concepts and the critically ill patient,* ed 2, Norwalk, CT, 1986, Appleton-Century-Crofts.

15. Roberts SL: Anxiety. *Nursing diagnosis and the critically ill patient,* Norwalk, CT, 1987, Appleton & Lange.

16. Roberts SL: Cognitive model of depression and the myocardial infarction patient, *Prog Cardiovasc Nurs* 4:61-70, 1989.

17. Roberts SL: Depression. *Behavioral concepts and the critically ill patient,* ed 2, Englewood Cliffs, NJ, 1985, Prentice Hall, Inc.

18. Roberts SL: Depression. *Nursing diagnosis and the critically ill patient,* Norwalk, CT, 1987, Appleton & Lange.

19. Roberts SL: Hopelessness. *Behavioral concepts and the critically ill patient,* ed 2, Englewood Cliffs, NJ, 1985, Prentice Hall, Inc.

20. Roberts SL: Hopelessness. *Nursing diagnosis and the critically ill patient,* Norwalk, CT, 1987, Appleton & Lange.

21. Roberts SL: Powerlessness. *Behavioral concepts and the critically ill patient,* ed 2, Englewood Cliffs, NJ, 1985, Prentice Hall, Inc.

22. Roberts SL: Powerlessness. *Nursing diagnosis and the critically ill patient,* Norwalk, CT, 1987, Appleton & Lange.

23. Roberts SL, White BS: Powerlessness and personal control model applied to the myocardial infarction patient, *Prog Cardiovasc Nurs* 5:84-94, 1989.

24. Rubin J: The emotion of anger: some conceptual and theoretical issues, *Prof Psychol Res Pract* 17:115-124, 1986.
25. Schneider J: Hopelessness and helplessness, *J Psychosoc Nurs Ment Health Serv* 23:12-21, 1985.
26. White BS, Roberts SL: Powerlessness and the pulmonary alveolar edema patient, *Dimens Crit Care Nurs* 12:127-137, 1993.

CHAPTER 4

Care of the Child in the Adult ICU

When a child is admitted to an adult intensive care unit (ICU), the nurse must be prepared to make necessary modifications in care. Rosenthal[39] proposed the "PEDS framework" to assist the adult intensive care nurse in the care of the child who is admitted to the adult ICU. The PEDS framework includes the following components:

*P*sychosocial and *p*hysical aspects
*E*nvironment and *e*quipment
*D*elivery of fluids, blood components, and medications
*S*afety issues

*P*SYCHOSOCIAL AND *P*HYSICAL ASPECTS

Psychosocial Issues

Like most adult patients, the child admitted to the ICU is in the presence of an unfamiliar and threatening ICU environment. For the adult ICU nurse, the care of the critically ill child may also be unfamiliar and threatening. Proactive assessment and planning for the child's and family's psychosocial and developmental needs are prerequisites to therapeutically and effectively communicating with the child and family. Important psychosocial skills for the nurse to incorporate into care include the following:

1. Integrating developmentally sensitive communication skills and behavioral assessment techniques into the nursing care of the child and family
2. Identifying concepts regarding family-centered care and methods of incorporating these concepts into the care of the child and family

Communication Skills and Behavioral Assessment Techniques

One of the essential elements of communication is establishing trust with the child and family. Demonstrating developmentally sensitive interaction with the child is important in gaining the family's sense of trust. Information from the admission history, such as cognitive and physical age of the child, and any history of chronic or previous acute illness requiring hospitalization may assist in individualizing care for the child and family.

As compared to the adult patient who may consciously screen most behaviors and the spoken word, the young child does not. The young child, subconsciously, communicates behaviorally through verbal, nonverbal (body language, behaviors), and abstract cues (play, drawing, storytelling) (Table 4-1) Although the child's behavior is more natural in

TABLE 4-1 Components of a Pediatric Behavioral Assessment

Verbal
    What is the child saying?
    Does the child understand what is being said?
    Do significant others understand the child?
    Does the verbal communication seem appropriate to the child's age?
Affective or nonverbal
    Posture
    Gestures
    Movements or lack of movement
    Reactions or coping style
    Facial expression (general, eyes, mouth)
Abstract
    Play or exploration or lack thereof
    Artistic expression through drawings or choice of color
    Storytelling
    Third-person techniques
Is there congruency among the types of behaviors?

Modified from Rosenthal CH: *Pediatric behavioral assessment for the adult ICU nurse,* Trends 1990 Conference, Philadelphia, 1990, SEPA Chapter, AACN.

the home or a familiar environment, cues such as disinterest in a favorite toy or crying that ceases when a parent approaches the bedside suggest how a child is feeling or perceiving an event or the presence of an individual.

In general, the child's normal behavior is more activity oriented and emotional than adult behavior. These qualities of a child's behavior should be viewed as normal in average healthy children and may be used as parameters to contrast the critically ill child (Table 4-2).

Children can be categorized into groups according to physical and cognitive age and common developmental capabilities, tasks, and fears. However, all hospitalized children share common fears despite their cognitive or physical age. These fears include loss of control, threat of separation, painful procedures, and communicated anxiety.[48]

When the child's physical and cognitive age are the same, the nurse can generally predict the child's expected social, self, language, thought, and physical development capabilities. If the child's physical and cognitive ages are discrepant, the assessment phase is critical to identify the level at which the child is functioning and to incorporate age-appropriate expectations and interventions into the plan of care.

In depth psychosocial and developmental assessment is beyond the scope of this reference. However, Table 4-3 summarizes specific age-group characteristics with common parental considerations and nursing interventions.

Family-Centered Care

The most essential concept regarding the family is to value, recognize, and support family members in the care of their child. See the box on p. 363. Involving parents in assessing the child's level of comfort or in scheduling daily activities such as bathing, feeding, or physical therapy exercises demonstrates a commitment to the family's involvement in the child's care. The family is the "constant" in the child's life and is ultimately responsible for responding to the child's emotional, social, developmental, physical, and health care needs.[43] Table 4-4 includes some suggested methods of incorporating the family in the care of a critically ill child.

Appropriate support and incorporation of parents in the health care delivery system have the benefit of buffering the threats of the ICU environment on the child. Parents may assist or influence the child's cognitive appraisal or evaluation

Text continued on p. 363.

TABLE 4-2   Contrasting Affective Nonverbal Behavioral Cues of the Healthy and the Critically Ill Child

Healthy	Critically ill
Posture	
Moves, flexes	May be loose, flaccid
	May prefer fetal position or position of comfort
Gestures	
Turns to familiar voices	Responds slowly to familiar voices
Movement	
Moves purposefully	Exhibits minimal movement, lethargy, or unresponsiveness
Moves toward new, pleasurable items	Shows increased movement, irritability (possibly indicating cardiopulmonary or neurological compromise, pain, or sleep deprivation)
Moves away from threatening items, people	
Reactions/coping style	
Responds to parents coming, leaving	Responds minimally to parent presence, absence
Responds to environment, equipment	Responds minimally to presence, absence of transitional objects
Cries and fights invasive procedures	Displays minimal defensive responses
Facial expressions	
Looks at faces, makes eye contact	May not track faces, objects
Changes facial expressions in response to interactions	Avoids eye contact or has minimal response to interactions
Responds negatively to face wash	Minimally changes facial expression during face wash
Blinks in response to stimuli	Has increase, decrease in blinking
Widens eyes with fear	Avoids eye contact
Is fascinated with mouth	Avoids, dislikes mouth stimulation
Holds mouth "ready for action"	Drools, has loose mouth musculature
	Displays intermittent, weak suck on pacifier

TABLE 4-3 Age-Specific Characteristics, Parental Concerns, and Associated Nursing Interventions

Age group characteristics	Identified parental considerations	Nursing interventions
Infants (birth to 12 mos)		
Develops sense of trust versus mistrust	Needs bonding	Recognize identifiable changes in status.
Is not able to provide self-care	Needs encouragement to do "passive physiotherapy" (range of motion, stroking)	Adhere to handwashing and screen visitors for contagious illnesses.
Requires expert respiratory management	Needs encouragement to do parental tasks: feeding, touching, holding, bathing, changing diaper	Converse in a quiet, unabrupt manner.
Requires strict adherence to infection control	Needs assistance with interpreting sibling responses to hospitalization of infant	Encourage presence of parents and siblings, and assistance with activities of daily living.
Needs stimulation through sight and sound	Needs information and support for decision regarding continuation of breastfeeding	Act as surrogate in absence of parents.
Requires active play with toys		Provide mobiles to look at and toys to hold.
Experiences separation anxiety at approximately 8 months and older		Establish and maintain immediately accessible oxygen and emergency airway equipment.
		Anticipate and assist in meeting needs of breastfeeding mother.
		Recognize need and establish plan for management of pain and anxiety.
Toddler (1 to 3 yrs)		
Has prime concern of sense of autonomy and fear of separation	Needs encouragement to provide comfort measures and communication	Encourage parental participation through demonstration.

Is a dependent person but has own mind and will	Needs encouragement in holding child at bedside	Offer explanations of thoughts child might feel but cannot express (e.g., pain, Mommy not here).
Begins speech, albeit limited in use and vocabulary	Needs encouragement to participate in parental tasks: feeding, touching, bathing	Suggest parents avoid participating in painful procedures; instead, offer comfort afterward by holding, stroking.
Is concerned about body integrity	Needs assistance with interpreting sibling response to brother's or sister's hospitalization	Use sedation and restraints as necessary for safety.
Protects self from environment through avoidance, escape, and denial	Needs education regarding safety measures	Demonstrate procedures and/or illness by dressing up toys and dolls, using puppets (child life worker).
Requires active play		Hold, stroke, spend time with child (especially at bedtime) if parents absent.
Requires safe environment for play		Assess level of comfort and establish plan for management of pain and anxiety.
Regards parents as most significant persons		Offer support to child through simple, short explanations and direction (e.g., "no more," mommy's here).
Becomes especially lonely at bedtime		Maintain developmentally appropriate bowel/bladder routines and foster skill development when appropriate.

Continued.

From Soupios M, Gallagher J, Orlowski JP: Nursing aspects of pediatric intensive care in a general hospital, *Pediatr Clin North Am* 27(3):628-629, 1980.

TABLE 4-3 Age-Specific Characteristics, Parental Concerns, and Associated Nursing Interventions—cont'd

Age group characteristics	Identified parental considerations	Nursing interventions
Preschool (3 to 6 yrs)		
Wants to maintain acquired skills of doing for self; immobility is frightening	Needs encouragement in offering explanations of procedures and events, based on established trust with child	Demonstrate and discuss procedures with parents/family using understandable adult vocabulary.
Has vivid imagination and sense of initiative	Needs encouragement to participate in parenting tasks; reading, game playing, activities based on limits of child's illness, holding, stroking, communication	Allow child to participate in acquired tasks.
Is acquiring language through limited use of words		Answer questions; understand parent(s) may respond with denial through withdrawal.
Imitates adult behavior with potential accompanying sense of guilt	Needs assistance with anticipating needs of siblings	Allow child to demonstrate fears through role playing (e.g., using dressed up toys).
Develops concept of self and nonself by exploring environment and body and by questioning		Facilitate and assist in preparation for sibling visitation when appropriate.
Regards family members as significant persons		Personalize the room/bedside with familiar toys, pictures, blanket, music.
		Assess level of comfort and establish plan for management of pain and anxiety.
		Use restraints only as necessary for safety.
		Encourage emotional ties with home by encouraging parents to bring in child's favorite toys, games, pictures of pets and siblings, tape recordings.

School age (6 to 12 yrs)

Needs recognition of accomplishment; has strong sense of duty	Needs encouragement to promote reading, game playing, activities based on limits of child's illness	Use rewards such as stickers and verbal praise.
Experiences inferiority through unattainable achievement, possibly depleting sense of identity	Needs encouragement to provide comfort measures; can act as go-between in communication for explanations and reinforcement	Ascertain child's level of understanding to identify and correct misconceptions and offer explanations at appropriate level.
Is capable of verbalizing pain		Permit child participation in progressive self-care.
May demand overabundance of love and attention from parent and regress	Needs encouragement to participate in parenting tasks: holding, stroking	Understand and offer comfort for parental separation.
Requires that limits be set to foster a sense of security	Needs assistance in reality orientation with news of school and home	Be aware of verbal, nonverbal indications for pain and anxiety.
Regards school and related events as main focus of significant persons		Use child life worker for play therapy.
		Utilize computer games, videos, etc., as diversional activities.
		Offer child choices whenever possible.

Continued.

TABLE 4-3 Age-Specific Characteristics, Parental Concerns, and Associated Nursing Interventions—cont'd

Age group characteristics	Identified parental considerations	Nursing interventions
Puberty adolescence (12 to 19 yrs)		
Seeks identity, independence, and clarification of role in society after separation from family	Needs to understand potential for regression	Treat as adult based on level of psychological adjustment.
Is especially vulnerable to depersonalization and regression	Needs encouragement to promote awareness of disease and prognosis	Recognize and foster independence through participation in care.
May experience loss of body control, destroying sense of pride in own sexuality	Needs encouragement to treat adolescent as an adult	Set limits but encourage decision making in planning of care.
Attempts to identify own sense of belonging, self-esteem	Encourage touching and communication	Encourage personal belongings at bedside.
Is concerned with body image change through surgery or illness	Needs assistance with anticipating needs of adolescent	Include peers in visiting policies, since relationships are moving away from family.
Regards peer group as significant persons		Use music, news of peer group and home events as comfort measures.

Elements of Family-Centered Care

Recognize that the family is the constant in a child's life and that the service systems and personnel within those systems fluctuate.

Facilitate parent/professional collaboration at all levels of health care.

Honor the racial, ethnic, cultural, and socioeconomic diversity of families.

Recognize family strength and individuality and respect different methods of coping.

Share with parents, on a continuing basis and in a supportive manner, complete and unbiased information.

Encourage and facilitate family to family support and networking.

Understand and incorporate the developmental needs of infants, children, and adolescents and their families into health care systems.

Implement comprehensive policies and programs that provide emotional and financial support to meet the needs of families.

Design accessible health care systems that are flexible, culturally competent, and responsive to family-identified needs.

From National Center for Family-Centered Care: *Key elements of family-centered care,* Bethesda, MD, Association for the Care of Children's Health, brochure.

of the environment, personnel, and events. The child often uses the reactions of the parent as a barometer in interpreting events from the range of threatening to beneficial.

The presence and participation of parents in the care of their critically ill child offer three kinds of support: emotional, tangible, and informational.[44]

Young friends or family members can also offer support by visiting the child hospitalized in the ICU. It is important to remember that the patient's needs and desire to have visitors, as well as the appropriateness of another child visiting the ICU, should be assessed and respected. The number of child visitors may increase when children are hospitalized in the adult ICU, necessitating a structured plan to address epidemiological issues and educational needs related to the child visitor. A child can be a carrier of organisms that pose a risk to pediatric and adult patients who are immunocompromised and/or critically ill. Rotavirus and respiratory syncytial virus

TABLE 4-4   Support Offered by Child's Parents, Suggested Activities, and Nursing Interventions

Support offered	Parent activity	Nurse intervention
Emotional	Parent presence	Support open visitation. Support parent and child while parent takes breaks. Assess parents' ability to care for themselves. Assess the status of siblings.
Tangible	Assist in physical care: bathing, turning, stroking, feeding Assist in diversional activities: playing, reading, music	Assist parent to revise role of a parent of a well child to the role of a parent of a sick child.
Informational	Provide facts and knowledge that will assist the child in coping Provide feedback that the child is secure and will recover	Keep parents informed regarding rationale of events and child's progress. Support parents in providing appropriate feedback to child.

(RSV) are seen in the adult population as secondary contacts from pediatric cases. Thus in a patient care setting with a mixed population, cross contamination must be prevented. To decrease this risk, a pediatric health screening tool (Figure 4-1) can be developed. The tool can provide an objective measure to determine if the visitor is eligible to enter the ICU, and it can be easily implemented by ICU staff.

Children who are visitors to the ICU may not know what to expect upon entering the ICU, nor what is expected of them while visiting their friend or relative. Polaroid pictures of the hospitalized child and the ICU environment can provide a visual explanation of what the visiting child can expect to

Health Screening Tool

Visitor's name: _____

Instructions: Interview the pediatric visitor or parent/caretaker of the prospective visitor. If any of the boxed answers are marked, the visitor is deemed ineligible to enter the patient care area.

Does the pediatric visitor have (or had in the past two weeks) any of the following symptoms:

	Yes	No
Fever	Yes ___	No ___
Cough	Yes ___	No ___
Sore throat	Yes ___	No ___
Runny nose	Yes ___	No ___
Conjunctivitis	Yes ___	No ___
Skin lesions/rash	Yes ___	No ___
Diarrhea/vomiting	Yes ___	No ___

Figure 4-1   An example of a health screening tool. (Critical Care Nursing Service, National Institutes of Health.)

Continued.

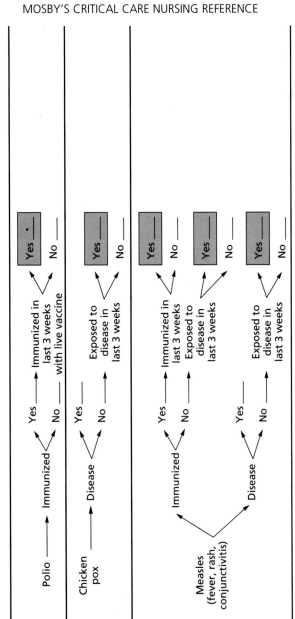

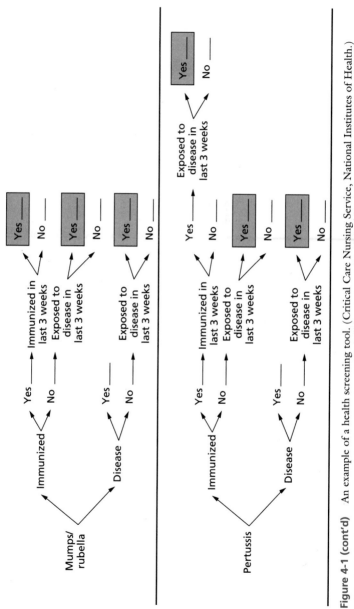

Figure 4-1 (cont'd)   An example of a health screening tool. (Critical Care Nursing Service, National Institutes of Health.)

see. The visiting child's response to the pictures can also help in determining the appropriateness of the visit or any additional preparation needed. It is important to educate the young visitor(s) about policies such as handwashing, identify "safe" places for them to stand or sit, and explain unusual sights and sounds. Structure the first visit based on the age and needs of both the hospitalized child and the visiting child. For example, the visiting child can count bandages, hold the patient's hand, give kisses, or simply hang a picture that the child has drawn. The visiting child should be accompanied by a supportive adult who is prepared to assist in meeting the needs of that child, and can provide explanations and a continuous physical presence throughout the visit.

PHYSICAL ASSESSMENT

Approaching the child in a therapeutic and age-appropriate manner will not only facilitate the assessment process but also lessen the threatening nature of the experience. The reader is encouraged to incorporate the essential psychosocial skills previously discussed into the physical assessment process. Important physical assessment skills include the following:

1. Interpreting vital signs based on age-appropriate norms as well as the child's present clinical condition
2. Modifying assessment techniques based on the anatomical and physiological differences and similarities of the child and adult
3. Recognizing the decompensating child using a quick examination approach

Interpreting Vital Signs

Although assessment of the child requires a knowledge base of normal physiological parameters (Table 4-5), it is imperative to note the importance of observing vital signs before stimulation. Most physiological parameters such as respiration, heart rate, and blood pressure will vary with the presence of a foreign or threatening stranger. Baseline parameters are the most useful and are obtained at rest or sleep if possible. As in the adult, expect that pain, fear, fever, and activity will normally increase the child's vital signs.

It is important to compare the child's vital signs to not only the age-appropriate "norms," but also to the present clinical condition. Normal vital signs may not be appropriate to the sick child. For example, the child who is ill should

TABLE 4-5   Pediatric Vital Signs

Age	Heart rate	Respirations	Systolic BP
Newborn	100-160	30-60	50-70
1-6 wk	100-160	30-60	70-95
6 mo	90-120	25-40	80-100
1 yr	90-120	20-30	80-100
3 yr	80-120	20-30	80-110
6 yr	70-110	18-25	80-110
10 yr	60-90	15-20	90-120
14 yr	60-90	15-20	90-130

Modified from Seidel JS, Henderson DP: *Prehospital care of pediatric emergencies,* Los Angeles Pediatric Society, California Chapter 2, Los Angeles, 1987, American Academy of Pediatrics.

compensate by increasing heart rate, respiratory rate, and temperature in the presence of pneumonia. Since a child's primary means of increasing cardiac output is by increasing heart rate, inability to increase heart rate or a slowing in heart rate may be a sign of decompensation, especially in the face of a worsening clinical picture. Trends in vital signs, rather than single parameters, are usually more reflective of the child's clinical course.

Anatomical and Physiological Differences in Children

An understanding of the anatomical and physiological differences in children is necessary to make appropriate modifications in assessment techniques and to interpret physical findings. The following are critical anatomical and physiological differences in the adult and child:
1. Neurological differences
   - Neurological functioning: at birth, the infant functions at a subcortical level composed primarily of brainstem functioning and spinal cord reflexes. Cortical development is 75% complete by 2 years of age.
   - Cranium: at birth, the child's cranial sutures are not completely fused. Complete fusion of the cranium is complete at 18 to 24 months of age, with posterior fontanel closing by 3 months and anterior fontanel closing at 9 to 18 months of age.
   - Rate of brain growth: brain growth is rapid during the first few years of life. The newborn's brain is 25% of

mature adult weight at birth, and at 2½ years, it has reached 75% of mature adult weight.

- Reflexes: in addition to intact protective reflexes, several newborn reflexes are present. Moro reflex is present until 6 months of age. Rooting reflex is present until 4 months of age. Grasp reflex is present until 3 months of age. Babinski's reflex is present until 9 to 12 months of age or at the time of walking.
- Motor ability: motor ability develops following the loss of newborn reflexes and the acquisition of voluntary motor skills.
- Meningeal irritation: in addition to nuchal rigidity and Kernig's and Brudinski's signs, the young child may display paradoxical irritability, which is heightened irritability in response to normally soothing interventions, such as cradling.
- Response to injury: in response to trauma, the child has a lower incidence of mass lesions[6] and a higher incidence of intracranial hypertension[27] and is more likely to develop "malignant brain edema."[6]

2. Cardiovascular differences
- Heart rate: the infant and young child have a higher heart rate than the adult. The higher heart rate assists the child in meeting the need for a higher cardiac output despite a smaller stroke volume. As in the adult, coronary artery filling time occurs during diastole; in the young child, diastolic filling time is shorter.
- Skin (end-organ perfusion): the child's skin is thinner than that of the adult's; therefore it will display color changes rapidly and easily. Skin color, texture, and temperature are of great significance during assessment of the child. However, the temperature of the environment and presence of warming devices should be considered.
- Peripheral perfusion: the presence and quality of peripheral pulses in the adult and young child are the same. Capillary refill is normally recorded in seconds rather than as brisk, normal, or slow. In an ambient temperature environment, normal capillary refill time in children is less than 2 seconds. However, the time of two seconds has not been scientifically validated.
- Circulatory blood volume: the child has an estimated blood volume that varies with age and weight. Despite

a higher ml/kg of body weight volume, the overall total circulating volume is small. A small amount of blood loss can be significant in the child.

- Blood pressure: the child can compensate for up to a 25% blood loss before the systolic blood pressure falls.

3. Respiratory differences

- Basal metabolic rate: the newborn's metabolic rate is almost twice that of the adult's in relation to body size. This increased metabolic rate leads to a higher minute volume secondary to an increased respiratory rate and increased oxygen consumption.
- Airway patency: due to the infant's large head (in proportion to body size), weak, underdeveloped neck muscles, and lack of cartilaginous support to the airway, poor head and neck position alone may compress or obstruct the airway. The narrowest part of the child's airway (until approximately 8 years of age) is at the level of the cricoid ring as opposed to the glottic opening in the adult.
- Airway size: the infant and young child's airways are smaller in diameter and in length and thus require smaller artificial airways. Airway compromise can be caused by the slightest amount of inflammation or edema, mucous plugs, and small foreign bodies or foods (such as popcorn or peanuts).
- Chest characteristics: the young child has a very thin, compliant chest wall that rises and falls easily with adequate ventilatory efforts. Due to the thin chest wall, breath sounds can be heard louder than breath sounds in the adult.
- Respiratory muscles: both the accessory muscles of the neck and back and the intercostal muscles are poorly developed in the young child. As in the adult, the major muscle of respiration is the diaphragm. However, the child is more diaphragm dependent due to the weak accessory and intercostal muscles.

4. Gastrointestinal differences

- Contour of abdomen: the abdomen of an infant and young child is normally soft and protuberant and becomes flat at approximately the time of adolescence.
- Stomach capacity: stomach capacities vary with the age of the child. A newborn's stomach capacity is 90 ml, a 1-month-old's is 150 ml, a 12-month-old's is 360 ml, and an adult's is 2000 to 3000 ml.

- Stomach emptying time: the infant and young child have a gastric emptying time of approximately 2½ to 3 hours, which lengthens to 3 to 6 hours in the older child. The infant has an immature cardiac sphincter and may experience reverse peristalsis, leading to regurgitation.
- Liver border: the position of the liver border beyond the costal margin varies with age. It is normally up to 3 cm below the costal margin in the newborn, 2 cm below the costal margin in a 1-year-old, and 1 cm below the costal margin in a 4- to 5-year-old.
- Bowel function: bowel function remains involuntary until 14 to 18 months of age, at which time myelination of the spinal cord is complete.
- Nutritional needs: the child has larger obligate energy needs because the major metabolic organs make up a larger percentage of body weight. The child also has lower macronutrient stores (proteins, fats, and carbohydrates). The lack of stores and high metabolic rate place the child at risk for protein calorie malnutrition. The child requires more calories per kilogram of body weight to meet these larger requirements.

5. Renal differences
- Urine output: the infant has less ability to concentrate urine and therefore has a normal urine output of 2 ml/kg/hr. For the child and adolescent, normal urine output is 1 ml/kg/hr and 0.5 ml/kg/hr, respectively.
- Body surface area (BSA): the infant and young child have a larger BSA in relation to body weight than the adult. Maintenance fluid requirements are precisely determined according to body weight or BSA.
- Fluid volume status: the child's extracellular fluid compartment consists of a higher percentage of body fluids than the adult's. In addition, the child has a higher insensible water loss because of the higher basal metabolic rate, higher respiratory rate, and larger BSA.

6. Endocrine differences
- Glucose metabolism: glucose production is increased in the neonate and the child up to 6 years of age (4 to 8 mg/kg/min), then slowly falls to adult levels (2 mg/kg/min). The infant and young child have smaller glycogen stores and an increased glucose demand because of the larger brain-to-body-size

ratio. Therefore hypoglycemia is a concern in this population.

7. Immunological differences
   - Inflammatory response: the newborn has fewer stored neutrophils and is less able to repeatedly replenish WBCs in the presence of overwhelming infection. Complement levels do not reach adult levels until 24 months of age, thus affecting chemotactic activity of phagocytes and opsonization of bacteria.
   - Humoral immunity: the newborn has a limited ability to differentiate B lymphocytes to mature plasma cells. Although the fetus and newborn synthesize small amounts of immunoglobulin, most is received via placental transfer from the maternal host. Physiological hypogammaglobulinemia occurs at approximately 4 to 5 months of age.
   - Cell-mediated immunity: although the infant/child has all the components to perform cellular immunity, the opportunity to refine abilities to respond to bacteria, viruses, and fungi is nonexistent.

Pediatric Head-to-Toe Assessment

Because of anatomical and physiological differences, assessment techniques must be modified. The following assessment is described in a systematic head-to-toe format; however, assessing the pediatric critically ill patient requires flexibility. Assuming the child's physical condition does not require immediate interventions, preforming the least invasive assessment techniques first may build trust with the child and family, as well as prevent disruption of the remaining assessment. As with the adult patient, the child's physical and psychological condition may dictate the priority and sequence in which the data are collected.

Neurological

LEVEL OF CONSCIOUSNESS

Level of consciousness is determined by assessing the state of arousal and orientation of the infant/child. (See Tables 4-1 and 4-2 to assess a child's behavior and interaction with the environment.)

Wakefulness or arousability is assessed in the same manner as in the adult and may vary from spontaneous arousability to no response to noxious stimuli. In fact, fear alone may be a noxious stimulus that arouses the child. If it is necessary to assess the child's response to pain, the intensity of the sternal pressure must be modified to avoid injury to the skin or chest wall. Orbital and nipple pressure is not recommended in the pediatric patient. If examining a young child's eyes, care should be taken to avoid injury to the thin and fragile eyelids.

Orientation can be assessed by using the age-appropriate Glasgow Coma Scale. The adult and infant Glasgow Coma Scales are presented for comparison in Table 4-6.

TABLE 4-6   Adult and Infant Glasgow Coma Scales*

Activity	Adult Best response	Points	Infant Best response
Eye opening	Spontaneous	4	Spontaneous
	To verbal stimuli	3	To speech
	To pain	2	To pain
	No response to pain	1	No response to pain
Motor	Follows commands	6	Normal spontaneous movements
	Localizes pain	5	Localizes pain
	Withdrawal in response to pain	4	Withdrawal in response to pain
	Flexion in response to pain	3	Flexion in response to pain
	Extension in response to pain	2	Extension in response to pain
	No response to pain	1	No response to pain
Verbal	Oriented	5	Coos, babbles
	Confused	4	Irritable crying
	Inappropriate words	3	Cries to pain
	Incomprehensible sounds	2	Moans to pain
	No verbal response	1	No verbal response

*Possible points of 3-15; score of <8 = coma.

CRANIAL NERVE ASSESSMENT

Cranial nerve physiology is the same in the adult and child. However, the assessment of cranial nerve function may be challenging in the young child. Moving toys and familiar objects across the field of vision and having a child stick out his or her tongue are ways to elicit cranial nerve function.

HEAD CIRCUMFERENCE

Because brain growth is rapid during the first few years of life, measurement of head circumference is important in the child up to 2 years of age. The circumference of the child's head is related to intracranial volume and estimates the rate of brain growth. A measuring tape is held securely over the child's occipital protuberance and the forehead, but it should not cover the ears. The measurement is recorded in centimeters. Table 4-7 reviews the average head circumference of children, although abnormal trends found in sequential measurements are more significant than an isolated measurement.

FONTANELS

Fontanels provide a useful parameter to assess hydration or potential increased intracranial pressure. Bulging fontanels

TABLE 4-7   Average Head Circumference

Age	Mean (cm)	Standard deviation (cm)
Birth	35	1.2
1 mo	37.6	1.2
2 mo	39.7	1.2
3 mo	40.4	1.2
6 mo	43.4	1.1
9 mo	45	1.2
12 mo	46.5	1.2
18 mo	48.4	1.2
2 yr	49	1.2
3 yr	50	1.2
4 yr	50.5	1.2
5 yr	50.8	1.4
6 yr	51.2	1.4
7 yr	51.6	1.4
8 yr	52	1.5

Modified from Lowrey GH: *Growth and development of children,* Chicago, 1986, Mosby.

may be seen with increased intracranial pressure or with fluid overload. Sunken fontanels may be seen with fluid deficit.

NEWBORN REFLEXES

The newborn reflexes most commonly assessed are the Moro, rooting, grasp, and Babinski's reflexes. The *Moro* reflex is tested by producing a loud noise such as hand clapping near the infant. The response should be abduction of the arm and shoulder; extension of the arm at the elbow; extension of the fingers, with a C formed at the thumb and the index finger; and later, adduction of the arm at the shoulder. In other words, in a normal response the infant moves the upper extremities out and then curls in as if to try and provide self-comfort.

The *rooting* reflex is tested by stroking one side of the infant's cheek. The normal response is for the infant to turn toward the stimulus and suck. The *grasp* reflex is tested by pressing a finger into the infant's palm. The normal response is for the infant to grasp the examiner's fingers. *Babinski's* reflex is tested by stroking the lateral aspect of the sole of the feet. The normal response in the infant is a fanning of the toes and dorsiflexion of the big toe.

MOTOR RESPONSE

Motor response can be assessed by evaluating muscle strength, tone, and coordination, as well as by using the Glasgow Coma Scale. If the infant/child moves the extremities spontaneously, movements should be of equal strength and tone. Although the expected findings are the same in the adult and child, the methods of assessment may be different. The infant/child may require a creative stimulus such as a favorite toy to reach for as an encouragement to move.

Cardiovascular

HEART RATE

Heart rate (see Table 4-5 for normal ranges), although an important indicator of cardiac function and fluid volume status, should not be assessed in isolation. *Tachycardia* is a nonspecific response to a variety of entities such as pain, anxiety, fever, shock, and hypoxemia. Bradycardia often produces significant changes in perfusion, since cardiac output is largely heart rate dependent. An acute event of *bradycardia* is most often caused by vagal stimuli, such as intubation, suctioning, nasogastric (NG) tube insertion, and defecation. Bradycardia in infants is a typical initial response to hypoxemia. However, older children will typically have a tachycardic compensatory response to hypoxemia. Bradycardia in the older child may indicate failure of compensatory mechanisms and impending arrest.

PERIPHERAL PERFUSION

Decreased perfusion to the skin is an early and reliable sign of shock. Before assessing the skin, the examiner should note the room temperature, since some findings may be a normal response to the environment (such as mottling in a drafty operating room). Mottling in a bundled infant or in a warm environment is reason for further investigation. Assess skin temperature as well as the line of demarcation between extremity coolness and body warmth. Coolness or the progression of coolness toward the trunk may be a sign of diminishing perfusion.

Skin and mucous membrane color may vary from pink, dusky, pale, to ashen grey. Cyanosis can be peripheral or central. Peripheral cyanosis is normal in newborns but an abnormal finding in young children, as in the adult. Central cyanosis is always an abnormal finding. Cyanosis is a sign of poor perfusion, but it is a late and unreliable indicator.

PULSES

Carotid, brachial, radial, femoral, dorsalis pedis, and posterior tibial pulses are readily palpable in healthy infants and children. Note differences between peripheral and central (carotid, femoral) pulses. Peripheral pulses may be decreased because of hypothermia or may be an early sign of decreased perfusion. A loss of central pulses is a late sign of diminished perfusion. A capillary refill time longer than 2 seconds is also an early sign of decreased perfusion.

BLOOD PRESSURE

Normal ranges for blood pressure can be found in Table 4-5. Blood pressure should not be used as the sole indicator of systemic perfusion because a child's blood pressure may be within the normal range even though a state of diminished perfusion exists (e.g., weak pulses, cool skin, capillary refill >2 seconds). Pulse pressure, an index of stroke volume, may be used to assess the adequacy of systemic perfusion. A decrease in pulse pressure or an increase in diastolic pressure may be detected before a drop in systolic blood pressure. However, clinical manifestations of decreased perfusion should alert the clinician of cardiovascular compromise despite the presence of a "normal" blood pressure. Hypotension is a late sign and may signal impending cardiac arrest. Hypertension is rare in the critically ill child unless renal or cardiac disease is present.

In the absence of renal or cardiac disease, hypertension may be an indicator of pain and anxiety.

Pulmonary

RESPIRATORY RATE

The higher basal metabolic rate in the child accounts for a higher respiratory rate. (See normal ranges in Table 4-5.) The infant and child will increase respiratory rates to compensate for increased oxygen demand. Tachypnea is often the first sign of respiratory distress. A slow respiratory rate in a sick child often indicates impending respiratory arrest. Associated conditions such as fever and seizure activity, which further increase the metabolic rate, will also increase oxygen requirements. These conditions can cause rapid deterioration in an already compromised child.

AIRWAY

The infant is an obligate nose breather until 6 months of age; thus obstruction of nasal passages can produce significant airway compromise and respiratory distress. Secretions, edema, inflammation, and poorly taped NG tubes or occluded nasal cannulas can cause obstructed nasal passages in the infant.

The child's airway is small and can easily become obstructed. Whether the child is breathing spontaneously or has an artificial airway in place, it is critical to check airway patency. In a child, the "sniffing" position is utilized to open the airway. Avoid overextending or overflexing the neck because the airways are easily collapsible. Note the position in which the child is maintaining airway patency. The child who needs to sit up and forward to breathe is experiencing significant airway obstruction.

In positioning the decompensating child for optimal airway patency, place a small roll horizontally behind the child's shoulders. This will place the head and neck in a neutral position. An ideal-sized roll for the infant or younger child is one or two adult pillow cases rolled up together or a folded baby blanket.

The infant's airway is short—3.6 to 6 cm as compared to the adult's airway length of 11 cm.[56] If intubated, the child's head should remain in the neutral, midline position because flexion, extension, or turning of the child's head can cause the endotracheal tube (ETT) to move. As the child is repositioned or turned side to side, it is important to maintain ETT positioning and monitor for any change in chest expansion or breath sounds. An ETT that is repositioned based on a chest radiograph taken while the child's head was not aligned properly can result in extubation or single lung ventilation.

THORAX

The thin, compliant chest wall normally allows for easy assessment of air entry. Air entry is assessed by observing the rise and fall of the child's chest. Unequal chest movement may indicate the development of a pneumothorax or atelectasis. Unequal chest movement may also indicate ETT obstruction or ETT displacement into the right mainstem bronchus.

Due to the child's flexible rib cage, which offers little stability to the chest wall, suprasternal, sternal, intercostal, and subcostal retractions may be seen in the child in respiratory distress. Assess for the presence, location, and intensity of retractions.

The accessory muscles in the infant and young child are poorly developed and cannot be relied on for respiratory effort. The infant and the child use abdominal muscles to assist with breathing. This gives the appearance of "seesaw" breathing, a paradoxical movement of the chest and abdomen. Seesaw breathing becomes more exaggerated with respiratory distress or airway obstruction. Nasal flaring and a "head-bob" movement with each breath may also signal severe respiratory impairment.

BREATH SOUNDS

Obstructed airways often produce sounds that are easily heard during assessment. Listen for expiratory grunting, inspiratory and expiratory stridor, and wheezing. Expiratory grunting is a sound produced in an attempt to increase physiological positive end-expiratory pressure (PEEP) to prevent small airways and alveoli from collapsing. As in the adult, stridor is usually heard with upper airway obstruction; wheezing is consistent with lower airway obstruction.

The infant and child's thin chest wall may allow the examiner to hear breath sounds over an area of pathology when sounds are actually being referred from another area of the lung. Listen for changes in the breath sounds as well as for their presence or absence. ETT placement should be visualized or confirmed with a chest radiograph if there is a sudden, unexplained change in ventilation or breath sounds.

Gastrointestinal

ABDOMEN

Although a protuberant abdomen is normal in the infant and young child, it is important to note if the abdomen is hard, firm, distended, or tender. Measure the abdominal girth at least every shift or more often if there is concern about abdominal distention. The measuring tape should be placed right above the umbilicus.

STOMACH

The stomach capacity of the infant and child is smaller than that of the adult (see p. 371), so caution must be taken when formulas or other fluids are instilled into the stomach. Bolus feedings should be of an appropriate amount, consistent with the child's stomach capacity. The volume of fluids used with diagnostic tests, such as barium swallows, should not exceed age-appropriate volumes. The fluid may need to be administered by feeding tube or NG tube in order to obtain an adequate volume in the necessary time.

Slower gastric emptying times must be taken into consideration with other nursing care activities. Allow an appropriate amount of time for absorption of formula before checking residuals. Caution should be used with large syringes or high pulling pressures with aspiration. Residuals of greater than half of the child's hourly feeding may necessitate further evaluation. If at all possible, residuals should be refed to the child. When the child is receiving chest physiotherapy, allow enough time or check the gastric contents before starting the procedure so that problems with reflux and aspiration will be minimized. It may be necessary to delay CPT, and adjust the feeding schedule to allow more time between feeds and CPT. Feeding tubes may be placed in the duodenum or jejunum to facilitate feeding in the child with impaired stomach function or difficulty with digestion.

Abdominal distention, secondary to retention of gastric contents or swallowed air, may restrict diaphragmatic excursion and place the child at risk for respiratory compromise. The stomach should be decompressed with a nasal or oral gastric tube, for example, to relieve distention that occurs with bag-valve mask ventilation.

LIVER BORDER

Determining the location of liver border should be part of the initial assessment and will establish a baseline for later comparison. The liver is normally not protected under the costal margin in the young child; thus when palpating the liver edge, it is wise to start at the iliac crest and move up until the liver border can be palpated.

If the liver extends 3 cm beyond the right costal margin, it may be an early sign of heart failure, tumor, or hepatitis.

Unlike adults, children sequester fluids in their liver during fluid overload, and liver enlargement may not be indicative of heart failure.

NUTRITION

The child has a high nutritional demand; therefore a thorough nutritional assessment is imperative. Table 4-8 lists the estimated nutrient needs per kilogram of body weight.

As in the adult, many parameters can be used to assess nutritional status in the child. Weight is a critical parameter. The child should be weighed daily at the same time and with the same scale. An unexplained weight loss of greater than 5% of the admission weight places the child nutritionally at risk. A weight loss of greater than 10% is associated with increased morbidity. A weight loss of greater than 30% is associated with increased mortality.[36]

Renal

URINE

Assessment of urine includes the amount, color, clarity, odor, specific gravity, pH and the presence of hemoglobin, ketones, glucose, protein, and bilirubin. Because the infant has less ability to concentrate urine, a low specific gravity does not necessarily mean that the infant is adequately hydrated.

HYDRATION

The child's kidneys are not as mature as the adult's and may not process fluid as efficiently. This makes the child less able to handle sudden large amounts of fluid and more prone to fluid overload.

A higher percentage of total body water and higher insensible water loss predisposes the child to dehydration. Carefully measure fluid intake and output (I & O), including weighing diapers and dressings. Sudden weight loss or gain indicates fluid imbalance (Table 4-9). An unexplained sudden change in weight could also indicate an error in weighing. Additional armboards, a wet diaper, or water in a ventilator tubing may significantly affect the weight of an infant or small child. Therefore it is important to record meticulous intake and output and make sure the change in weight correlates with the intake and output balance.

Signs of dehydration include dry mucous membranes, decreased urine output, increased urine concentration, sunken fontanels and eyes, and poor skin turgor. Circulatory decompensation accompanies severe dehydration. Fluid overload is evidenced by bulging fontanels, taut skin, edema (usually

TABLE 4-8 Recommended Dietary Allowances for Calories and Protein Based on Median Heights and Weights

Age	Wt (kg)	Ht (cm)	Kcal/kg	Kcal/day	Protein (g/kg)	Protein (g/day)
<6 mo	6	60	108	650	2.2	13
6-12 mo	9	71	98	850	1.6	14
1-3 yr	13	90	102	1300	1.2	16
4-6 yr	20	112	90	1800	1.1	24
7-10 yr	28	132	70	2000	1.0	28
11-14 yr (M)	45	157	55	2500	1.0	45
11-14 yr (F)	46	157	47	2200	0.8	44
15-18 yr (M)	66	176	45	3000	0.9	59
15-18 yr (F)	55	163	40	2200	0.8	44

M, male; F, female.
Modified from *Recommended dietary allowances*, Washington, DC, 1989, National Academy Press.

TABLE 4-9 Significant Weight Gain or Loss

Weight gain related to fluid overload	Weight loss related to dehydration
Infants	
>50 g/24 hr	Mild: 5% of body weight
	Moderate: 10% of body weight
	Severe: 15% of body weight
Children	
>200 g/24 hr	Mild: 3% of body weight
	Moderate: 6% of body weight
	Severe: 9% of body weight
Adolescents	
>500 g/24 hr	Mild: 3% of body weight
	Moderate: 6% of body weight
	Severe: 9% of body weight

periorbital and sacral), hepatomegaly, and other signs of heart failure.

Endocrine

GLUCOSE METABOLISM

The infant/young child's low glycogen stores and high glucose demand in average circumstances place the child at significant risk for hypoglycemia during states of psychological and physiological stress or prolonged fasting. Assessment of the length of the child's status without oral intake as well as quality and quantity of infusing intravenous (IV) fluids is paramount in assessing the child's risk for hypoglycemia. The presence of signs and symptoms of hypoglycemia should be noted, and serum glucose levels should be checked at regular intervals. (See box on p. 384.)

Immunological

INFECTION

Like the adult patient in the ICU, the pediatric patient is subjected to many situational aspects that carry the risk for infection. Admitting diagnosis, medical and nursing interventions, nutritional status, and stress may lead to an increased risk of infection. In addition, there are immunological, anatomical, and physiological differences that place the young child at risk. The infant experiencing an overwhelming infection may present

Signs and Symptoms of Hypoglycemia

Neonate	Infant/child
Pallor	Pallor, sweating
Tremors, jitteriness	Increased heart rate
Tachypnea	Nausea, vomiting
Feeding difficulties	Hunger, abdominal pain
Hypotonia	Irritability
Abnormal cry	Headache, visual disturbances
Apnea, cyanosis	Mental confusion
Convulsions	Convulsions, coma
Coma	

without the normal systemic signs, specifically fever and leuko-cytosis. Therefore it is extremely important for the nurse to be astute to the subtle signs of infection in the infant, such as changes in feeding behaviors, altered glucose metabolism, and altered temperature regulation (hypothermia).

Until the child's humoral and cellular immunity matures, the child is susceptible to numerous infections. The child is particularly susceptible to infections caused by viruses, *Candida* species, and acute inflammatory bacteria during the period of physiological hypogammaglobulinemia.

Assessment of Pain and Agitation

A number of assessment tools are available to assess pain in the child; however, assessment of pain and agitation in a child who is preverbal, or nonverbal secondary to pharmacological sedation or paralysis may be more difficult. Table 4-10 lists developmentally appropriate responses to pain and agitation in the infant and young child. However, children respond in a variety of ways and the nurse should involve the parents or caregivers in the assessment and relief of their child's pain.

Visual analogue scales or interactive tools may be used to assess pain if the child is alert, verbal, or at the appropriate cognitive level. Self report tools are appropriate for children older than four years of age; numerical rating scales may be used by children who are 8 or 9 years old. The Wong-Baker Faces Rating Scale is appropriate for 3- to 18-year-olds (Figure 4-2).

Behavior alone should be interpreted cautiously, since children may be coping with pain by watching TV, sleeping, playing, or lying still. A lack of response does not necessarily

Figure 4-2   Faces Pain Rating Scale. 1) Explain to the child that each face is for a person who feels happy because he or she has no pain (hurt, or whatever word the child uses) or feels sad because she or he has some or a lot of pain. 2) Point to the appropriate face and state, "This face is . . .": 0—"very happy because he or she doesn't hurt at all." 1—"hurts just a little bit." 2—"hurts a little more." 3—"hurts even more." 4—"hurts a whole lot." 5—"hurts as much as you can imagine, although you don't have to be crying to feel this bad." (Modified from Wong D: *Whaley and Wong's nursing care of infants and children,* ed 5, St Louis, 1995, Mosby. Wong-Baker FACES Pain Rating Scale: Available in Spanish, Portuguese, French, and Italian at no charge from The Purdue Frederick Company, 100 Connecticut Ave., Norwalk, CT 06850-3590; 203/853-0123, ext. 4010.)

TABLE 4-10   Developmentally Appropriate Responses to Pain or Agitation

	Motor movement	Communication
Newborn (0-3 months)	Generalized motor movements	Intermittent crying
Young infant (3 months)	Move/turn slowly	Sustained cry, moan, whimper
Infant (6 months)	Kick, pull away, wring hands, bite/pinch self	Anticipatory cry, fear cry
9 months	Push away, elevate, control limb	"Mommy"
12 months	Resist, tremors, bite towel	"Mommy"
18 months	Resist, tremors, bite towel	"Ow," "hurt"

mean lack of pain. Physiological indicators such as heart rate, blood pressure, and oxygen saturation are less sensitive indicators of pain and should be used as adjuncts to self report and behavioral observations such as facial expressions (e.g., wrinkled forehead, furrows between the brows, inability to elicit a smile) and body movements (e.g., clinging to parents, moving head from side to side, clenched fists). If the child is unwilling or unable to give a self report of pain, the parent's or caregiver's assessment of the child's pain should be used since they are the best individuals to potentially understand their child better than anyone else.

Recognizing the Decompensating Child

A quick and systematic examination that is congruent with the American Heart Association's pediatric advanced life support standards can be used to rapidly recognize a child in distress. Using this approach to conduct ongoing assessments of the critically ill child may prevent subtle clues of deterioration from being overlooked. Table 4-11 outlines extremes in critical physiological functioning that can be used to determine the degree of decompensation and the child's response to therapy.

ENVIRONMENT

Psychosocial Environment

The presence of pediatric patients in the adult ICU influences adult patients and their families, as well as fellow health care team members. It is a societal belief that children should not die and parents should outlive their offspring. Adult patients and staff who are exposed to the sights and sounds of the critically ill child may express a wide variety of emotions such as guilt, anger, and nontherapeutic empathy for the child and family. When another patient expresses concern for a crying child, it may be beneficial to offer a simple update, reassurance, or explanation for the sights and sounds.

Whether the nurse is an experienced pediatric clinician or an experienced adult clinician, approaching the bedside with confidence goes a long way in reinforcing the child's and family's level of trust in the care that they will receive. Small efforts to decrease anxiety such as sitting down or positioning yourself at the child's eye level when talking to the child can make a difference. A child's uneasy feelings may be in response to the parent's anxiety and the anxiety of the health care team members in the child's immediate environment. Interventions to relieve the anxiety of parents and fellow health team members will have a direct impact on the child's well-being. Interventions may include assisting parents/staff in anticipating the child's responses to therapy and illness and guiding parents/staff in therapeutic communication techniques.

TABLE 4-11 Quick Examination of a Healthy versus Decompensating Child

Assessment	Healthy child	Decompensating child
Airway		
Patency	Requires no interventions; child verbalizes and is able to swallow, cough, gag	Child self-positions; requires interventions such as head positioning, suctioning, adjunct airways
Breathing		
Respiratory rate	Is within age-appropriate limits	Is tachypneic or bradypneic compared to age-appropriate limits and condition
Chest movement (presence)	Chest rises and falls equally and simultaneously with abdomen with each breath	Has minimal or no chest movement with respiratory effort
Chest movement (quality)	Has silent and effortless respirations	Shows evidence of labored respirations with retractions Has asynchronous movement (seesaw) between chest and abdomen with respiratory efforts
Air movement (presence)	Air exchange is heard bilaterally in all lobes	Despite movement of the chest, minimal or no air exchange is noted on auscultation
Air movement (quality)	Breath sounds are normal intensity and duration per auscultation location	Has nasal flaring, grunting, stridor, wheezing, or retractions

Continued.

TABLE 4-11   Quick Examination of a Healthy versus Decompensating Child—cont'd

Assessment	Healthy child	Decompensating child
Circulation		
Heart rate (presence)	Apical beat is present and within age-appropriate limit	Has bradycardia or tachycardia as compared to age-appropriate limits and clinical condition
Heart rate (quality)	Heart rate is regular with normal sinus rhythm	Has irregular, slow, or very rapid heart rate; common dysrhythmias include supraventricular tachycardia, bradyarrhythmias, and asystole
Skin	Has warm, pink extremities with capillary refill ≤2 seconds; peripheral pulses are present bilaterally with normal intensity	Has pallor, cyanotic or mottled skin color; has cool to cold extremities; capillary refill time is ≥2 seconds; peripheral pulses are weak, absent; central pulses are weak
Cerebral perfusion	Is alert to surroundings, recognizes parents or significant others, is responsive to fear and pain, has normal muscle tone	Is irritable, lethargic, obtunded, or comatose; has minimal or no reaction to pain; has loose muscle tone (floppy)
Blood pressure	Has blood pressure within age-appropriate limits	Shows fall in blood pressure from age-appropriate limits (late sign)

All ICU patients, including the young child, may distort reality as a result of sensory overload or sleep deprivation. Interventions to reduce reality distortion in children are similar to interventions for the adult patient, (e.g., minimize the instances that the patient may be exposed to procedures or to the procedures experienced by other patients, manipulate the environment to reduce noise and lights, promote routine nap times, allow family visits, and allow the child's favorite stuffed animal or toy to be at his or her side).

Physical Environment

Planning a designated area

A specific area in the adult ICU should be designated and designed for the care of the child and family. The optimal solution is the design of glass-enclosed isolation rooms to physically separate the two populations of patients and to minimize the noise that is inherent in the care of children. Many adult ICUs allot a certain number of patient bedspaces in a specified location in the unit.

If a permanent designated space in the unit is not possible, modification of an individual bedspace may include the addition of a pediatric supply cart, limitation of extraneous bedside equipment, and placement of the child in a bedspace of the unit that facilitates a balance between low stimulation and adequate observation by nursing staff. Every effort should be made to create a nonthreatening "safe place" for the child and family that reduces exposure to sights and sounds of an open ICU environment.

Family support areas

Family support areas should be in close proximity to the unit. A waiting room, nutritional area, private consultation area, and sleeping accommodations are essential in meeting basic physical needs of families as they support their child through the ICU experience. If the physical environment is not conducive to supporting parents or significant others, it is extremely important that these needs be recognized and addressed daily with a professional resource person.

Pediatric supply cart

In the adult-pediatric ICU, it is difficult to predict the number and acuity of the patient census; therefore a mechanism to facilitate bedside equipment access and supply is important. The development of a pediatric supply cart consolidates the required equipment and allows routine intensive care delivery to the infant, child, and adolescent within an adult-oriented unit. Just as the adult equipment is maintained at the bedside ready for use, it is helpful to organize the same supplies in the appropriate sizes for pediatric use in a cart that may be rolled to any bedside depending on the circumstances of a pediatric admission. Some suggested items to include on the pediatric supply cart are listed in the box on pp. 391-392.

*E*QUIPMENT

Physical Assessment Supplies

Supplies to perform a physical assessment on a pediatric patient are essentially the same as those for an adult patient. The size of instruments is dependent on the size of the patient. Basic equipment for physical assessment includes a scale, stethoscope, blood pressure cuff, thermometer, measuring tape, and an otoscope with various size speculums.

Weighing devices

Because many therapies for the child, such as drug and fluid delivery, are weight specific, obtaining an accurate weight on or soon after admission is vital. Infant and adult scales should be available on the unit and should be able to measure in kilograms and grams, since the loss or gain of grams may be significant in a young child. (See Table 4-9.) If a weight cannot be determined, a pediatric resuscitation tape is available to assist in estimation of weight, drug dosages, and equipment size selection. Gram scales are also used to measure urine collected in a diaper or blood or body fluid loss on dressings and linen. The total weight of the diaper (g), minus the weight of a dry diaper, indicates the volume of urine (ml).

Stethoscope

Stethoscopes of any size can be used for auscultation; however, the small child has a more rounded chest wall, which may be auscultated more easily using a pediatric stethoscope with the smaller diaphragm and bell.

Blood pressure cuffs

The blood pressure cuff should be ⅔ to ¾ of the upper arm size, and the cuff bladder should completely encircle the child's arm only once. Various sizes should be readily available and used appropriately as determined by the size of the child. Table 4-12 reviews normal blood pressure cuff sizes in the pediatric patient.

Pediatric Supply Cart Contents

Drawer #1: reference cards and PALS guidelines

Broselow resuscitation tape or guidelines for selection of equipment based on size or weight

Drawer #2: intravenous therapy

20 ga 1'' IV catheter
22 ga 1'' IV catheter
24 ga ¾'' IV catheter
21 ga Butterfly needle
23 ga Butterfly needle
25 ga Butterfly needle
Extension set with T connector
Syringes (1, 3, and 6 ml)
Suture kits
Infant/child soft restraints
Bandages
Infant/child arm boards
Tongue blades
⁵⁄₁₆'' and ½'' penrose drains, rubber bands (infant/child tourniquets)
Safety pins (to secure restraints or armboards)
Cotton balls (to support/pad catheter hub)
IV site protection (commercially-made or medicine cup half)
Tape ½'' and 1''
Normal saline without preservative

Drawer #3: respiratory

Endotracheal tubes
Oxisensors (pediatric, infant)
Oral airways (4-5-6-7 mm)
Nasopharyngeal airways
Tracheostomy tubes (pediatric 00, 0, 1, 2, 3)
Pediatric or small oral suction device
Pediatric chest percussor (small, medium)
Junior or pediatric spirometer
Sterile tracheal suction catheters (5, 8, 10, 12, 14 Fr)
Bulb suction

Continued.

Pediatric Supply Cart Contents—cont'd

Drawer #4: cardiovascular

Small electrodes
BP cuffs (newborn, child, young adult)
Pediatric stethoscope
Sets of pediatric blood tubes
Sterile mosquito clamps
Sterile needle drivers (small)
Lancets or other device for fingersticks and heelstick

Drawer #5: GI/GU

Nasogastric tubes (8, 10, 12 Fr)
Feeding tube (5 Fr)
Measuring tape
Bottle
Nipple
Pacifier
Urine bags
Foley catheters (6*, 8, 10, 12 Fr)

Drawer #6

Pediatric chest drainage collection unit
Trocar catheters (10, 12, 14, 16)
Pediatric trach tray
Pediatric LP tray
Percutaneous line insertion tray
Central venous catheters (beginning with 4 Fr)
Suture (3.0, 4.0, 5.0 silk)
Intraosseous needles
IV tubing and buretrols, if used
Radiation shield
Baby blanket, medium-sized diapers

(*May use 5 Fr feeding tube if 6 Fr Foley not available.)

Noninvasive blood pressure

Blood pressure values obtained via the indirect method of mercury manometer and auscultation or palpation can be reliable. Repetitive measurements can be time-consuming; thus the use of automatic oscillometric monitors may be preferred. Research has determined that this device accurately measures blood pressure in the normotensive child. However, in the hemodynamically unstable child, the ability to accurately mea-

TABLE 4-12   Commonly Available Blood Pressure Cuffs

Cuff name*	Bladder width (cm)	Bladder length (cm)
Newborn	2.5-4	5-9
Infant	4-6	11.5-18
Child	7.5-9	17-19
Adult	11.5-13	22-26
Large arm	14-15	30.5-33
Thigh	18-19	36-38

*Cuff name does not guarantee that the cuff will be appropriate size for a child within that age range.
From Horan MJ: Task force on blood pressure control in children: report of the second task force on blood pressure control in children, *Pediatrics* 79(1):3, 1987.

sure acute pressure changes is questionable.[19] There is also some evidence that automatic oscillometric devices are less reliable in the lower pressure range, and may overestimate pressure in the infant experiencing hypotension.[9] It may be necessary to use doppler to assess blood pressure and peripheral pulses in the hemodynamically compromised child.

Temperature measurement

If using the standard glass thermometer, avoid obtaining the young child's temperature orally. There is a high risk of the child biting and breaking the instrument. In obtaining rectal temperatures, use only rectal-tipped thermometers to minimize the risk of perirectal damage. Rectal temperatures are avoided until a newborn passes the first meconium stool and when a child has diarrhea, rectal irritation, neutropenia, or thrombocytopenia. Tympanic thermometers offer a less invasive option of temperature measurement. The temperature obtained most closely correlates with core body temperature. Although the popularity and usage of this device is growing, the accuracy of the device in children with marked hypothermia and hyperthermia is still being validated. The device is not recommended for infants under three months of age. Consult the specific product information for specific age limitations. The accuracy of the tympanic thermometer directly correlates with the skill of the user and compliance with specific product usage guidelines. Core body temperature may be assessed using a Foley catheter with a bladder thermistor device, or using the thermistor of a pulmonary artery catheter that has been inserted for hemodynamic monitoring.

Measuring tape

A nonstretch measuring tape that has units in both centimeters and inches should be available to record head circumferences and abdominal girths. Head circumferences are generally measured in children less than 2 years of age.

Otoscope

Due to the high frequency of ear infections in the pediatric population, an otoscope with appropriate-sized speculum covers should be available.

Needles for Subcutaneous or Intramuscular Injection

Small, 30-gauge, ½-inch needles are available for uses such as subcutaneous injection of buffered lidocaine for local anesthesia. Issues regarding intramuscular medication delivery are discussed in the medication delivery section of this chapter.

Peripheral Intravenous Access

Intravenous catheter selection

The optimal IV catheter size is one that is the smallest gauge to achieve the intended therapy and not impair blood flow around the catheter once placed in the intended vessel. Catheter types are the same as those found for the adult population: butterfly needles and over-the-needle catheters. Table 4-13 reviews suggested catheter sizes according to patient age.

Site selection

Each site for IV catheterization has its advantages and disadvantages. As in the adult patient, the clinician should consider the condition of the vessels, the purpose for the IV infusion, and the projected duration of the IV therapy.

Scalp veins are easily found in infants, but they require shaving a portion of the child's head and may be aesthetically unpleasant to the parents. Preferably, upper extremity sites are used and include the dorsum of the hand and cephalic and median basilic veins. When selecting an upper extremity, the clinician should note the child's preference for right-sided or left-sided dominance and use the nondominant hand for the IV therapy. Antecubital veins are infrequently used because they limit the child's mobility and pose a greater risk for dislodgement. Lower extremity sites are usually avoided in the adult population because of venous stasis and increased risk for thrombosis. Compliance with this standard is attempted in

TABLE 4-13   Suggested Intravenous Catheter Sizes for Children

Age	Butterfly	Over-the-needle
Infant	25-27 ga	24 ga, range 22-26
Child	23-25 ga	22 ga, range 20-24
Adolescent	21-23 ga	20 ga, range 18-22

the pediatric population, especially if the child is near the age of walking. In the infant and toddler, veins such as the saphenous, median marginal, and dorsal arch are used if necessary.

IV access in the infant and young child may be time-consuming and difficult. A systematic approach should be in place to ensure efficient IV access in the event a pediatric patient requires resuscitation. According to PALS[7] recommendations, access is attempted in large peripheral veins three times or for a total of 90 seconds, whichever is less. If the child is over 6 years of age and initial peripheral access is unsuccessful, a percutaneous central venous access or saphenous vein cutdown should be attempted. If the child is 6 years of age or younger and initial peripheral access is unsuccessful, intraosseous (IO) access should be attempted.

Patient management

The process of insertion and maintenance of IV catheters is essentially the same in the pediatric and adult patient. Table 4-14 reviews the essential differences in the pediatric patient and the associated, necessary interventions.

Phlebotomy Issues

Blood volume requirements for laboratory analysis

It is essential to establish minimum blood volumes required for laboratory tests to minimize repeat testing and excessive blood loss. This determination should reflect a joint effort among existing general pediatric units, the hospital laboratory, the emergency department, and the ICU. Microtubes and/or pediatric blood tubes should be available along with reference sheets listing the required blood volumes for each test.

Blood loss

Blood loss associated with the blood drawn for laboratory analysis can be significant during a child's hospitalization. The amount of blood drawn from the patient should be

TABLE 4-14 Intravenous Catheter Insertion and Maintenance in Children

Difference	Result	Interventions
Cooperation	Difficulty is in accessing an uncooperative, moving target.	Explanation and preparation of infant is of minimal value, but prepare parent if present. Provide comfort and reassurance. Preparation of young child should be age-appropriate. Practice good positioning techniques of child (e.g., mummy wrap). Obtain assistance from another health care team member to hold child if necessary.
Security	Once IV is in place, difficulty is securing it due to small size of insertion site and frequent movement of child.	Prepare and use an arm board when necessary. For infant, make arm boards out of padded tongue blades. Select an IV site away from a joint or highly mobile area. Avoid dominant hand and feet, if ambulatory. Use soft restraints on affected extremity to minimize movement and risk of kinking or dislodging the catheter. Avoid circumferential taping. Use nonadhesive, easily removable, adherent wrap to stabilize IV without additional adhesive tape and potential skin breakdown.
Technique for venous distention	Because of young child's thin and sensitive skin, warm soaks may burn the patient and large tourniquets may be ineffective.	Obtain small latex drains or rubber bands for infants and small children or utilize a second person's hand to apply circumferential pressure above the insertion site. May use disposable diapers with warm water to wrap around extremity to dilate vessels, but keep the bed dry. Carefully check the temperature of any moist heat to avoid burning the child's thin skin.

documented in the fluid balance record. Estimating the child's circulatory blood volume (nl ~80 ml/kg) and comparing it with the total amount of blood withdrawn for analysis can assist the clinician in determining the severity of blood loss. When the volume of blood for analysis exceeds 5% to 7% of the circulatory blood volume, or if there is a significant decrease in hematocrit levels and accompanying symptomatology, blood replacement should be anticipated.[15]

Blood sampling

The majority of blood samples in the pediatric population are obtained through IV or intra-arterial lines, which increases the chance of sampling error secondary to contamination from intravenous fluids or flush solutions. An adequate discard volume should be withdrawn to clear the fluid from the sampling port of the catheter without contributing to excessive blood loss. Deadspace or the priming volume of the catheter is generally considered in determining the discard volume and the amount of flush solution used to clear the catheter once the blood sample is withdrawn. Discard volumes and flush volumes should be determined by each institution. The intravascular access should be "flushed" with each sampling and the amount of flush solution and discarded volume should be accurately measured and documented. The blood used to clear the line can be reinfused to minimize blood loss.

Intraosseous Access and Infusion

Description

Placing an access in the bone marrow cavity offers many advantages because the bone marrow functions as a rigid vein that does not collapse in the presence of hypovolemia or circulatory shock. The marrow sinusoids drain into the venous systems, where fluid or medication can be immediately absorbed into the general circulation. Blood products, fluids, and medications may be administered through the IO route, although it is recommended that hypertonic and alkaline solutions be diluted before infusion.[11,13] Complications of IO infusions have been reported in fewer than 1% of patients. (PALS) Potential complications include tibial fracture, compartment syndrome, skin necrosis, and osteomyelitis. Contraindications include osteogenesis imperfecta, osteoporosis, and a fracture in the extremity to be accessed.

The optimal site for IO placement during a resuscitative effort is the proximal tibia (Figure 4-3), which precludes

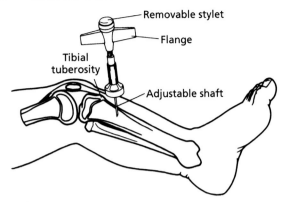

Figure 4-3 Intraosseous needle placement. Optimal insertion is in the medial, flat surface of the anterior tibia approximately 1 to 3 cm below the tibial tuberosity. The needle is directed at a 60- to 90-degree angle away from the growth plate to avoid the epiphyseal plate. (From Fiser D: Intraosseous infusion, *N Engl J Med* 322(22):1580, 1990.)

interference with ventilations and chest compressions. Reusable or disposable bone marrow needles, sizes 15 to 18 gauge, should be available.

Patient management

Once the IO access is in place, the needle should stand firmly upward without support, but it should be secured with tape and a sterile 2 × 2 to prevent dislodgement. As with any intravascular access, signs of extravasation and patency should be monitored. Heparin-saline flushes may discourage clotting of the access. The IO access is not meant to be a permanent access; therefore attempts should be made to acquire other IV access and discontinue IO needle as soon as possible.

ECG Monitoring

Continuous display of the child's electrocardiogram (ECG) and a system to accurately and clearly record a paper tracing are essential. The optimal pediatric ECG machine must be able to monitor and record rapid heart rates of 250 to 300 beats per minute. Because of the infant's irregular respiratory rate and the infant's and young child's propensity toward respiratory rather than cardiac arrest, the machine should also have the capability of monitoring respiratory rate and breathing pattern. Apnea alarm capability is an asset.

Electrodes should be smaller than adult electrodes to allow for sensitivity of the infant's and young child's thinner skin. The adhesive component of the electrode may be irritating to the skin if left in place for extended periods of time or if irritants, such as iodophor, are left in contact with the patch. To decrease the incidence of skin irritation, electrode patches and sites should be rotated on a regular basis. Skin preparation is essentially the same process as in the adult, and of equal importance in the pediatric patient. Electrode placement and chest landmarks are the same in the child and in the adult. If using the same system to monitor respiratory function, place the lower electrode on the abdomen to sense respiratory movement.

Pulse Oximeter

Pulse oximetry is essentially the same technique in the pediatric and adult patient, with a few exceptions. Because the skin is a reliable reflection of perfusion states, the child with poor peripheral perfusion is not an optimal candidate for pulse oximetry. In an impaired perfusion state the monitor will reflect inaccurate or unobtainable readings. In addition, the infant/young child tends to be more active, and movement of the extremity with the probe will lead to inaccurate readings. Site and size specific oximetry sensors are used. Alternative sites for the small infant or child include the hand area between the thumb and forefinger, or the medial aspect of the infant's foot. Skin under the sensor should be evaluated at least once every 8 hours. Sensor site may be rotated to prevent skin irritation from heat and pressure.

End Tidal CO_2 Monitoring

The indications and methods for end tidal CO_2 monitoring are the same in the adult and pediatric patient.

Peripheral Artery Catheterization

Indications and site selection

The indications and sites for arterial cannulation and monitoring are the same as for the adult patient. The selection of an arterial site for arterial cannulation is determined by the stability of the artery and the availability of sufficient collateral circulation. Radial artery cannulation is the most commonly used site after verification of collateral ulnar artery circulation using the Allen test. Other optional sites include femoral, pedal, posterior tibial, temporal, and axillary arterial sites.

Patient management

The most important issues regarding arterial lines in the child are patency and security of the line, regulation of the amount and pressure of the flush solution, setting of appropriate alarm limits, and monitoring for complications. It is recommended that arterial lines be sutured at the insertion site and luer lock connections used in the young child to minimize the risk of accidental dislodgement. There should be a continuous administration of heparinized intra-arterial solution to maintain patency. Consideration of the type of solution and need for heparinization and the amount of fluid that the child receives hourly and daily are important.

For infants and small children, it is recommended that the arterial line be placed on an infusion pump to regulate the flow and to avoid inadvertent administration of unnecessary fluid. Arterial lines should be slowly flushed using a manual flush method rather than the pigtail flush method, regardless of the size of the child. Manual flushing facilitates accurate intake assessment, avoids unnecessary pressures on small, fragile vessels, and limits retrograde embolization into the central circulation. Alarms for all hemodynamic lines should be set for age-appropriate limits and should remain on at all times.

Complications

Complications are similar to those found in the adult; however, children have an increased risk of vasospasm and thrombosis. Infusion of papaverine-containing solutions into arterial catheters has been shown to reduce the risk of catheter failure in pediatric patients.[20] However, its use is not recommended in neonates.

Central Venous Catheterization

Insertion and maintenance of these lines are the same in the child as in the adult. Commonly used sites include the femoral and the external and internal jugular veins. The subclavian vein can be used; however, there is a higher risk of complications associated with this location even by the expert clinician. This is due to the close proximity of the subclavian vein to the apex of the lung. Chest radiograph is required to confirm catheter position and evaluate for a potential pneumothorax.

Pulmonary Artery Catheterization

Description

Pulmonary artery catheters are indicated in children who are receiving the most aggressive therapies, such as high ventilator pressures, massive hemodynamic support, and/or barbiturate therapy for increased intracranial pressure. Pulmonary artery catheters are available in five sizes. Table 4-15 lists suggestions for the selection of a pulmonary artery catheter.

Insertion

Pediatric pulmonary artery catheters are much smaller in diameter than adult catheters, yet they are not much shorter. The femoral vein is a commonly used vessel because it can accommodate the entire length of the catheter and allows for correct placement of catheter ports. Adult pulmonary artery catheters may also have an additional port for infusion of fluids and medications, which pediatric catheters do not. The CVP port of the 5 Fr catheter is extremely small and clots easily; therefore it is not an optimal port for blood component administration.

Normal values

The pressures of the cardiac chambers and great vessels are the same in the child over 2 years of age as in the adult in the absence of congenital or acquired cardiac disease. Cardiac output varies greatly with size and body; therefore it is prudent to monitor cardiac index in children. The normal cardiac index ranges between 3.5 and 4.5 L/min/m².

Patient management

The same standards used for the management of arterial lines should be used for pulmonary artery lines (e.g., manual flushing, placing the catheters on infusion pumps for the infant or small child). In addition, the amount of solution used for cardiac output injectates is generally 3 or 5 ml rather than 10 ml and should be recorded as a part of the child's hourly intake. When using smaller volumes, iced injectate is recommended.

TABLE 4-15 Suggestions for Pulmonary Artery Catheter Sizes

Age	Size
Infant	4 Fr with no CVP port
1-3 yr	5 Fr with 10 cm CVP
3-8 yr	5 Fr with 15 cm CVP
8-14 yr	7 Fr with 20 cm CVP
≥14 yr	7 Fr with 30 cm CVP

CVP, central venous port.

Knowing the deadspace or priming volume of catheters is paramount to withdrawing the appropriate amount of discard blood and infusing the minimal amount of flush to clear the catheter. Table 4-16 shows an example of a reference that can be developed by clinicians to determine priming volumes of catheters commonly used in their institutions.

Assistive Respiratory Devices
Manual resuscitation bags

Unlike the adult 1 liter manual resuscitation bag, pediatric manual resuscitation bags are available in infant (250 ml) and pediatric (500 ml) sizes. The resuscitation bag should be capable of delivering one and one-half times the child's tidal volume (V_T), or 10 to 15 ml/kg, as well as 100% oxygen. For the pediatric bags to consistently deliver 100% oxygen at rapid respiratory rates, the manual resuscitation bag should have an oxygen reservoir.

TABLE 4-16   Priming Volumes of Central Catheters—Pediatric

Catheter type	Size/length	Capacity/lumen (ml)
Triple-lumen	5.5 Fr/8 cm	0.2
	5.5 Fr/13 cm	0.2
	5 Fr/8 cm	0.2
	5 Fr/12 cm	0.3
	5 Fr/15 cm	0.3
Double-lumen	4 Fr/5 cm	0.1
	4 Fr/8 cm	0.2
	4 Fr/13 cm	0.3
	4 Fr/30 cm	0.6
	3 Fr/8 cm	0.1
Swan-Ganz	5 Fr/75 cm	0.6 blue
	5 Fr/80 cm	0.5 blue
Introducer	6 Fr/7 cm	1.2
Manifold		0.1 proximal
		0.2 distal
Broviac	2.7 Fr	0.15
	4.2 Fr	0.3
	6.6 Fr	0.7

Developed by Uhlman L: 10D Adult/Pediatric ICU, National Institutes of Health, Bethesda, MD.

Most pediatric resuscitation bags are designed with a pop-off valve to prevent excessive pressure delivery with the average manual breath. Pop-off valves are normally activated with breaths requiring peak inspiratory pressures (PIPs) between 35 and 60 cm H_2O pressure, depending on the brand of resuscitation device. The pop-off valve is an operational device that reduces the incidence of barotrauma or gastric distention by releasing excessive pressure to the atmosphere rather than to the child. When manual ventilations are essential, this pop-off valve should be covered or deactivated to ensure maximal ventilation of the child, even if the lungs are stiff and require high PIPs. The pop-off valve is always open or activated unless covered with adhesive tape or the clinician's finger during manual breath delivery.

The infant's lung tissue is sensitive to high pressure ventilation. Pneumothoracies may be induced from aggressive manual or mechanical ventilation. A pressure manometer is connected in-line to the manual resuscitation bag to minimize excessive PIPs and to provide breaths similar in pressure to the mechanical breaths received from the ventilator. This is especially helpful in a unit that provides care to a variety of patient populations and may minimize the incidence of excessively high-pressure breaths being delivered. Although a pressure manometer can assist in minimizing pressure and the reservoir can assist in providing 100% oxygen, the only indicator to ensuring adequate V_T delivery is a clinical one. The adequate amount of V_T delivered during a mechanical resuscitation breath is the amount that causes an observable rise and fall of the child's chest.

Resuscitation masks

Like bags, resuscitation masks come in a variety of sizes ranging from neonatal to young adult. The ideal mask is one that covers the child's nose and mouth yet avoids pressure on the eyes. Clear masks are preferred so that the presence of vomitus or a change in lip color can be observed immediately. If absolutely necessary, the Laerdal face mask may be used upside down on the infant's face to completely cover the child's face while minimizing orbital pressure.

Artificial Airways

All pediatric airways are small compared to the overall body size of the patient. It is important to recognize that the smaller the airway, the more difficult it is to maintain position and patency.

Nasopharyngeal and oropharyngeal airways

The indications for the use of nasopharyngeal and oropharyngeal airways are identical in the pediatric and adult patient. The correct length for a nasopharyngeal airway in the infant or child is determined by measuring from the tip of the nose to the tragus of the ear. The diameter of the nasopharyngeal airway should be the largest size that easily inserts without causing blanching of the nares. The pediatric patient often has large adenoids and fragile nasal mucosa that can lacerate during the insertion process, causing significant nose bleeds. Nasopharyngeal airways should be maintained as patent as possible, since the infant is an obligate nose breather.

An oropharyngeal airway is particularly useful as an assistive device to bag-valve mask ventilations in the unconscious child. The proper size is estimated by placing the airway next to the child's face. The flange should be at the level of the central incisors, and the end should be approximately at the tip of the mandibular angle. Insertion is facilitated by using a tongue depressor to hold the tongue down onto the floor of the child's mouth. Because of the fragility of the child's oral mucosa, inserting the airway upside down and then rotating it 180 degrees is not recommended.

Endotracheal tubes

Unlike the adult patient, there are numerous sizes of ETTs available for the critically ill infant and child. To estimate the correct size of the ETT, choose a tube approximately the same size as the child's little finger, or use the following formula:

$$\text{Internal diameter} = \frac{16 + \text{age in yr}}{4}$$

It is important to recognize that both of these methods are estimations of the ETT size and that tubes one-half size (0.5 mm) larger and one-half size smaller should be available for immediate use. Generally, uncuffed ETTs are used in the child of less than 8 years of age because the narrow cricoid cartilage provides an anatomical cuff in the presence of physiologically normal lungs. Pediatric endotracheal cuffs are available in cuffed tubes and may be indicated in the patient with stiff, noncompliant lungs. To prevent accidental extubation, the ETT must be secured with adhesive tape, twill tape, or a commercially made tube holder, and the ventilator tubing must be secured in a position that allows the child to turn his or her head from side to side.

Pediatric intubation

Although the nurse is not primarily responsible for intubating the pediatric patient, an understanding of the procedure will help prepare the nurse to assist with this life-saving measure. Every effort should be made to intubate the child under controlled conditions using appropriately sized equipment to prevent unsuccessful intubation or airway damage (Table 4-17). Awake intubations should be considered only for resuscitation situations or when there is considerable question about whether the child can be ventilated by bag and mask when sedated and pharmacologically paralyzed. Rapid sequence sedation and paralysis with IV medications provide the clinician satisfactory visualization of the larynx in most cases. Cricoid pressure should be considered in all pediatric intubations to minimize aspiration.

Tracheostomy tubes

Tracheostomy tubes are available in neonatal and pediatric internal diameters. The difference between the neonate and pediatric sizes is in length of the airway. Pediatric-sized tracheostomy tubes are not available with cuffs unless the tube is custom ordered.

Patient management

HUMIDIFICATION

Humidity should always be provided with the use of any artificial airway. Respiratory distress can drastically increase the child's insensible water loss, increasing the vital significance of this intervention. Humidity will minimize insensible water loss, excessive drying of respiratory secretions, and the risk of occluding the artificial airway with mucous plugs. Humidity also prevents excessive drying and irritation of the airways.

SUCTIONING

Suctioning the child is the most common method used to determine patency of the artificial airway and to clear accumulated secretions.[56] Despite the frequency of this nursing intervention, care must be taken in the actual performance of the procedure to minimize complications.

Suction catheters are available in 5, 6, 8, 10, and 14 French sizes. The selected catheter should be large enough to obtain secretions without completely occluding the child's artificial airway. Suction catheters should be no more than

TABLE 4-17 Recommended Resuscitation Equipment for the Child

Age	0-6 mos	6-12 mos	1 yr	18 mos	3 yrs	5 yrs	6 yrs	8 yrs	10 yrs	12 yrs	14 yrs
Weight (kg)	3-5	7	10	12	15	20	20	25	30	40	50
Resus mask	0-1	1	1-2	2	3	3	3	3	3	4	4-5
Laryngoscope (Miller/Mac)	0	1	1	1	2	2	2	2	2	2	3
ETT	3	3.5	3.5	4	4.5	5	5.5	6	6	6.5	7
Suction (ETT/trach)	6	6	8	8	10	10	10	10	10	14	14
Suction (OP/NP)	10	10	10	10	14	14	14	16	16	16	16
Chest tube	10-12	10-12	16-20	16-20	16-20	20-28	20-28	20-28	28-32	28-32	32-42
NG/OG	8	8	8	8	10	10	10	10	12	12	14
Foley	6*	6*	8	8	10	10	10	10	12	12	14
Trach (ped)	00,0	1	1	1-2	2-3	3	3	4	4	5	6

*May use 5 Fr feeding tube.
Modified from Widner-Kolberg MR. Baltimore, 1989, Maryland Institutes for Emergency Medical Services Systems.

> ### Formula for Determination
> ### of Suction Catheter size
>
> **ETT size (mm) × 2 = suction catheter size (Fr)***
>
> **Example: 4.5 mm × 2 = 9 or**
> **= 8 Fr suction catheter**

*Round to next lowest size.

one-half the internal diameter of the ETT. See the box above for an easy formula to approximate suction catheter size.

Each pass of the suction catheter should not exceed 10 seconds. During suctioning, the wall suction pressure gauge should not exceed 100 mm Hg so that airway damage is minimized. Use of catheters with fixed markings that correspond with ETT markings alerts the clinician to the appropriate depth to suction and prevents mucosal damage. Another intervention to prevent mucosal damage that is practiced in some pediatric facilities includes measuring the suction catheter so that the catheter extends only beyond the end of the tracheostomy or ETT during the procedure. Once this measurement is determined, an example of the marked suction catheter should be posted at the child's bedside.

Mechanical Ventilation of the Child

The optimal ventilator

A ventilator must be able to deliver small but accurate V_Ts ($\leq$100 ml) against high airway resistance and low lung compliance because the young child has a higher basal metabolic rate, larger BSA, and a smaller airway diameter with higher airway resistance. Pediatric ventilators must be able to generate low and high inspiratory flow rates. A flow rate that is too high may result in the premature delivery of volume, the generation of unnecessary high pressures, and inadequate inspiratory/expiratory (I:E) ratios. A flow rate that is too low may not deliver the total V_T in the short inspiratory time available. Pediatric ventilators must have rapid response times or there will be poor coordination of the ventilator with the child's own breathing, thus increasing the child's work of breathing and the risk of not reversing the respiratory failure.

Modes of Mechanical Ventilation

Unlike the adult patient who is commonly ventilated using a volume-cycled ventilator, the pediatric patient may be ventilated using a variety of modes: volume cycled, pressure cycled, and time cycled.

Pressure-cycled ventilation is commonly used in the newborn or infant population because of the low V_Ts needed and because a continuous-flow system requires no extra energy to initiate a breath.

Pressure-controlled ventilation (using Siemens Servo C) is frequently used in the management of pediatric patients. This mode of ventilation permits airflow to reach a preset inspiratory pressure quickly in the inspiratory phase as opposed to near the end of the inspiratory phase (as occurs in pressure cycled). In pressure-controlled ventilation, the ventilator delivers breaths with a constant preset pressure at a preset rate. The pressure is maintained during the inspiratory effort. This mode may be advantageous because it encourages partially collapsed alveoli to open with sustained inspiratory pressure. This mode of ventilation may decrease the mean airway pressure in some patients.

Volume-cycled ventilation may be used to ventilate even small children if proper consideration is given to the compliance factor of the ventilator circuit. It is also important to assess whether the ventilator has a backup ventilation mode with parameters programmed that may be deleterious to the infant or child. For example, a machine with a backup ventilation mode that has a V_T of 500 ml could cause barotrauma in a child weighing 15 kg.

The choice of ventilator control may be critical to its success with a volume-cycled ventilator. Because small or weak children may have trouble opening the demand valve in the intermittent ventilation demand (IMV) circuit, hypoventilation is a real concern. Most current volume-cycled ventilators that are used in children have the options of assist control, IMV, synchronized IMV (SIMV), and pressure support. The use of SIMV with pressure support generally overcomes the problem of opening the demand valve and still allows the child the opportunity to breathe independently between ventilator breaths.

Time-cycled ventilation provides a continuous flow of gas in the respiratory circuit, which can decrease the work of breathing for the ill infant. In this situation the infant does not have to open a demand valve to access the next breath. The disadvantage to time-cycled ventilation is that the machine may have too low inspiratory flow capabilities and may not provide adequate flows for children who weigh more than 15 kg. Inspiration and expiration timing may be adjusted in an attempt to provide optimal ventilation. Sedation and paralysis may be required in order for the child to tolerate these adjustments.

Indications for Mechanical Ventilation

In addition to the broad, generic reasons for mechanical ventilation such as respiratory failure, pediatric patients commonly require mechanical ventilation to decrease the work and the oxygen cost of breathing.

Initial ventilatory settings

RATE

The ventilator rate is determined by the child's age-appropriate respiratory rate, taking into consideration the underlying pathophysiology as well as the desired V_T. For example, if the child is to receive a V_T on the low range of normal (10 ml/kg), the rate may be set higher. If the child is to receive a V_T on the high range of normal (15 ml/kg), the rate may be set lower. This allows the minute ventilation (V_E) to remain within a normal range.

TIDAL VOLUME

The standard V_T used in the pediatric patient is between 10 and 15 ml/kg. Although the ventilator may be set to deliver a V_T, the actual volume that the child receives may vary because of air leaks around the ETT or compressible volume in the ventilator circuit. With the use of predominately uncuffed ETT, a portion of the set V_T may be lost around the tube. Even if a cuffed tube is used (where it is standard to maintain a minimal leak), some volume will be lost. Therefore it is necessary to monitor the exhaled V_T or returned volume to estimate the delivered V_T.[29]

It is important to use pediatric ventilator circuitry (e.g., small bore with minimal compliance factor [compliance factors vary from 0.5 to 2 ml/cm H_2O]) because the adult circuitry may significantly alter the V_T the child actually receives.

PEAK INSPIRATORY PRESSURE

As in the adult patient, PIP is predetermined in the pressure-cycled and pressure-controlled modes of ventilation. It is a measured end product of V_T and inspiratory time in other modes of ventilation. It is important to recognize that the respiratory compliance is similar in all age groups, so it takes about the same PIP to ventilate the lungs of a normal infant, child, and adult.

Fraction of Inspired Oxygen (FIO_2)

As in adults, manipulations are made with various ventilation parameters to decrease the FIO_2 to below 0.40 whenever possible.

Positive End Expiratory Pressure

Normally, physiological PEEP assists in stabilizing alveoli and maintaining the functional residual capacity (FRC). The young child has a greater tendency to collapse the alveoli than the older child or adult because of the underdeveloped collateral ventilatory channels. As soon as a child is intubated, physiological PEEP is lost, leading to the general recommendation that the young child routinely receive 2 to 3 cm H_2O PEEP.[29] With acute lung injury syndromes in which the FRC is low, higher levels of PEEP may be used similar to adults with acute respiratory distress syndrome (ARDS).

Complications

A common complication of ventilation devices in both pediatric and adult patients is barotrauma with air leaks. Although the treatments are identical (e.g., chest tubes), the etiologies and identification of the problem may be different. The infant not only sustains mechanical barotrauma but may experience spontaneous pneumothorax. Identification of the presence of air leaks in the pediatric patient may be challenging. Their thin chest walls may lead to referred breath sounds over collapsed lung fields, and the ability of pediatric patients to maintain their blood pressures for prolonged periods despite a tension pneumothorax may mask the classic signs of pneumothorax. Table 4-18 shows the two most common complications found in the child receiving mechanical ventilation, the developmental or situational aspects placing the child at risk, and the associated interventions.

Resuscitation Equipment and Supplies

Table 4-17 provides a list of essential resuscitation equipment based on the age and weight of the child. These supplies are recommended as contents in a resuscitation cart serving pediatric patients. The items are suggested as additions to other equipment listed in the chapter and are not inclusive. Additional recommended supplies include infant and pediatric internal and external defibrillator paddles and an external pacemaker machine with appropriately sized pacer electrodes.

Drainage Devices

Chest drainage systems

The indications and uses of chest drainage systems are identical in the adult and pediatric patient. Two primary differences

TABLE 4-18 Complications of Mechanical Ventilation

Complication	Developmental/situational risks	Interventions
Extubation (inadvertent)	Infant/child is cognitively too immature to understand rationale for tube placement and security. Infant/child is more activity oriented. Infant/child is usually intubated with uncuffed tube. Although cuffed tube does not ensure security, it does assist in stability.	Use soft restraints or elbow restraints. Keep soft restraints for all extremities at the bedside. Provide adequate sedation and analgesia. Increase use of paralytic agents. Assess and document security of tube and markers at teeth/gums every hour. Consider nasotracheal intubation for long-term ventilation to increase stability and comfort. If using adhesive tape to secure ETT, utilize benzoin under tape to enhance adhesiveness.
Aspiration, gastric distention	Infant/child has delayed gastric emptying. Use of uncuffed ETTs is increased. Infant/child is prone to vomiting when extremely upset. Weak cardiac sphincter and large manual ventilation breaths increase the risk of introducing air into the stomach. Infant/child swallows air when upset and crying.	Place NG tube early. Facilitate gastric emptying with enteral medication delivery or feedings by placing patient on right side. Check residuals frequently. Assess stomach contents before upsetting procedures, Trendelenburg position, chest physiotherapy. Manually ventilate only with as much air that raises and lowers the child's chest.

include determining the size of the catheter and accurately measuring and interpreting the output. Various sizes are available to meet the needs of the different drainage purposes (air versus blood) and the size of the patient. (See Table 4-17.) Accurately measuring the hourly output from a chest drainage system is facilitated by numerical markings that are in small (1 to 2 ml) increments. It must be remembered that although the chest tube drainage may be small in absolute hourly output, it may be a significant proportion of the child's circulatory blood volume. A critical bleed following postoperative cardiac surgery is defined as 3 ml/kg of body weight for more than 2 hours and will require surgical intervention.[16]

Maintenance of chest tube patency is challenging in the presence of bloody drainage, since the lumen of these catheters are small. Chest tubes are not normally stripped because of the danger of creating excessively large negative intrathoracic pressures; however, in the presence of bloody chest drainage, gentle manipulation and stripping is imperative to maintain tube patency.

Gastrointestinal drainage devices

The indications and uses for gastrointestinal (GI) drainage devices are identical in the adult and pediatric patient but may have a greater significance in the pediatric patient because there is a greater incidence of aspiration and impedance to ventilatory efforts with abdominal distention. A variety of types and sizes of NG tubes are available. (See Table 4-17.) The smaller sized tubes, such as the 5 French, are referred to as *feeding tubes* because they are primarily used for this purpose. Polyurethane tubes are generally used for continuous or long-term feeding, but will collapse if aspiration is attempted. Movement of the contents in these tubes is generally left to gravity, and they are manually irrigated as needed. Levine tubes are available in a variety of sizes and do not have a vent lumen. The ordinary Salem sump tubes with a blue vent lumen are available in sizes 10, 12, and 14 French. These tubes may be connected to low intermittent wall suction, which should not exceed 100 mm Hg.

Due to the small lumen of the NG tubes, maintaining patency is challenging, especially if enteral medications are administered. Tube patency should be verified every 2 hours, and the tube should be irrigated if patency is questioned. Rather than irrigating with the standard 30 ml, it is wise to irrigate the pediatric NG tube with one and one-half times the deadspace volume of the tube, usually 5 to 10 ml to avoid excessive fluid administration to the child. All fluid entering and leaving the child's drainage system should be documented in the child's I & O record.

Urinary drainage devices

Urine output is an indicator of end-organ perfusion in the infant and young child and should be accurately measured every hour. Foley catheters are available in a variety of sizes. (See Table 4-17.) Sizes above a 6 French do not differ from adult Foley catheters other than the size of the lumen and the capacity of the balloon. Some 6 French Foley catheters use a stylet. The integrity and capacity of the balloon should be checked before insertion to avoid overdistending or breaking the balloon once in place. The double-lumen Foley used for continuous irrigation is not available in pediatric sizes. In the newborn or small infant, a 5 French feeding tube may be used as a urinary catheter. The catheter may be connected to a volufeeder or baby bottle for collection and measurement.

Urinary drainage bags or stoma bags may be used to collect urinary specimens or monitor urinary output. These devices are challenging to secure to the child, particularly the female patient. It is recommended that whatever urinary drainage device is chosen, a chux or diaper be placed under the child so that it can be weighed to determine any urine spillage or leakage. To test the specific gravity or pH of urine collected in a child's diaper, follow these steps:

1. Remove the top dry liner of the inside of the diaper to obtain urine-saturated fibers.
2. Place fibers into the barrel of a syringe.
3. Replace the plunger of the syringe and push the plunger, squeezing the urine from the syringe into a medicine cup.

Thermal Devices

Infants and young children have large BSAs in relation to body weight, which may place them at risk for hypothermia resulting in physiological instability. Infants cannot shiver to keep warm but rather undergo nonshivering thermogenesis to generate body heat. This is a limited capability because once the newborn burns brown fat, more cannot be generated. Furthermore, hypothermia shifts the oxyhemoglobin dissociation curve to the left, prevents the release of oxygen to the tissue, and increases oxygen consumption and glucose utilization in an effort to maintain the body's core temperature. The infant/young child who presents in respiratory distress may decompensate following exposure to the drafty ICU environment during invasive line placement. Thus it is important to provide a temperature-controlled environment and monitor body temperature closely, particularly in the newborn and young child patient population and those with head injury.

Over-the-bed radiant warmers

The radiant warmer can provide an environment that allows access to the child while maintaining the child's normal body temperature. It is recommended that the child remain uncovered and that the warmer be used in the mode in which the child's temperature regulates the amount of heat rather than the manual mode in which the machine delivers a certain percentage of power. Care should be taken to secure the skin temperature probe according to the manufacturer's directions and to frequently monitor both the skin probe temperature and the child's core temperature. The skin probe must be open to air for accurate temperature regulation. Clinicians and parents should avoid using oil-based solutions on the child while under the warmer, since this may lead to thermal burns similar to sunburn.

Hypothermia/hyperthermia devices and blood warmers

The indications, uses, and complications of thermal devices are the same in children and adults. Hyperthermia blankets are rarely used in the infant and young child because over-the-bed radiant warmers are so efficient. Cooling blankets are often helpful in controlling the body temperature of children who remain febrile despite antipyretic medications. If a thermal blanket is used, avoid placing the blanket on top of the child because the weight can impede ventilatory movement of the chest and abdomen. Cover the blanket with liners to avoid thermal tissue damage of unprotected skin. Airflow systems are available and easily adapted to accommodate the pediatric patient.

General indications for a blood warming device are the same as in the adult patient. Since blood warming devices are standardly equipped for large volume, rapid, gravity administration, it may be necessary to add an IV pump or manually draw the warmed blood into a 60 ml syringe and deliver it directly.

DELIVERY OF FLUIDS, MEDICATIONS, AND BLOOD

Fluid Management
Fluid requirements by weight

Each child is individually assessed for the amount and type of prescribed IV fluid. The average child maintenance fluid requirements may be determined by body weight (Table 4-19).

TABLE 4-19   Calculation of Daily Maintenance Fluid Requirements

Weight	Fluid requirement	Example
0-10 kg (>72 hr old)	100 ml/kg	Pt weight = 5 kg Pt wt (kg) × fluid requirement: 5 × 100 = 500 ml/day Hourly rate = 500 ÷ 24 = 21 ml/hr
11-20 kg	100 ml/kg for the first 10 kg or 1000 ml/day plus 50 ml/kg for each kg 11 through 20	Pt weight = 13 kg For the first 10 kg: 10 kg × 100 = 1000 ml For kg over 10 and ≤20 (total of 3): 3 kg × 50 = 150 ml $\quad$ 1000 ml $\quad$ +150 ml TOTAL 1150 ml/day Hourly rate = 1150 ÷ 24 = 48 ml/hr
21-30 kg	100 ml/kg for the first 10 kg or 1000 ml/day plus 50 ml/kg for each kg 11 through 20 plus 25 ml/kg for each kg 21 through 30	Pt weight = 26 kg For the first 10 kg: 10 kg × 100 = 1000 ml For kg over 10 and ≤20 (total of 10): 10 kg × 50 = 500 ml

Continued.

TABLE 4-19 Calculation of Daily Maintenance Fluid Requirements—cont'd

Weight	Fluid requirement	Example
		For kg over 20 and ≤30 (total of 6):
		6 kg × 25 = 150 ml
		1000 ml
		500 ml
		+150 ml
		TOTAL 1650 ml/day
		Hourly rate = 1650 ÷ 24 = 69 ml/hr
31-40 kg	100 ml/kg for the first 10 kg or 1000 ml/day	Pt weight = 32 kg
	plus 50 ml/kg for each kg 11 through 20	For the first 10 kg:
	plus 25 ml/kg for each kg 21 through 30	10 kg × 100 = 1000 ml
	plus 10 ml/kg for each kg 31 through 40	For kg over 10 and ≤20 (total of 10):
		10 kg × 50 = 500 ml
		For kg over 20 and ≤30 (total of 10):
		10 kg × 25 = 250 ml
		For kg over 30 and ≤40 (total of 2):
		2 kg × 10 = 20 ml
		1000 ml
		500 ml
		250 ml
		+20 ml
		TOTAL 1770 ml/day
		Hourly rate = 1770 ÷ 24 = 74 ml/hr

Fluid requirements by body surface area

The child's maintenance fluid requirements may also be calculated according to BSA. (To determine BSA, see nomogram in Appendix E.) Maintenance fluid requirements are 1500 ml/m^2/day. For example, a child weighing 8 kg who is 35 cm long and has a BSA of 0.43 m^2 requires 645 ml/day (1500 ml × 0.43 m^2 = 645 ml) at an hourly rate of 27 ml (645 ÷ 24 hr = 27 ml/hr).

Alteration in maintenance fluid requirements

Maintenance fluid requirements may be altered based on the child's disease state. Frequently, a child recovering from postoperative cardiac surgery, a neurological disorder, or a renal disorder is placed on restricted maintenance fluid requirements such as two-thirds maintenance fluid or replacement of insensible fluid loss only.

Accurate monitoring and delivery of fluid

It is imperative that fluid be administered accurately and safely to the critically ill child, since small fluid imbalances can be clinically significant. IV fluids are administered most commonly via an infusion device rather than by the gravity method. The gravity method is appropriate in very few instances due to the unreliability of the tubing clamps and patient and/or visitor exploration of the clamps. IV site should be observed for signs of infiltration at least every 1 to 2 hours.

Optimal pediatric infusion device

The optimal pediatric infusion device should have all the common safety alarms as well as the ability to accurately deliver small increments of fluid hourly (0.01 ml/hr). It is equally important, however, for the pediatric pump to deliver large, rapid fluid boluses (999 ml/hr). It is common for a nurse to use both macrorate and microrate devices at the bedside of a sick child.

Accompanying a pediatric infusion device should be the necessary IV tubing, small IV fluid containers, and buretrols, or solusets. Buretrols, or solusets, may not be used if another mechanism for controlled administration is available. IV tubing should ideally be microbore or contain the least amount of fluid as possible and have luer-locked connections. Attach an in-line buretrol so that the amount of fluid hanging at the child's bedside is not an inordinate amount. In case of pump malfunction or misprogram, the distal clamp of the buretrol will prevent delivery of the entire IV container to the child.

IV tubing should ideally contain the least amount of fluid as possible and have luer-locked connections.

Administration of Fluid Boluses

Fluid boluses include the intermittent delivery of either colloid or crystalloid fluid in an attempt to restore intravascular volume. For bolus fluid resuscitation therapy, pediatric advanced life support (PALS) standards recommend 20 ml/kg of isotonic crystalloid solution delivered as rapidly as possible (over approximately 20 minutes).

Important considerations regarding pediatric fluid boluses include (1) determination of the accurate amount and type of fluid, (2) rapid administration of fluid (given over 20 to 30 minutes), and (3) reevaluation of the patient for the need of another fluid bolus. Due to the small volumes of fluid and the small catheters with high resistances, gravity flow may not be sufficient to deliver a bolus efficiently. Fluid boluses are often drawn up in a 60 ml syringe and manually pushed. Dextrose-containing solutions are not recommended for fluid resuscitation because of the risk for hyperglycemia.

Blood Component Administration

The fundamental principles in blood component administration are the same in the adult and pediatric patient. The primary difference is the prescribed dose, which is determined by the child's weight. Table 4-20 reviews blood component therapy, suggested dose, and rates of administration.

Medication Administration

Dose determination

Since a child may be significantly smaller or larger than the average child in the associated age group, medications are prescribed on a microgram, milligram, or milliequivalent per kilogram of body weight basis rather than on a standard dose according to age. Confirming the weight (in kg) that is being used to determine drug dosages is important. This same weight should be used during the child's entire hospitalization unless the child substantially loses or gains lean muscle mass.

Route determination

The nurse should recognize that drug absorption can be erratic if topical, rectal, oral, subcutaneous, or intramuscular (IM) routes are used. Delayed gastric emptying, less subcutaneous

TABLE 4-20 Blood Component Administration in Children

Blood component	Usual dose	Rate of infusion	Comments
Whole blood	20 ml/kg initially	As rapidly as necessary to restore volume and stabilize the child	Administration is usually reserved for massive hemorrhage.
Packed RBCs	10-15 ml/kg	5 ml/kg/hr or 2 ml/kg/hr if heart failure develops	1 ml/kg will increase Hct approximately 1%. Infuse within 4 hr. If necessary, divide the unit into smaller volumes for infusion.
Platelets	0.1 unit/kg	Each unit over 5-10 min via syringe or pump	The usual dose will increase platelet count by 50,000/mm³.
Fresh frozen plasma	Hemorrhage: 15-30 ml/kg Clotting deficiency: 10-15 ml/kg	Hemorrhage: rapidly to stabilize the child Clotting deficiency: over 2-3 hr	Monitor for fluid overload.
Granulocytes	Dependent on WBC counts and clinical condition, 10 ml/kg/day initially	Slowly over 2-4 hr because of fever and chills, side effects commonly associated with infusion	Granulocytes have a short lifespan. Transfuse as soon after collection as possible.
Albumin 5%	1 g/kg or 20 ml/kg	1-2 ml/min or 60-120 ml/hr	Monitor for fluid overload. Type and crossmatch are not required.
Albumin 25%	1 g/kg or 4 ml/kg	0.2-0.4 ml/min or 12-24 ml/hr	Monitor for fluid overload. Type and crossmatch are not required.

fat, and less-developed muscle mass are a few factors that can affect drug absorption in the critically ill child. Thus, a greater number of medications are administered via the IV route.

Oral medications

For administration of oral medications to the young child, it is important to account for the child's developmental capabilities. The developmental level will determine the method of administering the oral medication (spoon, cup, nipple, or single-dose system with needleless syringe). Generally the child of less than 8 years of age is unable to swallow a pill. Many dosage forms cannot be crushed (e.g., sustained-released products); therefore it may be necessary to order the liquid dosage form.

Intramuscular medications

It is important to use the appropriate size syringe and needle to properly administer IM medications to the infant or young child. The amount of the medication, age of the child, and injection site are factors to consider (Tables 4-21 and 4-22). The gluteus maximus and deltoid muscles are avoided in the infant because these muscles are underdeveloped and nerves can be damaged. Seek assistance to restrain the toddler, pre-schooler, and school-aged child when an IM injection is required. Avoid asking the parent to restrain the child. Encourage the parent(s) to provide comfort and support during and after the procedure.

Continuous vasoactive infusions

For children weighing less than 40 kg, an easy method for preparing vasoactive continuous infusions in buretrols is listed in Table 4-23. In mixing the solution, it is important to

Text continued on p. 425.

TABLE 4-21   Intramuscular Injections According to Age Group

Age group	Needle length (in)	Needle gauge	Maximum volume (ml)
Infant	⅝	25-27	1
Toddler	1	22-23	1
Preschooler	1	22-23	1-1.5
School age	1-1.5	22-23	2
Adolescent	1-1.5	22-23	2

TABLE 4-22 Sites for Intramuscular Injections

Site	Landmarks	Interventions
Vastus lateralis: Preferred in children <3 yr (rectus femoris muscle also possibly used)	Greater trochanter and knee	Give injection in middle third of anterolateral aspect of thigh.

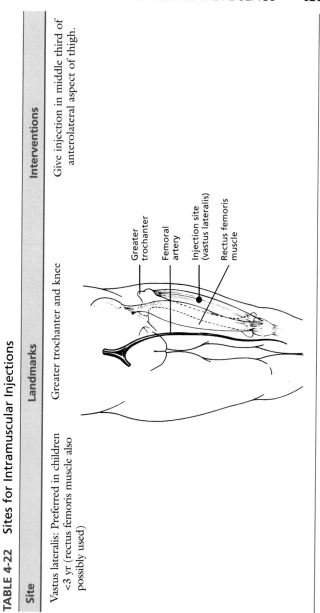

Greater trochanter

Femoral artery

Injection site (vastus lateralis)

Rectus femoris muscle

Continued.

TABLE 4-22   Sites for Intramuscular Injections—cont'd

Site	Landmarks	Interventions
Dorsogluteal: Preferred in children >3 yr and who have been walking over 1 yr	Posterosuperior iliac crest and greater trochanter	Give injection superior and lateral to imaginary line connecting landmarks.

Posterior superior iliac spine

Injection site

Greater trochanter

Sciatic nerve

Ventrogluteal: Use in children >3 yr and who have been walking over 1 yr

Greater trochanter, anterior iliac spine, and posterior edge of iliac crest

Give injection at center of **V** that is formed when the index finger is placed on anterior iliac crest, middle finger on posterior iliac crest while palm of the hand is resting on greater trochanter. Use right hand to find landmarks when injecting into left ventrogluteal site; use left hand to find landmarks when injecting into right ventrogluteal site.

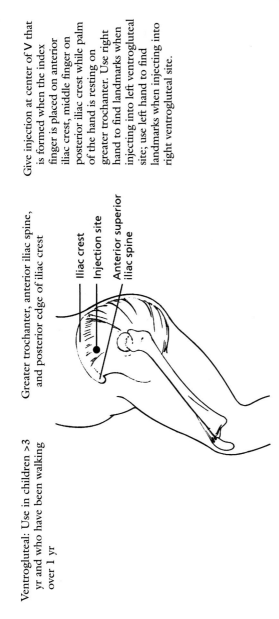

Iliac crest

Injection site

Anterior superior iliac spine

TABLE 4-23 Continuous Infusions (Based on 100 ml Solution)

Drug	Dose*	Final preparation**	Dosage range
Alprostadil PGE₁	0.6 × wt (kg)	1 ml/hr delivers 0.1 μg/kg/min	0.1-0.4 μg/kg/min
Dobutamine	6 × wt (kg)	1 ml/hr delivers 1 μg/kg/min	2-20 μg/kg/min
Dopamine	6 × wt (kg)	1 ml/hr delivers 1 μg/kg/min	2-20 μg/kg/min
Epinephrine	0.6 × wt (kg)	1 ml/hr delivers 0.1 μg/kg/min	0.1-1 μg/kg/min
Isoproterenol	0.6 × wt (kg)	1 ml/hr delivers 0.1 μg/kg/min	0.1-1 μg/kg/min
Lidocaine	60 × wt (kg)	1 ml/hr delivers 10 μg/kg/min	20-50 μg/kg/min
Nitroglycerin	6 × wt (kg)	1 ml/hr delivers 1 μg/kg/min	1-25 μg/kg/min
Nitroprusside	6 × wt (kg)	1 ml/hr delivers 1 μg/kg/min	1-8 μg/kg/min
Norepinephrine	0.6 × wt (kg)	1 ml/hr delivers 0.1 μg/kg/min	0.1-1 μg/kg/min

*Dose in mg added to the IV solution to make 100 ml. If preparing solution in a 60 cc syringe, divide the dose by 2, and add solution to make 50 ml.
**The concentration may be increased or decreased to accommodate needs of patient.

note that the dose of the vasoactive medication is added first, and then the syringe or buretrol is filled with the selected admixture to the total volume limit. Agitate the buretrol gently for several minutes to distribute the medication. When delivering small volumes, mixing the drug in a syringe and delivering the solution on a syringe pump may be advantageous. Drug wastage is minimized, and medications can be delivered at the closest port to the catheter for increased accuracy in medication delivery. If using a buretrol set-up, it is important that a clamp is placed between the admixture and the buretrol to avoid filling the buretrol with additional admixture and diluting the drug solution. A medication label should be placed on the syringe or buretrol rather than the admixture bag or bottle, to accurately label the infusion.

Pain Management

The bedside nurse must often act as an advocate for pain management in a young child. The child may be subject to painful procedures and/or postoperative pain. An analgesic and/or local anesthetic should be administered prior to a painful procedure in addition to the administration of an anxiolytic or sedative to reduce associated anxiety. Anxiolytics and sedatives do not relieve pain; thus analgesics should be administered to treat and prevent pain associated with diagnostic/therapeutic procedures.

Postoperative pain may be managed with opioid and non-opioid analgesics. Around-the-clock or continuous infusion is recommended. Intramuscular injections are painful and frightening and should be used under exceptional circumstances; the oral route is recommended as soon as the child can tolerate oral intake.

The primary difference between adult and pediatric management is the dosing. Table 4-24 is a table of usual dosages for analgesics and sedatives.

Physiological dependence (withdrawal) may develop with narcotic and benzodiazepine administration. A child may demonstrate increased irritability, wakefulness, tremors, tachypnea, refusal to eat, or diarrhea after 3 to 5 days of dosing. Steadily decreasing doses by a predetermined percentage, as opposed to abruptly stopping a medication, may prevent withdrawal syndrome.

Precalculated drug sheets

Pediatric dosages may be unfamiliar to the adult clinician; therefore a precalculated emergency drug sheet is very helpful.

TABLE 4-24 Usual Dosages for Children >6 Months and <50 kg

Drug	Oral dosage mg/kg		Parenteral dosage	
Acetaminophen	10-15	q4h		
Aspirin	10-15	q4h		
Ibuprofen	10	q6-8h		
Codeine	1	q3-4h		
Fentanyl			0.5-1.5 mcg/kg/hr	
Hydromophone	0.06	q3-4h	0.015 mg/kg	q3-4h
Levorphanol	0.04	q6-8h	0.02 mg/kg	q6-8h
Midazolam			0.05-0.1 mg/kg	q1-2h
			0.05-0.2 mg/kg/hr	
Nalbuphine			0.1-0.2 mg/kg	q1-2h
			0.1-0.4 mg/kg/hr	

All emergency medication doses are based on the child's weight (in kg). The emergency drug sheet should include the recommended resuscitation medication dosages, medication concentration, and final medication dose and volume the individual child is to receive. The recommended dosages should reflect the American Heart Association's PALS standards.

Some hospitals have successfully incorporated the drug sheet into their existing computer system so that the calculations are made after entering the child's name and weight into the computer. The target user of the emergency drug sheet (pediatric code team or pediatric ICU team versus adult code team or adult ICU team) should be identified during the development and implementation of the drug sheet. If the emergency sheet is to be used primarily by adult clinicians, the drug sheet should reflect the adult perspective as closely as possible.

If the drug sheet is manually calculated, two registered nurses should verify the mathematical calculations and document the sheet's accuracy by signing and dating the sheet. A listing of select pediatric drugs and dosages can be found in Table 4-25.

Medication pitfalls
SPECIAL CONSIDERATIONS
Several medications are available in multiple concentrations. For the child who weighs less than 20 kg, it is more efficient and accurate to use the lower concentration of the medication so that the dose in volume is not miniscule. Due to the mixed population of young children and adult patients, it

TABLE 4-25 Pediatric Drugs and Dosages*

Drug	Usual IV dose	Comments
Adenosine	0.1 mg/kg	Rapid IV push; maximum dose = 6 mg (child), 12 mg (adolescent).
Atropine	0.02 mg/kg	Maximum single dose: 0.5 mg (child); 1 mg (adolescent). May
	Minimum dose 0.1 mg	repeat dose after 5′; maximum total 1 mg child; 2 mg adolescent.
Bretylium	Initial: 5 mg/kg	
	Repeat: 10 mg/kg	
Calcium chloride 10%	20 mg/kg (0.2 ml/kg)	Give slowly.
Dextrose 50%	0.5–1 g/kg	Requires 1:1 dilution with NS (peripheral IV).
Diazepam	0.1 mg/kg	
Epinephrine	0.01 mg/kg (1:10,000)	For asystolic or pulseless arrest, IV doses as high as 0.2 mg/kg of 1:1000 may be effective.
Ketamine	1–2 mg/kg (normovolemia)	
	0.5 mg/kg (hypovolemia)	
Lidocaine	1 mg/kg	
Naloxone	0.1 mg/kg	Children >5 yrs may be given 2 mg. Give slowly and titrate to desired effect.
Phenobarbital	20 mg/kg	Use with NS. Do not exceed 50 mg/min.
Phenytoin	15 mg/kg	Do not exceed 50 mg/min.
Procainamide	5 mg/kg	Give slow IVP.
Propranolol	0.1 mg/kg	
Sodium bicarbonate	1 mEq/kg/or	If child <1 yr, dilute one to one with D_5W. Infuse only after adequate ventilation is achieved.
	0.3 × kg × base deficit	
Verapamil	0.1 mg/kg	Do not use if child <1 yr.

*Use central line if available; flush line after medication administration.

TABLE 4-26 Recommendations for the Use of Medications with Multiple Drug Concentrations in Children

Drug name	Neonate/child (<20 kg)	Child (>20 kg)
Naloxone	Neonatal 0.02 mg/ml	Adult 0.4 mg/ml
Digitalis	Neonatal 0.1 mg/ml	Adult 0.25 mg/ml
Ketamine	Pediatric 10 mg/ml	Adult 100 mg/ml
Sodium bicarbonate	4.2% (0.5 mEq/ml)	8.4% (1 mEq/ml)

may be necessary to have both concentrations available on the unit and code cart. Table 4-26 includes commonly used medications available in adult and pediatric concentrations.

DOSAGE CALCULATIONS

The risk for dosage calculation errors related to decimal point placement is greater when calculations are performed mentally. A calculator should be used to determine pediatric dosages.

Single-dose system

It is not uncommon for a nurse to administer a prescribed dose of a drug several times from the same syringe (e.g., 50 µg fentanyl from a syringe containing 200 mg) to an adult patient. A pediatric patient may require doses that are substantially smaller and thus more difficult to estimate from a multiple-dose syringe. Therefore a single-dose system is recommended for pediatric patients.

The *single-dose system* involves preparing one syringe to contain *only* the prescribed medication dose. The syringe should be properly labeled with the drug name and dose. The nurse administers the entire volume of the syringe to ensure that the prescribed dose has been given. The single-dose system prevents the nurse from overmedicating or undermedicating the patient, a hazard that can occur if a syringe containing a larger dose than prescribed is used.

After implementation of the single-dose system, it is important to realize that an unlabeled syringe can potentially contain any medication. *Nothing* should be administered to a child from an unlabeled syringe. All syringes must be labeled appropriately, including syringes of 0.9% sodium chloride used for flushing IV catheters.

Preparation of the first-line resuscitative medications

Administering medications during a resuscitative event using the single-dose system can be lengthy, especially for the inex-

---

Emergency Medications That May Be Delivered Via ETT

A tropine
L idocaine
I suprel
E pinephrine*
N aloxone

---

*Requires higher dose (0.1 mg/kg).
Dilute medications for administration, follow with 1-2 ml NS and several ventilations.

perienced pediatric clinician. Thus preparing and labeling syringes containing the child's first line resuscitative drugs such as epinephrine and atropine ahead of time can save time in the event of an emergency. These prepared syringes must be replaced every 24 hours because the medications contain no preservatives. Medications that can be delivered via an ETT create the acronym ALIEN. See the box above.

Sodium chloride flushes

Flushes (0.9% sodium chloride) are used to ensure delivery of medications. Manual flushing rather than gravity or pump-assisted flushing is preferred in the pediatric patient. The recommended volume for a flush should not exceed 3 ml for an infant and 5 ml for the child.[7] Flushes should be considered as intake and calculated in fluid intake totals.

SAFETY

Environmental Safety

In an environment that potentially contains critically ill patients of different ages and sizes, the importance of maintaining a safe and efficient environment cannot be overemphasized. It is recommended that a standard for an environmental safety check be developed and implemented. The box on p. 430 is an example of an environmental safety check standard adopted by the Critical Care Nursing Service, National Institutes of Health.

Soft Restraints

Soft restraints in the management of the adult ICU patient are most commonly used when the patient displays confusion, delirium, or combativeness. In an attempt to protect patient's civil rights, a medical order is required for the use of

Environmental Safety Check Standard

1. The safety check of the patient care environment will include verification of the following at the patient's bedside:
   a. Patient identification/allergy band present
   b. ECG, respiratory and hemodynamic monitor alarms activated with age-appropriate limits set
   c. Appropriate-sized manual resuscitation bag and oxygen-connecting tubing
   d. Appropriate-sized resuscitation mask
   e. Extra appropriate-sized artificial airways, if applicable
   f. Yankauer set-up with suction tubing and suction catheter
   g. Appropriate-sized blood pressure cuff
   h. Soft restraints at bedside
   i. Side rails positioned as appropriate to patient, safety tops on cribs when appropriate
   j. Patient call system in reach of patient/family
   k. Completed emergency drug sheet using child's dry weight in kilograms
   l. Bed in lowered position, as needed
   m. Bed or crib is free of sharp or small objects (e.g., needle caps, plastic bags, wrappers)
2. If any component of the safety check standard is missing or incorrect, it is the responsibility of the on-coming nurse assigned to the patient to rectify the situation.

soft restraints, and this medical order cannot be written as a "prn" order. In the pediatric critical care setting the availability and use of soft restraints is generally considered a safety measure and used at the discretion of the bedside nurse. In an effort to provide optimal safety without awkward positioning, the ties may be secured to the infant or small child's diaper. A confirmatory medical order for restraint(s) is required. The critically ill child is unable to understand the rationale and maintenance of invasive and noninvasive equipment, so the use of soft restraints is common to ensure the security of artificial airways and intravascular lines.

Parents often ask to loosen soft restraints stating that they will ensure restraint of the child's extremities. If parents were given this responsibility, they would feel an overwhelming sense of guilt if the child successfully pulled out a tube or catheter.

PREPARING THE CRITICALLY ILL CHILD FOR TRANSPORT

If a critically ill child must be transported to or from any critical care area within a hospital or to another health care facility, a safe transport must be planned. Optimal communication between hospital departments or the referring and receiving facilities is necessary for a successful transport. Guidelines and interventions that can be used for transporting the critically ill child include the following[53]:

1. Knowledge of the destination: to determine the length of time the patient will be at the alternate setting and what is needed, call ahead.
2. Evaluation of patient stability: determine the risk/benefit of transport. Assess the level of intervention the patient has needed in the last 2 to 4 hours.
3. Maintenance of the airway: anticipate potential emergencies and associated equipment needs. Secure ETT with tape that is well-anchored around the tube and face. Assign someone to manually hold the ETT while "bagging" and moving the patient.

   Disconnect the ETT from ambu bag when moving the patient to and from the stretcher.

   Suction the ETT just before leaving the unit. Take extra pediatric suction catheters and saline.

   Take a self-inflatable bag and correct size mask for all patients who have an ETT.

   Take an extra ETT, tape, and pediatric intubation equipment if the patient is going to an area that is not familiar with pediatric patients. Take an extra trach tube, ties, and scissors for all patients who have a tracheostomy tube. Full E-cylinder oxygen tanks should be used. Check the gauge on the tank, and take oxygen masks for delivery of supplemental oxygen.
4. Continuous monitoring: check battery on all portable ECG, respiratory, and pressure waveform monitors. Take vital signs every 5 minutes to ½ hour, including a check of neurological function. Monitor arterial pressure, intracranial pressure, or pulmonary artery pressure if applicable. Always take a blood pressure cuff and monitor pulse oximetry.
5. Maintenance of IV access: check for a blood return and check the skin around IV catheter site. Make sure IV is anchored to the skin and protected from dislodgement.

Have extra vascular volume expanders (NS, Lactated Ringers [LR], blood) for those patients who require frequent fluid boluses. IVs should be regulated by a pump if the patient is fluid restricted or has vasoactive medications (attach more than one IV pump to one IV pole).

6. Immobilization: immobilize combative or active patients to protect them from injury.

   For infants, use stockinette restraints for arms and legs. These can be safely pinned to the bedding, but detach them when transferring the infant out of the bed. For children, use arm and leg restraints (even on those patients who are recovering from anesthesia).

   Maintain C-spine precautions for all children with a suspected head or neck injury. For infants/toddlers, use two 10 lb sandbags, or liter bags of IV fluid, one on either side of the head, taping across the forehead to each bag. For older children, maintain neck collar placement.

   Utilize as many trained health care team members as needed to help move the patient. Secure drainage bags to the bed or stretcher. Avoid securing items to the side rail.

7. Temperature regulation: cover the child sufficiently with blankets. For infants, swaddle them in blankets and use head covering (stockinette caps). Have warming lights/blankets/radiant warmers ready on return from the transport. Use battery-powered warmed isolette for neonates.

8. Medications: emergency IV push medications include atropine, epinephrine 1:10,000, sodium bicarbonate, and 50% dextrose. Have a pediatric emergency drug card with drug doses calculated for the patient's weight, and have narcotics, sedatives, or anticonvulsants available.

REFERENCES

1. Ambuel B et al: Assessing distress in pediatric intensive care environments: the comfort scale, *J Ped Psychology* 17(1):95-109, 1992.
2. American Red Cross, Council of Community Blood Centers, American Association of Blood Banks: *Circular of information: for the use of human blood and blood components,* March, 1994.
3. Anand KJS, Hickey PR: Pain and its effects in the human neonate and fetus, *N Engl J Med* 317(21):1321-1327, 1987.
4. Bailey JM et al: Relationship between clinical evaluation of peripheral perfusion and global hemodynamics in adults after cardiac surgery, *Crit Care Med* 18(12):1353-1356, 1990.

5. Behrman RE, Vaughan VC, Nelson WE: *Nelson textbook of pediatrics,* ed 13, Philadelphia, 1994, W.B. Saunders.
6. Bruce DA: Head trauma. In Eichelberger MR, ed: *Pediatric trauma: prevention, acute care, and rehabilitation,* St Louis, 1993, Mosby.
7. Chameides L, Hazinski MF: *Textbook of pediatric advanced life support,* Dallas, 1994, American Academy of Pediatrics and American Heart Association.
8. Dickman CA, Rekate HL: Spinal trauma. In Eichelberger MR, ed: *Pediatric trauma: prevention, acute care, and rehabilitation,* St Louis, 1993, Mosby.
9. Diprose GK et al: Dinamapp fails to detect hypotension in the very low birthweight infants, *Arch Dis Child* 61:771, 1986.
10. Disabato J, Wulf J: Nursing strategies: altered neurologic function. In Foster R, Hunsberger M, Anderson J, eds: *Family centered nursing care of children,* Philadelphia, 1989, W.B. Saunders.
11. Eichelberger MA: *Pediatric trauma: prevention, acute care, and rehabiliation,* St Louis, 1993, Mosby.
12. Fields AI: Respiratory support and mechanical ventilation. *Pediatric critical care clinical review series: part I,* Fullerton, CA, 1989, Society of Critical Care Medicine.
13. Fiser DH: Intraosseous infusion, *N Engl J Med* 322(22):1579-1581, 1990.
14. Guyton AC: *Textbook of medical physiology,* ed 7, Philadelphia, 1991, W.B. Saunders.
15. Hazinski MF: Critical care of the pediatric cardiovascular patient, *Nurs Clin North Am* 16(4):671-697, 1981.
16. Hazinski MF: Hemodynamic monitoring in children. In Daily EK, Schroeder JS, eds: *Techniques in bedside hemodynamic monitoring,* ed 4, St Louis, 1989, Mosby.
17. Hazinski MF: *Nursing care of the critically ill child,* ed 2, St Louis, 1992, Mosby.
18. Hazinski MF: Understanding fluid balance in the seriously ill child, *Pediatr Nurs* 14(3):231-236, 1988.
19. Headrick CL: Hemodynamic monitoring of the criticially ill neonate, *J Pediatr Neonat Nurs* 5(4):58-67, 1991.
20. Heulitt M et al: Double-blind, randomized, controlled trial of papaverine-containing infusions to prevent failure of arterial catheters in pediatric patients, *Crit Care Med* 21(6):825-838, 1993.
21. Hunsberger M, Isseman R: Nursing strategies: altered digestive function. In Foster R, Hunsberger M, Anderson J, eds: *Family centered nursing care of children,* Philadelphia, 1989, W.B. Saunders.
22. Kennedy J: Renal disorders. In Hazinski MF, ed: *Nursing care of the critically ill child,* ed 2, St Louis, 1992, Mosby.

23. Kidder C: Reestablishing health factors influencing the child's recovery in pediatric intensive care, *J Pediatr Nurs* 4(2):96-103, 1989.

24. Kirsch CSB: Pharmacotherapeutics for the neonate and the pediatric patient. In Kuhn MM, ed: *Pharmacotherapeutics: a nursing process approach,* ed 2, Philadelphia, 1991, FA Davis Co.

25. Landier WC, Barrell ML, Styffe EJ: How to administer blood components to children, *MCN* 12(3):178-184, 1987.

26. Lowrey GH: *Growth and development of children,* ed 8, Chicago, 1986, Mosby.

27. Mayer T, Walker M: Emergency intracranial pressure monitoring in pediatrics: management of the acute coma of brain insult, *Clin Pediatr* 21:391, 1982.

28. McCaffery M, Beebe A: *Pain clinical manual for nursing practice,* St Louis, 1989, Mosby.

29. McWilliams BC: Mechanical ventilation in pediatric patients, *Clin Chest Med* 8(4):597-609, 1987.

30. Mills NM: Pain behaviors in infants and toddlers, *J Pain Symptom Manage* 4(4):184-190, 1989.

31. Moloney-Harmon PA: The pediatric trauma patient. In Welton RH, Shane K, eds: *Case studies in trauma nursing,* Baltimore, 1989, Williams & Wilkins, Inc.

32. Pain Management Guideline Panel, Agency for Health Care Policy and Research, US Health and Human Services: Clinician's quick reference guide to acute pain management in infants, children, and adolescents: operative and medical procedures, *J Pain Symptom Manage* 7(4):229-242, 1992.

33. Patel RI: Blood use and coagulation. In Eichelberger MR, ed: *Pediatric trauma: prevention, acute care, and rehabilitation,* St Louis, 1993, Mosby.

34. Petrillo M, Sanger S: *Emotional care of hospitalized children: an environmental approach,* ed 2, Philadelphia, 1980, J.B. Lippincott.

35. Pollack M: Nutritional failure and support in pediatric intensive care. In Shoemaker W et al, eds: *Textbook of critical care,* ed 2, Philadelphia, 1989, W.B. Saunders.

36. Pollack M et al: Malnutrition in critically ill infants and children, *JPEN* 6:20, 1982.

37. Reily MD: The renal system. In Smith JB, ed: *Pediatric critical care,* New York, 1983, John Wiley & Sons, Inc.

38. Rennick J: Re-establishing the parental role in the pediatric intensive care unit, *J Pediatr Nurs* 2:40-44, 1986.

39. Rosenthal CH: Immunosuppression in pediatric critical care patients, *Crit Care Nurs Clin North Am* 1(4):775-785, 1989.

40. Rosenthal CH: *Pediatric critical care nursing in the adult ICU: essentials of practice, National Conference on Pediatric Critical Care Nursing,* New York, 1990, Contemporary Forums.

41. Rossetti V et al: Difficulty and delay in intravascular access in pediatric arrests, *Ann Emerg Med* 13:406, 1984 (abstract).

42. Rubenstein J, Hageman J: Monitoring of critically ill infants and children, *Crit Care Clin North Am* 4:621, 1988.

43. Rushton CH: Family-centered care in the critical care setting: myth or reality? *Child Health Care* 19(2):68-78, 1990.

44. Schaefer C, Coyne JC, Lazarus RS: The health-related functions of social support, *Behav Med* 4:381-399, 1982.

45. Schechter NL, Allen DA, Hanson K: Status of pediatric pain control: a comparison of hospital analgesic usage in children and adults, *Pediatrics* 77(1):11-15, 1986.

46. Shelton T, Jeppson E, Johnson B: *Family centered care for children with special health care needs,* Washington, DC, 1987, Association of the Care of Children's Health.

47. Slota M: Pediatric neurological assessment, *Crit Care Nurse* 3:106, 1983.

48. Smith JB, ed: *Pediatric critical care,* New York, 1983, John Wiley & Sons, Inc.

49. Soupios M, Gallagher J, Orlowski JP: Nursing aspects of pediatric intensive care in a general hospital, *Pediatr Clin North Am* 27(3):621-633, 1980.

50. Sperhac AM, Harper J: Physical assessment. In Mott SR, James SR, Sperhac AM, eds: *Nursing care of children and families,* ed 2, Redwood City, CA, 1990, Addison-Wesley.

51. Susla GM, Dionne RE: Pharmacokinetics-pharmacodynamics: drug delivery and therapeutic drug monitoring. In Holbrook P, ed: *Textbook of pediatric critical care,* Philadelphia, 1993, W.B. Saunders.

52. Tietjen SD: Starting an infant's IV, *Am J Nurs* 90(5):44-47, 1990.

53. Tomkins J: Guidelines for intrahospital transport, *Pediatr Nurs* 16(1):50-53, 1990.

54. Trad PV: *Psychosocial scenarios for pediatrics,* New York, 1988, Springer-Verlag.

55. Tribett D, Brenner M: Peripheral and femoral vein cannulation, *Prob Crit Care* 2(2):266-285, 1988.

56. Turner BS: Maintaining the artificial airway: current concepts, *Pediatr Nurs* 16(5):487-489, 1990.

57. Van Lente F, Pippenger CE: The pediatric acute care laboratory, *Pediatr Clin North Am* 34(1):231-246, 1987.

58. Wofford LG: The pediatric patient. In Price MS, Fox JD, eds: *Hemodynamic monitoring in critical care,* Rockville, MD, 1987, Aspen Publishers, Inc.

CHAPTER 5

Diagnostic Tests and Patient Management

ANGIOGRAPHY

Clinical Brief

Angiography involves the injection of a contrast medium via a percutaneously inserted catheter in the area to be studied. Radiographs are then taken of the flow of the contrast material.

Digital subtraction angiography involves a computerized technique that subtracts images that block visualization of arteries.

Cardiac catheterization

Catheterization of the left side of the heart allows evaluation of mitral and aortic valvular function, ventricular function and structure, hemodynamics, and coronary artery patency. It also provides a means for interventional therapies such as percutaneous transluminal coronary angioplasty, intracoronary thrombolytic therapy, atherectomy, laser therapy, insertion of a stent, and valvuloplasty.

Catheterization of the right side of the heart allows for evaluation of tricuspid and pulmonic valvular function, the presence and degree of shunts, hemodynamics, and right ventricular function.

The contrast medium used to visualize cardiac structures and the great vessels can cause volume overloading, decreased contractility (thus increasing the risk for heart failure), renal toxicity, which can result in acute renal failure, as well as allergic reaction in some patients.

Aortography

Aortography allows visualization of the aorta—ascending, thoracic, and/or abdominal segments—to identify abnormalities such as aneurysms, coarctation, or dextraposition.

Cerebral angiography

Cerebral angiography allows for identification and evaluation of vascular abnormalities such as aneurysms, arteriovenous malformations (AVMs), vasospasm, atherosclerosis, and intracerebral hemorrhages. For suspected tumors, an angiogram can illustrate both the vascular supply to the tumor and the relationship of surrounding blood vessels to the mass.

Gastrointestinal angiography

Gastrointestinal angiography provides a view of the anatomical structures. It can be used to locate the source of GI bleeding, evaluate cirrhosis and portal hypertension, determine the extent of vascular damage to the liver and spleen after trauma, and locate tumors via selective celiac and superior mesenteric arteries. It can also be used to deliver chemotherapy or institute therapeutic measures such as introducing autologous clots and vasopressin to halt bleeding.

Pulmonary angiography

Pulmonary angiography allows visualization of pulmonary vessels and the measurement of pressures, cardiac output, and pulmonary vascular resistance. Angiography allows identification of abnormalities in pulmonary perfusion, aiding in the diagnosis of thrombi, aneurysms, or blood vessel defects. Angiography may also be performed for preoperative patient evaluation or after an inconclusive ventilation/perfusion lung scan.

Renal angiography

Renal angiography allows for visualization and identification of abnormalities of the renal circulation. It also provides a means for balloon dilation angioplasty or thrombolytic therapy to restore perfusion through the renal artery. Occasionally it is used for renal embolization to restore or maintain hemostasis after trauma or in patients with major renal vascular disorders.

▶ Complications and related nursing diagnoses

General	
Contrast reaction	Impaired skin integrity
	Decreased cardiac output
	Ineffective breathing pattern
	Impaired gas exchange
	Fluid volume deficit
Hematoma/hemorrhage/ pseudoaneurysm at catheter insertion site	Altered tissue perfusion: peripheral
	Decreased cardiac output
	Fluid volume deficit

Continued.

Arterial occlusion	Altered tissue perfusion: peripheral, cerebral, renal, gastrointestinal, cardiopulmonary
Renal failure	Altered urinary elimination
	Fluid volume excess
Osmotic diuresis	Altered urinary elimination
	Fluid volume deficit

Organ specific

Brain—cerebral embolism	Altered tissue perfusion: cerebral
Cardiac—myocardial ischemia	Pain
	Decreased cardiac output
Cardiopulmonary—dysrhythmias	Decreased cardiac output
Myocardial perforation/tamponade	Decreased cardiac output

Special Patient Management
Pretest

1. Obtain baseline VS and rhythm strip (if patient is on monitor).
2. Assess the quality of pulses and mark pulse sites.
3. Check for allergies to iodine and seafood.
4. Check for previous history of contrast reaction.
5. Check laboratory results for BUN and creatinine (renal function); INR/PT, PTT, platelets (coagulation), and Hgb, Hct (oxygenation).
6. Assess hydration status and ensure that the patient is well hydrated for angiography (if not contraindicated).
7. GI angiography may require bowel preparation.

Posttest
OUTCOME CRITERIA

1. HR 60-100 beats/min
2. SBP 90-140 mm Hg
3. Eupnea; RR 12-20/min
4. Hemostasis at catheterization insertion site
5. Peripheral pulses unchanged
6. Affected extremity warm
7. Absence of pulsatile mass at catheter insertion site
8. Urine output ≥25-30 ml/hr
9. Absence of systemic or pulmonary vascular engorgement
10. Alert and oriented; neurological examination unchanged
11. Absence of hives, flushing, diaphoresis

INTERVENTIONS

1. Keep patient on bed rest for 6 to 12 hours (or as ordered).
2. Prevent flexion of affected extremity.

3. Encourage fluids (if not contraindicated).
4. Monitor hemodynamic status:
   VS q15" × 2
   q30" × 2
   qlh until stable, then per unit routine
5. Check dressing with VS checks; if bleeding occurs, apply pressure to the site.
6. Assess for pulsatile groin mass, bruit, and/or complaint of acute tearing sensation.
7. Assess tissue perfusion with VS checks:
   Peripheral: for arterial puncture, assess the quality of the pulse (use Doppler if unable to palpate pulse), skin temperature, color, and sensation of the extremity. For venous puncture, assess for swelling, redness, pain, or any increase in skin temperature.
   Cerebral: assess the level of consciousness, motor strength and sensation, and speech.
   Renal: assess urine output hourly (profound diuresis, secondary to contrast medium, and electrolyte disturbances may occur). If dialysis access was studied, assess for thrill and bruit with VS checks.
8. Apply ice to the puncture site prn for pain and hematoma.
9. Observe for delayed hypersensitivity reaction: decreased BP, increased HR, flushing, diaphoresis, hives, decreased urine output.
10. Assess for complaints of flank pain. If associated with signs and symptoms of blood loss, suspect retroperitoneal bleeding.

CONSULT WITH PHYSICIAN

- Vascular insufficiency: cold, pale, mottled extremity, absent or diminished pulse, or sudden pain
- Allergic reaction: hives, flushing, diaphoresis, increased HR, and decreased BP
- Renal insufficiency: decreased urine output, increased BUN and creatinine
- Hemorrhage: uncontrolled bleeding at puncture site
- Dysrhythmias compromising CO: syncope, irregular rhythm, decrease in BP
- Cerebral ischemia: change in neurological status or worsening neurological deficits

If cardiac catheterization or pulmonary angiography performed:

- Cardiac tamponade: hypotension, tachycardia, pallor or cyanosis, JVD, decrease in pulse pressure, decrease in heart sounds, tachypnea

- Myocardial ischemia: severe chest discomfort, ST segment changes
- Heart failure: S_3, crackles, increased HR, decreased urine output

BARIUM ENEMA
Clinical Brief

A barium enema is used to examine the colon. Radiographic barium sulfate is instilled into the rectum and X ray films are taken. Barium and air, which produce a more clear picture of the integrity of the bowel lining, can also be used. This test should only be performed after all GI bleeding has stopped. A barium enema is routinely scheduled before an upper GI series. Other diagnostic tests such as ultrasonography or CT scans must be performed before any barium study. Abnormal findings will suggest areas of probable bleeding or tumors. A barium enema should not be performed if there is a possibility that a bowel perforation or obstruction exists.

▶ **Complications and related nursing diagnoses**

Retained barium	Constipation
Perforated bowel	Pain
	Risk for infection

Special Patient Management
Pretest

1. Ensure hydration.
2. Check to see that patient has received and responded to the bowel prep, and if ordered, has remained NPO since midnight.
3. Validate narcotic withholding, since narcotics may interfere with intestinal motility.
4. Validate routine medication administration of the patient when NPO.

Posttest
OUTCOME CRITERION

1. Barium will be evacuated

INTERVENTIONS

1. Administer laxatives after the test and assess bowel evacuation; barium should pass in 24 to 72 hours following the test.
2. Encourage fluids if not contraindicated.

CONSULT WITH PHYSICIAN

- Bowel perforation: abdominal pain, rigid abdomen, hypoactive bowel sounds

- Constipation: absence of stools, palpable mass in abdomen, hypoactive bowel sounds

BARIUM SWALLOW
Clinical Brief
A barium swallow is used to examine the mucous membranes of the esophagus, stomach, and small intestines. Barium is ingested and serial X-ray films are taken that may reveal areas of ulcerations, hiatal hernia, varices, strictures, polyps, foreign bodies, diverticula, tumors, or motility abnormalities. This test is contraindicated if the patient has an intestinal obstruction or is actively bleeding.

▶ Complications and related nursing diagnoses

Retained barium   Constipation

Special Patient Management
Pretest
1. Validate withholding anticholinergic agents and narcotics, since these agents affect motility.
2. Check to see that the patient has received and responded to bowel prep, and if ordered, has remained NPO.
3. Validate routine medication administration if the patient is NPO.

Posttest
OUTCOME CRITERION
1. Barium will be evacuated

INTERVENTIONS
1. Administer laxatives after the test and assess bowel evacuation; barium should pass in 24 to 72 hours following the test.
2. Encourage fluids if not contraindicated.

CONSULT WITH PHYSICIAN
- Bowel perforation: abdominal pain, rigid abdomen, hypoactive bowel sounds
- Constipation: absence of stools, palpable mass in abdomen, hypoactive bowel sounds

BIOPSY
Clinical Brief
A biopsy involves the percutaneous or surgical insertion of a needle, under the guide of ultrasound, fluoroscopy, or CT scan, to obtain tissue for analysis. Biopsies may also be obtained via

endoscopy using forceps or suction. *Bone* biopsies are used to evaluate developmental stages of blood cells and diagnose leukemia and anemias. *Liver* biopsies are used to diagnose parenchymal disorders of the liver and assess transplant functioning. *Pancreatic* biopsies are used to diagnose pancreatic cancer. *Endoscopic* biopsies are used to diagnose gastric mucosal abnormalities, gastric polyps, carcinoma, or gastric ulcers. *Renal* biopsies are used to diagnose or stage various renal disorders and to assess transplant functioning. Biopsy is contraindicated in the presence of severe coagulopathy or active bleeding.

▶ **Complications and related nursing diagnoses**

Hemorrhage	Decreased cardiac output
	Altered tissue perfusion

Special Patient Management
Pretest
1. Notify the physician if the patient has been on anticoagulant therapy, or taking aspirin or NSAIDs.
2. Check to see that the results of the patient's clotting studies are normal and that hemoglobin and hematocrit levels are stable.
3. Obtain baseline vital signs.
Posttest
OUTCOME CRITERIA
1. Hemostasis at insertion site
2. Patient is alert and oriented
3. SBP 90-140 mm Hg
4. HR 60-100 beats/min
INTERVENTIONS
1. Apply a pressure dressing to the biopsy site.
2. If bleeding occurs, apply pressure to the puncture site.
3. Monitor hemodynamic status: VS q15" × 2; q30" × 2; qlh until stable; check dressing with VS checks.
4. Keep the patient on bed rest. Renal biopsy—keep the patient lying supine for 24 hours (or as ordered); liver biopsy—keep the patient lying on the right side for 4 hours after the biopsy (or as ordered).
5. Monitor urine output after renal biopsy; urine should clear within 8 hours after biopsy.
CONSULT WITH PHYSICIAN
• Hemorrhage: uncontrolled bleeding at puncture site
• Abdominal and flank hematoma or pain

- Gross hematuria
- Decreasing BP or increasing HR

CHEST RADIOGRAPH
Clinical Brief
A chest radiograph is used to provide information about gross anatomical proportions and the location of cardiac structures, including the great vessels; to evaluate lung fields; and to confirm placement of airways, central venous catheters, pulmonary artery catheters, chest tubes, and transvenous pacemaker leads.

The least dense (air-filled) structures (e.g., lungs) absorb fewer x-rays and appear black on the radiographic film. Structures that are as dense as water (e.g., heart and blood vessels) appear gray. Bone and contrast materials are most dense and appear white on the radiograph.

Figure 5-1 depicts a normal chest radiograph with underlying structures outlines; Figures 5-2, 5-3, and 5-4 identify conditions commonly evaluated in ICU patients. Normal findings are identified in Table 5-1.

Serial assessments of endotracheal tube, central lines, and chest tube placement should be done. An endotracheal tube should be 2 to 3 cm above the carina. Table 5-2 lists abnormal radiographic findings common to ICU patients.

▶ **Complications and related nursing diagnosis**
None

Special Patient Management
None

COMPUTED TOMOGRAPHY (CT) OR COMPUTED AXIAL TOMOGRAPHY (CAT)
Clinical Brief
CT or CAT scans are used to obtain rapid and more definitive visualization of body structures than radiographs provide. X-ray beams are passed through substances of varying densities and a computer makes calculations to provide cross-sectional images of the specific body part being studied. A contrast medium, which enhances vascular areas, may or may not be used. White-appearing images reflect more dense substances such as bone; black-appearing images reflect less dense substances such as air or CSF. Soft tissue appears as shades of gray.

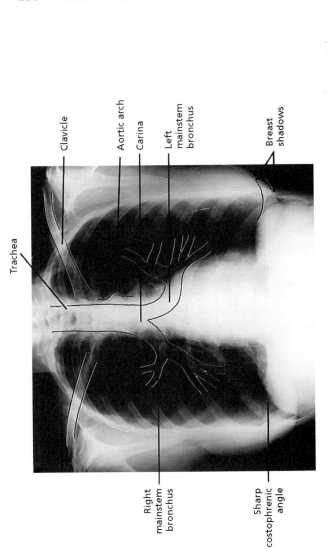

Figure 5-1 A, Location of structures on a chest radiograph. (From Talbot L, Meyers-Marquardt M: *Pocket guide to critical care assessment,* ed 2, St Louis, 1993, Mosby.)

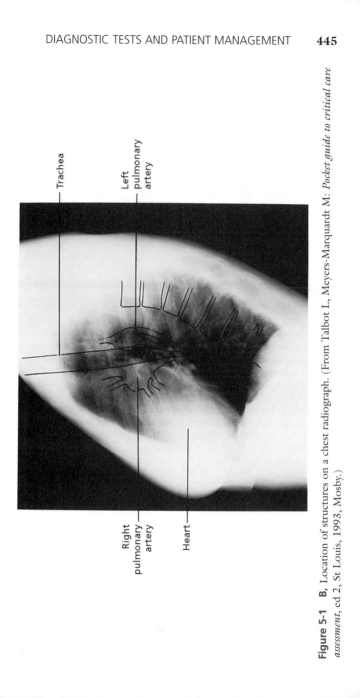

Figure 5-1 B, Location of structures on a chest radiograph. (From Talbot L, Meyers-Marquardt M: *Pocket guide to critical care assessment*, ed 2, St Louis, 1993, Mosby.)

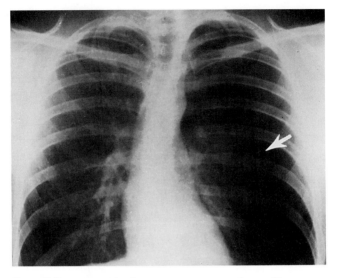

Figure 5-2 Radiograph of a spontaneous pneumothorax. (From Sahn SA: Pneumothorax and pneumomediastinum. In Mitchell RS, Petty TL, Schwarz MI, eds: *Synopsis of clinical pulmonary disease*, ed 4, St Louis, 1989, Mosby.)

▶ **Complications and related nursing diagnoses**   (contrast CT)

Reaction to contrast	Impaired skin integrity
	Ineffective breathing pattern
	Decreased cardiac output
	Altered urinary elimination

Special Patient Management
Pretest
1. Check for allergy to iodine or seafood.
2. Verify NPO status and need for bowel prep.
Posttest
OUTCOME CRITERION
1. Absence of contrast reaction: hives, skin rash, pruritis, nausea, wheeze, laryngospasm, hypotension, oliguria or change in level of consciousness, headache

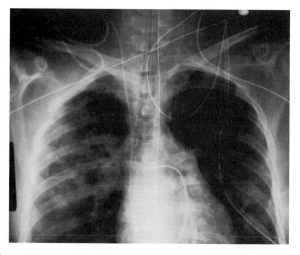

Figure 5-3   Radiograph of patient admitted with acute respiratory distress syndrome. (From Petty TL: Adult respiratory distress syndrome. In Mitchell RS, Petty TL, Schwarz MI, eds: *Synopsis of clinical pulmonary disease*, ed 4, St Louis, 1989, Mosby.)

INTERVENTIONS
1. Obtain VS.
2. Encourage fluids if not contraindicated.
3. Monitor for reaction to contrast.

CONSULT WITH PHYSICIAN
- Delayed contrast reaction: hives, skin rash, pruritis, nausea, wheeze, laryngospasm, hypotension, oliguria, change in level of consciousness, and headache
- Renal failure: decreased urine output, increased BUN and creatinine

ELECTROCARDIOGRAPHY: SIGNAL AVERAGED

Clinical Brief

The signal averaged ECG (SAE) is a simple, noninvasive diagnostic test used to identify patients prone to ventricular tachycardia (VT) and sudden death. Information necessary for signal averaging is gathered via the standard Frank X, Y, and Z leads. Signal averaging, done by a computer, allows detection of low amplitude waveforms that are normally masked by noise. These low amplitude late potentials are associated with increased

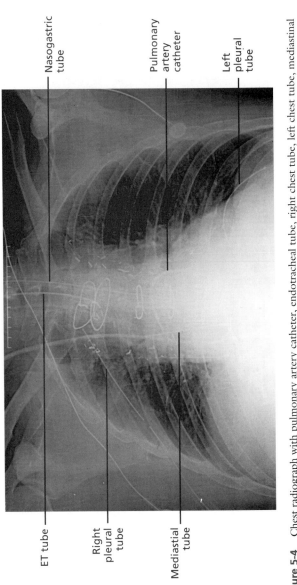

Figure 5-4 Chest radiograph with pulmonary artery catheter, endotracheal tube, right chest tube, left chest tube, mediastinal tube, and nasogastric tube.

TABLE 5-1 Normal Findings on Chest Radiograph

Assessed area	Usual adult findings
Trachea	Midline, translucent, tubelike structure found in the anterior mediastinal cavity
Clavicles	Equally distant from the sternum
Ribs	Thoracic cavity encasement
Mediastinum	Shadowy-appearing space between the lungs that widens at the hilum
Heart	Solid-appearing structure with clear edges visible in the left anterior mediastinal cavity; cardiothoracic ratio should be less than half the width of the chest wall on a PA film; cardiac shadow appears larger in an AP film
Carina	Lowest tracheal cartilage at the bifurcation
Mainstem bronchus	Translucent, tubelike structure visible approximately 2.5 cm from the hilum
Hilum	Small, white, bilateral densities present where the bronchi join the lungs; left should be 2 to 3 cm higher than the right
Bronchi	Not usually visible
Lung fields	Usually not completely visible except for "lung markings" at periphery
Diaphragm	Rounded structures visible at the bottom of the lung fields; right side is 1 to 2 cm higher than the left; costophrenic angles should be clear and sharp

Adapted from Talbot L, Meyers-Marquardt M: *Pocket guide to critical care assessment,* ed 2, St Louis, 1993, Mosby.

TABLE 5-2 Abnormal Radiographic Findings

Finding	Possible diagnosis
Nondistinct or widened aortic knob	Aortic dissection
Silhouette sign (loss of border visibility)	Infiltrates or consolidation of RML or lingula
Enlarged cardiac silhouette	HF, pericardial effusion, pulmonary edema
Blackened area without tissue markings	Pneumothorax
Patchy infiltrates or streaky densities	Pneumonia, atelectasis
Fluffy infiltrates (Kerely B lines)	Pulmonary edema
Loss of costophrenic angle sharpness	Pleural effusion

incidence of VT. Patients with a history of dilated cardiomyopathy, MI, unexplained syncope, or VT may be candidates for SAE. Identification of patients prone to VT increases the chance of appropriate intervention to prevent sudden death.

▶ **Complications and related nursing diagnosis**
None

Special Patient Management
None

ELECTROCARDIOGRAPHY: TWELVE-LEAD

Clinical Brief
Twelve-lead ECG is used as a diagnostic tool in determining overall electrical functioning of the heart and can aid in identifying pathological conditions. Normal and abnormal activity, as evidenced by examining individual waves, deflections, intervals, and segments, can be evaluated.

Twelve leads
The 12 leads are either bipolar or unipolar. The precordial leads (V_1 to V_6) are unipolar and provide information about anterior, posterior, right, and left electrical forces. The bipolar limb leads (I, II, III) consist of a + and − electrode and compose Einthoven's triangle. Leads aV$_R$, aV$_L$, and aV$_F$ are unipolar limb leads representing augmented vector right, left, and foot. The limb leads provide information about vertical electrical forces as well as left and right forces.

Deflections
Deflections signify individual cardiac cycle events and their electrical direction in relation to a positive electrode. When the electrical current moves in the general direction of a positive electrode, an upward or positive deflection is recorded. Conversely, a downward or negative deflection signifies movement away from the positive electrode. Major deflections are referred to as the P, Q, R, S, T, and U waves.

Waves, intervals, and segments
See Table 5-3 for components of a normal ECG.

Electrical axis
An imaginary line drawn between two electrodes is called the axis of the lead. A vector signifies a quantity of electrical force that has both a given magnitude and direction. When the cardiac vector is parallel to the axis of the lead recording it, the ECG deflection is either the most upright or the most negative (Figure 5-5). When the direction of the electrical activity

TABLE 5-3 Components of Normal ECG

Component	Criteria	Comment
Rhythm	Atrial and ventricular are same; R-R and P-P intervals vary ≤0.12 sec	
Rate	Atrial and ventricular rates are equal; 60-100 cycles/min	
P-wave	Present; only one P for each QRS	
Direction	Upright in I, II, aV$_F$, and V$_4$ to V$_6$; inverted in aV$_R$; biphasic, flat or inverted in III, V$_1$ and V$_2$	Upright and notched in I, II, V$_4$ to V$_6$ suggests left atrial abnormality; Tall and peaked in II, III, aV$_F$ suggests right atrial abnormality
Shape	Rounded, symmetrical, without notches, peaks	
Amplitude	<3.0 mm	
Width	1.5-2.5 mm (0.06-0.10 sec)	
Axis	0 to +90 degrees	
PR interval	0.12-0.20 sec	>0.20 = AVB ≥0.12 = BBB
QRS interval	0.06-0.10 sec	V$_1$ V$_2$ are best to measure QRS
QT interval	< Half the preceding R-R interval in normal rates $QTc = \dfrac{QT \text{ (measured)}}{\sqrt{R - R \text{ interval(s)}}}$ Normal ≤0.39 (men) ≤0.44 (women)	Prolonged QT interval is associated with torsade de pointes

Adapted from Kinney M, Packa D, Dunbar S: *AACN's clinical reference for critical-care nursing*, New York, 1993, Mosby.

Continued.

TABLE 5-3   Components of Normal ECG—cont'd

Component	Criteria	Comment
QRS complex Configuration	Follows each P qRs Rs qR rSR' QS	Uppercase and lowercase letter indicate the relative sizes of the QRS components
Q wave	Width: <0.039 sec Depth 1-2 mm in I, aV_L, aV_F, V_5 and V_6; deep QS or Qr in aV_R and possibly in III, V_1 and V_2	Significant if 0.04 sec wide or 25% the height of the R wave
Amplitude	>5 mm and <25 mm in limb leads; 5 to 30 mm in V_1 and V_6; 7 to 30 mm in V_2 and V_5; 9 to 30 mm in V_3 and V_4	
R progression	Progressive increase in R wave amplitude from V_1 to V_6	
Axis	-30 to +110 degrees	
Transition	V_3 or V_4	
Intrinsicoid deflection	≤0.02 sec in V_1; ≤0.04 sec in V_6 V_6	Delayed in BBB and chamber enlargement

ST segment	Isoelectric, but may be elevated ≤1 mm in limb leads and ≤2 mm in some precordial leads	Elevation associated with vasospasm or acute injury; depression suggests ischemia
	Not depressed more than 0.05 mm	
	Curves gently into proximal limb of T wave	
T wave		
Direction	Upright in I, II, and V_3 to V_6; inverted in a V_R; and varies in III, aV_L, aV_F, V_1 and V_2	Tall T wave is associated with hyperkalemia, ischemia
Shape	Slightly rounded and asymmetrical	
Height	≤5 mm in limb leads; ≤10 mm in precordial leads	
Axis	Left and inferior	
U wave		
Direction	Upright	
Amplitude	0.33 mm in precordial leads (average); 2.5 mm (maximum)	Increases in amplitude in hypokalemia
Width	≤0.24 sec	

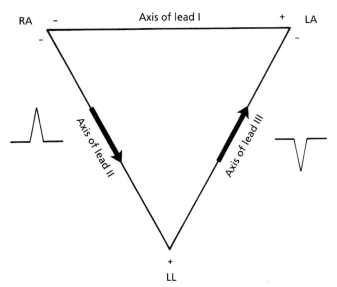

Figure 5-5 Axis. When a mean vector is parallel to the axis of a lead, the tallest (electrical current flowing toward the positive lead) or the deepest (electrical current flowing away from the positive lead) complex will result in that lead.

is perpendicular to the axis of the lead recording it, an equiphasic deflection will be recorded.

Hexaxial reference system

The mean vector, or axis of the heart, can be measured in degrees using the hexaxial reference system. A normal QRS vector should lie between -30 and +110. Left axis deviation can be caused by left anterior hemiblock, left bundle branch block, left ventricular hypertrophy, obesity, or inferior myocardial infarction. Right axis deviation can be caused by left posterior hemiblock, right ventricular hypertrophy, limb lead reversal, dextrocardia, or lateral myocardial infarction.

Quick method to axis determination

See Figure 5-6

ECG pattern associated with ischemia

Reduced blood supply is characterized by inverted T waves, transient ST depression during anginal episodes due to a fixed lesion, and transient ST elevation during anginal episodes that are due to vasospasm (Figure 5-7).

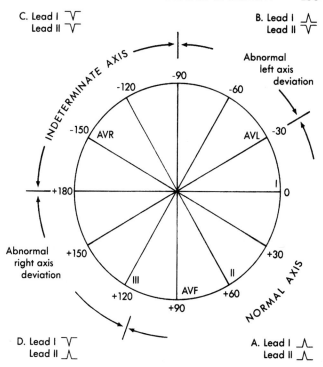

Figure 5-6 Estimating axis using leads I and II. **A,** If the QRS is upright in both I and II, the axis is normal. **B,** If the QRS is upright in I and down in II, left axis deviation is present. **C,** If the QRS is down in both I and II, indeterminate axis is present. **D,** If the QRS is down in I and upright in II, right axis deviation is present.

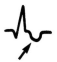 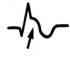

Ischemia
Symmetrically
inverted T waves

Injury
ST elevation
(indicates acuteness)

Infarction
Diagnosed by large
Q wave—0.04 sec wide
or 25% the height
of the R wave

Figure 5-7 ECG changes with infarction.

ECG pattern associated with injury

Acuteness of an infarction is represented by ST segment elevation. ST segment elevation is one of the earliest changes characteristic of infarction. ST segment depression is characteristic of non-Q-wave infarction.

ECG pattern associated with Q-wave infarction

Indicative changes, significant Q waves, ST elevation, and T-wave inversion can be found in leads over infarcted myocardium:

- Anterior MI—leads V_1-V_4
- Lateral MI—leads I, aVL, and V_5 and V_6
- Inferior MI—leads, II, III, and aVF
- Posterior MI—reciprocal changes in anterior leads (e.g., tall R wave, ST depression, and tall symmetrical T wave in V_1-V_4)

Right ventricular infarction is represented by lead V_{4R} and will exhibit ST elevation >1 mm.

Wellen's Syndrome—Critical stenosis of proximal LAD

Signs associated with critical stenosis of the proximal LAD and impending infarction include unstable angina; little or no cardiac enzyme elevation; little or no ST elevation in V_2 and V_3; ST segment turning down into a deeply inverted and symmetrical T wave in V_2 and V_3; and no significant Q waves in precordial leads (Figure 5-8).

Differentiating bundle branch block

LBBB characteristics include a mainly negative QRS in V_1 and an R wave with no Q or S wave in leads I, aVL, and V_6. RBBB characteristics include an upright QRS in V_1; intrinsicoid deflection 0.07 sec or later in V_1; and small Q wave and broad S wave in leads I, aVL, and V_6. See Figure 5-9 for quick identification of BBB.

Chamber enlargement

Table 5-4 outlines changes on ECG indicative of chamber enlargement.

Ventricular ectopy versus aberrant ventricular conduction

Wide QRS complexes with bizarre morphology generally signify either ventricular ectopy or aberrant ventricular conduction. Ventricular ectopy has its origin in the ventricle and indicates increased ventricular irritability. Aberrant ventricle conduction is caused by a supraventricular impulse (e.g., PAC) arriving at the ventricle too early; the ventricles are not totally repolarized so the impulse is conducted abnormally or aberrantly.

V_2- V_3

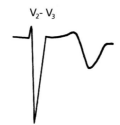

Figure 5-8   ECG changes associated with Wellen's Syndrome. (From Conover MB: *Pocket guide to electrocardiography*, St Louis, 1990, Mosby.)

A $V_1 V_2$

B

$V_5 V_6$

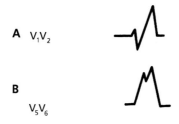

Figure 5-9   Right and left bundle branch block (BBB). **A,** Check right precordial leads (V_1, V_2) for RR', suggesting RBBB. **B,** Check left precordial leads (V_5, V_6) for RR', suggesting LBBB.

Both ventricular ectopy and aberrant conduction present as a wide QRS. Differential diagnosis is important because treatment is different.

Characteristics favoring aberrancy include: QRS 0.12 to 0.14 sec; P waves (if identifiable) are associated with the QRS. Characteristics favoring ectopy include: QRS >0.14 sec; P waves (if identifiable) independent of the QRS. Additional diagnostic clues are seen in Figure 5-10.

Wolff-Parkinson-White Syndrome (WPW)

WPW is a form of ventricular preexcitation characterized by a short PR and a prolonged QRS due to a delta wave (initial slurring of the QRS). An anomalous or accessory pathway between the atrium and ventricle allows the atrial impulse to bypass the AV node and therefore reach the ventricle earlier than normal. The patient with WPW is predisposed to PSVT and atrial fibrillation. The tachydysrhythmias usually have a

TABLE 5-4 Chamber Enlargement

Chamber	Changes
RA	Tall peaked P wave (>2.5 mm) in II, III, aVF; low or isoelectric P wave in I; P waves in V_1, V_2 may be upright with increased amplitude
LA	P-wave duration >0.12 sec, P wave notched and upright in I, II, V_4-V_6; wide, deep, negative component to P wave in V_1
RV	Right axis deviation, R/S ratio >1 in V_1; ST segment depression and T-wave inversion in V_1 or V_2
LV*	Increased voltage; R or S wave in limb leads >20 mm or S wave in V_1 or V_2 >30 mm or R wave in V_5 or V_6 >30 mm, 3 points
	ST changes; with digitalis, 1 point; without digitalis, 2 points
	LA enlargement, 3 points
	Left axis deviation, 2 points (-30 or more)
	QRS duration ≥0.09 sec, 1 point
	Intrinsicoid deflection in V_5 or V_6 ≥0.05 sec, 1 point

*4 points, LVH likely; 5 points, LVH present.

narrow QRS (orthodromic); however, a wide QRS tachycardia (antidromic) may occur and be confused with VT.

Systematic approach to twelve-lead electrocardiogram
Review all 12 leads to determine (1) underlying rhythm; (2) patterns of ischemia, injury, or infarction; (3) chamber enlargement; and (4) ventricular axis.

1. Determine rate.
2. Examine P-P and R-R intervals for regularity in rhythm.
3. Analyze P waves in each lead.
4. Measure PR, QRS, and QT intervals.
5. Analyze QRS complex.
6. Identify leads having significant Q waves.
7. Determine presence of R-wave progression and identify lead associated with transition.
8. Measure intrinsicoid deflection.
9. Determine axis.
10. Identify leads displaying ST segment elevation or depression.
11. Analyze T wave for increased amplitude.
12. Identify presence of U wave.

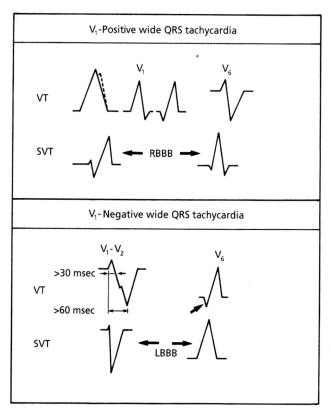

Figure 5-10 Differential diagnosis in wide QRS tachycardia (From Conover MB: *Pocket guide to electrocardiography*, ed 3, St Louis, 1994, Mosby.)

▶ **Complications and related nursing diagnosis**
None

Special Patient Management

None

ELECTROENCEPHALOGRAPHY (EEG)

Clinical Brief

Electroencephalography is used to detect and/or localize abnormal electrical findings, which may be caused by hemorrhage, tumor, abscess, or infarction. EEG can also help identify seizure types and aid in the diagnosis of brain death. Electrodes are placed over the scalp and connected to a main recording system that provides a printout of the electrical activity of the brain.

▶ **Complications and related nursing diagnosis**
None

Special Patient Management

Verify withholding anticonvulsants, stimulants, (e.g., cola, tea, coffee), depressants, or tranquilizers prior to the test, since these drugs can affect electrical activity of the brain.

ELECTROPHYSIOLOGICAL STUDY: CARDIAC (EPS)

Clinical Brief

An EPS involves positioning multipolar catheter electrodes, via right and/or left heart catheterization, at various sites within the heart for the purpose of recording electrical activity and/or stimulating the atria or ventricles. The procedure can be performed to diagnose dysrhythmias and their mechanisms, to evaluate the effectiveness of drug therapy on tachyarrhythmias, to terminate a tachycardia by pacing, or to ablate an accessory pathway involved in a reentrant tachycardia.

▶ **Complications and related nursing diagnoses**

Cardiac perforation	Decreased cardiac output
Thrombus formation on catheter and emboli	Altered tissue perfusion: peripheral, cerebral, renal, coronary, pulmonary
Hematoma/bleeding at catheter insertion site	Pain Altered tissue perfusion: peripheral Fluid volume deficit
Lethal dysrhythmia	Decreased cardiac output

Special Patient Management
Pretest
1. Obtain baseline VS and rhythm strip.
2. Verify withholding antidysrhythmic medication with physician.

Posttest
OUTCOME CRITERIA
1. Absence of life-threatening dysrhythmias
2. Patient is alert and oriented

3. SBP 90-140 mm Hg
4. Hemostasis at catheter insertion site

INTERVENTIONS

1. Keep patient on bed rest for 6-12 hours as ordered.
2. Prevent flexion of affected extremity.
3. Monitor hemodynamic status:
   VS q15" × 3
   q30" × 3
   qlh until stable, then per unit routine
4. Check dressing with VS checks; if bleeding occurs, apply pressure.
5. Assess tissue perfusion: level of consciousness, urinary output, peripheral pulses.
6. Check for thrombophlebitis of affected extremity: swelling, redness, pain, or any increase in skin temperature.
7. If pacer catheters are left in place, ground ends of pacer wires to protect against electrical injury.

CONSULT WITH PHYSICIAN

- Dysrhythmias compromising CO: syncope, decreased BP
- Cardiac perforation: hypotension, tachycardia, pallor/cyanosis, JVD, decreased pulse pressure, diminished heart sounds, tachypnea
- Emboli: chest pain, change in level of consciousness, dyspnea, diminished pulses
- Thrombophlebitis: swelling, redness, pain, increased skin temperature
- Bleeding at site of catheter insertion: hematoma, swelling, pain, blood

ENDOSCOPY

Clinical Brief

Endoscopy is used to visualize an organ, structure, or system via a rigid or flexible scope. *Esophagogastroduodenoscopy,* or *panendoscopy,* refers to visualizing the esophagus, stomach, and duodenum. *Proctoscopy* and *sigmoidoscopy* visualize the rectum and sigmoid colon. *Colonoscopy* involves the visualization of the large intestine. *Endoscopic retrograde cholangiopancreatography* (ERCP) is a contrast procedure visualizing the pancreatic duct and hepatobiliary tree. *Bronchoscopy* refers to visualization of the trachea and bronchi.

Ulcers, sites of hemorrhage, or neoplasms can be confirmed with GI endoscopy. Pancreatic, gallbladder, and liver disorders such as stones, strictures, and tumors or growths can often be visualized with ERCP. Tumors, sites of hemorrhage, and lesions can be visualized with bronchoscopy.

Endoscopy also allows a means to remove specimens or foreign bodies, cauterize or sclerose bleeding vessels, and obtain biopsies.

▶ Complications and related nursing diagnoses
General

Perforation of the GI/respiratory tract	Pain
	Risk for infection
Postprocedural bleeding	Decreased cardiac output
	Fluid volume deficit
Oversedation	Risk for injury
	Ineffective breathing pattern
	Risk for aspiration
Cardiac dysrhythmias	Decreased cardiac output

Bronchoscopy, ERCP, panendoscopy

Aspiration	Risk for infection
	Impaired gas exchange

Bronchoscopy

Laryngospasm/bronchospasm	Impaired gas exchange
	Ineffective breathing pattern

ERCP

Pancreatitis	Hyperthermia
	Pain
Sepsis	Increased cardiac output
	Altered tissue perfusion
Cholangitis	Hyperthermia
	Pain

Special Patient Management
Pretest
1. Obtain baseline VS.
2. Check clotting studies.
3. If a proctoscopy, sigmoidoscopy, or colonscopy is to be performed, check to see whether the patient has received and responded to the bowel prep, if it was ordered.
4. Check to see that the patient has remained NPO at least 6 hours.

Posttest

OUTCOME CRITERIA

1. Patient is pain free
2. SBP 90-140 mm Hg
3. HR 60-100 beats/min
4. Absence of bleeding
5. Patient is alert and oriented
6. Gag reflex present (following bronchoscopy, panendoscopy, ERCP)
7. Lungs clear to auscultation

INTERVENTIONS

1. Assess VS for fever, hemodynamic instability, and respiratory compromise.
2. Determine presence of gag reflex (after the appropriate test) and keep the patient NPO until the reflex returns.
3. Monitor for bleeding or perforation.

CONSULT WITH PHYSICIAN

- Perforation or bleeding: decreased BP, increased HR, pain, fever, abdominal tenderness, difficulty breathing
- Oversedation: inability to arouse, decreased respirations

GI BLOOD LOSS SCAN

Clinical Brief

A GI blood loss scan is used to detect and localize the site of bleeding. Once the radioactive material is injected, imaging is begun. Delayed repeated imaging may be performed if the patient exhibits clinical signs of active bleeding and results of the initial scan were negative.

▶ Complications and related nursing diagnosis
None

Special Patient Management

Determine whether the patient has received barium in the last 24 hours, since barium may interfere with imaging and obscure the site of bleeding.

INTRAVENOUS PYELOGRAM (IVP)

Clinical Brief

An intravenous pyelogram is used to assess the renal system structure and excretory function. Contrast medium is injected intravenously, followed by serial radiographs; CT may also be done. Radiographs can be taken after the patient voids to assess residual urine volume. A retrograde pyelogram involves cystoscopy to inject dye through catheters placed into the ureters.

▶ **Complications and related nursing diagnoses**

Contrast reaction	Impaired skin integrity
	Ineffective breathing pattern
	Decreased cardiac output
	Altered urinary elimination
Osmotic diuresis secondary to contract medium	Fluid volume deficit
Infection from catheterization	Risk for infection

Special Patient Management
Pretest
1. Check for allergy to iodine or seafood.
2. Check to see that the patient has received and responded to bowel prep and, if it was ordered, has remained NPO for 4 to 6 hours before the procedure.
3. Check BUN; IVP is contraindicated if levels are >40 mg/dl.
Posttest
OUTCOME CRITERIA
1. SBP 90-140 mm Hg
2. Urine output >30 ml/hr
3. Absence of contrast reaction; hives, rash, pruritis, wheeze, hypotension, oliguria
INTERVENTIONS
1. Obtain VS and measure urine hourly.
2. Encourage fluids if not contraindicated.
3. Monitor for reaction to contrast.
CONSULT WITH PHYSICIAN
- Reaction to contrast medium: hives, rash, difficulty breathing, decreased BP
- Renal failure (new onset): decreased urine output, increasing BUN and creatinine
- Urinary tract infection: cloudy urine, pain with voiding, increased temperature

LAPAROSCOPY

Clinical Brief
Laparoscopy allows direct visualization of structures and organs within the abdominal cavity and biopsy of suspicious

abdominal tissue. It is indicated for evaluation of hepatic disease (exclude malignancy, assess benign disease, follow up on abnormal hepatic imaging) and peritoneal disease, and for staging lymphomas.

▶ Complications and related nursing diagnoses

Hemorrhage	Decreased cardiac output
	Altered tissue perfusion
Perforation	Pain
	Risk for infection
	Decreased cardiac output
Ileus	Pain
	Ineffective breathing pattern
Oversedation	Risk for injury
	Ineffective breathing pattern
	Risk for aspiration

Special Patient Management
Pretest
1. Check to see that patient has received and responded to the bowel prep, and has remained NPO since midnight.
2. Check to see that the results of the patient's clotting studies are normal and that hemoglobin and hematocrit levels are stable.
3. Obtain baseline vital signs.

Posttest
OUTCOME CRITERIA
1. Hemostasis at insertion site
2. Patient is alert and oriented
3. SBP 90-140 mm Hg
4. HR 60-100 beats/min
5. Patient is pain free

INTERVENTIONS
1. Assess VS for fever, hemodynamic instability, and respiratory compromise.
2. Assess for pain, particularly shoulder or subcostal discomfort.
3. Assess GI function: bowel sounds, abdominal pain; signs and symptoms of peritonitis: rigid abdomen, distention.
4. Determine presence of gag reflex and keep the patient NPO until the reflex returns.

CONSULT WITH PHYSICIAN
- Perforation or bleeding: decreased BP, increased HR, pain, fever, abdominal tenderness, difficulty breathing
- Oversedation: inability to arouse, decreased respirations

LIVER/SPLEEN SCAN

Clinical Brief

A liver/spleen scan is used to evaluate size, shape, and position of the liver, gallbladder, common bile duct, and spleen. Space-occupying lesions, metastatic disease, infarctions, and damage to organs can be determined. These studies are performed in conjunction with computed tomography to provide a three-dimensional view of the radioactive material distribution.

▶ Complications and related nursing diagnosis

None

Special Patient Management

Determine whether the patient has received barium within the last 24 hours, since barium may interfere with imaging.

MAGNETIC RESONANCE IMAGING (MRI)

Clinical Brief

MRI is a noninvasive technique used to obtain biochemical information from body tissues and produce tomographic images without the use of ionizing radiation. The hydrogen atom is the proton studied. Hydrogen reflects water content of tissue; thus the varying densities of hydrogen atoms and their interactions with other tissues can be made. Images are generated as hydrogen atoms change alignment of their nuclei when exposed to radio waves and are generally displayed in one of three planes: axial, sagittal, or coronal. MRI is most beneficial in evaluating body structures that have little or no motion; it is superior to radiographs and ultrasonography because distortion from surrounding bone is nonexistent. A hazard does exist if some types of metal are present in the environment, necessitating careful screening of patients.

Brain/Spinal cord

MRI visualizes cerebral lesions such as brain abscesses, brainstem tumors, and small hemorrhages not evident on CT scans, identifies areas of infarction within a few hours of the incident, localizes lesions in white matter and identifies cerebral and spinal cord edema, arteriovenous malformations, degenerative diseases (e.g., multiple sclerosis, Alzheimer's disease), and congenital anomalies. *Magnetic Resonance Angiography (MRA)* is a special computer MRI program that highlights the cerebral vasculature. It is quick and noninvasive.

Cardiac

In cardiac evaluation, MRI has had limited usefulness thus far.

Renal

MRI can be used to identify renal structures and differentiate such abnormalities as cyst contents, tumor stages, and the status of renal transplants.

▶ Complications and related nursing diagnosis

None

Special Patient Management

Screen the patient for metallic implants such as a pacemaker, an implantable defibrillator, prosthetic heart valves, neurostimulators, aneurysm clips, cochlear implants, an insulin pump, or metal bullet fragments. Hip implants, dental fillings and braces, sternal wire sutures, and intrauterine devices are not dangerous for the study.

MULTIPLE GATED ACQUISITION SCAN (MUGA) AND FIRST PASS SCAN

Clinical Brief

These blood pool imaging tests use Technetium-99m pyrophosphate to tag red blood cells. A special camera records the movement of the radiotracer through the heart and a computer creates images of the heart and its function throughout the cardiac cycle. The "first pass" technique analyzes the radiotracer as it first passes through the right heart, lungs, and the left heart. The "gated" technique analyzes radiotracer volume within a given cardiac chamber over 200 to 300 cardiac cycles, estimating chamber performance. "Gated" scans are frequently obtained after first passes and can better estimate chamber volumes, left and right ventricular ejection fractions, and rates of ventricular filling. These scans can be performed with or without exercise "stress" testing. The normal left ventricular response to exercise is for the ejection fraction to increase by at least 5%. Failure to accomplish this and/or the development of one or more regional wall abnormalities may indicate significant coronary artery disease.

▶ **Complications and related nursing diagnosis**
None

Special Patient Management

If stress testing is performed, monitor VS and ECG as per protocol. MI, sustained VT, or cardiac arrest may occur during the stress test.

MYELOGRAPHY

Clinical Brief

Myelography is used to visualize the spinal canal and nerve roots. A contrast material is injected through a lumbar or cisternal puncture, and areas in question are visualized on radiographs or by CT scanning. Lesions that block subarachnoid space (e.g., herniated intervertebral disks, spinal cord tumors or vascular anomalies) can be identified.

▶ **Complications and related nursing diagnoses**

Contrast reaction	Impaired skin integrity
	Ineffective breathing pattern
	Decreased cardiac output
	Altered urinary elimination
Headache	Pain
Seizures	Risk for injury

Special Patient Management

Pretest

1. Obtain baseline VS and neurological assessment.
2. Verify the type of contrast material to be used; patients who are receiving water-soluble contrast should be well-hydrated.

Posttest

OUTCOME CRITERIA

1. SPB 90-100 mm Hg
2. Neurological assessment appropriate for patient
3. Absence of seizures, headache, nausea, backache, and neck stiffness

INTERVENTIONS

1. Obtain VS every 30" for 2 hrs, every 60" for 2 hrs, then every 4 hrs for 24 hrs.
2. If a *water-soluble contrast* is used, maintain patient upright at 30- to 45-degree angle for first 12 to 24 hrs.

Increase fluids if not contraindicated. Avoid pheno-thiazines for nausea and vomiting, since these agents can increase symptoms of toxicity.

3. If an *oil-based contrast* is used, keep the patient flat for 6 to 24 hrs and force fluids. Headache is a common complication and is aggravated by an upright position.

4. In both *water-soluble and oil-based contrast*, observe the patient for nausea, vomiting, back pain, muscle spasms, elevated temperature, difficulty voiding, and nuchal rigidity

5. Administer analgesics as ordered.

CONSULT WITH PHYSICIAN
- Nausea/vomiting
- Severe headache, change in level of consciousness, or seizure activity

MYOCARDIAL INFARCT IMAGING

Clinical Brief

Myocardial infarct imaging is useful when standard methods of diagnosing infarction (enzymes, ECG, history) yield questionable data. Technetium-99m pyrophosphate is the isotope used because it binds with calcium within damaged myocardial cells. Necrotic areas are visualized as "hot spots"; normal, healthy cells do not take up the isotope so do not appear in the scanned image. Cardioversion or chest wall trauma may result in false-positive uptake.

▶ **Complications and related nursing diagnosis**
None

Special Patient Management

If stress testing is performed, monitor VS and ECG as per protocol. MI, sustained VT, or cardiac arrest may occur during the stress test.

MYOCARDIAL PERFUSION IMAGING

Clinical Brief

Myocardial perfusion imaging is used to identify areas of stress-induced ischemia or old infarction. Myocardial uptake of thallium-201, which concentrates in normal tissue (not ischemic or infarcted tissue), is analyzed after intravenous injection. Normal myocardial imaging should result in a homogeneous appearance of all structures. Ischemic or scarred areas have a lessened uptake of thallium-201, resulting in a "cold spot." If exercise stress testing is performed with this technique, a 4-hour postinjectate image is typically obtained to ascertain whether "cold spots" begin to appear normal, which could indicate transient ischemia rather than infarction.

Myocardial perfusion imaging with exercise stress testing is more sensitive and specific than exercise stress testing alone and can be useful in detecting ischemia in patients with exercise-induced ECG changes that are difficult to interpret. For those patients unable or unwilling to exercise in conjunction with myocardial perfusion imaging, pharmacologic stress testing is an alternative. Agents such as dipyridamole or adenosine can be used to dilate the coronary arteries (rather than exercise) so that perfusion can be assessed.

▶ Complications and related nursing diagnosis
None

Special Patient Management

If stress testing is performed, monitor VS and ECG as per protocol. MI, sustained VT, or cardiac arrest may occur during stress test.

PULMONARY FUNCTION TESTS
Clinical Brief

Spirometry is used to measure lung volumes, capacities, and flow rates to quantify the performance of the respiratory system. Spirometry can be performed at the bedside or in the pulmonary function laboratory. More sophisticated tests, such as body plethysmography and gas dilution techniques, require testing in the pulmonary function laboratory; these tests measure lung volumes and diffusion capacities.

Pulmonary function tests can be used to predict the need for mechanical ventilation and the likelihood of success at weaning a critically ill patient from mechanical ventilation. A commonly measured lung volume is the vital capacity (VC), which correlates with the patient's ability to deep breathe and cough. A vital capacity of ≥10 to 12 ml/kg is generally needed for spontaneous breathing. Another useful test to predict successful weaning is the negative inspiratory force (NIF). A negative inspiratory force of at least -20 cm H_2O is necessary to maintain spontaneous ventilation.

Other measurements that provide an assessment of lung function in the mechanically ventilated patient include maximal voluntary ventilation (MVV), which is reflective of muscle strength, lung mechanics, and patient effort; the V_D/V_T ratio, which represents wasted ventilation; and compliance, or the stiffness of the lungs and chest wall, which is often decreased in the presence of air flow obstruction, increased lung stiffness, or limited chest wall mobility. A discussion of the mechanically ventilated patient can be found in Chapter 7. Pulmonary function tests are also used to differentiate obstructive from restrictive lung disorders and to assess patient response to therapy (e.g., before and after use of a bronchodilator). Restrictive lung disorders have little or no effect on air flow; however, lung volumes and capacities are decreased. Restrictive defects are commonly caused by chest wall deformity (e.g., scoliosis) and neuromuscular weakness. Patients with obstructive lung disorders, which affect the patient's ability to exhale, have decreased flow rates with normal or decreased lung volumes and capacities. The most common obstructive diseases leading to respiratory failure are emphysema and chronic bronchitis.

Pulmonary function tests can also be used to assess high-risk patients undergoing thoracic or abdominal surgery. Patients who smoke or experience pulmonary symptoms or who will undergo thoracic or abdominal surgery are at a high risk for developing postoperative pulmonary complications, such as atelectasis, pneumonia, and prolonged ventilation. Assessing lung function in these patients is helpful to identify patients who will benefit from intense respiratory care. A patient with an FEV_1 less than 2 L has little respiratory reserve and, if not supported meticulously, is at risk for developing respiratory failure. Table 5-5 lists pulmonary function assessment parameters.

▶ Complications and related nursing diagnosis
None

Special Patient Management
Monitor for development of bronchospasm.

RENAL SCAN
Clinical Brief
A renal scan is used to assess perfusion to and functioning of the kidneys; it is especially helpful to differentiate acute tubular necrosis (ATN) from rejection in transplanted kidneys.

▶ Complications and related nursing diagnosis
None

TABLE 5-5 Pulmonary Function Assessment Parameters

Parameter	Description
Tidal volume (V_T)	Volume of gas inspired or expired with each quiet breath; normally ~500 ml
Inspiratory reserve volume (IRV)	Additional volume of gas that can be inspired after a normal tidal volume inspiration; normally ~3000 ml
Inspiratory capacity (IC)	Maximum volume of gas inspired after a normal exhalation; includes V_T + IRV; normally ~3500 ml
Expiratory reserve volume (ERV)	Additional volume of gas that can be forcefully exhaled after a normal expiration; normally ~1000 ml
Vital capacity (VC)	Maximum volume of gas exhaled after a maximal inspiration; includes V_T + IRV + ERV; normally ~4500 ml
Residual volume (RV)	Volume of gas remaining in the lungs after a maximal expiration; normally ~1500 ml
Functional residual capacity (FRC)	Volume of gas remaining in the lungs after a normal expiration; includes RV + ERV; normally ~2500 ml
Total lung capacity (TLC)	Sum of all of the lung volumes, which includes IRV + V_T + ERV + RV; normally ~6000 ml

Forced vital capacity (FVC)

Maximum volume of gas forcibly and rapidly exhaled after a forceful inspiration; normally ~4500 ml

Forced expiratory volume (FEV)

Amount of FVC that has been exhaled at a timed measurement

FEV_1

Amount of gas exhaled in the first second during maximal exhalation; most commonly used test to measure obstruction; also expressed as a ratio: FEV_1/FVC; a ratio <75% indicates airway obstruction

$FEF_{25\%-75\%}$

The forced expiratory flow between 25% and 75% vital capacity; reflects small airways function

Maximal voluntary ventilation (MVV)

Volume of gas exhaled during a specified time (usually 1 min) while performing repetitive maximal efforts; normally ~50-250 L/min

Minute ventilation (V_E)

Volume of gas inhaled and exhaled during quiet breathing per minute: (V_T) × respiratory rate per minute; normally ~6 to 7 L/min

Deadspace (V_D)

Volume of gas that never reaches the alveoli; normally ~1 ml/lb

Deadspace to tidal volume ratio (V_D/V_T)

Amount of V_T used to ventilate areas of the lung that do not participate in gas exchange; normally ~<0.4

Compliance (Δ Volume/Δ Pressure)

Increase in volume for a given pressure change; normally ~50-100 ml/cm H_2O

Negative inspiratory force (NIF)

Pressure the respiratory muscles must generate to maintain spontaneous ventilation; normally ~-20 cm H_2O or greater

Special Patient Management

Check that the patient is adequately hydrated prior to test. Encourage patient to empty bladder immediately after the test to reduce radiation exposure to the bladder wall.

SKULL AND SPINE RADIOGRAPHS

Clinical Brief

X-ray films of the skull are used to evaluate the head-injured patient for skull fractures and detect air-fluid levels in the skull or sinus, which may indicate a possible CSF leak. Spine radiographs are helpful to evaluate trauma patients for any fractures/subluxation of the cervical, thoracic, and lumbar regions.

▶ Complications and related nursing diagnosis
None

Special Patient Management

Patients should be maintained in a neutral position. Prevent any movement that could result in further neurological deterioration until the initial spine films have been read.

ULTRASONOGRAPHY

Clinical Brief

Ultrasonography is a noninvasive procedure in which high-frequency sound waves are reflected off tissue to produce images of internal organs. Structure and function of organs can be visualized and evaluated.

Carotid ultrasonogram

Carotid ultrasound is used to detect stenosis of the extracranial carotid arteries.

Echocardiogram

An echocardiogram is used to assess ventricular function, cardiac wall abnormalities, and valvular function. Currently four methods can be used. (1) M-mode echocardiography involves a single beam to sweep across cardiac structures. Valvular mobility, chamber size, pericardial effusions, and septal size can be evaluated. (2) Two-dimensional (2D)(cross-sectional) echocardiography involves an ultrasonic beam that oscillates across viewed cardiac structures. Valvular vegetations, septal defects, wall motion, chamber size, the presence of a pericardial effusion, valve motion, and wall thickness can be evaluated. (3) Doppler echocardiography analyzes blood flow velocity and turbulence. Cross-valvular pressure gradients, blood flow patterns, and specific valve orifices can be evaluated. (4) Transesophageal echocardiography (TEE) uses the 2D and Doppler modes to visualize the heart via an endoscope positioned in the esophagus against the left atrium. Signal quality is improved because ultrasound waves are not impeded by lung or fat tissue. In additional to visualizing the heart, TEE is also sensitive enough for diagnosing aortic dissection.

Gastrointestinal ultrasonogram

A GI ultrasonogram is useful for confirming gallbladder, pancreas, or liver disease; differentiating obstructive versus nonobstructive jaundice; localizing tumors and hematomas; and guiding biopsies and drainage of abscesses. A gaseous filled bowel or a dehydrated state may render this test inconclusive.

Renal ultrasonogram

Renal ultrasonography is used to identify and locate renal structures and abnormalities such as ureteral leaks, abscesses, and obstructions; to differentiate cysts from solid masses (tumors); and to guide biopsies, aspiration, and drain insertion.

Transcranial Doppler flow study

Doppler flow studies are used to assess velocity of cerebral blood flow and the degree of stenosis, occlusion, collateral blood flow, and vasospasm of the internal carotid, anterior cerebral, middle cerebral, posterior cerebral, and occasionally the basilar arteries. Flow rates are increased in cases of vasospasm or vessel disease because the vessel lumen is narrowed.

Normal velocity rates are as follows:

ICA 40-60 cm/sec
ACA 20-40 cm/sec
MCA 60-80 cm/sec
PCA 20-40 cm/sec

▶ Complications and related nursing diagnoses (TEE)

Perforation of esophagus	Pain
Oversedation	Risk for injury
	Ineffective breathing pattern
	Risk for aspiration

Special Patient Management (GI, Renal Ultrasonograms)

Patients should be adequately hydrated before ultrasonograms are performed.

Special Patient Management (TEE)
Pretest
1. Verify NPO for 4-6 hours.
2. Give sedation if ordered.
During test (may be done at bedside)
1. Monitor VS, cardiac rhythm, SaO_2, and patient tolerance to procedure.
2. Verify suction equipment and code cart are readily available.
Posttest
OUTCOME CRITERIA
1. SBP 90-140 mm Hg
2. HR 60-100 beats/min
3. Gag reflex present
4. Patient is pain free (mild sore throat is expected)
INTERVENTIONS
1. Assess VS for hemodynamic instability or respiratory compromise.
2. Determine presence of gag reflex. Keep patient NPO until reflex returns.
3. Monitor for persistent or unusual stomach discomfort (esophageal perforation/bleeding).
4. Maintain bedrest with side rails up until effects of sedation wear off.
CONSULT WITH PHYSICIAN
1. Esophageal perforation/bleeding: persistent or unusual throat or stomach discomfort
2. Oversedation: inability to arouse, decreased respiration

VENTILATION-PERFUSION SCAN (V/Q SCAN)
Clinical Brief
A ventilation-perfusion scan is used to diagnose pulmonary emboli. After a radioactive material is injected intravenously, pulmonary vascular supply and air flow movement in the lungs are elevated. The V/Q scan is compared with the chest radiograph. A high probability of pulmonary emboli is present if the V/Q scan has a perfusion defect larger than the radiograph or multiple segmental or lobar mismatch defects.
▶ Complications and related nursing diagnosis
None

Special Patient Management
None

XENON CEREBRAL BLOOD FLOW

Clinical Brief

This study is used to estimate cerebral blood flow. Xenon-133 is inhaled and brain tissue is monitored for isotope clearance. Probes that are externally positioned around the head provide information to a computer, which calculates blood flow. Conditions of increased or decreased blood flow are evaluated (e.g., injured brain, vasospasm). Normal cerebral blood flow is 50 to 75 ml/100 g/min.

▶ **Complications and related nursing diagnosis**
None

Special Patient Management

None

REFERENCES

1. Ahrens TS: Pulmonary data acquisition. In Kinney MR, Packa DR, Dunbar SB, eds: *AACN's clinical reference for critical care nursing,* ed 3, St Louis, 1993, Mosby.
2. Allison MC: Investigation of the colon. In Misiewicz JJ, Pounder RE, Venables CW, eds: *Diseases of the gut and pancreas,* ed 2, Boston, 1994, Blackwell Scientific Publication.
3. Bell TE et al: Transcranial doppler: correlation of blood velocity measurement with clinical status in subarachnoid hemorrhage, *Neurosci Nurs* 24(4):215-219, 1992.
4. Bontozoglou N et al: Three-dimensional display of the orifice of intracranial aneurysms: a new potential application for magnetic resonance angiography, *Neuroradiology* 36:346-349, 1994.
5. Borkowski GP: Hepatobiliary and pancreatic imaging. In Achkar E, Farmer RG, Fleschler B, eds: *Clinical gastroenterology,* ed 2, Philadelphia, 1992, Lea & Febiger.
6. Brown L: Transesophageal echocardiography: implications for the critical care nurse, *Crit Care Nurse* 14(3):55-59, 1994.
7. Cherryman GR: Magnetic resonance angiography, *Br J Hosp Med* 52(2-3):68-69, 1994.
8. Chesnut RM: Computed tomography of the brain: a guide to understanding and interpreting normal and abnormal images in the critically ill patient, *Crit Care Nurs Q* 17(1):33-50, 1994.
9. Conover M: Diagnosis and management of arrhythmias associated with Wolff-Parkinson-White syndrome, *Crit Care Nurse* 14(3):30-41, 1994.
10. DeMarco JK et al: Prospective evaluation of extracranial carotid stenosis: MR angiography with maximum intensity projections and multiplanar reformation compared with conventional angiography, *AJR* 163:1205-1212, 1994.

11. Hearns P: Differentiating ischemia, injury, infarction: expanding the 12-lead electrocardiogram, *Dimens Crit Care Nurs* 13(4):172-178, 1994.

12. Keeffe EB, Schrock TR: Complications of gastrointestinal endoscopy. In Sleisenger MH, Fordtran JS, eds: *Gastrointestinal disease: pathophysiology/diagnosis/management,* ed 5, Philadelphia, 1993, W.B. Saunders.

13. Kelly-Heidenthal P, O'Connor M: Nursing assessment of portable AP chest xrays, *Dimens Crit Care Nurs* 13(3):127-132, 1994.

14. Mancini D et al: Prognostic value of an abnormal signal-averaged electrocardiogram in patients with nonischemic congestive cardiomyopathy, *Circulation* 98(4):1083-1092, 1993.

15. Marchiondo K: Pharmacologic stress testing: an alternative to exercise, *Crit Care Nurse* 14(6):41-45, 1994.

16. McKinley M: Electrocardiographic monitoring. In Logston Boggs R, Wooldridge-King M, eds: *AACN procedure manual for critical care,* ed 3, Philadelphia, 1993, W.B. Saunders.

17. Morady F: Who is a good candidate for electrophysiologic testing? *J Crit Illn* 8(4):520-536, 1993.

18. Rotello L et al: MRI protocol for critically ill patients, *Am J Crit Care* 3(3):187-190, 1994.

19. Sahn SA: Pneumothorax and pneumomediastinum. In Mitchell RS, Petty TL, Schwarz MI, eds: *Synopsis of clinical pulmonary disease,* ed 4, St Louis, 1989, Mosby.

20. Schrier RW, Gottschalk CG, eds: *Diseases of the kidney,* Boston, 1993, Little, Brown & Co.

21. Sheldon RL: Clinical application of the chest radiograph. In Wilkins RL, Sheldon RL, Krider SJ, eds: *Clinical assessment in respiratory care,* St Louis, 1994, Mosby.

22. Shorvon PH, Loft D: Radiology and endoscopy of the stomach and duodenum. In Misiewicz JJ, Pounder RE, Venables CW, eds: *Diseases of the gut and pancreas,* ed 2, Boston, 1994, Blackwell Scientific Publications.

23. Society of Gastroenterology Nurses and Associates: *Gastroenterology nursing: a core curriculum,* St Louis, 1993, Mosby.

24. Stiesmeyer J: Unstable angina associated with critical proximal left anterior descending coronary artery stenosis, *Am J Crit Care* 2(3):248-253, 1993.

25. Sugawa C, Joseph AL: Endoscopic interventional management of bleeding duodenal and gastric ulcers, *Surg Clin North Am* 72(2):317-334, 1992.

26. Talbot L, Meyers-Marquardt M: *Pocket guide to critical care assessment,* St Louis, 1993, Mosby.

27. Thompson E: Adenosine thallium imaging: pharmacodynamics and patient monitoring, *Dim Crit Care Nurs* 13(4):184-193, 1994.

28. Thompson E: Transesophageal echocardiography: a new window on the heart and great vessels, *Crit Care Nurse* 13(5):55-66, 1993.
29. Underwood M: Nuclear cardiology stress testing, *Nursing 94*, 24(10):63-64, 1994.
30. Urden LD, Davis JK, Thelan LA: *Essentials of critical care nursing*, St Louis, 1992, Mosby.
31. Worthley LIG: *Synopsis of intensive care medicine*, London, 1994, Churchill Livingstone.

CHAPTER 6

Monitoring the Critically Ill Patient

ARTERIAL BLOOD GAS ANALYSIS

Clinical Brief

Arterial blood gas analysis is done to assess the acid-base balance of the body, the adequacy of oxygenation and/or ventilation, and the adequacy of circulation, and to detect metabolic abnormalities.

Indications

Arterial blood gas analysis may be done in any of the following clinical situations: (1) serious respiratory problems or prolonged weaning from mechanical ventilation, (2) cardiac dysfunction associated with decreased CO, and (3) shock states.

Description

A sample of blood (1 to 3 ml) is drawn from an artery and analyzed; the partial pressures of oxygen (Pao_2) and carbon dioxide ($Paco_2$) are determined, as well as the pH and bicarbonate ion levels and oxygen saturation.

The pH measures hydrogen ion concentration, which is an indication of acid-base balance. The body maintains a normal pH by keeping bicarbonate ion (a function of the kidneys) and $Paco_2$ (a function of the lungs) in a constant ratio of 20:1. When there is a disturbance in acid-base balance, there will be compensation by the system (respiratory or renal) *not* primarily affected to return the pH to normal. If the disturbance is respiratory, the kidneys compensate by altering bicarbonate excretion in order to return the pH to normal; however, the kidneys are slow to respond to changes in pH and compensation may take days. If the disturbance is metabolic, the respiratory system will compensate by increasing or decreasing ventilation (and CO_2 removal) to return the pH to normal; the lungs respond to changes in pH within minutes.

The Paco$_2$ level is adjusted by the rate and depth of ventilation: hypoventilation results in *high* Paco$_2$ levels, whereas hyperventilation results in *low* Paco$_2$ levels.

The Pao$_2$ reflects the amount of oxygen dissolved in arterial blood. Pao$_2$ does not directly influence the acid-base balance, although hypoxemia with anaerobic metabolism can lead to lactic acidosis.

Oxygen saturation reflects the amount of oxygen combined with hemoglobin that is carried in arterial blood. The oxygen-hemoglobin dissociation curve demonstrates the relationship between Pao$_2$ and O$_2$ saturation. As tissues utilize the oxygen dissolved in arterial blood, oxygen dissociates from the hemoglobin, causing a decrease in saturation. Significant changes in oxygen saturation occur when the Pao$_2$ falls below 60 mm Hg. Various conditions can affect the oxygen-hemoglobin affinity and thus affect oxygen availability for tissues (Figure 6-1).

The bicarbonate ion level represents the renal component of acid-base regulation. The kidneys adjust the level of bicarbonate ion by changes in the excretion rate.

Values

Normal
pH 7.35-7.45
Paco$_2$ 35-45 mm Hg

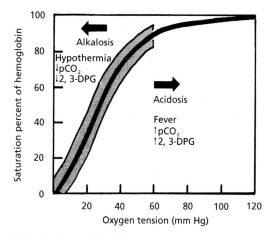

Figure 6-1   Oxyhemoglobin dissociation curve.

PaO_2 80-100 mm Hg
O_2 saturation 95%-99%
Serum bicarbonate (HCO_3) 22-26 mEq/L

Significance of abnormal values

pH <7.35: acidosis, pH >7.45: alkalosis. It is impossible to determine the cause (respiratory or renal) of acidosis or alkalosis by looking at the pH alone.

$PaCO_2$ <35 mm Hg: respiratory alkalosis, caused by hyperventilation (may be secondary to ventilatory support, central nervous system disease, fever, liver disease, heart failure, pulmonary embolism).

$PaCO_2$ >45 mm Hg: respiratory acidosis, caused by hypoventilation (may be secondary to impaired alveolar ventilation, respiratory depressants, intracranial tumors).

PaO_2 <80 mm Hg: hypoxemia, with inadequate O_2 to meet tissue needs. If hypoxemia is left untreated, anaerobic metabolism and acidosis will result.

PaO_2 >100 mm Hg: hyperoxemia, usually a result of excessive concentration of oxygen. FIO_2 should be lowered to produce PaO_2 >60 to 70 mm Hg or O_2 saturation ≥95%.

O_2 saturation <95%: hypoxemia.

HCO_3 <22 mEq/L: metabolic acidosis (may be secondary to renal failure, lactic acidosis, diabetic ketoacidosis, diarrhea).

HCO_3 >26 mEq/L: metabolic alkalosis (may be secondary to vomiting, ingestion of diuretics, nasogastric suction, steroid therapy, hyperaldosteronism, hyperadrenocorticism).

Steps to Interpret ABGs

1. Look at pH to determine whether imbalance is acidosis or alkalosis.
2. Look at $PaCO_2$ and compare with pH; they are inversely proportional, so if the pH and $PaCO_2$ are moving in opposite directions, the imbalance is the result of a respiratory problem.
3. Look at HCO_3 and compare with pH; they are directly proportional, so if the pH and HCO_3 are moving in the same direction, the imbalance is the result of a metabolic problem.
4. Compare $PaCO_2$ and HCO_3 with each other; if they are moving in the same direction, one system is attempting to compensate for a disturbance in the opposite system. If they are moving in the opposite direction, a mixed imbalance is present. Usually the value that deviates most from normal is the primary disturbance.

5. Look at Pao_2 and O_2 saturation and determine whether they are decreased, normal, or increased; low values indicate the need for improved oxygenation and/or ventilation, and high values indicate the need to decrease the delivered concentration of oxygen.

Examples

1. pH 7.6 (increased)
   $Paco_2$ 25 mm Hg (decreased)
   HCO_3 24 mEq/L (normal)
   Disturbance: respiratory alkalosis, no compensation
2. pH 7.20 (decreased)
   $Paco_2$ 38 mm Hg (normal)
   HCO_3 15 mEq/L (decreased)
   Disturbance: metabolic acidosis, no compensation
3. pH 7.32 (decreased)
   $Paco_2$ 66 mm Hg (increased)
   HCO_3 28 mEq/L (increased)
   Disturbance: respiratory acidosis with kidneys trying to compensate (Note: Compensation is not complete until pH is within normal limits.)
4. pH 7.56 (increased)
   $Paco_2$ 32 mm Hg (decreased)
   HCO_3 38 mEq/L (increased)
   Disturbance: mixed metabolic and respiratory alkalosis

ARTERIAL PRESSURE MONITORING

Clinical Brief

Direct arterial pressure monitoring provides a continuous display of the arterial blood pressure waveform and digital readings of the systolic, diastolic, and mean pressures. Mean arterial pressure (MAP) is the average pressure throughout the cardiac cycle; it is an important indicator of tissue perfusion. MAP is determined by cardiac output and systemic vascular resistance. MAP can be calculated using the following formula:

$$MAP = \frac{\text{Systolic BP} + 2\,(\text{Diastolic BP})}{3}$$

When a pressure monitoring system is used, the bedside monitor displays the MAP, and it does not have to be calculated.

An indwelling arterial line also provides continuous access to arterial blood for sampling, such as for blood gas analysis and/or serum laboratory tests.

Indications

Arterial pressure monitoring may be used for the following: to monitor patients with unstable BP, to measure trends and evaluate the efficacy of vasoactive drugs, to obtain frequent arterial blood gases when weaning from mechanical ventilation, to obtain blood samples in the burn patient with limited vascular access through intact skin, or to monitor BP in shock states where conventional cuff BP may be difficult to determine. In addition, direct arterial pressure monitoring allows easy determination of MAP, an indicator of tissue perfusion.

Description

An arterial catheter, usually a Teflon catheter over a needle, is inserted into an artery through a percutaneous or cutdown method. The radial artery is preferred because of its accessibility, although the axillary, femoral, brachial, or pedal arteries can be used. The catheter is then attached to a pressure transducer setup with a continuous flush of heparinized saline. When the pressure bag is inflated to 300 mm Hg, 3 ml/hr will be delivered through the line, thus promoting patency of the line. The pressure transducer is connected to the monitor, and a continuous waveform is displayed on the oscilloscope. Digital display of the pressure is also available.

Values

Normal

Systolic blood pressure 90-140 mm Hg
Diastolic blood pressure 60-80 mm Hg
Mean arterial pressure 70-105 mm Hg

Significance of abnormal values

Systolic blood pressure values can be abnormal from changes in stroke volume (e.g., hypervolemia, hypovolemia, or heart failure), changes in wall compliance (e.g., arteriosclerosis and hypertension), changes in the rate of ejection of blood from the left ventricle (e.g., sympathetic nervous system stimulation and some vasoactive drugs) or when there is aortic insufficiency (elevated systolic blood pressure) or aortic stenosis (lowered systolic blood pressure).

Diastolic blood pressure may be elevated as a result of increased stroke volume or systemic vascular resistance; it may be lowered as a result of hypovolemia, peripheral dilation of blood vessels, or aortic insufficiency.

Changes in mean arterial pressure are caused by changes in cardiac output and/or changes in systemic vascular resistance.

Patient Care Management
Preinsertion
Before insertion of a radial arterial line, an Allen test should be performed to assess adequacy of collateral circulation to the hand (Figure 6-2).

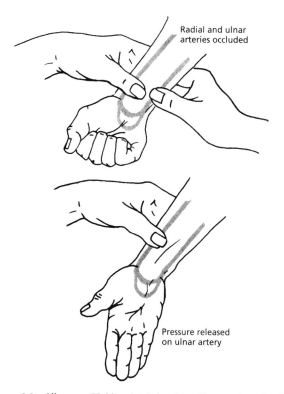

Figure 6-2   Allen test. Hold patient's hand up. Have patient clench and unclench hand while occluding the radial and ulnar arteries. The hand will become pale. Lower the hand and have the patient relax the hand. While continuing to hold the radial artery, release pressure on the ulnar artery. Brisk return of color (5 to 7 seconds) demonstrates adequate ulnar blood flow. If pallor persists for more than 15 seconds, ulnar flow is inadequate and radial artery cannulation should not be attempted. (From Stillwell S, Randall E: *Pocket guide to cardiovascular care,* ed 2, St Louis, 1994, Mosby.)

The insertion of the arterial catheter is done under aseptic conditions. Zero the transducer after connecting it to the monitor and prior to arterial cannulation. Attach the transducer to the pressure tubing so that the waveform is immediately visible upon cannulation of the artery.

▶ **Complications and related nursing diagnoses**

Hemorrhage   Fluid volume deficit

Hemorrhage can occur if the arterial catheter inadvertently becomes disconnected from the transducer. To prevent this, the alarm system must be activated at all times, and Luer-Lok connections should be used at all connections in the pressure setup. If the patient is restless or confused and is at risk for accidental dislodgement of the tubing or catheter, sedation or restraint should be considered.

Clot formation   Altered tissue perfusion: peripheral

Clot formation can occur at the insertion site or at the tip of the catheter. Patients with peripheral vascular disease or arteriosclerosis are particularly prone to clot formation and embolization. Use of the femoral artery is associated with a higher incidence of distal embolic complications than other sites. To prevent clot formation, a continuous infusion (3 ml/hr) of heparinized saline is connected to the arterial catheter. After the blood sample is obtained, the line must be flushed thoroughly to clear the catheter of blood. The tracing on the monitor must be observed frequently for loss of amplitude, which may be caused by clot formation. Assess capillary refill, and color and temperature of the skin, as well as sensation and movement of the extremity distal to the cannulation site at least every 2 hours. Signs of decreased circulation that result from embolization of a clot include pain, pallor, and cyanosis in the distal extremity.

Infection   Risk for infection

Infection can occur with any invasive monitoring line; it can occur within the system setup, at the cannulation site, or with the catheter. Flush solution containing glucose should be avoided to decrease the risk of bacterial growth. Strict aseptic technique is used during the system setup and catheter insertion, as well as during blood sampling procedures and dressing changes. Sterile deadend caps should be placed on all open ports of the stopcocks. The site should be inspected daily for redness, swelling, or exudate. The flush solution should be changed every 24 hours; the tubing, stopcocks, deadend caps, and dressing should be changed every 48 to 72 hours (or per facility protocol) and when contamination is suspected.

Vessel damage   Risk for injury

Vessel damage results from trauma to the vessel at the time of cannulation or from friction of the catheter in the vessel. The catheter should be handled gently at all times to minimize the friction on the wall of the vessel. If a clot is suspected, it should be aspirated instead of flushed into the artery. Vessel spasm can occur if too much force is used during blood sampling procedures; only minimal pressure should be used to draw blood into the syringe. If a radial catheter is used, support the patient's wrist on an armboard or other supportive device to prevent flexion and movement of the catheter.

Air embolus   Risk for injury
                                                           Altered tissue perfusion

Air that is trapped in the tubing can be inadvertently flushed into the artery and the systemic circulation. All air must be purged from the tubing during the setup of the system. Also, the tubing should be frequently inspected for air, especially before fast-flushing the line. Observe the arterial waveform for decreased amplitude, which may indicate air in the line or in the transducer. Any detected air needs to be aspirated.

Electric shock   Risk for injury

Electric shock is a potential risk with any fluid-filled monitoring system. It can occur if current leaks from an electrical device to the fluid-filled catheter, which provides a low resistance pathway directly to the heart. All electrical equipment used in patient rooms should be adequately grounded and have three-pronged plugs. Electrical devices used in the critical care unit should be checked by the biomedical department at regular intervals.

Postinsertion

With centrally located catheters (such as the femoral artery), the air reference port of the transducer should be leveled with the tip of the catheter, which is approximately at the level of the right atrium. This landmark, the *phlebostatic axis* (Figure 6-3), is the intersection of the fourth intercostal space and midanterior posterior chest. By leveling the air reference port of the transducer in this manner, the effects of hydrostatic pressure within the fluid-filled system are eliminated. Mark the phlebostatic axis with ink or tape on the patient's skin and use this same point for taking readings; failure to do so will result in inaccurate readings.

When the arterial catheter is located peripherally (such as the radial artery), it is more accurate to place the air reference port of the transducer at the level of the tip of the catheter (e.g., the patient's wrist); this eliminates the effects of hydrostatic pressure within the fluid-filled column and provides an accurate measurement of the static pressure within the artery itself.

Alarm parameters should be set (usually 10 to 20 mm Hg above and below the patient's baseline pressure) and activated. The alarms should be maintained at all times so that sudden changes in pressure and/or disconnection of the line is immediately noted.

Be aware that blood pressures obtained by direct monitoring methods (e.g., arterial line) will not necessarily be the same as those derived by indirect methods (e.g., cuff) that are flow dependent. The routine practice of comparing cuff and arterial line pressure should be discouraged. More important is evaluation of each patient situation to determine the most appropriate method for assessing BP.

Obtaining accurate measurements

Relevel the transducer every time the patient or transducer is moved, including each time the bed height or head elevation is changed, as well as with any significant change in the patient's

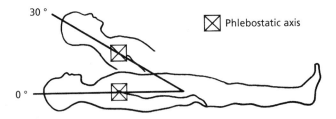

Phlebostatic axis

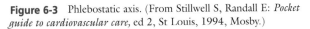

Figure 6-3 Phlebostatic axis. (From Stillwell S, Randall E: *Pocket guide to cardiovascular care,* ed 2, St Louis, 1994, Mosby.)

hemodynamic variables. Prevent kinks in the catheter by stabilizing securely. Observe the line frequently for air, which may damp the waveform. Flush the line thoroughly each time blood is drawn. Peripheral arterial catheters are often positional, and the waveform may be damped if the extremity is flexed. Use of an armboard or splint will eliminate this.

Waveform interpretation

Systole is apparent on the waveform as a sharp rise in pressure; this is the anacrotic limb, and it signifies the rapid ejection of blood from the ventricle through the open aortic valve. If there is a delay in this rapid rise, it could suggest a decrease in myocardial contractility, aortic stenosis, or damped pressure secondary to catheter position or clot formation. A steep rate of rise along with a high peak systolic pressure and a poorly defined dicrotic notch may be seen with aortic insufficiency.

Diastole follows closure of the aortic valve (seen as the dicrotic notch on the waveform) and continues until the next systole. The location of the dicrotic notch should be one third or greater the height of the systolic peak; if it is not, suspect a decreased cardiac output (Figure 6-4). Table 6-1 offers methods for troubleshooting invasive hemodynamic monitoring lines.

Obtaining a blood sample

1. Observe universal precautions.
2. Follow unit policy/manufacturer's recommendations for specific system in use.
3. Assure return of arterial waveform on monitor.

Removal of arterial catheter

1. Turn the stopcock off to the patient and disconnect the transducer from the monitor.
2. Remove the arterial line dressing from the site and remove any sutures.

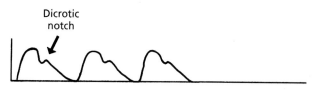

Dicrotic
notch

Figure 6-4   Arterial waveform. Dicrotic notch represents closure of the aortic valve.

TABLE 6-1 Troubleshooting Invasive Hemodynamic Monitoring Lines

Problem	Cause	Solution
Blood backup into tubing	Loose connections	Tighten connections
	Stopcock off to flush system	Open stopcock
	Inadequate pressure in bag	Inflate pressure bag to 300 mm Hg
Damped pressure tracing	Air bubbles in system	Purge air from system
	Clot formation	Aspirate blood from catheter and briefly flush system*
	Loose connections	Tighten connections
	Compliant tubing	Use stiff (high-pressure) tubing
	Change in patient condition	Assess and treat patient
	Inadequate pressure in bag	Inflate pressure bag to 300 mm Hg
No waveform	Transducer not open to catheter	Check system
	Transducer not connected to monitor	Connect transducer to monitor
	Incorrect scale selection	Select appropriate scale for physiological pressure
	Kink in catheter	Reposition catheter; use armboard to prevent wrist flexion
Inaccurate readings	Change in transducer reference level:	Keep transducer at phlebostatic axis or catheter tip level when obtaining readings
	Transducer *above* reference point results in false low readings	
	Transducer *below* reference point results in false high readings	
	Air or clotting within system	Check system: aspirate air or clots from system
Noise or fling in pressure waveform ("whip")	Excessive catheter movement: occurs when catheter in large vessel	Reposition catheter; use damping device to remove fling from waveform
	Excessive tubing length	Eliminate excessive tubing

*Do *not* flush ICP, LAP.

3. Gently withdraw the catheter from the artery and apply direct, firm pressure above the puncture site with sterile gauze while continuously assessing the circulation of the distal extremity. Maintain pressure for a minimum of 5 minutes or until bleeding stops.
4. Apply a pressure dressing to the site.
5. Assess the dressing for signs of bleeding and the distal extremity for evidence of impaired circulation.
6. Remove the dressing 8 hours after the removal of the catheter.

CAPNOMETRY
Clinical Brief
Capnometry is a continuous, noninvasive method for evaluating the adequacy of CO_2 exchange in the lungs.
Indications
Capnometry is useful in the mechanically ventilated patient who requires frequent blood gas sampling or who has an unstable respiratory status where minute-to-minute assessment of gas exchange is necessary. Patient response to different modes of ventilation and tolerance to weaning can be assessed using capnometry.
Description
Capnometry is the measurement of CO_2 concentration in respired gas. This concentration varies with the respiratory cycle; the inspired concentration is lowest, whereas the end tidal (P_{ETCO_2}) concentration is highest and is assumed to represent alveolar gas. End-tidal CO_2 can be used to estimate the pressure of CO_2 in arterial blood (Pa_{CO_2}), thus allowing the clinician to evaluate adequacy of CO_2 exchange in the lung. CO_2 concentration can be displayed digitally or as a capnogram (a recorded tracing of the waveform).

Values

Normal
P_{ETCO_2} is usually 1 to 4 mm Hg below Pa_{CO_2} in normal individuals.
Significance of abnormal values
The gradient between Pa_{CO_2} and P_{ETCO_2} is increased in patients with ventilation-perfusion mismatching and chronic obstructive pulmonary disease. Increased P_{ETCO_2} suggests an increase in Pa_{CO_2}, perhaps as a result of hypoventilation, while decreased P_{ETCO_2} suggests hyperventilation. Changes

in PETCO$_2$ should prompt the nurse to assess the patient and obtain arterial blood gases when a deterioration in respiratory status is suspected.

CENTRAL VENOUS PRESSURE MONITORING

Clinical Brief

Intermittent or continuous central venous pressure (CVP) monitoring is used to evaluate right-sided heart function and to assess efficacy of fluid replacement therapy.

Indications

CVP monitoring may be used to assess (1) volume replacement therapy, (2) right-sided heart failure (acute left ventricular failure will eventually elevate the CVP but pulmonary edema is already well-established), and (3) response to intravenous vasoactive drugs.

Description

The CVP catheter is inserted into a large vein by percutaneous or cutdown method. The catheter may be single lumen, or it may be a multilumen catheter that allows the infusion of several different or incompatible drugs or fluids simultaneously. The most common sites for insertion are the jugular (internal or external), subclavian, basilic, or femoral veins. Once the catheter is inserted, it is placed so that the tip is located in the superior vena cava, approximately 2 cm above the right atrium. The pressure waveform and digital value are displayed on the monitor.

Values

Normal

2-6 mm Hg

The waveform has systolic (positive) and diastolic (negative) variations, but the fluctuations are small (since the right atrium is a low-pressure chamber); thus the *mean* pressure is monitored.

Significance of abnormal values

Increased CVP may be caused by increased vascular volume, tricuspid or pulmonic valvular disease, ventricular septal defect with left-to-right shunting, constrictive pericarditis, right ventricular infarction, myocarditis, cardiac tamponade, chronic obstructive lung disease, pulmonary embolus, pulmonary hypertension, or *chronic* left ventricular failure.

Decreased CVP may be caused by hypovolemia, excessive diuresis, or systemic venodilation secondary to sepsis, drugs, or neurogenic causes.

Patient Care Management
Preinsertion
The patient is placed in the Trendelenburg position if the subclavian or jugular approach is to be used; this will facilitate filling of the vessel and will diminish the risk of air embolism. In addition, the patient should be instructed to hold a breath at peak expiration at the moment of catheter insertion. This will increase the intrathoracic pressure and diminish the risk for an air embolism.

▶ ## Complications and related nursing diagnoses
Similar to arterial pressure monitoring, CVP monitoring can result in air embolism, clot formation, hemorrhage, electrical shock, and infection (interventions to prevent these are the same as those described in Arterial pressure monitoring: patient care management, p. 485). Additionally, the following complications may occur with CVP monitoring:

Catheter tip migration   Decreased cardiac output

The tip of the catheter may move forward to the right ventricle and irritate the endocardium, causing ventricular dysrhythmias. If the tip migrates far enough that the heart wall is perforated, cardiac tamponade can result due to bleeding into the pericardial sac.

Postinsertion
Following the subclavian or jugular insertion of the catheter, both lung fields must be auscultated for symmetrical breath sounds since pneumothorax or hemothorax can occur. A chest radiograph is obtained to verify catheter placement and to rule out pneumothorax. A hydrothorax can occur if large amounts of fluids are infused through the catheter before a radiograph rules out the possibility of a pneumothorax.

A sterile occlusive dressing is applied to the site. The dressing should be changed every 48 hours, and the site should be inspected for signs of infection or phlebitis. The flush solution should be changed every 24 hours; the tubing should be changed every 48 to 72 hours (or per facility protocol). During tubing changes, place the patient in Trendelenburg position and instruct the patient to hold a breath to prevent air from entering the catheter.

The waveform should be monitored continuously or at regular intervals to ensure that the catheter tip has not migrated into the right ventricle; this would be apparent by a much taller waveform associated with higher pressures (25 to 30 mm Hg). Additionally, the ECG waveform must be monitored for ventricular dysrhythmias.

Alarm parameters should be set and maintained at all times.

Obtaining accurate measurements

Zero the transducer prior to obtaining the first reading. Level the transducer each time the patient/transducer is moved. The transducer should be kept at the level of the phlebostatic axis during readings (the phlebostatic axis should be marked with ink or tape on the patient's skin to ensure consistency). The waveform may fluctuate with respirations; readings should be taken at end-expiration to minimize the influence of intrathoracic pressure. (See Pulmonary artery pressure monitoring: obtaining accurate measurements, p. 524.)

Waveform interpretation

The CVP waveform (Figure 6-5) has positive waves and negative descents. The *a* wave indicates right arterial systole; it is followed by the *x* descent, which indicates the drop in pres-

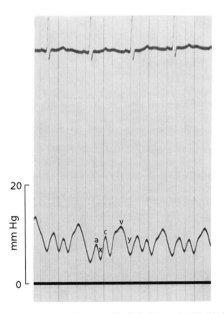

Figure 6-5 CVP waveform. (From Daily EK, Schroeder JS: *Techniques in bedside hemodynamic monitoring*, ed 4, St Louis, 1989, Mosby.)

sure that occurs during the right atrial relaxation. The *c* wave, which may not be distinguishable on the waveform, is caused by bulging of the closed tricuspid valve into the atrium during right ventricular systole; the *x'* descent follows the *c* wave. The *v* wave indicates right atrial diastole, when blood is filling the atrium; it is followed by the *y* descent, which indicates passive right atrial emptying of blood into the right ventricle through the open tricuspid valve.

Various changes in the CVP waveform can indicate pathophysiological changes in the heart and pulmonary vasculature. An elevated *a* wave is seen with tricuspid stenosis, right ventricular hypertrophy secondary to pulmonic valve stenosis, or pulmonary hypertension, constrictive pericarditis, and cardiac tamponade, all of which impede right atrial emptying. Tricuspid insufficiency, with backflow of blood into the right atrium during ventricular systole, will cause increased pressure and an elevated *v* wave on the right atrial waveform. Tricuspid insufficiency can also cause an absence of the *c* wave on the waveform, since the valve is incompetent and will not bulge back into the right atrium during ventricular systole.

Cannon waves (combined *a* and *c* waves) occur whenever the atrium contracts against a closed valve; for example, when junctional or ventricular beats occur, or with AV dissociation seen in complete heart block and ventricular tachycardia.

Troubleshooting

Table 6-1 offers troubleshooting suggestions for invasive hemodynamic monitoring lines.

Removal of CVP catheter

1. Place the patient flat or in Trendelenburg position to prevent air embolism during the catheter removal from the jugular or subclavian veins.
2. Turn the stopcock off to the patient and disconnect the transducer from the monitor.
3. Remove the dressing and remove the sutures.
4. Instruct the patient to hold a breath at full inspiration and remove the catheter slowly; inspect the tip to ensure the catheter is intact.
5. Apply pressure to the site until the bleeding has stopped, being careful not to compress any arteries (e.g., carotid) and impair blood flow.
6. Apply a sterile occlusive dressing to the site and leave in place for 24 hours.
7. Observe the site frequently for bleeding or hematoma.

ECG MONITORING

Choosing a Lead
Three-lead system

1. Lead II (Figure 6-6): This is a common lead used in cardiac monitoring. An advantage of this lead is that it allows observation of QRS axis changes associated with left anterior hemiblock.

2. Modified chest lead (MCL₁) (Figure 6-7): This lead is a preferred monitoring lead for identifying type of bundle branch block and differentiating ventricular ectopy from aberrant ventricular conduction.

3. Lewis lead (Figure 6-8): This lead is especially useful for identification of P waves.

4. MCL₆ lead (Figure 6-9): The use of this lead enables the clinician to switch from viewing MCL₁ to MCL₆ (V_6) by moving only the positive electrode. It is a useful lead in those patients with a median sternotomy.

Five-lead system (Figure 6-10)

This system allows the clinician to place the chest lead on select sites on the chest for ECG monitoring.

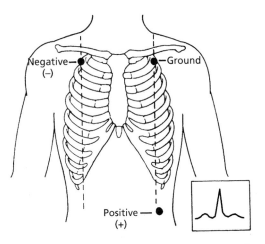

Figure 6-6   Lead II. Positive electrode—left leg; negative electrode—right arm. (From Stillwell S, Randall E: *Pocket guide to cardiovascular care,* ed 2, St Louis, 1994, Mosby.)

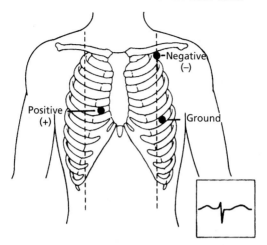

Figure 6-7   Lead MCL$_1$. Positive electrode—fourth intercostal space, right sternum; negative electrode—beneath left midclavicle. (From Stillwell S, Randall E: *Pocket guide to cardiovascular care*, ed 2, St Louis, 1994, Mosby.)

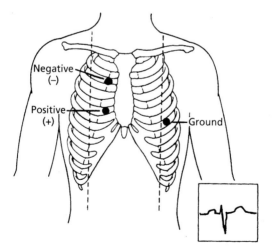

Figure 6-8   Lewis Lead. Positive electrode—fourth intercostal space, right of sternum; negative electrode—second intercostal space, right of sternum. (From Stillwell S, Randall E: *Pocket guide to cardiovascular care*, ed 2, St Louis, 1994, Mosby.)

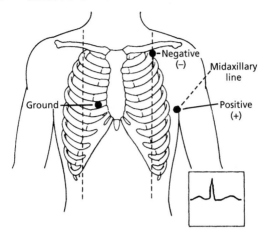

Figure 6-9 MCL$_6$ lead. Positive electrode—left fifth intercostal space, midaxillary line; negative electrode—below left clavicle. (From Stillwell S, Randall E: *Pocket guide to cardiovascular care*, ed 2, St Louis, 1994, Mosby.)

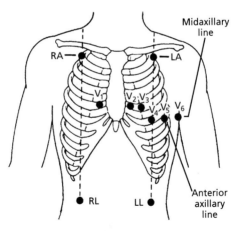

Figure 6-10 Five-lead system. RA electrode—below right clavicle, midclavicular line. LA electrode—below left clavicle, midclavicular line. RL electrode—right abdomen, midclavicular line. LL electrode—left abdomen, midclavicular line. Chest lead—place chest lead on V$_1$, V$_2$, V$_3$, V$_4$, V$_5$, or V$_6$ position. (From Stillwell S, Randall E: *Pocket guide to cardiovascular care*, ed 2, St Louis, 1994, Mosby.)

Rhythm Strip Analysis
Heart rate determination
Standard ECG paper is made up of a series of 1 mm squares, with each millimeter equal to 0.04 seconds. Each group of five small squares is marked by a darker line, so that one large square (5 mm) equals 0.20 seconds (Figure 6-11).

See Figures 6-12 and 6-13 for determining heart rate.

Rhythm determination
To determine whether the rhythm is regular, measure the R-R or P-P intervals and determine whether the length of the intervals is constant. The rhythm is regular if the length of the shortest and longest interval varies by less than or equal to 0.12 seconds. If the rhythm is irregular, it should be determined whether there is any kind of pattern to the irregularity or if it is totally erratic.

In addition to the rate and regularity of the rhythm, the PR and QRS intervals must be determined, as well as the relationship of atrial activity (P waves) to ventricular activity

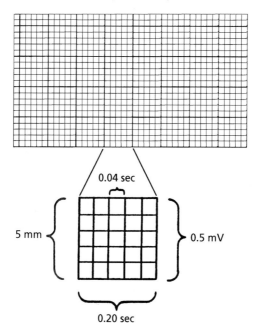

Figure 6-11   ECG paper.

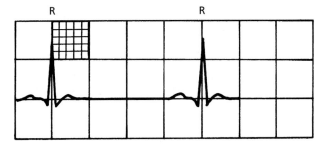

Figure 6-12 Heart rate determination with regular rhythm. Rate can be determined by dividing 300 by the number of large squares between cardiac cycles (300/4) or by dividing the number of small squares between cardiac cycles into 1500 (1500/20 = 75 beats/min). (From Stillwell S, Randall E: *Pocket guide to cardiovascular care,* ed 2, St Louis, 1994, Mosby.)

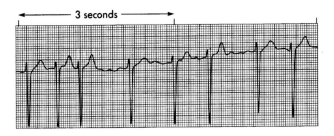

Figure 6-13 Heart rate determination with irregular rhythm. Heart rate can be approximated by multiplying the number of cardiac cycles in a 6-second period by 10; the heart rate is approximately 80. (From Stillwell S, Randall E: *Pocket guide to cardiovascular care,* ed 2, St Louis, 1994, Mosby.)

(QRS complex). Normal PR interval is 0.12 to 0.20 seconds in duration and normal QRS interval is up to 0.10 seconds in duration. QT interval is usually less than half the preceding R-R interval. (See Table 5-3.)

Dysrhythmias
Sinus bradycardia (Figure 6-14)
1. Determinants
   Rhythm: Regular
   Rate: <60

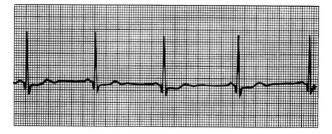

Figure 6-14 Sinus bradycardia. (From Conover MB: *Pocket guide to electrocardiography,* ed 3, St Louis, 1994, Mosby.)

P waves: Present, same morphology
PR interval: 0.12-0.20 seconds
QRS: ≤0.10 seconds, same morphology
2. Treatment: If the patient is asymptomatic, none. If the patient is symptomatic (i.e., hypotensive, syncopal), the treatment is atropine, pacemaker. If possible, the underlying cause also needs to be treated.

Sinus tachycardia (Figure 6-15)
1. Determinants
Rhythm: Regular
Rate: >100
P waves: Present, same morphology
PR interval: 0.12-0.20 seconds
QRS: ≤0.10 seconds, same morphology
2. Treatment: Treat the cause (e.g., stress/anxiety, fever, HF, pain, hypoxia, hyperthyroidism).

Sinus arrhythmia (Figure 6-16)
1. Determinants
Rhythm: Irregular, varies by >0.12 seconds
Rate: variable; increases with inspiration, decreases with expiration
P waves: Present, same morphology
PR interval: 0.12-0.20 seconds
QRS: ≤0.10 seconds, same morphology
2. Treatment: None

Premature atrial complex (Figure 6-17)
1. Determinants
Rhythm: Irregular due to ectopic beats
Rate: That of underlying rhythm
P waves: Present, same morphology except for ectopic beat

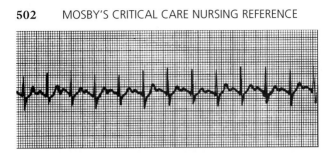

Figure 6-15   Sinus tachycardia. (From Conover MB: *Pocket guide to electrocardiography,* ed 3, St Louis, 1994, Mosby.)

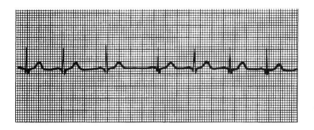

Figure 6-16   Sinus arrhythmia. (From Conover MB: *Pocket guide to electrocardiography,* ed 3, St Louis, 1994, Mosby.)

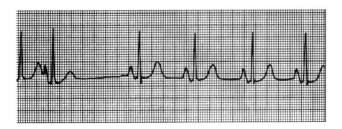

Figure 6-17   Premature atrial complex. (From Conover MB: *Pocket guide to electrocardiography,* ed 3, St Louis, 1994, Mosby.)

PR interval: 0.12-0.20 seconds (PR interval of the ectopic beat may vary from the others)

QRS: ≤0.10 seconds, same morphology

2. Treatment: Usually none

Atrial tachycardia with block (Figure 6-18)

1. Determinants

Rhythm: Regular

Rate: Atrial rate 130-250, ventricular rate may be less than atrial rate due to lack of conduction through the AV node

P waves: Present, same morphology

PR interval: 0.12-0.20 seconds

QRS: ≤0.10 seconds, same morphology

2. Treatment: Identify and treat the cause (e.g., if caused by digitalis toxicity, discontinue digoxin).

Atrial flutter (Figure 6-19)

1. Determinants

Rhythm: Atrial rhythm is regular; ventricular rhythm regular or irregular, depending on the AV conduction pattern

Rate: Atrial rate 230-350; ventricular rate usually <150 (depends on AV conduction)

P waves: Absent; replaced by flutter waves, which have a sawtooth appearance

PR interval: None

QRS: ≤0.10 seconds, same morphology

2. Treatment: If symptomatic, synchronized cardioversion; may also be treated with β blockers, calcium channel blockers, digitalis, or radiofrequency ablation.

Atrial fibrillation (Figure 6-20)

1. Determinants

Rhythm: Irregular

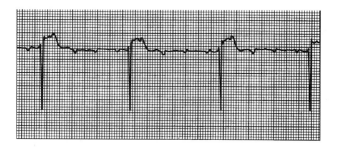

Figure 6-18   Atrial tachycardia with block. (From Conover MB: *Pocket guide to electrocardiography,* ed 3, St Louis, 1994, Mosby.)

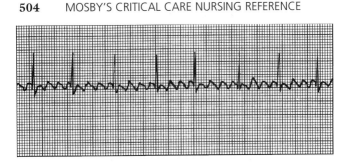

Figure 6-19 Atrial flutter. (From Conover MB: *Pocket guide to electocardiography,* ed 3, St Louis, 1994, Mosby.)

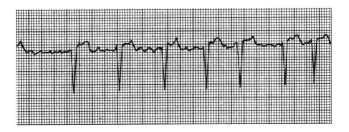

Figure 6-20 Atrial fibrillation. (From Conover MB: *Pocket guide to electrocardiography,* ed 3, St Louis, 1994, Mosby.)

Rate: Atrial rate >350; ventricular rate is variable
P waves: None; fibrillatory waves create a wavy, undulating baseline
PR interval: None
QRS: ≤0.10 seconds, normal morphology
2. Treatment: If symptomatic, synchronized cardioversion; may also be treated with beta blockers, calcium channel blockers, digitalis, anticoagulants to decrease risk of stroke; if any accessary pathway (e.g., WPW) is involved, digitalis is contraindicated; procainamide, synchronized cardioversion, or radiofrequency ablation are options.

Paroxysmal supraventricular tachycardia (Figure 6-21)
1. Determinants
Rhythm: Regular; occurs in bursts that begin and end abruptly

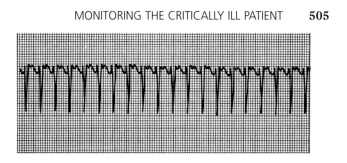

Figure 6-21 Paroxysmal supraventricular tachycardia. (From Conover MB: *Pocket guide to electrocardiography,* ed 3, St Louis, 1994, Mosby.)

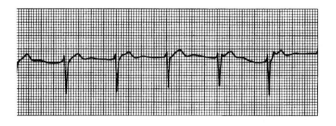

Figure 6-22 Accelerated idiojunctional rhythm. (From Conover MB: *Pocket guide to electrocardiography,* ed 3, St Louis, 1994, Mosby.)

Rate: 150-250
P waves: Cannot be clearly identified; may distort the preceding T wave
PR interval: None measurable
QRS: 0.10 seconds, same morphology
Ratio: Unable to determine
2. Treatment: Treat underlying cause. If symptomatic, cardioversion. (See Appendix A.)
Junctional rhythm (Figure 6-22)
1. Determinants
Rhythm: Regular
Rate: escape 40-60
accelerated 62-99
tachycardia 100-140
P waves: absent, negative in II, III, aVF; may be dissociated from QRS

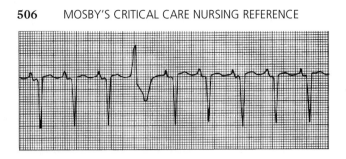

Figure 6-23 Premature ventricular complex. (From Conover MB: *Pocket guide to electrocardiography,* ed 3, St Louis, 1994, Mosby.)

PR: NA

QRS: ≤.10 seconds, same morphology

2. Treatment: If asymptomatic, none. If symptomatic due to decreased HR, atropine or pacemaker may be indicated. If junctional tachycardia occurs in a patient taking digitalis, stop digitalis.

Premature ventricular complex (PVC) (Figure 6-23)

1. Determinants

Rhythm: Irregular due to the ectopic beat(s)

Rate: Varies with the underlying rhythm

P waves: Present (except for the ectopic beat; same morphology

PR interval: 0.12-0.20 seconds

QRS: ≤0.10 seconds except for the ectopic beat (wide and bizarre morphology)

2. Treatment: None if benign; if greater than 6/min, couplets, multifocal, or PVCs that fall on the preceding T wave, treat with lidocaine, procainamide, bretylium

Accelerated idioventricular rhythm (Figure 6-24)

1. Determinants

Rhythm: Regular

Rate: 40-100 beats/min

P waves: Absent

PR interval: None

QRS: Wide (>0.12 seconds), bizarre appearance with same morphology

2. Treatment: None unless hemodynamically unstable, then treat as with other bradydysrhythmias (atropine and/or pacemaker)

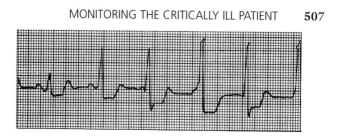

Figure 6-24   Accelerated idioventricular rhythm. (From Conover MB: *Pocket guide to electrocardiography,* ed 3, St Louis, 1994, Mosby.)

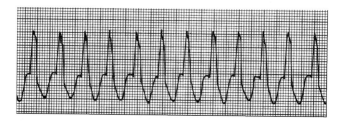

Figure 6-25   Ventricular tachycardia. (From Conover MB: *Pocket guide to electrocardiography,* ed 3, St Louis, 1994, Mosby.)

Ventricular tachycardia (Figure 6-25)

1. Determinants
   Rhythm: Regular or slightly irregular
   Rate: 100-250
   P waves: Usually not seen; if present, will be dissociated from ventricular rhythm
   PR interval: None measurable
   QRS: Wide (>0.12 seconds) and bizarre morphology
2. Treatment: If conscious with a pulse: cardiovert if unstable or administer lidocaine if the patient is stable. If the patient is unconscious without a pulse, defibrillate. (See Appendix A.)

Ventricular fibrillation (Figure 6-26)

1. Determinants
   Rhythm: Irregular, chaotic baseline
   Rate: Unable to measure
   P waves: None
   PR interval: None
   QRS: None

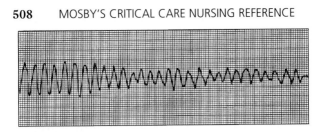

Figure 6-26 Ventricular flutter fibrillation. (From Conover MB: *Pocket guide to electrocardiography,* ed 3, St Louis, 1994, Mosby.)

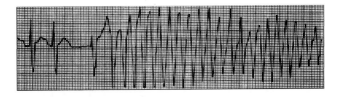

Figure 6-27 Torsade de pointes. (From Conover MB: *Pocket guide to electrocardiography,* ed 3, St Louis, 1994, Mosby.)

2. Treatment: CPR until defibrillator available, then rapid defibrillation beginning at 200 joules; defibrillation may be repeated two times at successively higher levels if restoration of rhythm does not occur. (See Appendix A.)

Torsade de pointes (Figure 6-27)

1. Determinants
   Rhythm: Regular or slightly irregular
   Rate: 200-250
   P waves: Usually not seen; if present, will be dissociated from ventricular rhythm
   PR interval: None measurable
   QRS: Wide (>0.12 seconds) and bizarre morphology; QRS complexes appear to be constantly changing and twist in a spiral pattern around the baseline
2. Treatment: IV magnesium sulfate or magnesium chloride; temporary overdrive pacing. Identify and treat cause: antidysrhythmic agents (e.g., quinidine, procainamide, amiodarone, sotalol); hypokalemia, hypocalcemia, hypomagnesemia, phenothiazines, or tricyclic antidepressants.

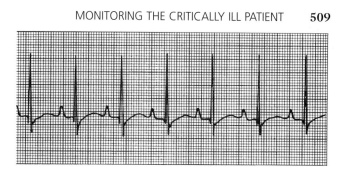

Figure 6-28   First-degree AV block. (From Conover MB: *Pocket guide to electrocardiography,* ed 3, St Louis, 1994, Mosby.)

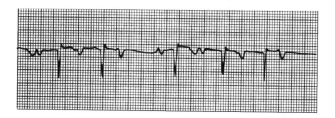

Figure 6-29   Second-degree AV block, type I. (From Conover MB: *Pocket guide to electrocardiography,* ed 3, St Louis, 1994, Mosby.)

First-degree AV block (Figure 6-28)
1. Determinants
   Rhythm: Regular
   Rate: 60-100
   P waves: Normal, same morphology
   PR interval: >0.20 seconds
   QRS: ≤0.10 seconds, same morphology
2. Treatment: Usually none unless associated with symptomatic bradycardia

Second-degree AV block (Type I, Wenchebach) (Figure 6-29)
1. Determinants
   Rhythm: Irregular
   Rate: Atrial rate 60-100; ventricular rate is slower as a result of dropped beats
   P waves: Normal, same morphology

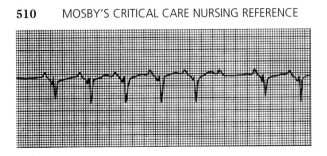

Figure 6-30   Second-degree AV block, type II. (From Conover MB: *Pocket guide to electrocardiography,* ed 3, St Louis, 1994, Mosby.)

PR interval: Progressive lengthening with each beat until a QRS is dropped; the PR interval is reset to normal with the dropped beat and the cycle of PR lengthening begins again

QRS: ≤0.10 seconds, same morphology

2. Treatment: Usually none.

Second-degree AV block (Type II) (Figure 6-30)

1. Determinants

   Rhythm: Irregular

   Rate: Atrial 60-100; ventricular rate is slower due to dropped beats

   P waves: Normal, same morphology

   PR interval: 0.12-0.20 seconds and fixed, except where beat is dropped

   QRS: Normal or wide, same morphology

2. Treatment: Careful monitoring; there is a high tendency to progress to complete heart block; if the patient is symptomatic, a pacemaker may be required.

Third-degree heart block (complete heart block) (Figure 6-31)

1. Determinants

   Rhythm: Regular

   Rate: Atrial 60-100; ventricular depends on site of escape rhythm, usually 20-60

   P waves: Normal, same morphology

   PR interval: Not measurable; no association between atrial rhythm and ventricular rhythm

   QRS: Normal (≤0.10 seconds) if from AV junction; widened (>0.12 seconds) if from below bundle of His

2. Treatment: Usually pacemaker is required.

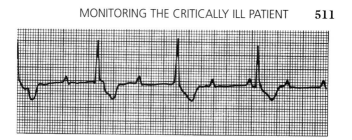

Figure 6-31   Third-degree AV block (complete heart block). (From Conover MB: *Pocket guide to electrocardiography,* ed 3, St Louis, 1994, Mosby.)

INTRACRANIAL PRESSURE MONITORING
Clinical Brief
Intracranial pressure (ICP) monitoring is used to measure the pressure within the brain and to evaluate cerebral compliance so that changes can be detected early and effects of various medical and nursing interventions can be evaluated. The traditional clinical signs of increased ICP (decreasing level of consciousness, increased systolic blood pressure and widening pulse pressure, bradycardia, and slow irregular respirations) do not actually reflect early increases in ICP and in fact may occur too late for intervention and treatment to be effective.

ICP monitoring also provides the necessary data to calculate cerebral perfusion pressure (CPP); this is measured by subtracting mean ICP from the mean arterial blood pressure. Adequate cerebral circulation is ensured if the CPP remains approximately 70 to 90 mm Hg.

A pressure transducer setup is connected, using sterile normal saline (without preservative) to provide a fluid column between the CSF within the ventricles and the transducer. The pressure is transmitted to a monitor, and the pressure waveform and digital readings are displayed. A continuous flush device is *not* used on any ICP monitoring system, because it may contribute to further increased intracranial pressure.
Indications
The Monroe-Kellie hypothesis states that the volume of the intracranium is equal to the volume of the brain plus the volume of the blood within the brain plus the volume of the cerebrospinal fluid (CSF) within the brain. Therefore any condition that results in an increase in the volume of one or

more of these will increase the ICP, unless there is a concomitant decrease in one or more of the components.

Description

The *intraventricular catheter* is placed via a burr hole, in the lateral ventricle of the nondominant hemisphere. When ICP is severely elevated, CSF can be drained using this type of system. This is the most invasive method of monitoring ICP, yet it is also the most accurate, because the catheter is placed directly into the ventricle.

The *subarachnoid screw/bolt* is inserted into the subarachnoid space. This system is unreliable in patients with elevated ICP because the device becomes obstructed by brain tissue.

The *epidural sensor* is a transducer placed between the skull and dura. It is less invasive than the intraventricular catheter and the subarachnoid screw, so it may be less accurate. Once it is placed, recalibration is not necessary. Drainage of CSF cannot be performed with this system.

The *fiberoptic transducer-tipped catheter* can be placed in the ventricle, subarachnoid or subdural spaces, or in the parenchyma. With ventricular placement, CSF can be drained. Once it is placed, it cannot be recalibrated.

Values

Normal

0-15 mm Hg

Significance of abnormal values

Consistently elevated ICP suggests that the compensatory mechanisms of cerebral autoregulation (arterial constriction and dilation) have failed. Patients usually become symptomatic with an ICP of 20 to 25 mm Hg, and a sustained ICP greater than 60 mm Hg is usually fatal. Factors that increase ICP include hypercapnea ($PaCO_2$ greater than 42 mm Hg); hypoxia (PaO_2 less than 50 mm Hg); excessive fluid intake; head, neck, and extreme hip flexion; head rotation of 90 degrees to either side; Valsalva maneuver (straining, coughing); and continuous activity without adequate rest. Additionally, arousal from sleep, REM sleep, emotional upset, and noxious stimuli such as suctioning are known to increase ICP.

Patient Care Management

Preinsertion

The patient is placed in a supine position with the head of the bed elevated 30 to 45 degrees for insertion. A twist drill is used to insert the device. Strict aseptic technique is essential, as is a sterile environment during the procedure.

▶ Complications and related nursing diagnoses

Infection of the central nervous system   Risk for infection

The entire pressure transducer setup must remain a closed system to prevent contamination. Strict aseptic technique must be followed during insertion of the device and while manipulating the pressure line and changing dressings. Risk factors that influence infection rate include the insertion environment and technique, type of device used, duration of monitoring, and patient factors such as age and state of immunosuppression.

Postinsertion

The ICP waveform should be continuously displayed on the monitor, and alarms should be set to coincide with the patient's clinical status. The ICP should be monitored and recorded as ordered, and the mean arterial blood pressure should be monitored to determine CPP.

It is imperative that strict aseptic technique be maintained during the care of the insertion site, pressure line and during dressing changes. Assess for signs of infection, drainage, swelling, or irritation. The site must be kept clean and dry and should be covered with an occlusive dressing at all times.

The patient should be positioned with the head of the bed elevated 15 to 30 degrees (unless contraindicated) and maintained in a neutral position with minimal hip and knee flexion to facilitate venous drainage from the brain and prevent further increases in ICP.

Additional measures to prevent sustained intracranial hypertension should be taken: avoid hypothermia and hyperthermia; keep $Paco_2$ at 28 to 30 mm Hg; instruct the patient to avoid Valsalva's maneuver; and restrict fluids as ordered.

Obtaining accurate measurements

1. Zero the transducer by opening the transducer to air and adjusting the monitor to read zero; this eliminates the pressure contributions from the atmosphere, and only pressures within the chamber being monitored will be measured. Check with the manufacturer's recommendations for routine zeroing. Epidural sensors and fiberoptic devices are only zeroed before insertion.

2. Level the air reference port of the transducer to the foramen of Monro (Figure 6-32) with each position change, a change in waveform, and after any manipulation of the

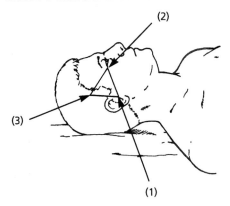

Figure 6-32 Location of foramen of Monro for transducer placement. Map an imaginary equilateral triangle from the external auditory meatus *(1)* to the outer canthus of the eye *(2)* to behind the hairline *(3)*. Point 3 is the location of the foramen of Monro.

system. Epidural and fiberoptic devices do not require leveling after insertion.
3. Check the fluid-filled systems frequently for air, since this will alter readings.
4. Obtain ICP readings at end-expiration to avoid the effects of thoracic pressures on the cerebral venous system.

Waveform interpretation

The ICP waveform (Figure 6-33) is very similar in appearance to that of the central venous pressure. It has small systolic and diastolic fluctuations, but the *mean* is monitored, since the ventricles of the brain are relatively low-pressure chambers. The waveform consists of at least three peaks (Figure 6-33), although additional peaks may be present in some individuals. An increase in ICP will cause an increase in all waveform components initially; as ICP progresses, there is an elevation of P_2.

A P_2 equal to or higher than P_1 suggests decreased compliance, which may precede an actual increase in ICP. This signifies that compensatory mechanisms are failing and that a small increase in the volume can increase ICP significantly.

The intraventricular catheter and subarachnoid screw may develop a damped waveform as a result of tissue, blood, or debris blocking the transmission of the pressure. The line is irrigated only when ordered by a physician (Table 6-2).

Removal

The ICP monitoring device is removed by a physician. A wrench is required for the bolt. Sterile technique is used to

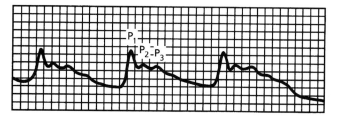

Figure 6-33   ICP waveform.

TABLE 6-2   Troubleshooting Intracranial Pressure Monitoring Lines

Problem	Cause	Solution
ICP waveform damped or absent	Air in transducer system	Eliminate air
	Loose connections	Tighten connections
	Occlusion of monitoring device	Flush device only as directed by physician
False high-pressure reading	Transducer too low	Place transducer at level of foramen of Monro and zero balance
	Air in transducer system	Eliminate air
False low-pressure reading	Transducer too high	Place transducer at level of foramen of Monro and zero balance
	Air in transducer system	Eliminate air

prevent contamination of the insertion site. A sterile dressing is applied to the site for at least 24 hours; after this, the site is left open to air. If there is evidence of a CSF leak, additional sutures may be required.

LEFT ATRIAL PRESSURE MONITORING

Clinical Brief

Left atrial pressure (LAP) is monitored to evaluate left-sided heart pressures (LVEDP) following open-heart surgery.

Indications

LAP monitoring can be used for the perioperative and post-operative assessment of left ventricular function and cardio-vascular status and to assess the hemodynamic response to vasoactive drugs or fluids.

Description

The LA catheter is inserted into the left atrium during cardiac surgery; it is threaded through the superior pulmonary vein into the left atrium and the external end is brought out through a small incision at the inferior end of the mediastinal incision. The catheter is connected to a pressure transducer setup, and the waveform is monitored continuously.

Values

Normal

4-12 mm Hg

Significance of abnormal values

Since the catheter is positioned in the left atrium, it indirectly reflects the LVEDP. Therefore the same factors that cause an increase or decrease in PAD and PAWP will cause abnormal LAP values. (See Pulmonary artery pressure monitoring: significance of abnormal values, p. 521.)

Patient Care Management

Preinsertion

The LA catheter is inserted during open-heart surgery, and the line will be in place when the patient arrives in the critical care unit.

▶ Complications and related nursing diagnoses

The potential risks of LAP monitoring are the same as those listed for CVP monitoring: air embolus, clot formation, infection, cardiac tamponade, and electrical hazards. (See Central venous pressure monitoring: complications and related nursing diagnoses, p. 493.) However, since the LA line provides direct access to the systemic circulation, the risk of air embolus is more threatening than with the CVP or PA lines. To decrease this risk, an in-line air filter should be used, and the line should never be irrigated or flushed.

Bleeding or pericardial tamponade following removal	Decreased cardiac output Fluid volume deficit

Bleeding and pericardial tamponade can occur following removal of the LA catheter. The mediastinal tubes should be left in place for at least 2 hours after the removal of the LA line so that blood does not collect in the mediastinum.

Postinsertion

The LA line should *never* be irrigated or flushed. The remainder of the postinsertion care is the same as that described with the CVP and PA lines (see pp. 493, 524).

Obtaining accurate measurements

The air port of the pressure transducer must be leveled with the phlebostatic axis during pressure readings. Readings should be taken at end-expiration and obtained from a calibrated strip chart recording if respiratory variation is present. The transducer should be leveled each time the patient or transducer has been moved. The patient should not be removed from the ventilator or PEEP during readings.

Waveform interpretation

The LAP waveform closely resembles that of the PAWP, and the mean pressure is monitored (Figure 6-34). The waveform has *a* and *v* waves, as well as *x* and *y* descents; these correlate

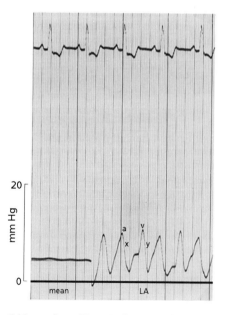

Figure 6-34 LAP waveform. (From Daily EK, Schroeder JS: *Techniques in bedside hemodynamic monitoring,* ed 5, St Louis, 1994, Mosby.)

to the same mechanical events of the cardiac cycle as the waves and descents of the PAWP waveform (see p. 525).

If large *a* and *v* waves appear on the waveform, it may be the result of catheter migration to the left ventricle; if this occurs, notify the physician at once and monitor the patient for ventricular dysrhythmias.

Troubleshooting
Basic troubleshooting of the LA line is similar to that of other hemodynamic lines (see Table 6-1 on troubleshooting invasive hemodynamic monitoring lines), *except* that the LA catheter is *never* flushed. If damping of the waveform occurs and clot formation is suspected as the cause, attempt to aspirate the clot. If the line cannot be aspirated or if the line remains damped, then the catheter needs to be discontinued.

Removal
The LA catheter is removed by a physician or nurse, depending on the institutional protocol. It is usually removed after 24 to 48 hours because of the increased risk for air embolus. The procedure for removal is the same as that for a CVP catheter (see p. 495). The site is covered with sterile occlusive dressing and must be observed frequently for bleeding. Following removal of the LA catheter, the patient must be monitored closely for signs of pericardial tamponade (jugular vein distention; cyanosis; elevation of CVP, PAD, and PAWP; pulsus paradoxus; decreased systolic blood pressure).

PULMONARY ARTERY PRESSURE MONITORING

Clinical Brief
The pulmonary artery (PA) catheter is used to continuously monitor right intracardiac and pulmonary artery pressures. The pulmonary artery end-diastolic pressure can reflect left-sided heart pressures; left ventricular end-diastolic pressure (LVEDP) can be estimated and the hemodynamic response to fluid or drug therapy can be assessed. The PA catheter also allows for the sampling of mixed venous blood from the pulmonary artery in order to measure oxygen saturation. (See discussion under Svo_2 monitoring, p. 528.) Finally, the PA catheter enables the measurement of cardiac output via the thermodilution technique.

Indications
The PA catheter may be used in the following clinical situations: (1) left-sided heart failure, (2) valvular disease, (3) titration of vasoactive drugs, or fluids, (4) severe respiratory failure,

and (5) perioperative and postoperative monitoring of surgical patients with cardiovascular or pulmonary dysfunction.

Description

The PA catheter usually has four ports: (1) the proximal lumen ends in the right atrium and is used for infusion of fluids or monitoring of right atrial pressure, and the injection of a bolus of fluid to measure cardiac output; (2) the distal lumen ends in the pulmonary artery, allowing measurement of PA pressures and left-sided heart pressures reflected across the pulmonary vasculature; (3) the balloon port leads to an inflatable balloon at the tip of the catheter; when the balloon is inflated it blocks pressures behind it (the right side of the heart) and senses pressures through the pulmonary vasculature from the left side of the heart; and (4) the thermodilution port terminates 4 to 6 cm proximal to the tip of the catheter and senses temperature changes during cardiac output measurement. Some PA catheters have additional ports for the infusion of fluids or for insertion of a temporary pacing wire; some have a sensor to continuously measure venous oxygen saturation. Other features include measurement of right-ventricular volumes and ejection fractions and continuous measurement of CO.

The catheter is inserted into a large vein (the same sites as those used for CVP catheters) via percutaneous or cutdown method. Upon entry into the right atrium, the balloon is inflated and the catheter is flow-directed into position in the pulmonary artery. Continuous pressure monitoring of the waveform during insertion shows the anatomical location of the tip of the catheter, based on the characteristic waveforms of the right atrium, the right ventricle, and the pulmonary artery (Figure 6-35). Once the pulmonary artery has been reached, the balloon tip "wedges" into a small branch of the pulmonary artery.

Values

Normal

RA: 2-6 mm Hg. See normal CVP values, p. 492.

RV: 15-28/0-8 mm Hg. Right ventricular pressure is measured during catheter insertion only; this value provides information about the function of the right ventricle as well as the tricuspid and pulmonic valves.

PAS: 15-30 mm Hg. The pulmonary artery systolic pressure indicates the pressure in the pulmonary artery during right ventricular contraction, when the pulmonic valve is open.

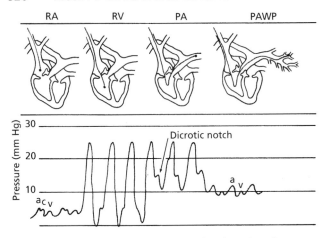

Figure 6-35 Pressure waveforms during PA catheter insertion.

PAD: 5-15 mm Hg. Pulmonary artery diastolic (PAD) pressure reflects the resistance to flow by the pulmonary vasculature. It indirectly measures the LVEDP, because the pulmonic valve is closed during diastole (thereby eliminating right heart pressure influences) and the mitral valve is open, so that the catheter "sees" the pressure in the left atrium and the left ventricle. PAD can be used in place of the pulmonary artery wedge pressure (PAWP) to estimate LVEDP when there is no pulmonary vascular obstruction, thereby decreasing the number of balloon inflations and potential patient risk. The PAD is normally 1 to 4 mm Hg higher than the PAWP because of the slight resistance to forward blood flow from the pulmonary vasculature; when the catheter is "wedged" there is no forward flow distal to the catheter tip and the effects of pulmonary vascular resistance do not affect the PAWP reading. The PAD/PAWP gradient is greater anytime there is increased pulmonary vascular resistance (pulmonary embolus, hypoxia, chronic lung disease). Neither PAD nor PAWP accurately reflects LVEDP in the presence of mitral valve disease because the pressure is increased by the altered blood flow between the atrium and the ventricle.

PAWP: 4-12 mm Hg. PAWP, also known as pulmonary artery occlusive pressure (PAOP), reflects the LVEDP most accurately because the pressures from the right side of the

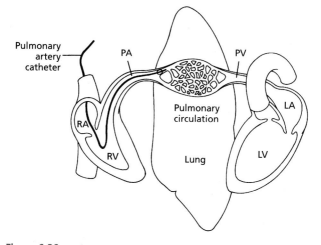

Figure 6-36   Pulmonary artery catheter in the wedged position. Balloon inflation allows for recording of pressures in the left heart as it "sees" the left atrium.

heart are blocked by the inflated balloon so that the tip of the catheter (distal to the balloon) senses pressures only forward of the catheter (Figure 6-36). The PAWP waveform has small fluctuations similar to the CVP waveform; thus the *mean* pressure is monitored.

Significance of abnormal values

RA: See abnormal CVP values, p. 492.

RV: Right ventricular systolic pressures may be elevated as a result of pulmonic stenosis, pulmonary hypertension, pulmonary vascular volume overload, ventricular septal defect with left-to-right shunting, chronic lung disease, pulmonary embolism, hypoxemia, or acute respiratory distress syndrome (ARDS). Decreased right ventricular systolic pressures may be the result of right ventricular failure secondary to infarction or ischemia, as a result of myopathy, or secondary to hypovolemia.

Right ventricular diastolic pressure may be elevated because of pulmonic valve insufficiency, right ventricular failure, pulmonary hypertension, cardiac tamponade, constrictive pericarditis, or intravascular volume overload. Decreased right ventricular diastolic pressure occurs with hypovolemia.

PAS: Pulmonary artery systolic pressure may be elevated due to increased pulmonary blood volume or increased pulmonary vascular resistance secondary to pulmonary embolism, hypoxemia, lung disease, or ARDS. Decreased pulmonary artery systolic pressure occurs with hypovolemia or vasodilation.

PAD: Pulmonary artery diastolic pressure is elevated in the same circumstances as the PA systolic pressure, as well as left heart dysfunction (from any cause), mitral stenosis/insufficiency, cardiac tamponade, or increased intravascular volume. Hypovolemia or vasodilation causes a decrease in pulmonary diastolic pressure.

PAWP: Pulmonary artery wedge pressure is increased in any situation in which there is left ventricular dysfunction: mitral stenosis/insufficiency, left ventricular failure, decreased left ventricular compliance, increased systemic vascular resistance, cardiac tamponade, or fluid volume overload. Decreased pulmonary artery wedge pressure is seen with hypovolemia or vasodilation with resulting decreased afterload.

Patient Care Management
Preinsertion
The patient is prepared in the same manner as for CVP insertion. Prior to insertion, the inflated balloon is tested for integrity by submerging it in saline and checking for air leaks. The transducer must be zeroed prior to catheter insertion, thereby ensuring accurate waveforms and pressure readings during catheter placement. (See Figure 6-35.) The pressures of the right atrium, right ventricle, and pulmonary artery are documented during insertion. It is important to monitor for ventricular dysrhythmias during insertion, especially during passage through the right ventricle.

▶ Complications and related nursing diagnoses
Pulmonary artery pressure monitoring is associated with the risk of developing the same complications as those seen with arterial and central venous pressure monitoring (air embolus, clot formation, hemorrhage, electrical shock, infection, and catheter tip migration [see pp. 486, 493]). Additional complications may occur with pulmonary artery pressure monitoring.

Perforation of the pulmonary artery by the catheter	Risk for injury

Perforation of the pulmonary artery can occur during catheter positioning; it is for this reason that the balloon should be inflated anytime the tip is repositioned, since the balloon provides some protection to the wall of the vessel.

Pulmonary artery infarction, hemorrhage, or embolism	Risk for injury Impaired gas exchange

Pulmonary artery infarction or hemorrhage can occur if the balloon is inadvertently left inflated or if the catheter spontaneously wedges, blocking blood flow to that branch of the vessel. The PA waveform must be monitored continuously so that inadvertent wedging of the catheter can be recognized immediately. If the PA waveform spontaneously develops a wedge appearance, the catheter has likely migrated forward into a smaller branch of the pulmonary artery. To regain a PA waveform, the line should be aspirated, then flushed; if the problem continues, have the patient cough and/or turn to the side because this may help the catheter move back into a larger branch of the pulmonary artery. The catheter may have to be pulled back slightly if these measures do not correct the problem. Pulmonary embolism can occur if a clot breaks off the tip of the catheter.

Ventricular dysrhythmias	Decreased cardiac output

Ventricular dysrhythmias, secondary to irritation of the ventricular wall by the catheter tip, can occur during insertion of the catheter or if the catheter falls back into the right ventricle after placement in the pulmonary artery. If this occurs, the catheter should be floated into the pulmonary artery by a physician or designee or it should be removed.

Balloon rupture	Risk for injury

The balloon of the catheter can rupture and cause an air embolus. The balloon should never be overinflated, and deflation should be passive (pulling back the air may damage the balloon). If balloon rupture is suspected (no resistance is felt during injection of air, failure to obtain wedge waveform, bleeding back into balloon port) the balloon port should no longer be used, and should be labeled appropriately.

Bundle branch block	Decreased cardiac output

Right bundle branch block may occur during manipulation of the catheter in the right ventricle. Generally this is not a problem unless the patient also has left bundle branch block, in which case complete heart block could result.

Postinsertion

A chest radiograph must be obtained to rule out pneumothorax and to verify correct placement. Fluids should not be infused directly into the distal lumen of the PA catheter.

Alarm parameters should be set and maintained at all times.

Obtaining accurate measurements

Zero the transducer before obtaining the first reading. Level the transducer with the phlebostatic axis every time the patient or transducer is moved. The head of the bed can be elevated up to 45 degrees for readings, but the patient should be supine.

Because the heart is subject to the same intrathoracic pressures as the lungs, there may be respiratory variation in the hemodynamic waveforms. When respiratory variation is present, there will be a decrease in the waveform during spontaneous inspiration and a rise in the waveform during expiration. The opposite occurs with positive-pressure ventilation—the waveform rises with inspiration and falls with expiration. When the patient is receiving intermittent mandatory ventilation, the waveform will peak and trough at different times during the respiratory cycle, depending on whether the breath is spontaneous or mechanically induced. Pressure readings should be taken at end-expiration because at this point the intrathoracic pressure is constant and the pressure waveform is most stable. The digital display is often inaccurate when respiratory variation is present, so the reading should be taken from a calibrated strip chart recording at end-expiration.

In patients receiving positive pressure ventilation or PEEP, the pressure reading should be taken without removing the ventilator so that the effects of positive pressure on the patient's hemodynamic status can be realized. In patients with normal lung compliance, the following equation can be used to estimate the effects of PEEP on PAWP.

$$PAWP \text{ (corrected)} = \text{Measured PAWP} - 0.5 \text{ (PEEP)}$$

In patients with ARDS or other conditions that decrease lung compliance, the following equation can be used to estimate the effects of PEEP on PAWP:

$$PAWP \text{ (corrected)} = \text{Measured PAWP} - 0.5 \text{ (PEEP} - 10)$$

The balloon should be inflated slowly when PAWP readings are taken, and inflation should cease as soon as the PAWP waveform is displayed. When obtaining a PAWP reading, do not leave the balloon inflated for more than 15 seconds; inflation longer than this can result in ischemia of the lung segment distal to the catheter. *Never* use more than the balloon capacity indicated by the manufacturer on the shaft of the catheter. Be sure that the PA waveform returns following passive deflation of the balloon.

PAD can be used to estimate LVEDP if the difference between PAD and PAWP is less than 5 mm Hg, there is no pulmonary vascular obstruction, and the heart rate is less than 130 beats per minute.

When obtaining thermodilution cardiac output (CO) readings, it is important to use the correct computation constant (provided in the catheter package insert). If the wrong computation constant is inadvertently used, the following equation can be used to correct the obtained reading:

$$\text{Correct CO} = \text{Wrong CO} \times \frac{\text{Correct computation constant}}{\text{Wrong computation constant}}$$

To obtain a cardiac output, iced or room temperature solution (usually 10 ml) is injected via the proximal port of the PA catheter; generally three consecutive measurements are obtained and averaged to determine CO. Injection should be smooth, take less than 4 seconds, and produce a CO curve on the monitor that has a smooth and even upstroke (Figure 6-37).

Once CO has been determined, most bedside monitors have the ability to calculate parameters such as CI, SI, SVRI, PVRI, LVSWI, and RVSWI. Formulas for hand calculating are found in Appendix F.

Other technology for determining CO and calculated parameters include continuous CO catheters and a noninvasive method using thoracic electrical bioimpedance (TEB) monitoring. Also available is a thermodilution ejection fraction/volumetric PA catheter that allows bedside assessment of RV systolic and diastolic volumes including RV ejection fraction.

Waveform interpretation

The pulmonary artery waveform looks similar to that seen with arterial pressure monitoring. The systolic pressure is seen as a steep rise as blood is ejected from the right ventricle. The diastolic component of the waveform occurs after the closure of the pulmonic valve, seen as the dicrotic notch.

The PAWP waveform is similar in appearance to the CVP waveform. The *a* wave on the PAWP tracing indicates left

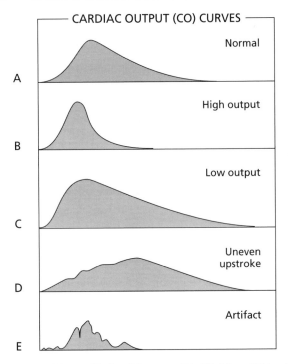

Figure 6-37 Thermodilution CO curves. (Modified from Tilkian A, Daily EK: *Cardiovascular procedures,* St Louis, 1986, Mosby.)

atrial contraction; it is followed by the *x* descent, which indicates left atrial relaxation. The *c* wave is rarely seen in the PAWP tracing. The *v* wave represents left atrial filling, and the *y* descent following it represents the decrease in atrial pressure when the mitral valve opens.

Elevated *a* waves on the PAWP tracing can be indicative of mitral stenosis or left ventricular failure. Elevated *v* waves, on the other hand, indicate mitral insufficiency. Elevation of both *a* and *v* waves simultaneously indicates severe left ventricular failure.

Troubleshooting

Table 6-1 offers suggestions for troubleshooting invasive hemodynamic lines.

Additional problems that may be encountered with the PA catheter are spontaneous wedging of the balloon, migration of the catheter tip to the right ventricle, and right bundle branch block. (See Complications, p. 522.)

If the catheter does not wedge and balloon rupture is not the cause, then the catheter may need to be advanced by the physician or designee. The chest radiograph should be used as a guide in determining correct placement.

Obtaining mixed-venous blood gases

The procedure for drawing mixed-venous blood gases is similar to that of drawing arterial blood gases. (See Arterial pressure monitoring: obtaining a blood sample, p. 489.) However, mixed-venous gases are drawn from the distal lumen of the PA catheter. It is important to be sure the balloon is deflated during the aspiration of the sample; otherwise, only highly oxygen-saturated blood from "down-stream" of the catheter tip will be drawn, causing erroneous results. Similarly, it is important to draw the sample slowly (not faster than 1 ml/20 sec), or arterialized blood from the pulmonary capillaries that is highly oxygenated will be drawn into the syringe and cause erroneously high readings. Following completion of the procedure, ensure the return of the PA waveform.

Removal

Before removing the PA catheter, actively deflate the balloon. The procedure is similar to that of CVP catheter removal (see Central venous pressure monitoring: removal, p. 495), except that the catheter should be rapidly pulled back to decrease the risk of ventricular dysrhythmias. If at any time resistance is felt, do *not* continue pulling and notify the physician immediately. The site should be covered with a sterile, occlusive dressing. If the introducer with side port is left in place for central venous access, cap the introducer or insert an obturator.

PULSE OXIMETRY

Clinical Brief

Pulse oximetry (SpO_2) is a noninvasive method of monitoring arterial oxygen saturation. It provides an early and immediate warning of impending hypoxemia.

Indications

Pulse oximetry may be used in any of the following clinical situations: (1) recovery from anesthesia; (2) assessment of adequacy of oxygen therapy or ventilatory management; and (3) any patients who are at risk for hypoventilation or respiratory arrest (such as those receiving epidural anesthesia, neurologically damaged patients, or those who are receiving high doses of narcotics).

Description

The pulse oximeter is a noninvasive optical method of measuring oxygen saturation of functional hemoglobin. The amount of arterial hemoglobin that is saturated with oxygen is determined by beams of light passing through the tissue. The sensor with the light source is placed on the finger or the bridge of the nose; the saturation is displayed on the monitor, and visual and audible alarms can be set to alert the clinician of changes in oxygenation.

Values

Normal

SpO_2 $\geq 95\%$

Significance of abnormal values

When the arterial saturation falls below 95%, it could be the result of a variety of causes. It may signify that the respiratory effort or oxygen delivery system is inadequate to meet the tissue needs, or that CO is impaired resulting in tissue hypoxia. If arterial flow to the sensor is impaired for any reason, it could result in an erroneously low reading while tissue oxygenation is adequate; therefore, it is important to correlate the reading with other assessment parameters.

Patient Care Management

Obtaining accurate measurements

Place the sensor on clean, dry skin (finger or bridge of nose). If the heart rate displayed on the pulse oximeter and the patient's heart rate are within 5 beats/min, the reading is accurate. If readings are consistently inaccurate, change the sensor or the site. The sensor should not be on the same extremity that has an automatic blood pressure cuff, since this reduces arterial blood flow distally and will alter readings. The patient and extremity should be kept as still as possible to reduce artifact and interference with the signal. If severe peripheral vasoconstriction interferes with measurements from a finger site, the sensor should be placed more centrally (e.g., the bridge of the nose).

SvO_2 MONITORING

Clinical Brief

Continuous monitoring of mixed-venous oxygen saturation (SvO_2) provides ongoing information about the balance between oxygen supply and demand. The blood in the pulmonary artery is a mixture of blood returned from the superior and inferior vena cavae, as well as the coronary sinus; the oxygen saturation of this blood returning from all perfused body parts indirectly reflects the amount of oxygen extracted systemically. The balance between oxygen supply and demand is affected by cardiac output, arterial oxygen saturation, amount of hemoglobin available to carry oxygen, and tissue oxygen consumption. When provided with an immediate warning that an imbalance exists, the clinician may be able to determine the cause of the imbalance and intervene appropriately.

Indications

Svo_2 monitoring may be used in any of the following clinical situations: cardiogenic shock, following open-heart surgery, acute myocardial infarction, concomitant with IABP therapy, acute respiratory distress syndrome, cardiac tamponade, vasoactive drug therapy, and heart failure. Additionally, Svo_2 monitoring is useful for early recognition of hemodynamic compromise, since a decrease in Svo_2 often occurs before changes in other parameters. Patients with an unstable hemodynamic or respiratory status may require fewer cardiac output or arterial blood gas measurements with the use of the Svo_2 monitor. Finally, the Svo_2 monitor is useful in assessing patient response to routine nursing interventions such as suctioning and repositioning.

Description

A thermodilution pulmonary artery catheter with a fiberoptic light is used. Reflection spectrophotometry is the technique by which oxygen saturation of venous blood is measured. The light reflected by the blood is transmitted to a photodetector, where it is converted to electrical signals and the oxygen saturation is computed and displayed. The Svo_2 is updated every second and is displayed on the digital screen as well as on a strip chart recording. The catheter has all other capabilities of the conventional PA catheter: right atrial, pulmonary artery, and pulmonary wedge pressure monitoring; thermodilution cardiac output; and infusion of intravenous fluids. Alarms can be set so that if the Svo_2 is outside the high and low limits, the clinician is immediately alerted.

Values

Normal

60%-80%

Significance of abnormal values

A decreased (<60%) Svo_2 can be caused by (1) an increase in oxygen consumption secondary to shivering, seizures, pain, activity, hyperthermia, or anxiety or (2) a decrease in oxygen delivery secondary to decreased cardiac output, dysrhythmias, hypoxemia, or anemia. An increased (80% to 95%) Svo_2 can be caused by (1) a decrease in oxygen consumption by the tissues secondary to hypothermia, anesthesia, sepsis, or alkalosis or (2) an increase in oxygen delivery secondary to hyperoxia and left-to-right shunting.

Patient Care Management
Preinsertion
See Pulmonary artery pressure monitoring: preinsertion, p. 522.

▶ Complications and related nursing diagnoses
There are no complications associated with fiberoptic monitoring of mixed venous oxygen saturation. However, the same complications that are associated with the PA catheter pertain to the use of the Svo_2 catheter. (See Pulmonary artery pressure monitoring: complications, p. 522.)
Postinsertion
See Pulmonary artery pressure monitoring: postinsertion, p. 524.
Obtaining accurate measurements
To maintain accuracy of the system, the oximeter should be calibrated daily to an in vivo measurement of mixed venous blood. The connection between the optical module and the catheter must remain intact; if for any reason the system becomes disconnected, an in vivo calibration should be performed. If fibrin develops on the tip of the catheter, it will interfere with the light intensity and accuracy of the readings; therefore, it is important to maintain patency of the catheter and to flush the line if there is a damped waveform or poor signal from the processor.

Changes of $\geq 10\%$ in the Svo_2 reading or decreases in Svo_2 below 60% are significant and should be followed by examination of other variables (cardiac output, arterial blood gases, hemoglobin level) to determine the cause of the change.

REFERENCES
1. Ahrens T, Penick J, Tucker M: Frequency requirements for zeroing transducers in hemodynamic monitoring, *Am J Crit Care* 4(6):466-471, 1995.
2. Anderson F et al: Indirect blood pressure measurement: a need to reassess, *Am J Crit Care* 2(4):272-279, 1993.

3. Baer CL: Acid base balance. In Kinney MR, Packa DR, Dunbar SB, eds: *AACN's clinical reference for critical care,* ed 3, St Louis, 1993, Mosby.

4. Boggs RL, Wooldridge-King M: *AACN procedure manual for critical care,* ed 3, Philadelphia, 1993, W.B. Saunders.

5. Bryan-Brown C, Dracup K: Doing the thing right: assumptions and assessment in hemodynamic monitoring, *Am J Crit Care* 2(4):269-271, 1993.

6. Bucher N: A safer way to get hemodynamic data, *RN* 55(11):56-62, 1992.

7. Conover MB: *Pocket guide to electrocardiography,* ed 3, St Louis, 1994, Mosby.

8. Daily E.K, Schroeder JS: *Techniques in bedside hemodynamic monitoring,* ed 5, St Louis, 1994, Mosby.

9. Diebel L et al: End-diastolic volume: a better indicator of preload in the critically ill, *Arch Surg* 127(7):817-822, 1992.

10. Doering L: The effect of positioning on hemodynamics and gas exchange in the critically ill: a review, *Am J Crit Care* 2(3):208-216, 1993.

11. Gardner P: Pulmonary artery pressure monitoring, *AACN Clin Issues Crit Care Nurs* 4(1):98-119, 1993.

12. Gilman P: Continuous measurement of cardiac output: a milestone in hemodynamic monitoring, *Focus Crit Care* 19(2):155-158, 1992.

13. Guzzetta C, Dossey B: *Cardiovascular nursing holistic practice,* St Louis, 1992, Mosby.

14. Hess D: Capnography: technical aspects and clinical applications. In Kacmarek RM, Hess D, Stoller JK, eds: *Monitoring in respiratory care,* St Louis, 1993, Mosby.

15. Kern L: Hemodynamic monitoring. In Logston Boggs R, Wooldridge-King M, eds: *AACN procedure manual for critical care,* ed 3, Philadelphia, 1993, W.B. Saunders.

16. Kinney M et al: *AACN's clinical reference for critical-care nursing,* ed 3, St Louis, 1993, Mosby.

17. McCarthy K et al: Pulse oximetry. In Kacmarek RM, Hess D, Stoller JK, eds: *Monitoring in respiratory care,* Philadelphia, 1993, Mosby.

18. Neagley SR: The pulmonary system. In Alspach JG, ed: *Core curriculum for critical care nursing,* ed 3, Philadelphia, 1991, W.B. Saunders.

19. Ostrow C et al: The effect of Trendelenburg and modified Trendelenburg positions on cardiac output, blood pressure, and oxygenation: a preliminary study, *Am J Crit Care* 3(5):382-386, 1994.

20. Pesola G et al: Room-temperature thermodilution cardiac output: proximal injectate lumen vs proximal infusion lumen, *Am J Crit Care* 2(2):132-133, 1993.

21. Renner L, Meyer L: Effect of position on selected hemodynamic parameters in postoperative cardiac surgery patients, *Am J Crit Care* 3(4):289-299, 1994.

22. Renner I, Meyer L: Injectate port selection affects accuracy and reproducibility of cardiac output measurements with multiport thermodilution pulmonary artery catheters, *Am J Crit Care* 3(1):55-61, 1994.

23. Sageman W, Amundson D: Thoracic electrical bioimpedance measurement of cardiac output in postaortocoronary bypass patients, *Crit Care Med* 21(8):1139-1142, 1993.

24. Shoemaker W: Monitoring and management of acute circulatory problems: the expanded role of the physiologically oriented critical care nurse, *Am J Crit Care* 1(1):38-53, 1992.

25. Smith M: Noninvasive hemodynamic monitoring with thoracic electrical bioimpedance, *Crit Care Nurse* 14(5):56-59, 1994.

26. Urban N: Integrating the hemodynamic profile with clinical assessment, *AACN Clin Issues Crit Care Nurs* 4(1):161-179, 1993.

27. Urden LD, Davie JK, Thelan LA: *Essentials of critical care nursing*, St Louis, 1992, Mosby.

28. Waldo A, Wit A: Mechanisms of cardiac arrhythmias, *Lancet* 341(8854):1189-1193, 1993.

29. Wood S, Ogusthorpe S: Cardiac output determination, *AACN Clin Issues Crit Care Nurs* 4(1):81-97, 1993.

CHAPTER 7

Therapeutic Modalities

Miscellaneous Modalities

AUTOTRANSFUSION

Clinical Brief

Autotransfusion is a technique that allows for the collection, filtration, and transfusion of the patient's own blood. Autologous transfusions have several advantages: they are readily available, eliminate the risk of transfusion reactions, and eliminate the risk of blood-transmittable diseases.

Autotransfusion can be performed preoperatively and saved for future use, intraoperatively to replace blood loss, and postoperatively to replace blood shed (e.g., mediastinal chest drainage). It can also be used in the trauma patient with massive intrathoracic bleeding when banked blood is not readily available.

Contraindications include blood that is contaminated by bacteria, bile, amniotic fluid, urine, or feces; AIDS, cancer, or sickle cell anemia; or in patients with wound blood greater than 6 hours old.

▶ Complications and related nursing diagnoses

Coagulopathies	Rick for injury: excessive bleeding
Sepsis	Risk for infection Altered tissue perfusion
Emboli	Altered tissue perfusion

Patient Care Management Guidelines
Patient assessment
1. Obtain pretransfusion baseline laboratory data: CBC, platelet count, INR/PT, PTT, hemoglobin, hematocrit, and electrolytes.
2. During the transfusion, obtain T, HR, RR, and BP q30min; measure urine output and hemodynamics (PAP, PAWP, CVP), hourly or more frequently if patient condition warrants.
3. Observe the patient for signs and symptoms of excessive bleeding: tachycardia, hypotension, decreased peripheral pulses, cool, clammy skin, decrease in CVP, PA pressures, PAWP, hematuria, hematemesis, increase in wound drainage, or chest tube drainage.
4. Observe the patient for signs and symptoms of emboli: SOB, change in LOC, absent or decreased pulses.

Patient management
1. Ensure optimal functioning of autotransfusion system. Follow manufacturer's instructions and maintain aseptic technique during the procedure.
2. Document the type and amount of anticoagulant used on the salvaged blood and note any clot formation.
3. Note any foam forming in the blood, which suggests increased hemolysis.
4. Accurately measure and record the amount of collected blood and infuse as directed.
5. Anticipate administration of blood products (platelets, FFP) if more than 6 L of salvaged blood have been infused.
6. Monitor CBC, platelet count, INR/PT, PTT, Hgb, Hct, and electrolytes during and after the infusion.

Critical observations
Consult with the physician for the following:
1. Suspected blood hemolysis or clots in salvaged blood
2. Embolic phenomenon
3. Thrombocytopenia
4. Increasing temperature, unstable BP
5. Excessive bleeding
6. Electrolyte imbalance

BLOOD ADMINISTRATION
Clinical Brief
Multiple blood components are available for transfusion therapy in the critically ill patient. Despite advances to maximize

the safety of blood, adverse reactions and the risk of transmitting infection still occur. Hepatitis can be transmitted by all forms of red cell products, plasma, cryoprecipitate, platelets, and coagulation concentrates. HIV can be transmitted by all forms of red cell transfusion, plasma, platelets, cryoprecipitate, and nonheated coagulation concentrates. CMV can be transmitted via blood products that contain white blood cells in which the virus is harbored.

Whole blood: used to replace volume in acute massive hemorrhage.

Packed red blood cells (PRBCs): used to increase the oxygen-carrying capacity with less risk of fluid overload.

Leukocyte-poor (washed) RBCs: contains PRBCs with leukocytes and platelets removed. Used to transfuse patients who have had more than one febrile transfusion reaction, patients who are likely to require multiple transfusions (leukemia), and patients who are immunocompromised and at risk for organisms that can be transmitted via leukocytes.

Platelets: used to restore platelets in patients who have a platelet defect and are bleeding; improve hemostasis in the thrombocytopenic patient who has received a massive transfusion, has undergone cardiac bypass surgery, or is in DIC. Prophylactic platelet transfusion is controversial.

Granulocytes: used to treat patients with decreased WBC count secondary to radiation or chemotherapy. Febrile reactions are common.

Fresh frozen plasma (FFP): used to treat patients with deficient coagulation factors (e.g., DIC, severe liver disease, massive transfusions).

Cryoprecipitate: contains factor VIII, factor XIII, and fibrinogen. Used to treat von Willebrand's disease, hypofirinogenemia, and to correct factor XIII deficiency.

Factor VIII concentrate: contains factor VIII. Used to replace factor VIII in hemophilia A patients.

Factor IX concentrate: contains factor IX. Used to supply factor IX in hemophilia B patients.

Albumin: used to expand intravascular volume or replace colloids. Available in 5% solution, used to correct colloid loss. Available in 25% solution, used to correct profound hypoalbuminemia.

Plasma protein fraction (Plasmanate): contains albumin and globulins. Used to expand intravascular volume or correct colloid loss.

▶ Complications and related nursing diagnoses

Hemolytic reaction	Altered tissue perfusion
	Hyperthermia
	Impaired gas exchange
Febrile reaction	Hyperthermia
	Pain: lumbar/headache
Anaphylactic shock	Altered tissue perfusion
	Impaired gas exchange
Circulatory overload	Fluid volume excess
Allergic reaction	Impaired skin integrity
	Ineffective breathing pattern

Patient Care Management Guidelines
Patient assessment
1. Obtain pretransfusion vital signs, and assess them again 15 minutes after initiating the transfusion. Obtain T, HR, RR, and BP q30min until the transfusion is completed. If transfusing granulocytes, measure VS q15min until the transfusion is complete.
2. Observe the patient for hemolytic reaction: high fever (39° C, 102.2° F); rigors; pain in the chest, loin, neck, or back; hematuria; oliguria; hypotension.
3. Observe the patient for an anaphylactic reaction: wheezing, edema of the tongue, larynx, and pharynx; stridor, hypotension, cardiopulmonary arrest.
4. Observe the patient for a febrile reaction: fever (38.3° C; 100.4° F), chills, flushed skin, headache or backache, hypotension, cough, dyspnea, nausea, and vomiting.
5. Observe the patient for fluid overload: SOB, tachycardia, hypotension, increased CVP, cough, crackles, distended neck veins, and S_3.
6. Observe the patient for an allergic reaction: pruritus, urticaria, headache, edema.
7. Assess the patient's response to therapy; check hemoglobin, hematocrit, prothrombin time, platelet count, sodium, potassium, and calcium levels.
8. Assess the patient for citrate toxicity if the patient is receiving a massive transfusion: tingling of extremities, hypotension, dysrhythmias, carpopedal spasm.

Patient management
1. Inspect the blood product for clots, bubbles, and discoloration.

2. Only NS can be used to prime or flush the blood administration set or to infuse simultaneously with the blood.

3. Do not administer medications through a blood infusion line.

4. Change blood filters if the infusion rate cannot be maintained, and per manufacturer's recommendations.

5. Use a blood warmer if large amounts of cold blood products are expected to be given over 4 hours or less, to postoperative hypothermic patients, and for patients with cold agglutinins. Warm blood to body temperature and monitor blood and body temperature throughout the infusion. Do not warm blood >42° C.

6. Verify the patient and blood product according to institution protocol. Generally another licensed professional is required to identify the patient and blood product. Information on the patient's ID bracelet, transfusion request, and blood product label should match. Do not administer the product if there is not a precise match. Be sure to check the expiration date of the blood product.

7. Ensure patency of the IV. Most blood products can be infused through an 18-gauge catheter.

8. Administer the blood product at a rate of 1 to 2 ml/min during the first 15 minutes and stay with the patient. Signs of anaphylaxis or a hemolytic reaction usually occur after a small amount of blood has been infused.

9. If no reaction occurs, increase the infusion rate based on the patient's condition and the type of the blood product (Table 7-1). Monitor patients with cardiovascular, renal, or liver disease for fluid volume overload.

10. Discontinue the transfusion if the patient manifests any signs and symptoms of a reaction. Save the blood product and tubing for the blood bank, and follow institution protocol.

Critical observations

Consult with the physician for the following:

1. Allergic reaction
2. Hemolytic reaction
3. Anaphylactic reaction
4. Febrile reaction
5. Volume overload

TABLE 7-1 Blood Component Administration Guidelines

Blood component	Infusion rate	Filter	Volume	Comment
Whole blood	2-4 hrs Max: 4 hrs	Required	500 ml	Rapid infusion if need is urgent
Packed red blood cells	2-4 hrs Max: 4 hrs	Required	250 ml	Hgb rises 1 g/dl; Hct rises 3% after 1 unit
Leukocyte-poor red blood cells	2 hrs	Required	Variable	
Fresh frozen plasma	1-2 hrs, rapidly if bleeding	Use component filter	250 ml	Notify blood bank—takes 20 min to thaw; infuse immediately after thawing
Platelets	Rapidly as patient tolerates	Use component filter	35-50 ml/unit	Usually 6-10 units are ordered. Request that blood bank pool all units
Albumin	1-2 ml/min in normovolemic patients	Special tubing	Varies	Comes in 5% and 25%; can increase intravascular volume quickly; infuse cautiously
Cryoprecipitate	30 min	Use component filter	10 ml/unit	Usually 6-10 units ordered Request that blood bank pool units
Granulocytes	2-4 hrs	Use component filter	300-400 ml	VS q15min during infusion

EPIDURAL ANALGESIA

Clinical Brief

Epidural analgesia is employed to provide pain relief to postoperative patients without adversely affecting the patient's mentation and respiratory function, as is associated with intravenous or intramuscular administration of narcotics. A narcotic can be administered by intermittent bolus, continuous infusion, and PCA pumps into a catheter placed in the epidural space: narcotics bind to spinal cord opioid receptors and thus interfere with pain transmission without causing blockade of sensory motor, or sympathetic nerve fibers.

Narcotics commonly used are morphine (Duramorph) and fentanyl (Sublimaze). Fentanyl is 100 times more potent than morphine. It has an immediate onset with a duration of 12 hours, whereas the onset of morphine is within 1 hour and has a duration of 24 hours. Therefore patients must be monitored closely for adverse effects 6 hours (fentanyl) to 24 hours (morphine) after the epidural infusion has been discontinued. Solutions containing an anesthetic (e.g., bupivacaine) along with the narcotic may also be used.

Patients with a history of allergy to narcotics, increased ICP, coagulopathy or on anticoagulant therapy, bacteremia, infection at the proposed puncture site, and prior laminectomy (if the dura was opened) are not candidates for epidural analgesia.

▶ Complications and related nursing diagnoses

Migration of catheter	Risk for injury
Respiratory depression	Ineffective breathing pattern
	Impaired gas exchange
Side effects of narcotics:	
• Nausea/vomiting	Fluid volume deficit
• Pruritus	Impaired skin integrity
• Urinary retention	Urinary retention
• Hypotension	Decreased cardiac output
Infection	Hyperthermia
Headache following dural puncture	Pain
Neurological sequelae:	Impaired physical mobility
• Paresthesia	
• Motor deficit	

Patient Care Management Guidelines

Patient assessment

1. If a bolus of narcotic is administered, monitor VS q15min × 4; q1h × 12; q2h × 12; then q4h.
2. Assess respiratory status q1h during epidural infusion. Count respirations for 1 full minute—note the rate and depth of respirations, skin color, and LOC. Monitor respiratory status closely for at least 6 hours after fentanyl is discontinued and 24 hours after morphine is discontinued.
3. Assess pain control q2 to 4h using a pain scale. (See Figure 1-1.) An increase in pain rating may indicate catheter occlusion.
4. Assess level of sedation (wide awake, drowsy, dozing intermittently, mostly sleeping, awakens only when aroused).
5. Check motor strength and sensation, since neurological changes can be caused by epidural hematoma or abscess. Numbness and weakness may occur if the solution contains an anesthetic.
6. Monitor temperature q4h; assess for signs and symptoms of meningitis.
7. Assess voiding; check for bladder distention or discomfort q4h.
8. Assess condition of catheter site and dressing. An enlarged hardened area at the site may indicate hematoma. A wet dressing may indicate catheter migration.

Patient management

1. Isolate the infusion pump if possible and label the pump and IV tubing with "Epidural Precautions."
2. Tape all ports on the IV tubing to prevent accidental injection of substances.
3. Dressing changes can increase the risk for catheter dislodgement. Check the institution protocol for how often and who is responsible for dressing changes. A wet dressing can be reinforced with a dry sterile 4 × 4 gauze.
4. Examine the catheter for kinks or loose connections. Maintain sterility when manipulating the catheter or dressing. If the catheter becomes disconnected, cover the end of the catheter with a sterile 4 × 4 gauze and notify the physician.

5. If >1 ml of clear fluid can be aspirated from the catheter and tests positive for glucose, migration of the catheter to the subarachnoid space should be suspected. If blood is aspirated, the catheter may be in an epidural vein. Catheter placement can be confirmed with a test dose of a local anesthetic containing epinephrine. If the HR or BP increases, the catheter tip is in the epidural vein. If a loss of sensory or motor function occurs in the lower extremities, and a decrease in BP occurs over 1 to 5 minutes, the catheter tip is in the intrathecal space. NOTE: an inability to aspirate or a negative test dose does not guarantee correct catheter placement.

6. *Avoid* using alcohol or iodine to clean connections; these substances can be toxic to the nervous system.

7. Verify the solution with another nurse to ensure the correct medication concentration and that the solution is *preservative-free.*

8. Check the infusion rate and verify correct dosage.

9. Ensure a patent emergency IV access during the infusion, 6 hours after fentanyl is discontinued, and 24 hours after morphine is discontinued.

10. Place the patient on a pulse oximeter and an apnea monitor during the infusion, 6 hours after fentanyl is discontinued, and 24 hours after morphine is discontinued.

11. Keep naloxone (Narcan) and a syringe at the bedside during the infusion, for 6 hours after fentanyl is discontinued, and 24 hours after morphine is discontinued.

12. If respiratory depression develops, follow institutional policy. Generally, if the rate is less than 8/min, SpO_2 less than 95%, or apnea greater than 10 sec, give 2 to 3 ml of a diluted (0.4 mg in 9 ml NS) naloxone IV q2 to 3 min until the desired effect is achieved.

13. If hypotension develops, place the patient flat and stop the epidural infusion; a fluid challenge may be needed.

14. A urinary catheter may be necessary for the duration of the epidural analgesia. Low-dose (0.1 mg IV or IM) naloxone may be given for urinary retention.

15. Diphenhydramine (Benadryl) 25 mg IM may be given for pruritus. For severe pruritus, low-dose (0.1 mg) naloxone may be given.

16. Promethazine (Phenergan) 6.25 to 12.5 mg IV or IM may be given for nausea or vomiting. Metoclopramide (Reglan) 10 mg IV or droperidal (Inapsine) 0.25 to 0.625 mg IV may also be used to relieve nausea or vomiting.

17. Consult with the physician before attempting to ambulate the patient receiving a solution containing a local anesthetic. The patient may be at risk for paresthesia and motor deficits.

CATHETER REMOVAL

1. Removal of the catheter is done by the anesthesiologist, nurse anesthetist, and in some institutions, the critical care nurse.

2. After the catheter has been removed, check the tip of the catheter and note the presence of a colored mark. The colored mark denotes an intact catheter. Document this finding in the chart.

3. Check the site for infection. Do not clean the site with alcohol. Apply a sterile dressing to the site.

Critical observations

Consult with the physician for the following:

1. Respiratory rate <10/min
2. Sustained SpO_2 <95%
3. Hypotension
4. Inadequate analgesia
5. Oversedation
6. Persistent side effects (e.g., n/v, pruritus, urinary retention)
7. Signs of infection
8. Dislodged epidural catheter
9. Presence of paresthesia or motor deficits
10. Inability to remove epidural catheter
11. Absence of colored mark on catheter tip, or a broken or sheared catheter on removal

NEUROMUSCULAR BLOCKADE IN THE CRITICALLY ILL

Clinical Brief

Neuromuscular blocking agents (NMBAs) are used as a "chemical restraint" when maximal sedation is not effective and there is risk of the patient injuring himself or herself; to reduce metabolic demands particularly in shock states; to prevent ventilator asynchrony in patients with acute respiratory distress syndrome;

and to stabilize cerebral blood flow in patients with elevated intracranial pressure. NMBAs produce muscle paralysis by blocking the receptor sites at the neuromuscular junction. The goal of neuromuscular blockade is to have less than a 100% block, and to use the least amount of drug to achieve the prescribed clinical end-points (e.g., no movement, no spontaneous ventilation, no ventilator asynchrony).

The depth of paralysis is monitored with a peripheral nerve stimulator (PNS). Patients should be comfortably sedated prior to initiating the NMBA. Prior to administering the NMBA and once the patient is sedated, a baseline neuromuscular response should be assessed. Train-of-four monitoring is commonly used to monitor the degree of block of the neuromuscular junction. This involves recording the number of twitches in response to four stimuli. If four twitches are observed/palpated, there is less than a 75% block; three twitches correspond to a 75% block; two twitches correspond to an 80% block; and no twitches correspond to a 100% block. A 100% blockade is not desirable because all receptor sites would be occupied and some receptor sites must be available for a reversal agent to be effective should reversal be desired. In addition, if all receptor sites were occupied, continued administration of the drug would cause the drug to be stored. This would lead to prolonged paralysis once the drug therapy was discontinued.

Neuromuscular blockade is not without its complications. Patients can experience complications related to immobility, side effects of the agent being used, and prolonged weakness after discontinuing the agent.

Neuromuscular blocking agents do not affect consciousness—patients are able to hear, feel, and think. It is important to keep the patient pain-free and anxiety-free with analgesics and anxiolytics through the duration of neuromuscular blockade, since the inability to move and communicate can be a frightening experience.

▶ Complications and related nursing diagnoses

Overdosage of NMBA	Risk for injury
Paralysis:	Risk for disuse syndrome
Inadequate airway/ventilation	Altered protection
Inadequate sedation/analgesia	
Skin breakdown	
Retention of secretions	
Corneal damage	
Disuse atrophy	

Patient Care Management Guidelines
Patient assessment
1. Prior to NMBA, obtain baseline neuromuscular response with PNS.
2. After drug initiated, assess depth of paralysis with PNS. Desired blockade is usually 1 to 2 twitches in the train-of-four mode. With intermittent dosing, check the response before and 15 minutes after the dose. With continuous infusion of the NMBA, check response every 4 hours while the patient's temperature or pH is changing, or if there is a change in concurrent drug therapy.
3. Inspect skin, pressure points, and cornea for dryness, ulceration.
4. Auscultate lungs and assess respiratory effort. Validate ventilator settings and alarms. Assess end tidal CO_2 if available.
5. Assess oxygenation status with continuous SpO_2 monitoring and ABG results and compare results to the prescribed parameters.
6. Assess fluid volume status and hemodynamic parameters: PA pressures (if available), BP, intake and output, weight, creatinine and BUN levels.
7. Assess vital signs: T, P, R, and BP.

Patient management
1. Titrate NMBA to prescribed goal; monitor with PNS after any titration in drug dose. Note that any changes in the patient's temperature, pH, or drug therapy can alter the effects of the NMBA.
2. Prevent complications associated with immobility: reposition patient frequently, maintain patient in proper body alignment, provide ROM exercises, prevent undue pressure on peroneal and ulnar nerves, apply antiembolic hose.
3. Prevent corneal drying/abrasions: administer an ophthalmic ointment as prescribed; keep eyelids closed with transpore tape (avoid dressings over the eyes).
4. Provide pulmonary hygiene: suction as necessary, reposition patient frequently.
5. Administer round-the-clock sedation and analgesics. Administer pain medication prior to any painful procedure.
6. Address the patient and family and explain what is going on around them. Reassure the patient and

family that the paralysis is temporary. Encourage the family to talk to the patient as if the patient was awake.

7. Reorient the patient every time you approach the bed.
8. Consider the use of relaxing music.
9. Place a sign at the head of the bed to communicate to other health care workers that the patient is receiving a NMBA but can still feel pain and hear.
10. Plan uninterrupted periods of rest and promote sleep/awake cycle.
11. After the NMBA is discontinued, slowly taper sedation and analgesic agents.
12. Have atropine and pharmacologic reversal agents available (e.g., pyridostigmine, neostigmine, edrophonium).

Critical observations

Consult with the physician for the following:

1. Inadequate oxygenation/ventilation
2. Hypotension, tachycardia
3. Inadequate neuromuscular blockade

SEDATION IN THE CRITICALLY ILL

Clinical Brief

A loss of control, disorientation, and the inability to communicate may potentiate fear and anxiety in the critically ill patient. Agitation increases oxygen consumption, increases the risk for accidental removal of monitoring equipment and invasive catheters, and interferes with diagnostic procedures or therapies that may feel unnatural or are uncomfortable. Sedating a patient in the ICU can provide comfort from frightening situations, relieve mental distress, improve oxygenation, and protect the patient from injury. The goal of sedation is to keep the patient calm, comfortable, and communicative. Patients should not drift too deep into a sedative state. All members of the health care team should be aware of the level of sedation prescribed for the patient. Monitoring this level can be performed with a sedation scale such as the Ramsay scale or modified Ramsay scale (Table 7-2). Sedative-hypnotics include the benzodiazepines (e.g., diazepam, lorazepam, and midazolam) and propofol, a nonbarbiturate anesthetic agent (Table 7-3). Narcotics that may be used for sedation in addition to their analgesic properties include morphine and fentanyl. Haloperidol, an antipsychotic drug, is used to treat delirium.

TABLE 7-2   Ramsay Scale

Level	Description
I	Anxious and agitated
II	Cooperative, oriented, tranquil
III	Responds only to verbal commands
IV	Asleep with brisk response to light stimulation
V	Asleep with sluggish response to stimulation
VI	Asleep without response to stimulation

TABLE 7-3   Commonly Used Sedatives for Continuous Intravenous Administration

Drug	Dose	Administration guides
Lorazepam (Ativan)	Bolus: 0.05 mg/kg Infusion: 0.5 mg/hr	Mixture: 10 mg lorazepam in 100 ml D_5W. Increase infusion rate 2-3 mg/hr to achieve desired sedation level. Use lowest rate necessary to maintain level of sedation. Change IV bag after 12 hours.
Midazolam (Versed)	Bolus: 0.1 mg/kg Infusion: 0.05-0.1 mg/kg/hr	Mixture: 100 mg Midazolam in 100 ml D_5W
Propofol (Diprivan)	Infusion: 5 mcg/kg/min	Mixture: propofol comes in a solution of 10% intralipids. Titrate infusion by 5-10 mcg/kg/min increments to desired level of sedation. Use least amount of propofol to maintain the desired level of sedation. Change bottle and tubing every 12 hours. Use strict aseptic technique. Do not administer any other solution or medication in the same line.

▶ **Complications and related nursing diagnoses**

Oversedation	Impaired physical mobility
	Inability to sustain spontaneous ventilation
	Impaired gas exchange
	Ineffective breathing pattern
	Decreased cardiac output
	Altered protection
	Risk for injury
	Impaired verbal communication
	Risk for impaired skin integrity

Patient Care Management Guidelines
Patient assessment
1. Identify the pathologic cause of agitation (e.g., hypoxia, hypercarbia, inadequate pain control, electrolyte disorder, increased intracranial pressure).
2. Assess for the presence of pain in the sedated patient. Pain should be treated with analgesics; anxiety and agitation should be treated with sedative agents.
3. Be alert for possible paradoxical agitation in the elderly.
4. Assess volume status prior to administering sedatives; changes in heart rate and blood pressure can be minimized if hypovolemia is corrected.
5. Monitor hemodynamics; be alert for changes in blood pressure, heart rate, and development of dysrhythmias.
6. Monitor respiratory function; sedatives abolish the hypoxic stimulus. Be alert for hypoventilation and decreased respiratory rate.
7. Monitor oxygen saturation with pulse oximetry.
8. Assess airway management in the nonintubated patient.
9. Assess sedation level with the Ramsay scale or other available sedative scale.

Patient management
1. Establish at least one other patent IV access.
2. Patients receiving continuous IV sedation should be mechanically ventilated.
3. Administer continuous infusion of the agent via an IV infusion pump, unless the drug is administered by IV bolus for short-term use (e.g., an unpleasant procedure may be treated with a dose of benzodiazepine or propofol).

4. Painful procedures should be treated with an analgesic agent.
5. Titrate the sedative agent to the prescribed level of sedation.
6. Prevent complications by repositioning the patient, provide meticulous skin care, pulmonary hygiene, and preventing the patient from injury.
7. See Chapter 8 for information on a specific drug.

Critical observations

Consult with the physician for the following:
1. Hemodynamic instability: bradycardia, hypotension, dysrhythmias
2. Inadequate oxygenation/ventilation
3. Inability to maintain prescribed level of sedation
4. See adverse effects of a specific drug in Chapter 8

THERMAL REGULATION

Clinical Brief

Cooling and rewarming methods are used to control body temperature. Common thermoregulation disorders treated in the critical care units include hyperpyrexia (fever) and postoperative hypothermia, although heat stroke, malignant hyperthermia, and hypothermia resulting from burns or accidental exposure are also seen in the critical care setting.

External cooling methods can be used alone or in combination with antipyretic therapy. Rewarming methods are generally used in patients who have undergone elective hypothermia (e.g., cardiovascular, thoracic, and neurosurgical surgeries).

Cooling methods are used to treat hyperthermia. Hyperthermia refers to a body temperature greater than 37.2° C (99° F) and is classified as (1) *mild*—37.2° C to 38.8° C (99° F to 102° F); (2) *moderate*—38.8° C to 40° C (102° F to 104° F); (3) *critical*—≥40.5° C (≥105° F); and (4) *malignant*—0.5° C/15 min to 42.7° C (1° F/15 min to 109° F).

Rewarming methods are used to treat hypothermia. Hypothermia refers to a body temperature less than 37° C (98.6° F) and is classified as (1) *mild*—34° C to 36° C (93.2° F to 96.8° F); (2) *moderate*—30° C to 34.5° C (86° F to 93.2° F); (3) *severe*—<30° C (86° F); and (4) *profound*—<16.5° C (<61.7° F).

▶ Complications and related nursing diagnoses

External cooling methods

Vasoconstriction/decreased heat loss	Hyperthermia
Frostbite	Impaired skin integrity
Overshoot	Hypothermia

Rewarming methods

Shock	Altered tissue perfusion
Burns	Impaired skin integrity
Overshoot	Hyperthermia

Patient Care Management Guidelines

COOLING METHODS

Patient assessment

1. Measure core temperature q15 to 30min during initial therapy. Anticipate an increase in HR, BP, and RR on initiation of therapy.
2. Assess LOC, presence of peripheral pulses, capillary refill, and skin temperature and condition.
3. Observe for shivering, which can cause an increase in metabolic rate and oxygen consumption. Tensing or clenching of the jaw muscles is an early sign of shivering. An ECG artifact associated with muscle tremor may also be observed.

Patient management

1. Maintain the environmental temperature at about 70° F (21° C); fans may be required to keep the room cool.
2. Use a wet sheet to cover the patient's torso; tepid baths may be given to lower the patient's temperature. Avoid cold baths, since shivering may occur.
3. A cooling blanket may be used:
   a. Precool the blanket if at all possible.
   b. Avoid layers of blankets; a single layer should be used to absorb perspiration.
   c. Turn the patient at least q2h and massage the skin. Keep the blanket in contact with patient during position changes.
   d. Monitor for drift (T change >1° C in 15 min). Avoid overshoot (continual temperature reduction after device is turned off) by stopping the cooling blanket when the core temperature is 39° C (102.2° F).
4. For prolonged moderate hyperthermia (38.8° C to 40° C; 101.8° F to 104° F) or critical hyperthermia (≥40.5° C; 104.9° F):
   a. Ice packs can be applied to major artery sites or ice baths may be given.
   b. Gastric, bladder, and rectal irrigations with iced isotonic solution may be required.
5. Administer antipyretics as ordered; neuroleptic agents may be required to control shivering.

Patient Care Management Guidelines

REWARMING METHODS

Patient assessment

1. Measure core temperature q15 to 30min during initial therapy. Anticipate increase in HR, BP, and RR on initiation of therapy. A drop in BP during rewarming may signal peripheral vasodilation, decreased venous return, and decreased CO (rewarming shock).
2. Continuously monitor ECG for dysrhythmias.
3. Assess LOC (hearing returns at ~34° C; 93.2° F); observe for signs of gastritis or ulceration, fluid volume excess, and thermal injury to skin.

Patient management

1. Minimize drafts and maintain room temperature; give warm fluids orally if the patient is alert and a gag reflex is present.
2. Apply a bath blanket and cover the head; peripheral vasodilation may occur with use of a hyperthermia blanket.
3. An external hyperthermia blanket may be used; turn the device off when core body temperature is within 1 to 2° of desired temperature. Monitor for drift (temperature drift may occur after the device is turned off).
4. In severe and profound hypothermia (<30° C; 86° F) active rewarming methods may be used: gastric, peritoneal, rectal, or bladder irrigations with heated isotonic solutions, or extracorporeal circulation may be required.
5. If cardiopulmonary arrest occurs, raise the core temperature to 32° C to 33° C (92° F) to optimize conditions for defibrillation.
6. Monitor the patient for "bolus effect" of pharmacological agents given during a hypothermia episode, as vasodilation occurs with rewarming.
7. Maintain extremities below heart level until vasodilation and hemodynamic stability have been achieved. Cardiac dysrhythmias may result from venous return of acidemic peripheral blood when arms or legs are raised.
8. Do not exceed a rate of 2° C/hr to rewarm the patient.
9. If blood transfusions are required, use a blood warmer.

Critical observations

Consult with the physician for the following:

1. Hypothermia or hyperthermia unresponsive to therapeutic interventions
2. Excessive shivering

3. Hypotension
4. Dysrhythmias
5. Fluid and electrolyte disturbances
6. Hypoxemia and acid-base imbalance
7. Seizures
8. Cardiopulmonary arrest

VENOUS ACCESS DEVICES

Clinical Brief

Selection is based upon the osmolality of solution, expected duration of therapy, and patient need. These devices can be temporary peripheral and central venous catheters, tunneled central venous catheters, or implanted ports. Catheters also come in single and multilumen capacities. See Table 7-4 for types and characteristics of commonly used central venous devices.

▶ Complications and related nursing diagnoses

Air emboli	Ineffective breathing pattern
	Impaired gas exchange
	Pain: chest pain
Local or systemic infection	Risk for infection
	Impaired skin integrity
Loss of catheter function:	Risk for injury
• Catheter occlusion	
• Catheter dislodgement	
• Catheter migration	
• Catheter tear	

Patient Care Management Guidelines

Patient assessment

1. Review initial and serial chest radiographs to verify catheter placement.
2. Assess skin integrity at the catheter insertion site or exit site each shift. Note any redness, tenderness, swelling, skin breakdown, fluid leakage, or purulent drainage at the site.
3. Monitor vital signs q4h, noting any trend in increase in temperature.
4. Assess for air embolus (increased risk occurs during tubing changes or with procedures requiring exposed catheter hub): chest pain, tachycardia, tachypnea, cyanosis, hypotension.

TABLE 7-4 Characteristics of Central Venous Devices

Device	Use	Volume	Heparinization*	Comment
Centrally placed catheter				
Single and multilumen	Short-term	0.5-0.6 ml/lumen	Required	Distal port can be used for CVP monitoring; distal port is 16 gauge; middle and proximal ports are 18 gauge; can be inserted at bedside
Peripherally inserted central catheter (PICC)				
Single/multilumen Groshong PICC Per-a-Cath	Moderate-long-term	0.1-0.4 ml/lumen	Required	Inserted into the basilic or cephalic vein with the tip advanced to the SVC or subclavian veins
Implantable port				
Porta-cath Medi-port	Long-term	2 ml port 2 ml lumen	Required	OR insertion required

Tunneled			
Hickman	Long-term	1.8 ml/lumen	Required	OR insertion required; catheter is tunneled subcutaneously and contains a dacron mesh cuff to stabilize catheter
Broviac	Long-term	1.0 ml/lumen	Required	See Hickman
Groshong	Long-term	1.8 ml/lumen	Required	OR insertion required; catheter is tunneled subcutaneously; contains a three-position valve

*For catheter lumens not used for continuous infusions.

5. Monitor for any increased trend in WBC or blood glucose levels, which may signal infection.

Patient management

All catheters: (Implantable ports, see p. 556)

Prevent infection:

1. Use strict aseptic technique while manipulating catheters (e.g., dressing changes, accessing ports, changing injection caps). Povidone-iodine can be used as an antiseptic to cleanse the site and injection ports.
2. Change dressing as per protocol—more frequently if the dressing becomes soiled, wet, or loose.
3. Change injection caps per protocol.

Prevent catheter dislodgement/disconnection:

1. Secure catheter and extension tubings to prevent catheter dislodgement or disconnection. Document catheter position, using markings on the catheter (except totally implanted ports). Have a clamp (without teeth) available. If an air embolus is suspected, clamp the catheter, turn the patient to the left side, and lower the HOB. Administer oxygen.

Catheter malfunction:

1. If unable to aspirate blood from the catheter, raise the patient's arm or have patient C & DB. Try flushing the catheter gently with NS. Catheter placement may need to be verified by a chest radiograph.
2. If unable to infuse IV fluid or medication, try flushing the catheter gently with NS—*do not use force*. Catheter placement may need to be verified by a chest radiograph. If a clot is suspected, urokinase may be ordered; follow institution protocol. Generally 1 ml (5000 U/ml) is injected using a tuberculin syringe; wait 5 to 10 minutes and aspirate. The procedure can be repeated twice. If catheter patency has been achieved, withdraw 5 ml of fluid from the catheter and discard. Flush the catheter with NS and resume previous fluid administration. If a medication precipitate is suspected, 0.1 normal hydrochloric acid may be used to clear the catheter of drugs with a low pH; sodium bicarbonate may be used with drugs with a high pH; and 70% ethyl alcohol may be effective if the occlusion is due to fat accumulation from lipids administration.

Obtaining blood samples: PICC and CVC

1. To obtain blood samples, turn off IV solution(s) for 1 minute; attach a syringe to the hub of the catheter; discard 3× the volume of the catheter lumen (see Table 7-4); and withdraw the amount of blood needed. Flush the lumen and resume IV fluids; if the lumen is not in use, flush and heparinize the lumen.

Catheter repair:

1. Inspect the catheter for cracks or tears—fluid and blood will leak from the damaged site.
2. For temporary repair, clamp the catheter between the site of insertion and the damaged section of the catheter. Cut the damaged section using sterile scissors. Insert a blunt-end needle of the appropriate gauge into the end of the catheter. Cap the needle and heparinize the catheter. An angiocath may be used; however, pull back on the stylet to avoid puncturing the catheter when inserting the angiocath into the catheter. A tongue blade can be used to splint or support the repaired area.
3. Permanent repair for long-term catheters should be done with the manufacturer's repair kit as soon as possible. Short-term multilumen catheters should be changed as soon as possible.

CATHETER REMOVAL: TEMPORARY CVC

1. If catheter insertion is in a neck vein, place the patient in the Trendelenburg position (to prevent air embolus).
2. Using aseptic technique, remove sutures and steadily pull the catheter back. Apply pressure to the insertion site and apply a sterile occlusive dressing. Check to see if the catheter is intact.

CATHETER REMOVAL: PICC

1. Remove dressing.
2. Gently tug on the catheter; if there is resistance, place tension on the catheter, tape it down, and try again in a few minutes.

SINGLE/MULTILUMEN CATHETERS

Patient management

1. Tape piggybacked intermittent infusion lines securely to prevent inadvertent disconnection.
2. Flush the catheter lumen with heparinized saline q8 to 12h (or according to institution protocol) when not in use. Flush the catheter lumen with 2 ml NS before infusing intermittent medications. After the infusion is complete, flush with NS and heparinize the lumen.

3. To reduce the risk of introducing air into the catheter, draw up 3 ml of the normal saline or heparinized solution but inject only 2 to 2.5 ml. To prevent a backflow of blood into the catheter tip, withdraw the needle from the injection port while continuing to inject the solution (do not completely empty the syringe). Discard remaining NS or heparinized saline.

BROVIAC CATHETER
Patient management
See single/multilumen catheters.

HICKMAN CATHETER
Patient management
See single/multilumen catheters.

PICC
Patient management
1. Do not draw blood or take BP in the arm with the line inserted.
2. See single/multilumen catheters.

GROSHONG
Patient management
1. Maintain a sterile occlusive dressing to exit site.
2. Change dressing q72h or more frequently if the dressing becomes soiled, wet, or loose.
3. Change injection caps q7days or more frequently (e.g., if blood is in the cap or cap is perforated excessively).
4. Tape piggybacked intermittent infusion lines securely to prevent inadvertent disconnection.
5. Flush catheter vigorously with 5 ml normal saline after completion of intermittent infusions.
6. Flush the catheter lumen with 10 ml NS after blood infusions or obtaining blood samples.
7. Inject 20 ml NS before aspirating a blood sample following an infusion of TPN.
8. A Groshong catheter requires no clamping because of its specially designed valve.

IMPLANTABLE PORTS
Patient management
1. Use aseptic technique when accessing the implanted port. Stabilize the port with thumb and index finger. If port moves freely, suspect dislodgement.
2. Cannulate the port using a Huber needle and extension tubing flushed with NS. A 90-degree-angled needle is recommended with continuous infusions for patient comfort and ease of dressing applications.

3. Push the Huber needle through the port until it touches the back of the port (to ensure that it is not in the rubber septum).
4. Aspirate for a blood return and flush the system with NS to confirm patency before initiating the infusion.
5. Flush the catheter with 5 ml NS after a bolus injection; follow with 5 ml heparinized saline.
6. Flush catheter with 20 ml NS after a blood sample has been withdrawn or blood has been administered.
7. Maintain a sterile dressing over the needle and port when in use; otherwise no dressing is required.
8. Change Huber needles q3 to 7 days during continuous infusion.
9. Check the site for irritation or ulceration around the needle; rotate the insertion site prn; the skin area over the port is ~1 inch × 1 inch.

Critical observations

Consult with the physician for the following:
1. Patient becomes febrile
2. Unable to inject fluid into or withdraw blood from catheter
3. Patient develops chest pain, dyspnea, cyanosis
4. Site is inflamed, tender, or is draining fluid or pus
5. Catheter tears/cracks
6. Implantable port is dislodged

BARBITURATE COMA

Clinical Brief

The use of barbiturates in treating cases of malignant ICP (sustained ICP >20 mm Hg) has remained controversial in its wide range of clinical applications. While barbiturates have been used for patients with severe head injury, there have been other opportunities for its use in the acute care setting. These include cases of intractable seizures, sagittal sinus thrombosis, Reye's syndrome, and ischemic stroke.

The mechanism of barbiturate action is not fully understood, but it is believed to play a role in the reduction of cerebral blood flow, oxygen demand, and cerebral metabolism, thereby reducing ICP. The use of barbiturates may also reduce swelling and promote resolution of cerebral edema.

In patients whose ICP has not responded well to CSF drainage, hyperventilation, or osmotic therapy and in whom there is no surgical lesion, barbiturate coma may be instituted. Since the clinical examination is not reliable during the drug-induced coma, a surgical lesion must be removed before barbiturate coma is instituted.

Serial EEG recordings guide induction of the coma and adjustments in dosage maintenance of barbiturate infusion.

Contraindications to barbiturate therapy include those patients whose ICP is normal or those patients who respond promptly to CSF drainage, hyperventilation, and/or osmotic therapy. Patients who suffer from cardiac disease, especially heart failure, are not candidates for barbiturate coma because of the myocardial depressive effects of barbiturates.

▶ Complications and related nursing diagnoses

Hypotension	Decreased cardiac output
	Altered tissue perfusion
Hypostatic pneumonia	Impaired gas exchange
Aspiration	Risk for infection
	Impaired gas exchange
Hypothermia	Hypothermia

Patient Care Management Guidelines
Patient assessment
1. Continuously monitor arterial BP and MAP; assess the patient for hypotension and tachycardia.
2. Obtain ICP readings and calculate cerebral perfusion pressure.
3. Continuously monitor oxygen saturation with pulse oximetry and PETCO$_2$ with capnometry (if available). Review ABGs to evaluate oxygenation and acid-base status.
4. Obtain PA and wedge pressures as well as CO/CI to evaluate the hemodynamic response to barbiturate coma.
5. Closely monitor body temperature; barbiturates reduce metabolism and can cause hypothermia.
6. Assess neurological status to evaluate degree of coma.

Patient management
1. Intubation and mechanical ventilation are required. Anticipate NG tube placement to maintain gastric decompression and prevent the risk of aspiration.
2. Portable EEG monitoring or compressed spectral analysis (CSA) will be necessary to monitor the patient's response to the loading dose and to adjust maintenance dosing. Obtaining hourly EEG printouts is recommended.
3. A loading dose of pentobarbital is 5 to 10 mg/kg IV at a rate no faster than 100 mg/min. Designate one IV line for pentobarbital infusion only. Have phenylephrine HCl 50 mg/250 ml D$_5$W available in case the patient becomes hypotensive; dopamine (ACLS concentration: Patient's wt in kg × 15 = Amount in 250 ml) may also be prepared and ready to infuse during the loading dose of pentobarbital. Maintain MAP >70 mm Hg and cerebral perfusion >60 mm Hg.
4. The maintenance dose is usually 1 to 3 mg/kg/hr and may be given hourly as a bolus or as a constant infusion. The dosage is adjusted according to electrical activity recorded on EEG or CSA.
5. During the first several hours of pentobarbital infusion, assess neurological function. The patient will become nonresponsive and flaccid; corneal, cough, gag, swallow, and/or pupillary reflexes will decrease or become absent; and spontaneous respirations will cease.
6. Osmotic therapy and CSF drainage may continue as needed for intermittent ICP control during barbiturate coma.

7. Once the ICP has been lowered and remains stable for greater than 48 hours, a slow taper of barbiturates may begin. Osmotic diuretics and CSF drainage may continue prn. If ICP does not respond to diuretics and CSF drainage (i.e., ICP >20 mm Hg), barbiturate therapy may be resumed.

Critical observations
Consult with the physician for the following:
1. ICP unresponsive to barbiturate administration
2. CPP <60 mm Hg
3. Hypotension
4. O_2 sat <95%
5. Hypothermia
6. Suspected aspiration
7. Unilateral change in pupil size

CAROTID ENDARTERECTOMY

Clinical Brief
Carotid surgery can be performed to repair traumatic injuries to the artery or to improve cerebral circulation in patients with occlusive vascular disease.

Carotid endarterectomies are usually performed to remove atherosclerotic plaques that have significantly reduced the lumen of the artery or have become ulcerative and are the source of emboli. The symptoms in carotid disease are caused by a significant reduction in cerebral blood flow resulting from an area of tight stenosis or by transient ischemic attacks (TIAs) resulting from embolization of plaque fragments, platelet clumps, or small blood clots from the ulcer in the atheroma. The objective of endarterectomy is to remove the embolism source and improve cerebral circulation.

▶ Complications and related nursing diagnoses

Embolic stroke	Altered tissue perfusion: cerebral
	Risk for disuse syndrome
Cranial nerve impairment	Ineffective airway clearance
	Risk for aspiration
	Risk for injury: dysrhythmia
	Sensory/perceptual alteration: visual

Patient Care Management Guidelines

Patient assessment
1. Assess neurological status hourly and compare findings with baseline assessment. Note the integrity of the

cough and gag reflexes, and visual fields and motor and sensory integrity. Monitor speech for comprehension and quality. Ask the patient to report signs and symptoms of TIAs.

2. Assess the patency of the carotid artery by palpating the superficial temporal artery and note the presence, quality, strength, and symmetry of pulses.

3. Assess vital signs hourly and carefully note BP: hypotension can occur secondary to carotid sinus manipulation during surgery; hypertension can occur secondary to surgical denervation of the carotid sinus.

4. Assess respiratory status: note rate and depth of respirations; observe respiratory pattern and note patient's ability to handle secretions (gag, cough, swallowing reflexes). Assess for hematoma or swelling at the operative site, which may adversely affect airway patency; note the presence of any tracheal deviation. Continuously monitor oxygen saturation via pulse oximetry (SpO_2).

5. Continuously monitor ECG for dysrhythmias secondary to intraoperative manipulation of carotid sinus.

6. Examine the surgical dressing for bloody drainage. Note any swelling or hematoma formation at the incision site.

Patient management

1. Keep HOB at 30 degrees unless hypotensive events occur, then lower HOB to enhance cerebral blood flow.

2. Maintain a dry, occlusive dressing at the incision site. Keep firm pressure over the dressing if bleeding occurs.

3. Administer analgesics as ordered and evaluate the effectiveness of medication.

4. Administer vasopressors and/or antihypertensive agents as necessary to maintain BP within set parameters.

5. Turn and position the patient to prevent airway obstruction and aspiration. Provide incentive spirometry and C & DB the patient. Keep the patient NPO until the gag and swallow reflexes return to normal.

Critical observations

Consult with the physician for the following:

1. Symptoms reported by the patient that suggest TIAs
2. Hemiparesis/hemiplegia, pupillary irregularity, aphasia
3. Difficulty in breathing
4. Excessive bleeding at incision site
5. Dysrhythmias, hypotension, or hypertension

CRANIOTOMY

Clinical Brief

A craniotomy provides a "bone window" through which to evacuate hematomas, clip or ligate aneurysms or feeding vessels of an AVM, resect tumors, and biopsy the brain. Craniotomies are also used in the surgical treatment of epilepsy (i.e., intraoperative electroencephalography and resection of the cortex areas responsible for seizure activity). Pituitary tumors may be approached either transcranially through a craniotomy (especially when the tumor has a large suprasellar component) or by the transnasal transsphenoidal route.

Possible complications depend on the reason the surgery was performed, the location of the pathological condition, and underlying medical conditions.

NEURO

▶ Complications and related nursing diagnoses

Cerebral hemorrhage, edema, ischemia	Altered tissue perfusion: cerebral
	Decreased adaptive capacity: intracranial
CNS infection	Risk for infection
CSF leak	Risk for infection
Diabetes insipidus (DI)	Fluid volume deficit
Hydrocephalus	Decreased adaptive capacity: intracranial
Syndrome of inappropriate ADH (SIADH)	Fluid volume excess

Patient Care Management Guidelines

Patient assessment

1. Assess pupil size, reactivity, and visual fields, LOC, quality and comprehension of speech, and sensorimotor function. Test gag, swallow, and corneal reflexes.
2. Observe for signs and symptoms of meningitis: lethargy, severe headache, photophobia, nuchal rigidity, positive Kernig's sign.
3. Assess trends in ICP; initial readings may be required q15 to 30 min. Calculate and record cerebral perfusion pressure (CPP) readings (normal is 60 to 100 mm Hg) q1h. Note effects of patient and nursing activities on CPP and plan care accordingly. See p. 511 for information on ICP monitoring.

4. Obtain BP and MAP; CPP depends on adequate BP. Obtain CVP and PA pressures (if available) to determine imbalances in volume status that can adversely affect cerebral perfusion pressure.

5. Measure I & O hourly and determine fluid balance q8h. Measure specific gravity at least q8h and review serum electrolyte levels. If urine output <30 ml/hr or >200 ml/hr for two consecutive hours, suspect SIADH or DI.

6. Assess for CSF leaks. For transsphenoidal and transoral surgical approaches, question the patient about a feeling of a postnasal drip down the back of the throat. Apply moustache dressing to check for CSF leaks from either nostril (transsphenoidal approach). Assess patient's posterior pharynx for any signs of CSF leak (transoral approach).

7. Assess respiratory function. Monitor airway patency, oxygen saturation via pulse oximeter, and the patient's ability to handle secretions (i.e., gag/swallow reflex). Note rate, depth, and pattern of respirations and assess the lungs for adventitious sounds.

8. Examine the surgical dressing for bloody drainage or possible CSF drainage (CSF drainage will test positive for glucose).

Patient management

1. Administer analgesics as ordered and evaluate the effectiveness of medication. Maintain a quiet environment and provide uninterrupted rest periods.

2. Administer oxygen as ordered and monitor ABGs; hypoxia and hypercarbia are disturbances that can cause an increase in ICP. Promote pulmonary hygiene to prevent atelectasis and pneumonia.

3. Fluid management depends on the type of surgery and potential complications. Generally hypotonic solutions are avoided, since they may cause an increase in ICP.

4. Keep HOB at 30 to 45 degrees or as ordered to promote cerebral venous drainage. Maintain the patient's head and neck in proper alignment; teach the patient to avoid the Valsalva maneuver; hyperoxygenate the patient's lungs before and after suctioning secretions, and limit suctioning to 15 seconds.

5. Pharmacological agents such as chlorpromazine may be needed to reduce shivering; paralytics may be needed to prevent posturing; and anticonvulsants may be needed to control seizures.

6. Vasoactive agents may be required to control BP since CPP depends on an adequate BP. For hypotension, a dopamine or phenylephrine infusion may be titrated to the desired BP. For hypertension, labetalol or hydralazine HCl may be ordered.

7. If a ventriculostomy is being used, drain CSF according to established parameters (generally to maintain ICP <20 mm Hg). Keep the CSF drainage system at the level ordered to prevent inadvertent collapse of the ventricles.

8. If a shunt was placed, avoid pressure on the shunt mechanism; keep head in neutral alignment to prevent kinking or twisting of shunt catheter.

9. H_2 blocking agents may be ordered to decrease gastric acid secretion. If an NG tube is in place, sucralfate may be ordered to reduce the risk of ulcer formation.

10. Nutritional needs may be met when the patient is alert and awake. If the patient is comatose or unable to take food/fluids orally, a feeding tube may be required or parenteral nutrition may be indicated.

11. Patients who have undergone transsphenoidal surgery may develop episodes of diabetes insipidus (DI) in the first 72 hours. Maintenance IVs plus replacement fluid and/or administration of aqueous pitressin may be ordered. Carefully measure urine output hourly; specific gravity measurements may be required q2h.

12. Patients who have developed subarachnoid hemorrhage from a ruptured aneurysm preoperatively are continued on calcium channel blocking agents postoperatively. If the patient develops neurological deficits, secondary to vasospasm, hypervolemic hemodilution therapy may be initiated. To increase intravascular volume and decrease hematocrit levels, crystalloid infusions may be used to maintain a PA diastolic pressure at 14 to 16 mm Hg or CVP at 10 to 12 mm Hg. Hypertensive therapy (e.g., dopamine, phenylephrine) may be employed to raise SBP 25% to 40% in an effort to enhance cerebral blood flow during vasospasm.

13. See pp. 237 and 260 for information on SIADH and DI.

Critical observations

Consult with the physician for the following:

1. Change in LOC, pupillary inequality, hemiparesis or hemiplegia, visual changes, onset or worsening of aphasia, or any deterioration in neurological functioning
2. A loss of the gag or swallow reflexes
3. ICP >15 mm Hg and unresponsive to ordered therapy
4. Suspected CSF leak
5. Urine output >200 ml/hr for 2 hours (without diuretic) or urine output <30 ml/hr
6. Hypernatremia or hyponatremia
7. Sudden bloody drainage from ventriculostomy
8. Signs of meningitis: altered mental status, nuchal rigidity, Brudzinski's sign, Kernig's sign

HYPERVENTILATION THERAPY

Clinical Brief

Cerebral edema resulting from head injury, brain tumors, or cerebrovascular accidents raises ICP. The use of chronic hyperventilation therapy to lower $PaCO_2$ has been shown to be a useful adjunct in the treatment of increased ICP. The patient is chemically sedated, paralyzed, and placed on a mechanical ventilator to maintain a $PaCO_2$ of 28 to 30 mm Hg by controlling the rate of respirations.

Hypercarbia produces cerebral vasodilation and consequently increases intracranial pressure. Hypocarbia, induced by hyperventilation, produces vasoconstriction of the cerebral capillaries, which restricts venous blood pooling and decreases ICP. In the initial phase (24 to 36 hours) of therapy, ICP may be reduced as much as 25% to 30% with up to a 10 mm Hg drop in $PaCO_2$.

The use of acute hyperventilation (manually ventilating the patient at a rapid rate to "blow off" CO_2) is rare. Manually ventilating a patient too rapidly can cause increased intrathoracic pressure, which can decrease venous return. This results in a decreased cardiac output and cerebral perfusion.

▶ **Complications and related nursing diagnoses**

Respiratory alkalosis	Impaired tissue perfusion: systemic
Hypotension	Decreased cardiac output

Patient Care Management Guidelines
Patient assessment
1. Obtain ICP readings to assess the patient's response to hyperventilation therapy. Calculate CPP (normal is 60 to 100 mm Hg). The inability to reduce ICP with hyperventilation is a poor prognostic indicator. See p. 511 for information on ICP monitoring.
2. Monitor $PETCO_2$ with capnometry to evaluate the patient's response to hyperventilation therapy. Generally $PaCO_2$ levels are maintained at 28 to 30 mm Hg. If $PaCO_2$ drops below 20 mm Hg, cerebral hypoxia can occur as a result of severe vasoconstriction.
3. Review ABGs to assess oxygenation and acid-base balance. Respiratory alkalosis can occur as a result of hyperventilation therapy. Hypoxemia (PaO_2 <50 mm Hg) can lead to cerebral vasodilation.
4. Monitor body temperature. Hypothermia can shift the oxyhemoglobin dissociation curve to the left. This causes hemoglobin and oxygen to be more tightly bound and reduces oxygen availability to the tissues.
5. Continuously monitor blood pressure and MAP; monitor CVP and PA pressures (if available).
6. Monitor fluid volume status: measure intake and output hourly; determine fluid balance q8h.

Patient management
1. Sedatives and paralytics may be used to reduce ICP caused by agitation. Monitor LOC carefully.
2. Ensure airway patency; suction secretions only when necessary.
3. Inotropic or vasoactive agents may be ordered to maintain a MAP that results in a CPP of at least 60 mm Hg.

Critical observations
Consult with the physician for the following:
1. ICP unresponsive to maximum hyperventilation
2. CPP <60 mm Hg
3. O_2 sat <95%
4. Systolic blood pressure <90 mm Hg
5. pH consistently >7.45

Pulmonary Modalities

CHEST DRAINAGE

Clinical Brief

Chest tubes (CT) drain blood, fluid, or air that has accumulated in the thorax to restore negative intrapleural pressure. Intermittent drainage can be accomplished via thoracentesis. A pleural CT is inserted for a pneumothorax, hemothorax, hemopneumothorax, empyema, or pleural effusion. In post-op cardiothoracic surgeries, mediastinal tubes may be placed to prevent the accumulation of fluid around the heart, which could lead to cardiac tamponade.

A chest tube drainage system must have two components—a collection container and a water seal. The water seal prevents air from entering the chest on inspiration. A three-bottle system contains a drainage bottle, a water seal bottle, and a third bottle that is attached to a suction and serves as a pressure regulator. Suction is used to increase air flow from the pleural space. Disposable systems are available in either the one-bottle or three-bottle systems (Figure 7-1).

A flutter (Heimlich) valve has been developed that may be used in place of a drainage system to prevent air from entering the chest on inspiration. This valve opens on expiration, allowing air to escape from the chest, and collapses on inspiration to prevent air from entering the thorax (Figure 7-2). The Heimlich valve is useful during patient transport and for increasing patient mobility.

▶ Complications and related nursing diagnoses

Pain	Pain related to chest tube
	Ineffective breathing pattern
Occluded chest tube	Impaired gas exchange
	Ineffective breathing pattern
Infection	Impaired skin integrity
	Hyperthermia

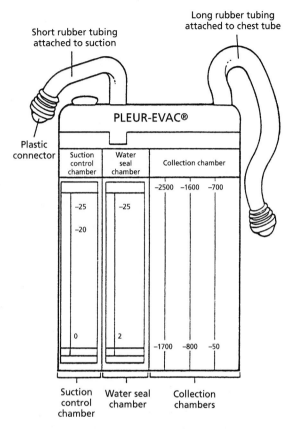

Figure 7-1 Disposable chest drainage system: Pleur-Evac. The **collection chamber** provides fluid collection. The **water seal chamber** provides the one-way valve that prevents air from being drawn into the thorax on inspiration. The **suction control chamber** controls the amount of negative pressure in the system. (From Thompson JM et al: *Mosby's clinical nursing,* ed 3, St Louis, 1993, Mosby.)

Patient Care Management Guidelines

Patient assessment

1. Assess respiratory status: note rate and rhythm and ease of respiration, auscultate breath sounds, and palpate for subcutaneous emphysema. An obstruction or kinked tube can

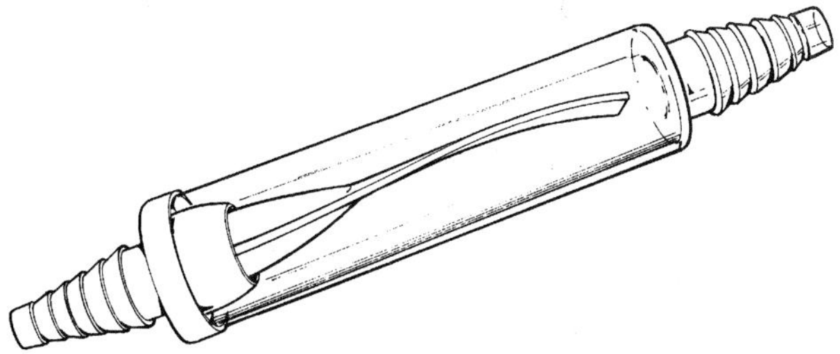

Figure 7-2   Heimlich valve.

cause a tension pneumothorax; a defect in the system can cause recurrence of hemothorax or pneumothorax.
2. Assess CT drainage on insertion and hourly thereafter until the patient's condition is stabilized. Document the type, color, and amount of drainage. A sudden change in the amount of drainage or a CT output of 200 ml/hr may indicate the need for surgical intervention. Sudden drainage cessation may indicate tube obstruction.

Patient management
1. Ensure that the water seal is at an appropriate level for the system being used and that all connections are tight. Ensure the patency of the tube. The water level should rise on inspiration and fall during expiration. The opposite occurs with mechanical ventilation. Monitor for the development of bubbling in the water seal chamber (see Figure 7-1), which indicates a leak either at a connection or the tracheobronchial tree. No bubbling or fluctuation should be observed in the water seal chamber when mediastinal CTs are used.
2. To assess for a tracheobronchial leak when the water seal chamber bubbles, clamp the CT close to the patient's chest; if the bubbling continues, the source is external. Caution must be taken, since a tension pneumothorax can quickly develop when bubbling CTs are clamped. *Do not* clamp CTs with known tracheobronchial leaks.
3. Verify that suction is at the prescribed amount; refill the suction water chamber as needed.
4. If the patient is being transported or if suction is not being used, leave the suction tubing open to air.

5. If the CT becomes disconnected from the drainage system, reconnect the tube—*do not* clamp the CT. If there is an air leak from the lung (e.g., bubbling in the water seal), more air will accumulate in the chest if the tube is clamped. A patient with a mediastinal tube may develop tamponade if the CT is clamped. Keep a 250 ml bottle of sterile saline available; if the chest drainage system breaks, submerge the CT 2 to 4 cm in sterile saline.

6. Stripping of CTs is a controversial issue because it creates large negative pressures in the thorax. Milking of chest tubes does not create pressures as high as does stripping, so it is more acceptable. Suction applied to the chest drainage system usually makes stripping or milking of chest tubes unnecessary. With large amounts of drainage or clots the physician may still prescribe stripping or milking to prevent an obstruction. A patient with a mediastinal tube may develop tamponade if the CT is obstructed.

7. Should the CT accidentally be pulled out, apply a dressing to the site to prevent air from entering the chest. If an occlusive dressing is used, monitor the patient for the development of a tension pneumothorax. If a three-sided dressing is used, air is allowed to escape on expiration.

Chest tube removal

CTs can be removed when drainage and air leaks have ceased. Trial clamping of the CT may be done before CT removal; closely monitor the patient for respiratory distress. Chest radiographs are reviewed to ensure that the lung is reexpanded. Necessary equipment includes a suture set, plain or petroleum gauze, 4 × 4s, and adhesive tape. The tube is removed quickly once the patient is asked to take a deep breath and hold it.

Critical observations

Consult with the physician for the following:

1. Respiratory rate >28/min
2. PaO_2 <60 mm Hg
3. Signs of hypoxia: restlessness, ↑ HR, dyspnea
4. CT drainage ≥200 ml/hr
5. New bubbling in underwater seal chamber not related to loose connections
6. Dislodged/obstructed CT
7. Deviated trachea
8. Unequal breath sounds

EXTRACORPOREAL MEMBRANE OXYGENATION (ECMO)

Clinical Brief

An extracorporeal circuit is used to remove blood from a patient with severe respiratory insufficiency that is unresponsive to conventional therapy, to infuse oxygen and extract carbon dioxide, and to return the blood to the patient. Generally a perfusionist is responsible for maintaining the ECMO circuit, although the critical care nurse may have this responsibility in some institutions.

▶ **Complications and related nursing diagnoses**

Thrombus formation	Altered tissue perfusion
Cannula malposition	Risk for injury: hemorrhage
	Impaired gas exchange
Sepsis	Decreased cardiac output
	Hyperthermia
Hemorrhage	Risk for injury: hemorrhage
	Decreased cardiac output
	Altered tissue perfusion
	Fluid volume deficit

PULM

Patient Care Management Guidelines

Patient assessment

1. Obtain PA pressures, BP, and CO/CI often if titrating pharmacological agents or if patient condition warrants. An increase in PA systolic pressure may be secondary to hypoxia.

2. Assess respiratory status: auscultate breath sounds at least q2h and note rate and rhythm; monitor oxygenation using pulse oximetry (SpO_2) and SvO_2 with fiber optics (if available). Review serial chest radiographs to assess improvement or worsening in condition.

3. Assess for hemorrhage: obtain vital signs q1h; an increased heart rate may be the first indication. Check cannula site as well as incisions and invasive line sites; observe for changes in LOC, onset of abdominal tenderness or distention; check for bloody sputum, hematuria, or coffee-ground nasogastric drainage. Guaiac-test NG aspirate, urine, and stool. Review serial Hct results for a decreasing trend.

4. Assess peripheral circulation q1h; note skin temperature and color, pulses, and capillary refill.

5. Measure and record hourly urinary output. Decreased urinary output may signify decreased renal perfusion secondary to decreased cardiac output.

6. Assess for signs and symptoms of infection: monitor temperature q4h; assess catheter site for redness, swelling, or drainage; and review serial WBC counts.

Patient management

1. Maintain the ECMO circuit as ordered with the assistance of a perfusionist.

2. Systemic anticoagulants are administered to prevent thrombus formation and are based on ACTs. Activated clotting times are usually maintained between 200 to 240 sec (normal <180 seconds). An initial heparin dose of 100 to 200 U/kg followed by a maintenance dose between 20 to 50 U/kg/hr may be required.

3. Administer fluids and vasoactive drugs as ordered to maintain MAP of at least 80 mm Hg. Carefully monitor the patient for fluid overload or CI <2.5 L/min/m².

4. Provide pulmonary hygiene with gentle suctioning, chest physiotherapy, and turning q2h.

5. Use strict aseptic technique with all procedures: change the cannula dressing daily using a povidone-iodine solution on the site.

6. Administer analgesics, sedatives, and paralytics as ordered.

7. Use pressure-reducing or pressure-relieving devices, since these patients are susceptible to pressure ulcers related to decreased tissue perfusion. Reposition the patient frequently and assist with passive range of motion exercises.

Critical observations

Consult with the physician for the following:

1. PaO_2 <60 mm Hg
2. SvO_2 <60% or >80%
3. SBP <90 mm Hg
4. CI <2.5 L/min/m²
5. Decreased LOC (independent of sedation)
6. Unilateral diminished breath sounds
7. Diminished/loss of pulses in extremity (in arterial cannulation)
8. Obvious bleeding: catheter site, invasive lines, sputum
9. Positive occult blood in NG drainage, urine, or stool
10. Urine output <20 ml/hr for 2 hours
11. Decreasing trend in Hct

12. T >38.5° C (101.3° F)
13. Redness, swelling, drainage at catheter site, invasive lines, or incision
14. ACT out of therapeutic range

LUNG TRANSPLANT
Clinical Brief
Single lung transplantation is performed for patients with end-stage restrictive or obstructive lung disease. Evaluation and criteria for lung transplantation differs among centers. Criteria usually include: end-stage disease with projected life expectancy less than 2 years or New York Heart Association Class III or IV. Contraindications include: age >50 for heart-lung and age >60 for single/bilateral lung, ventilator dependency, corticosteroid dependency, IDDM, active infection, malignancy, renal or hepatic failure, positive HIV, substance abuse, and psychological instability. Double lung transplants are recommended for patients with cystic fibrosis or septic pulmonary diseases since the native, diseased lung would contaminate the transplanted lung. Heart-lung transplantation is reserved for irreversible pulmonary or cardiac diseases associated with pulmonary hypertension. Single lung transplantation is performed through a lateral thoracotomy incision and utilizes single lung ventilation. The native lung is excised and the donor lung implanted with bronchial, left atrial, and pulmonary artery anastomoses. Double lung transplantation technique incorporates bilateral thoracotomy incisions with a transverse sternotomy. The donor lungs are implanted with single tracheal anastomosis since initial surgeries utilizing the block technique lead to airway problems. In the heart-lung transplant, the donor heart and lungs are implanted together en bloc through a median sternotomy incision utilizing cardiopulmonary bypass.

PULM

▶ Complications and related nursing diagnoses

Hemorrhage	Decreased cardiac output
	Altered tissue perfusion: cardiac, pulmonary, renal, cerebral
Organ rejection	Decreased cardiac output
	Altered tissue perfusion
	Impaired gas exchange
	Altered urinary elimination
	Activity intolerance
	Hyperthermia

Infection	Hyperthermia
Adverse effects of immunosuppressive therapy	Risk of infection
	Altered body image
	Altered urinary elimination
	Risk for injury: GI bleeding

See Thoracic surgery, p. 585, for other complications and nursing diagnoses.

Patient Care Management Guidelines

See Thoracic surgery, p. 585, for guidelines for the general thoracic surgery client.

Patient assessment

1. Continuously monitor SpO_2 and SvO_2 (if available); review serial ABGs and auscultate lungs q1 to 2h. Note any adventitious lung sounds and increased work of breathing. Assess cough and secretions. Be aware of the potential for pulmonary edema development. Monitor airway pressures and tidal volumes when mechanically ventilated. Increased airway pressures can cause barotrauma.

2. Assess tissue perfusion; note level of mentation, skin color and temperature, peripheral pulses, and capillary refill.

3. Continuously monitor ECG for dysrhythmias that may result from electrolyte imbalance, hypoxemia, and/or hemorrhage.

4. Monitor CVP, PA pressures, CO/CI, HR, BP, and MAP. Note trends and patient response to therapy. Monitor PVRI and SVRI and note trends and patient response to therapy. Calculate LVSWI and RVSWI to evaluate contractility in the heart-lung transplant.

5. Assess for bleeding: chest tube drainage >200 ml/hr; decrease in Hgb and Hct; abnormal coagulation studies.

6. Assess temperature. Patients may be hypothermic on returning from surgery. Monitor for signs of infection; consider IV sites, wound sites, the urinary tract, lungs, and mucous membranes as potential sites of infection.

7. Monitor pulmonary function tests to evaluate lung function.

8. Monitor sputum cultures, WBC count, and titers for presence of infection.

9. Monitor immunosuppressive serum levels for therapeutic range.

10. Monitor renal function: BUN and creatinine and urine output.

11. Assess patient for side effects of immunosuppression therapy: hypertension, hyperkalemia, gingival hyperplasia, leukopenia, hyperglycemia.

12. Assess neurological status. Potential side effects of cyclosporine include confusion, cortical blindness, seizures, encephalopathy, quadriplegia, and coma.

Patient management

1. Position patient with single lung transplant with operative side up to promote gravitational drainage and reduce postsurgical edema. Double lung transplant patients can be turned side-to-side and prone to mobilize secretions.

2. Because the patient is immunosuppressed, isolation protocols may be instituted. All dressing changes should be completed with strict aseptic technique. Intravenous access sites and dressings should be changed according to institutional protocol. Vigorous pulmonary toilet should be initiated and maintained at least q4h. Administer prophylactic antibiotics to prevent opportunistic infections.

3. Administer prophylactic IV cimetidine or ranitidine and oral antacids as ordered to prevent GI bleeding, which can result from corticosteroids. Test all stools and emesis for occult blood.

4. Cardiac function may be hampered postoperatively. Hemodynamic instability may be treated with vasoactive and inotropic agents. Titrate the infusion to achieve the desired hemodynamic response.

5. Determine level of comfort by using a visual analogue scale (see Figure 1-1) or other pain measuring tool. See Acute pain, p. 30.

6. See the information on mechanical ventilation below.

Critical observations

Consult with the physician for the following:

1. Signs and symptoms of impaired oxygenation
2. Signs and symptoms of rejection
3. Signs and symptoms of infection
4. Signs and symptoms of adverse effects of immunosuppression
5. Signs of acute renal failure

MECHANICAL VENTILATION

Clinical Brief

Various methods of mechanical ventilation can be used to improve alveolar ventilation, arterial oxygenation, lung volumes, and to prevent/treat atelectasis or reduce the work of

PULM

breathing in the critically ill patient who cannot effectively meet the body's metabolic needs. In addition, mechanical ventilation can decrease oxygen consumption, decrease intracranial pressure, and stabilize the chest wall. A variety of positive and negative pressure ventilators are available.

Negative pressure ventilators apply external subatmospheric pressure to the thorax, decreasing intrathoracic pressure and allowing air to enter the lungs. Examples include the iron lung, chest cuirass, and poncho wrap.

Positive pressure ventilators include time-cycled, pressure-cycled, or volume-cycled models; all of these apply positive pressure to the airways, causing air to enter the lungs.

The type of positive pressure ventilator is classified according to the physical parameter responsible for terminating inspiratory flow.

Time-cycled: Inspiratory flow ceases at a preset time regardless of the tidal volume delivered.

Pressured-cycled: Inspiratory flow is delivered until a preset airway pressure is reached.

Volume-cycled: Inspiratory flow is delivered until a preset tidal volume is reached, unless peak pressures are exceeded; then the delivery of tidal volume is terminated to prevent possible barotrauma.

Ventilator settings: positive pressure ventilation

FIO_2: The FIO_2 is adjusted to maintain a PaO_2 of at least 60 mm Hg and an SaO_2 ≥90%.

PEEP: When patients require FIO_2 >0.60 to maintain an adequate PaO_2. PEEP can be added to decrease the FIO_2. It is desirable to decrease the FIO_2 to nontoxic levels (0.40) to prevent oxygen toxicity.

Tidal volume: Tidal volume is calculated to be 8 to 10 ml/kg.

Rate: The rate is adjusted to maintain the patient's normal $PaCO_2$. Initially, rates may be set at 10 to 15/min.

Inspiratory flow: The speed of air flow is usually set at 40 to 60 L.

Sigh: Sigh ventilations, if used, are set at 1.5 to 2 times the tidal volume. If PEEP or large tidal volumes are being used, sigh ventilations are unnecessary. Sigh is also undesirable in a patient with COPD or any patient with poor compliance because of the increased risk of barotrauma.

High-frequency ventilation is a special positive pressure ventilation used in some patient conditions. The various modes of high-frequency ventilation are listed in Table 7-5. Other modes of mechanical ventilation are discussed in Table 7-6.

Independent lung ventilation (ILV) is a technique that allows each lung to be ventilated separately. It is used predominantly in patients with unilateral lung disease. ILV requires intubation with a double lumen tube (Carlens, White, Bryce-Smith, Robertshaw, Broncho-cath) and one or two ventilators. The special endobronchial tube is generally placed in the mainstem bronchus of the affected lung. The unaffected lung is ventilated through a side port located on the opposite side of the tube.

Indications

Suggested parameters for ventilatory support are listed in the box below. In patients with acute respiratory failure, mechanical

TABLE 7-5   Modes of High-Frequency Ventilation

Type	Description
HF positive pressure ventilation (HFPPV)	Extremely short inspiratory times with V_T equivalent to deadspace at a rate of 60-100 cycles/min
HF jet ventilation (HFJV)	Small volumes, ≤ anatomical deadspace, are pulsed through a jet injector catheter at rates of 100-600 cycles/min
HF oscillation (HFO)	Small volume of gas is continually vibrated in the airways at rates up to 4000 cycles/min

Guidelines for Ventilatory Support

RR	>35/min
Pao_2 (mm Hg)	<70 (on supplemental oxygen)
$Paco_2$ (mm Hg)	>55 (except chronic lung disease)
Vital capacity	<15 ml/kg body weight
FEV_1	<10 ml/kg body weight
Negative inspiratory force	<−25 cm H_2O
Compliance	<25 ml/cm H_2O
V_D/V_T	>0.6
Qs/Qt	>20%
$P(a-A)o_2$	>450 torr

TABLE 7-6 Modes of Ventilatory Support

Type	Description
Assist-controlled mode ventilation (ACV)	Patient triggers a breath and the ventilator delivers a preset volume; the control model takes over at a preset backup rate if patient becomes apneic
Bilevel CPAP (BiPAP)	Positive pressure applied during spontaneous breathing that allows the inspiratory positive airway pressure (IPIP) and expiratory positive airway pressure (EPEP) to be independently adjusted
Continuous positive airway pressure (CPAP)	Positive pressure applied during spontaneous breathing and maintained throughout the entire respiratory cycle; decreases intrapulmonary shunting
Controlled mandatory ventilation (CMV)	Ventilator delivers a preset tidal volume at a fixed rate regardless of the patient's efforts to breathe
Intermittent mandatory ventilation (IMV)	Patient may be able to breathe spontaneously but receives intermittent ventilator breaths at a preset rate and tidal volume; tidal volume stacking can occur
Inverse-ratio ventilation	Provides inspiratory time greater than expiratory time, thereby improving distribution of ventilation and preventing collapse of stiffer alveolar units
Positive end-expiratory pressure (PEEP)	Positive pressure applied during machine breathing and maintained at end-expiration; decreases intrapulmonary shunting
Pressure support ventilation (PSV)	Clinician-selected amount of positive pressure applied to airway during patient's spontaneous inspiratory efforts; PSV decreases work of breathing caused by demand flow valve, IMV circuit, and narrow inner diameter of ETT
Synchronized IMV (SIMV)	Intermittent ventilator breaths synchronized to spontaneous breaths to reduce competition between ventilator and patient

ventilation is required continuously. Nocturnal positive pressure ventilation may be indicated in patients with chronic disorders. The ventilator decreases the work of breathing and provides some rest for the respiratory system in patients with COPD or neuromuscular weakness. In patients with sleep apnea, nocturnal ventilation prevents apneic periods. A face mask or nasal mask can be used for nocturnal positive pressure ventilation.

▶ Complications and related nursing diagnoses

Tracheal tube obstruction	Impaired gas exchange
• Mucous plug	
• Kinked tube	
• Cuff herniation	
Decreased venous return	Decreased cardiac output
Pulmonary barotrauma	Ineffective breathing pattern
	Impaired gas exchange
Auto-PEEP	Decreased cardiac output
	Ineffective breathing pattern
Infection	Ineffective airway clearance
	Hyperthermia
Fluid/electrolyte imbalance	Fluid volume excess
	Impaired gas exchange
GI bleeding	Risk for injury: stress ulcer
Oxygen toxicity	Impaired gas exchange
Increased ICP	Altered tissue perfusion: cerebral

Patient Care Management Guidelines
Patient assessment

1. Assess placement of the endotracheal tube (ETT): auscultation of breath sounds should be done when intubation has been completed, a minimum of every shift, and with respiratory distress. Auscultate breath sounds bilaterally to assess presence and equality. NOTE: Gurgling heard over the epigastric region on auscultation may indicate esophageal intubation. Unilateral breath sounds may indicate that the endotracheal tube may be inserted too far into a mainstem bronchus (usually the right mainstem). If the patient coughs repeatedly, one should suspect that the endotracheal tube is placed against the carina. A chest radiograph should be obtained and reviewed to confirm proper placement of the ETT. (See Figure 5-4.) Once placement is confirmed, document tube placement by

using the endotracheal tube markings. EXAMPLES: 25 cm at the lips or 23 cm at the nares. Reconfirm placement each shift and review serial chest radiographs for definitive confirmation.

2. Assess oxygenation status: auscultate breath sounds and also note rate and depth of respirations. Monitor for signs that may indicate hypoxemia: a change in LOC, tachypnea, tachycardia, or dysrhythmias. Cyanosis is a late sign. NOTE: Breath and heart sounds will be difficult to assess because of the small tidal volumes being delivered and the sound generated by the jet ventilator.

Patient management

1. Check ventilator settings. A patient's discomfort (e.g., cough or air hunger) may be related to the inspiratory gas flow rate. Verify the I:E ratio. An increase in peak inspiratory pressure and increased plateau pressure suggests a change in lung compliance. An increase in peak pressure without a change in plateau pressure suggests an increase in airway resistance (e.g., bronchospasm, secretion, kinking of ETT).

2. Continuously monitor oxygen saturation with pulse oximetry (SpO_2). Monitor ventilation with capnography (if available). The $PETCO_2$ is 1 to 4 mm Hg lower than $PaCO_2$. $P(a/A)O_2$ ratio can also be used to monitor oxygenation.

3. Monitor airway cuff pressure to prevent an alteration in tissue integrity resulting from high pressure. Endotracheal tubes have a pilot balloon and port to measure the pressure. A cuff manometer is used to determine that the pressure of the cuff is less than the tracheal capillary pressure; cuff pressure should not exceed 20 mm Hg. A cuff pressure <15 mm Hg increases the risk of aspiration, although a properly inflated cuff does not prevent aspiration.

4. Prevent pressure ulcers to the lip or tongue by rotating tube placement daily. Caution should be taken so that the tube is not displaced or the patient is inadvertently extubated.

5. Talk with and reassure the patient, or if necessary, sedate the patient when anxious and "fighting" the ventilator. Provide the patient with a communication board to make needs known.

6. Ensure that the ventilator alarms are on and functional. Table 7-7 lists possible causes for ventilator alarming. Manually ventilate the patient's lungs with 100% oxygen if the cause of ventilator malfunction cannot be quickly identified or corrected.

7. Review ABGs at the beginning of the shift and periodically during the shift to ensure that the ventilator settings are appropriate and the patient's lungs are being properly ventilated. Allow 30 min after ventilator changes before drawing ABGs to ensure equilibration between alveolar ventilation and arterial blood.

Arterial oxygenation is based on the individual, however. Generally $Sao_2 \geq 90\%$ is clinically acceptable using an Fio_2 that is also acceptable. Patients with chronic respiratory acidosis should have alveolar ventilation titrated to pH not $Paco_2$.

Permissive hypercapnea may be employed as a strategy to limit the distending forces on the lungs, therefore avoiding lung injury.

8. Assess fluid balance q8h; note the condition of skin and mucous membranes; and compare serial weights. Ventilated patients are at risk for fluid volume excess due to increased secretion of ADH, which may reduce urine production.

9. If PEEP or CPAP is being used, do not remove the patient from the ventilator to obtain hemodynamic

TABLE 7-7   Summary of Ventilator Alarms

Alarm	Possible causes
High pressure	Secretion buildup, kinked airway tubing, bronchospasm, coughing, fighting the ventilator, decreased lung compliance
Low exhaled volume	Disconnection from ventilator, loose ventilator fittings, leaking airway cuff
Low inspiratory pressure	Disconnection from the ventilator, loose connections, low ventilating pressure
High respiratory rate	Anxiety, pain, hypoxia, fever
Apnea alarm	No spontaneous breath within preset time interval

PULM

pressure readings; patients may desaturate rapidly when the ventilator is disconnected.

10. Suctioning can lead to airway trauma and infection. To decrease the likelihood of complications, sterile technique is used and suctioning is performed only when rhonchi are auscultated. Ensure that the suction device is not set higher than 120 mm Hg and is applied only when the catheter is being withdrawn. Patients requiring high-frequency jet ventilation will have increased amounts of tracheobronchial and oral secretions. Monitor for possible aspiration and airway plugging. Two nurses will be needed to suction the secretions of patients requiring high-frequency jet ventilation.

11. Administer H_2 antagonists, antacids, or cytoprotective agent as ordered to raise gastric pH.

WEANING AND EXTUBATION

The box below lists weaning criteria. There are no criteria that guarantee a successful weaning, since many factors can affect the outcome. The patient's psychological state is important, as well as the circumstances surrounding the respiratory problem (e.g., a longstanding problem versus respiratory failure that has resolved quickly). In addition, malnutrition can adversely affect the diaphragm and other muscles of respiration, making weaning more difficult. Other conditions that have been implicated in failure to wean include bronchospasm, cardiovascular dysfunction, excessive secretions, small diameter ETT, hypophosphatemia, hypomagnesemia, and hypothyroidism.

POSTEXTUBATION

Close observation of the patient is essential. Observe for signs of respiratory distress and increased patient effort: diaphoresis, restlessness, respiratory rate >30/min or <8/min, or increase

---

Weaning Criteria

Vital capacity >10-15 ml/kg body weight
Spontaneous tidal volume 2-5 ml/kg
Resting minute ventilation <10 L/min and ability to double during MVV maneuver
Negative (maximal) inspiratory pressure >−20 cm H_2O
Adequate Pao_2 for the patient
RR <25/min
$Paco_2$ 35-45 mm Hg
$P(a/A)o_2$ ratio >0.25

of 10 respirations from starting respiratory rate; increase or decrease in HR by 20 beats/min or <60 beats/min; increase or decrease in BP by 20 mm Hg; PAWP >20 mm Hg; nasal flaring, recession of suprasternal and intercostal spaces, paradoxical motion of rib cage and abdomen; tidal volume <250 to 300 ml; minute ventilation increase of 5 L/min; SaO_2 ≤90%, PaO_2 <60 mm Hg, increase in $PaCO_2$ with a fall in pH <7.35.

Critical observations

Consult with the physician for the following:

1. Unequal or absent breath sounds
2. Respiratory distress/increased patient effort
3. SaO_2 ≤90%, PaO_2 <60 mm Hg, $PaCO_2$ >45 mm Hg with pH <7.35
4. Excessive coughing
5. Persistent cuff leak
6. High peak airway pressures
7. SBP <90 mm Hg
8. Fluid imbalance
9. GI bleeding

THORACIC SURGERY

Clinical Brief

Various procedures are performed to repair or explore abnormalities of the thorax. Indications include congenital or acquired deformities, traumatic injuries, lesions, and drainage of infectious processes (Table 7-8). Traditionally, the open incisional approach has been utilized for these procedures. However, biopsies and procedures such as pleurodesis, thoracic sympathectomy, empyema evacuation, and wedge resection can be performed via a closed approach (e.g., thoracoscopy).

The patient's medical condition and the size of lesion, as well as the surgeon's expertise, will determine if the open or closed approach is used.

▶ **Complications and related nursing diagnoses**

Pain	Pain related to incision, chest tube Ineffective breathing pattern
Hemorrhage	Fluid volume deficit Altered tissue perfusion
Dysrhythmias	Decreased cardiac output
Hypoxia	Impaired gas exchange Altered tissue perfusion
Infection	Risk for infection Hyperthermia

PULM

TABLE 7-8 Thoracic Procedures

Thoracic procedure	Definition	Indications
Segmental resection	Removal of segment of pulmonary lobe	Chronic, localized pyogenic lung abscess Congenital cyst or bleb Benign tumor Segment infected with pulmonary tuberculosis or bronchiectasis
Wedge resection	Excision of small peripheral section of lobe	Small masses that are close to pleural surface of lung (e.g., subpleural granulomas, small peripheral tumors [benign primary tumors])
Lobectomy	Excision of one or more lobes of lung tissue	Cancer Infections such as tuberculosis Miscellaneous benign tumors
Pneumonectomy	Removal of entire lung	Malignant neoplasms Lung almost entirely infected Extensive chronic abscess Selected unilateral lesions
Decortication of lung	Removal of fibrinous, reactive membrane covering visceral and parietal pleura	Restrictive fibrinous membrane lining visceral and parietal pleura that limits ventilatory excursion; "trapped lung"
Thoracoplasty	Surgical collapse of portion of chest wall by multiple rib resections to intentionally decrease volume in hemithorax	Closure of chronic cavitary lesions, empyema spaces, recurrent air leaks Reduction of open thoracic "dead space" after large resection

Thymectomy	Removal of thymus gland	Primary thymic neoplasm, myasthenia
Correction of pectus excavatum ("funnel chest")	Depression of sternum and costal cartilage corrected by moving sternum outward and realigning cartilage-sternal junction	Cosmesis and relief of cardiopulmonary compromise
Repair of penetrating thoracic wounds, drainage of hemothorax	Drainage of pleural cavity and control of hemorrhage	Hemorrhage produced by injury to thoracic vessels that causes blood loss as well as compression of lung tissue and mediastinum, resulting in cardiopulmonary compromise
Excision of mediastinal masses	Removal of masses/cysts in upper anterior/posterior mediastinum	Mediastinal tumors (benign or malignant), cysts, abscesses
Tracheal resection	Resection of portion of trachea, followed by primary end-to-end reanastomosis of trachea	Significant stenosis of tracheal orifice, usually related to mechanical pressure of cuffed tracheal tube; pressure produces tracheal wall ischemia, inflammation, and ulceration, leading to formation of granulation tissue and fibrosis, which narrow tracheal orifice; tumors
Esophagogastrectomy	Resection of part of esophagus and at least cardial portion of stomach with primary anastomosis of proximal esophagus to remaining stomach	Carcinoma of esophagus anywhere from neck to esophagogastric junction Severe reflux esophagitis producing hemorrhage Extensive alkali burns of esophagus

Continued.

PULM

From Johanson BC et al: *Standards for critical care*, St Louis, 1988, Mosby.

TABLE 7-8 Thoracic Procedures—cont'd

Thoracic procedure	Definition	Indications
Bullectomy	Removal by excision of cysts or pockets in lung, which result from confluence of many alveoli	Failure of medical therapy such as antibiotics and chest physiotherapy to control infection associated with such cysts or pockets Severe compression of tissue adjacent to pulmonary cysts or pockets
Closed thoracostomy	Insertion of chest tube through intercostal space into pleural space; chest tube is attached to water seal system, with or without suction	Provision of continuous aspiration of fluid from pleural cavity Prevention of accumulation of air in chest from leaks in lung or tracheobronchial tree
Open thoracostomy	Partial resection of selected rib or ribs, with insertion of chest tube into infected material to provide for continuous drainage	Drainage of empyemas when pleural space is fixed

Patient Care Management Guidelines
Patient assessment
1. Obtain BP and HR q15min until stable, hourly for the first 4 hours, then q2h. Hospital protocols may vary. Assess capillary refill (normal <3 sec) and quality of peripheral pulses. Calculate MAP; a MAP <60 mm Hg adversely affects cerebral and renal perfusion.
2. Assess oxygenation status: continuously monitor SpO_2. Review serial ABGs to evaluate oxygenation and acid-base status. Monitor PA systolic pressure (if available), since hypoxia can increase sympathetic tone and increase pulmonary vasoconstriction. During the weaning process assess the patient for respiratory distress and increased patient effort. (See Weaning, p. 584.)
3. Monitor fluid volume status: record chest drainage, urinary output, and fluid intake hourly; determine fluid balance q8h. PA pressures and CVP reflect the capacity of the vascular system to accept volume and can be used to monitor for fluid overload and pulmonary edema. PAWP <4 mm Hg, CVP <2 mm Hg, and tachycardia suggest fluid volume deficit. Crackles, S_3, PAWP >20 mm Hg, and CVP >10 mm Hg suggest fluid overload.
4. Continuously monitor ECG to detect dysrhythmias. Hypoxia, acidosis, and electrolyte imbalance are risk factors.
5. Check dressing q1h for bleeding.

Patient management
1. Administer crystalloids or blood products as ordered to replace volume from blood loss.
2. Potassium 10 to 15 mEq/hr may be required to replace depleted levels from blood loss.
3. Reinforce the dressing as needed.
4. Record chest tube drainage q1h. Note the patency of tubes. Milking or stripping of chest tubes may be necessary to maintain patency. (See Chest drainage, p. 569.)
5. Elevate the HOB with the operative side up to facilitate lung expansion. Pneumonectomy patients should be positioned with the "good side" up, since drainage contamination from leaking suture lines or a tension pneumothorax may occur when the operative side is up.
6. Administer analgesics as ordered. Thoracic surgery can cause severe pain, which can result in hypoventilation.

PULM

Encourage incentive spirometry and C & DB the patient. Provide chest physiotherapy and postural drainage to mobilize secretions.

7. If the patient is intubated and mechanically ventilated, see p. 577.

Critical observations

Consult with the physician for the following:

1. Tracheal deviation
2. Dysrhythmias
3. SBP <90 mm Hg
4. CT drainage ≥200 ml/hr
5. Urine output ≤20 ml/hr for 2 hours
6. O_2 sat <90%
7. PaO_2 <60 mm Hg
8. SvO_2 <60% or >80%
9. Potassium <3.5 mEq/L
10. Decreasing trend in Hgb and Hct
11. Development of air leak: bubbling in water seal chamber or subcutaneous emphysema
12. Possible pneumothorax: restlessness, SOB, increased respiratory rate, decreased compliance

Cardiovascular Modalities

CARDIAC SURGERY
Clinical Brief

Generally the purpose of cardiac surgery is to optimize cardiac function. Cardiac surgery is employed when medical management and less invasive interventions fail or no longer control symptoms. For all of the cardiac surgeries detailed in this section, general anesthesia and a sternotomy (vertical midsternal incision) approach is used. The anterior surface of the heart is accessed and the patient is placed on cardiopulmonary bypass (CPB) via cannulation of the aortic root and vena cava or right atrium. Proximal to the cannulation, the aortic root is clamped in order to ensure a bloodless environment. A cold, potassium-rich solution is infused into the coronary arteries to stop the heart and provide a quiet field plus dramatically reduce myocardial oxygen demand. Once the surgical procedure is complete, the aorta is unclamped, the heart is warmed, and the patient is weaned from the CPB machine. Epicardial wires may be placed for pacing, and chest tubes are inserted to drain the mediastinum and/or pleural space(s).

The purpose, indications, and description of the various cardiac surgeries are detailed in the box on pp. 592-593. Contraindications for cardiac surgery include inability to tolerate general anesthesia and terminal illness.

▶ **Complications and related nursing diagnoses**
(Common following cardiac surgery)

Perioperative myocardial infarction	Decreased cardiac output
Excess bleeding	Decreased cardiac output Altered tissue perfusion Fluid volume deficit
Cardiac tamponade	Decreased cardiac output Altered tissue perfusion
Increased afterload/ hypertension	Risk for injury Pain
Decreased preload/ hypovolemia	Decreased cardiac output Fluid volume deficit

Dysrhythmias	Decreased cardiac output: brady-cardia/SVT/VT/asystole/atrial fibrillation
Fluid and electrolyte imbalance	Fluid volume excess Fluid volume deficit
Acid/base imbalance	Impaired gas exchange Altered tissue perfusion
Renal failure	Altered tissue perfusion Fluid volume excess
Respiratory failure	Impaired gas exchange
Cerebral vascular accident	Altered tissue perfusion: cerebral

Cardiovascular Surgeries

- *Type:* Coronary Artery Bypass Graft Surgery (CABG)
  Purpose: To restore adequate blood flow to the myocardium distal to the coronary artery stenosis
  Indications: Myocardial ischemia refractory to medical management. Lesions must be discrete and not amenable to PTCA (e.g., triple vessel disease, diffuse disease, proximal lesions with a large amount of myocardium at risk).
  Description: Saphenous vein grafts (SVGs) are harvested from the lower extremities, and/or the internal mammary artery (IMA) is stripped down from the anterior chest wall. The SVGs are anastomosed to the aortic root at one end and the other end of the graft is anastomosed to the coronary artery distal to the stenosis. If the IMA is used, the distal end is anastomosed to the coronary artery distal to the stenosis. Another graft option is the gastric artery.
- *Type:* Valvular Repair/Replacement (VR)
  Purpose: To restore normal or near-normal function to a valve that is stenotic and/or incompetent
  Indications: Critical tricuspid, pulmonic, mitral, or aortic stenosis and/or incompetence. The patient must also be a candidate for major surgery.
  Description: Access is gained by an atrial incision or aortic/pulmonic artery root incision. During valvuloplasty the fused commissures may be split via incision. Leaflets may be sewn to repair tears or stretching. During VR the dysfunctional valve is removed and replaced with a mechanical or bioprosthetic (tissue) valve.

Cardiovascular Surgeries—cont'd

- *Type:* Atrial/Ventricular Septal Defect Repair
  Purpose: To repair left to right shunts that are a result of congenital defects or septal perforation related to acute myocardial infarction
  Indications: Congenital septal defects or acute septal perforation related to myocardial infarction. Surgical repair is reserved for hemodynamic instability secondary to the defect.
  Description: An incision is made in the atrium or ventricle. The defect is patched with a synthetic graft; the incision is closed.
- *Type:* Ventricular Aneurysm Repair
  Purpose: To remove scar tissue that has formed as a result of myocardial infarction and to improve pump function
  Indications: Ventricular aneurysm. Surgical repair is performed when the aneurysm is large enough to put the patient at high risk for ventricular rupture or there is evidence of significant thrombus formation.
  Description: The aneurysm is excised and the healthy muscle is brought back together and sutured.
- *Type:* Myotomy/Myomectomy
  Purpose: To restore an adequate left ventricular outflow tract
  Indications: Symptomatic obstructive hypertrophic cardiomyopathy
  Description: Access to the left ventricle is gained via the aortic valve orifice or a ventricular incision. Excess myocardium is shaved from the surface to create an adequate outflow tract. The aortic or mitral valve may be replaced as necessary.
- *Type:* Maze Procedure
  Purpose: To improve cardiac hemodynamics and decrease risk of thromboembolism by restoring sinus or AV synchronized rhythm
  Indication: Atrial fibrillation in a patient with intact SA node function who cannot or will not take antidysrhythmic medication
  Description: Multiple atrial incisions are used to interrupt reentry circuits that allow perpetuation of atrial fibrillation.
- *Type:* Cardiomyoplasty
  Purpose: To improve ventricular function as a bridge to transplantation and/or long-term alternative to transplantation
  Indication: Refractory end-stage heart failure
  Description: Skeletal muscle is wrapped around the heart and electrically stimulated to contract in synchrony with cardiac systole.

CV

Patient Care Management Guidelines

Patient assessment

1. A thorough assessment should be completed on the patient on arrival in the recovery area. The patient should be assessed frequently because of the instability often present in the early postoperative period.
2. The cardiovascular system should be assessed q15min until stable and then per unit protocol, and include VS, CVP, PA pressures, cardiac rhythm, incision/dressing appearance, hourly chest tube drainage, quality of peripheral pulses, and hourly urinary output. Heart sounds should be assessed for changes in quality and intensity of murmurs (VR and VSD/ASD repairs) and muffled tones.
3. A cardiac profile including CO, CI, and SVRI, and LVSWI should be done on admission, q8h, and with any significant changes in hemodynamic status.

Patient management

1. Restlessness as the patient is waking up from anesthesia is often associated with profound hypertension and hemodynamic instability. Restlessness may require the use of sedatives such as IV diazepam (Valium), midazolam (Versed), or lorazepam (Ativan). Pain can be managed with intravenous morphine sulfate; give IVP in 2 mg increments q5min to relieve symptoms. Dilute with 5 ml NS and administer over 4 to 5 min.
2. It is recommended to keep systolic blood pressure less than 140 mm Hg to prevent damage to the anastomoses or the fresh suture lines in patients who have had CABG surgery. Furthermore, a MAP of >70 mm Hg is desirable in these patients to prevent the acute collapse of the grafts.
3. Increased afterload occurs often postoperatively and is usually managed via intravenous administration of sodium nitroprusside and/or nitroglycerin. Nitroglycerin may be administered IV to gain desired response: start with an infusion of 5 µg/min; titrate to desired response or to maintain SBP >90 mm Hg. Increase dosage q5 to 10 min by 5 to 10 µg/min. If hypotension occurs, raise the patient's legs and stop the infusion. Sodium nitroprusside may be administered by IV infusion to maintain systolic BP to 100 mm Hg. Dose may range from 0.5 to 10 µg/kg/min. Do not administer more than 10 µg/kg/min or the patient may exhibit signs and symp-

toms of cyanide toxicity: tinnitus, blurred vision, delirium, and muscle spasm.

4. Decreased preload occurs often postoperatively and is usually secondary to hypovolemia. This relative hypovolemia is usually the result of CPB, diuretics administered while weaning from CPB, postoperative bleeding, and postoperative warming of the patient.

   Blood products and colloids are usually the most effective in correcting hypovolemia due to their longer intravascular half-life.

5. ST, T-wave changes may indicate myocardial ischemia and/or infarction, resulting in potential decreased CO with subsequent hypotension and increased dysrhythmias. Ensuring adequate oxygenation, administration of topical or intravenous nitroglycerin, and administration of sublingual nifedepine as per protocol may prove effective in relieving ischemia. Serial ECGs will reveal effectiveness of interventions. Decreased CO can be treated with inotropic agents such as dobutamine or milrinone administered as per protocol. Dobutamine can be administered via continuous IV infusion, initially at 0.5 μg/kg/min and up to 10 μg/kg/min. Milrinone is given as an initial bolus of 50 mcg/kg over 10 minutes followed by an infusion of 0.5 mcg/kg/min.

6. Chest tube drainage in excess of 150 ml/hr for 2 hours may indicate bleeding at graft anastomoses and may require emergent thoracic reexploration. Excess bleeding may also be a result of coagulopathy. Serium coagulation profiles (e.g., INR/PT, PTT, platelet count, fibrinogen) may reveal deficits requiring replacement with fresh frozen plasma, platelets, cryoprecipitae, and clotting factors. Anemia associated with excess bleeding can lead to relative hypoxemia and requires prompt replacement with packed RBCs.

7. PEEP may be used to decrease intrapulmonary shunting and improve gas exchange. As PEEP is increased, venous return may decrease, adversely affecting blood pressure and CO.

8. Dysrhythmias are common occurrences and can include atrial fibrillation, SVT, VT, junctional tachycardia, complete heart block, asystole, and ventricular standstill. Dysrhythmias should be treated as per ACLS protocol. Postoperatively, patients are prone to hypokalemia. Hypokalemia should be treated promptly and serum potassium levels monitored frequently. A temporary

CV

pacemaker should be available to use with epicardial pacing leads in the event of asystole, ventricular standstill, or hemodynamically unstable bradycardia.

9. Cardiac tamponade usually occurs as a result of excessive intrathoracic bleeding and/or ineffective draining of chest tubes. Signs of cardiac tamponade include narrowing pulse pressure, increasing and equalizing CVP and PAD/PAWP, increase in size of cardiac silhouette on chest radiograph, and muffled heart sounds. Treatment includes inotropic agents and increasing intravascular volume replacement until thoracic reexploration can be performed.

Critical observations

Consult with the physician for the following:

1. Acute drop in or trend of decreasing cardiac output
2. Inability to control blood pressure (sustained hypotension or hypertension)
3. Sudden cessation of chest tube drainage
4. Excessive chest tube drainage
5. New onset of ST, T-wave changes
6. Muffling of heart sounds

CARDIAC TRANSPLANT

Clinical Brief

Cardiac transplantation is reserved for patients with end-stage cardiac disease who are unresponsive to medical or interventional therapy. The surgical procedure involves a sternotomy incision, hypothermia induction, and initiation of CPB. The recipient's heart is removed, leaving the posterior walls of the atria; the inferior and superior vena cava and pulmonary veins are left intact. The donor's atria are anastomosed to the recipient's atria walls, and pulmonary artery and aorta are then anastomosed. Epicardial pacing wires are placed in the event of bradycardia and the chest tube inserted to drain the mediastinum. As a result of this procedure the heart is denervated and does not respond to ANS stimulation (heart rate changes in response to stressors).

▶ Complications and related nursing diagnoses

Organ rejection	Decreased cardiac output
	Altered tissue perfusion: cardiac, pulmonary, renal, cerebral
	Impaired gas exchange
	Altered urinary elimination
	Activity intolerance
	Hyperthermia

Infection

Adverse effects of
   immunosuppressive therapy

Hyperthermia

Risk for infection
Altered body image
Altered urinary elimination
Risk for injury: GI bleeding

See Cardiac surgery, p. 591, for other complications and
nursing diagnoses.

Patient Care Management Guidelines
Patient assessment

1. Monitor CVP, PA pressures, CO/CI, HR, BP, and
   MAP. Note trends and patient response to therapy.
   Monitor PVRI and SVRI and note trends and patient
   response to therapy. Calculate LVSWI and RVSWI to
   evaluate contractility.
2. Assess tissue perfusion; note level of mentation, skin color
   and temperature, peripheral pulses, and capillary refill.
3. Continuously monitor ECG for dysrhythmias that may
   result from electrolyte imbalance, hypoxemia, and/or
   hemorrhage.
4. Assess for bleeding: chest tube drainage >200 ml/hr or
   development of cardiac tamponade; decrease in Hgb
   and Hct; abnormal coagulation studies. A donor heart
   may be smaller than the native heart, which can result
   in a larger pericardial space and potential reservoir for
   bleeding and tamponade.
5. Monitor HR and cardiac rhythm. The denervated heart
   has no increase in heart rate in response to decreased cardiac output. The donor sinus node stimulates electrical
   conduction; however, the recipient P waves may be seen
   on ECG. Monitor for junctional rhythm with AV block.
6. Continuously monitor SpO_2 and SvO_2 (if available);
   review serial ABGs and auscultate lungs q1 to 2h. Note
   any adventitious lung sounds and increased work of
   breathing. Assess cough and secretions.
7. Assess temperature. Patients may be hypothermic on
   returning from surgery. Monitor for signs of infection;
   consider IV sites, wound sites, the urinary tract, lungs,
   and mucous membranes as potential sites of infection.
8. Monitor immunosuppressive serum levels for therapeutic range.
9. Monitor sputum cultures, WBC count, and titers for
   presence of infection.

10. Monitor renal function: BUN, and creatinine and urine output.
11. Assess patient for side effects of immunosuppression therapy: hypertension, hyperkalemia, gingival hyperplasia, leukopenia, hyperglycemia.
12. Assess neurological status. Potential side effects of cyclosporine include confusion, cortical blindness, seizures, encephalopathy, quadriplegia, and coma.

Patient management
1. Hemodynamic instability may be treated with fluids, isoproterenol, prostaglandins, dobutamine, and dopamine. Isoproterenol is used to enhance contractility and decrease PVR. Prostaglandins may be used to decrease elevated PVR. Dobutamine and dopamine may be used to increase myocardial contractility. Dopamine is often used to enhance renal output. Titrate the infusion to achieve desired hemodynamic response. Diuretics and digitalis may be prescribed for heart failure.
2. Be prepared to pace the patient for bradycardia or heart block. NOTE: Atropine has no effect on the denervated heart.
3. Isolation protocols should be followed. Dressings should be completed with aseptic technique. IV sites should be changed according to institutional protocol. Catheters and other invasive equipment should be removed as soon as possible. The patient should be weaned from the ventilator as soon as possible. Vigorous pulmonary toilet should be initiated.
4. Administer IV cimetidine or ranitidine and oral antacids as prescribed to prevent GI bleeding. Test all stools and emesis for evidence of occult blood.
5. Administer blood products that are seronegative for CMV as prescribed.
6. Be prepared to administer OKT3 or ATGAM as prescribed to treat acute rejection.
7. See Cardiac surgery, p. 591, for other patient management guidelines.

Critical observations
Consult with the physician for the following:
1. Bleeding; chest tube >200 ml/hr, cardiac tamponade, abnormal coagulation studies
2. Signs and symptoms of myocardial dysfunction: decreased CO, heart failure, dysrhythmias, hemodynamic instability

3. Adverse effects of immunosuppression: GI bleeding, hyperglycemia, hyperkalemia
4. Signs of renal failure: rising BUN and creatinine, decreased urine output
5. Signs of infection: elevated temperature, abnormal WBC, incisional drainage, purulent sputum

IMPLANTABLE CARDIOVERTER DEFIBRILLATOR (ICD)
Clinical Brief
The ICD is an effective treatment option for patients with recurrent ventricular dysrhythmias at risk for sudden death. ICD components include (1) a pulse generator (generally placed subcutaneously in the left periumbilical area), which contains the battery and capacitors and (2) leads or electrodes that monitor heart activity and deliver electrical therapy. ICD implantation originally required a median sternotomy or thoracotomy; newer models have leads that can be implanted transvenously and subcutaneously, thus avoiding major surgery. New models also offer programmability of more features including bradycardia back-up pacing, and antitachycardia pacing, as well as low energy cardioversion and high energy defibrillation therapy. Predicted battery life is 3 to 5 years.

▶ Complications and related nursing diagnoses
(for the implantable defibrillator)
(See Complications and management guidelines, p. 591, for cardiac surgery.)

Malfunction	Risk for injury:
• Inappropriate shock	dysrhythmias/sudden death
• Failure to shock	

Patient Care Management Guidelines
Patient assessment (see Cardiac surgery, p. 591)
1. Monitor heart rhythm and patient response before, during, and after ICD therapy. As long as the ICD continues to respond and the patient is stable, no intervention is necessary.
2. Assess the patient's risk factors for a lethal event (e.g., hypoxemia, electrolyte imbalances).
Patient management
1. Be aware of the specific device implanted and how it is programmed (e.g., is the device on or off, what is the tachycardia detection rate?). Place a sign with this information at the head of the bed.

2. Emergency care of the patient with an ICD should follow ACLS protocol.
3. When the ICD discharges, individuals touching the patient can receive up to a 2 joule shock. If VT/VF continues, initiate CPR and countershock. (Use of an external defibrillator does not damage ICD.)
4. Inappropriate discharge of the ICD may occur infrequently (patient shocked while in NSR). Be alert to this complication. Inactivate the ICD; depending on institutional policy, nurses may or may not use a magnet to inactivate the ICD.
5. Monitor for signs of infection after implantation of the ICD. Monitor temperature q4h. Note any drainage, redness, and increased tenderness at the surgical site.
6. Patient and family teaching must be done to prepare them to live with an ICD. The patient should be instructed to avoid 60-cycle interference, because it may temporarily or permanently render the defibrillator nonfunctioning. Magnetic resonance imaging is contraindicated.

Critical observations

Consult with the physician for the following:
1. Inappropriate discharge of ICD
2. Failure (of ICD) to discharge
3. Evidence of wound infection: T >38.3° C (101° F), redness, drainage

INTRAAORTIC BALLOON PUMP (IABP) COUNTERPULSATION

Clinical Brief

The purpose of the IABP is to increase coronary artery perfusion and decrease myocardial oxygen consumption. Counterpulsation permits an increased aortic pressure during diastole (balloon inflation), augmenting coronary perfusion, and a decreased aortic pressure during systole (balloon deflation), decreasing afterload. Consequently, counterpulsation produces the following effects:

Increased supply	Decreased demand
↑ MAP/SI/CI	↓ LVEDP/PAWP (preload)
↑ Renal perfusion	↓ SVRI (afterload)
↑ Cerebral perfusion	↓ MVO_2
↑ Coronary artery perfusion	↓ HR

Indications for IABP include cardiogenic shock related to acute MI or following cardiac surgery, noncardiogenic shock, ventricular septal defect, papillary muscle dysfunction, unstable angina that is unresponsive to medical management, and prophylactically for high-risk CV patients undergoing coronary angiography or general anesthesia.

Contraindications include irreversible brain damage, end-stage cardiac disease, aortic regurgitation, dissecting aortic aneurysm, and significant peripheral vascular disease.

Description

The IABP device consists of a balloon-tipped catheter and power console that permits inflation and deflation of the balloon during diastole and systole, respectively. The patient generally receives anticoagulation therapy. The catheter is inserted in the femoral artery via a percutaneous approach and advanced through the aorta. Correct placement of the catheter should be confirmed in the descending aorta distal to the left subclavian artery and proximal to the renal arteries. Inflation and deflation of the IAB is most often triggered from the ECG; timing is fine-tuned from the arterial waveform (Figure 7-3). The balloon inflation causes an increase in diastolic aortic pressure and coronary artery pressure and improves coronary artery blood flow. This period is called *diastolic augmentation*. Rapid deflation of the balloon is timed to occur just before systole. Proper deflation of the balloon decreases the aortic pressure dramatically and allows the ventricle to empty more completely. Initially, the IABP is usually set to augment every cardiac cycle or every other cycle (Figure 7-4).

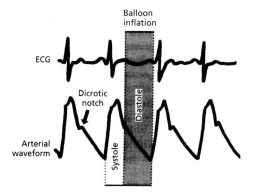

Figure 7-3 IABP period of balloon inflation. Balloon inflation occurs during diastole and should begin at aortic valve closure (dicrotic notch); balloon deflation should occur just before the aortic valve opens. (From Stillwell S, Randall E: *Pocket guide to cardiovascular care,* ed 2, St Louis, 1994, Mosby.)

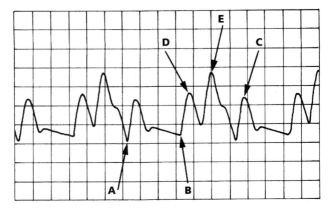

Figure 7-4 IABP timing 1:2 assist mode. *A*, Balloon-assisted aortic end diastolic pressure; *B*, patient aortic end diastolic pressure; *C*, balloon-assisted systole; *D*, patient systole; *E*, peak diastolic augmented pressure.

▶ Complications and related nursing diagnoses

Poor IABP augmentation
• Balloon leak
• Incorrect timing
• ↑ HR
• ↓ MAP/SI/SVRI
• Incorrect balloon size
• Incorrect balloon position

Decreased cardiac output

Balloon migration
• Subclavian/carotid artery obstruction
• Renal artery obstruction

Altered tissue perfusion: cerebral, renal

Bleeding
• Thrombocytopenia
• Related to anticoagulation

Decreased cardiac output
Fluid volume deficit

Hematoma formation at percutaneous access site

Pain in groin area secondary to hematoma
Decreased cardiac output

Loss of peripheral pulses related to thrombus formation at access site

Altered tissue perfusion: peripheral
Pain in affected extremity

Embolization

Altered tissue perfusion: cerebral, renal, peripheral

Infection	Hyperthermia
	Risk for injury: sepsis
Aortic dissection	Decreased cardiac output
	Altered tissue perfusion: peripheral, renal

Patient Care Management Guidelines
Patient assessment

1. The cardiovascular (CV) system should be assessed q15 to 30 min until stable after IABP insertion and then per unit protocol; include VS, CVP, PA pressures, and cardiac rhythm; urine output should be monitored hourly.

2. A cardiac profile including CO/CI, SVRI, and LVSWI should be done on admission, q8h, and with any significant changes in hemodynamics.

3. Assess peripheral pulses (both pedal and posttibial pulses) for strength and equality q15min for 1 hour and then q2 hours. Radial and brachial pulses in the left arm should also be assessed during these times to check for possible catheter migration, which would result in a diminished or absent pulse in this extremity. Verify that the skin color remains pink, the skin is warm to the touch, and that capillary refill is equally brisk bilaterally. If a change in quality of pulses is noted, a Doppler device should be employed to attempt to identify pulses.

4. Assess the percutaneous insertion site for oozing, ecchymosis, or hematoma formation q15 to 30 min for 4 to 6 hours after IABP insertion. Assess coagulation status via ordered laboratory tests.

5. Augmentation of IABP should be assessed hourly and as needed. Balloon-assisted systolic pressure should be lower than the patient's systolic pressure. Balloon migration should be ruled out with the development of poor IABP augmentation, changes in LOC (possible subclavian artery occlusion), a diminished radial pulse in the left arm, or a decrease in urinary output (possible renal artery occlusion). A stat chest radiograph is crucial to verify placement. The radiopaque catheter tip should be just distal to the aortic arch in the 2nd to 3rd intercostal space.

6. If pain occurs at the groin percutaneous access site, assess the area for hematoma formation and administer analgesics as per protocol.

CV

Patient management

1. Maintain proper functioning of the balloon pump according to the manufacturer's guidelines. Maintain airtight seals on all connections between the pump and the patient.
2. The inflation of the balloon should be timed to occur at the dicrotic notch and to deflate just before the next systole. (See Figure 7-3.) Instruct the patient to keep the affected leg immobilized and do not elevate the HOB >30 degrees.
3. Inflation and deflation timing are usually adjusted via slide bars. The goal of the adjustment is to achieve maximum diastolic augmentation and minimum aortic end diastolic pressure.
4. Red or brownish discolorations inside the balloon connecting tubing indicates balloon leak. The IABP should be placed on stand-by and the physician called immediately to remove the balloon.
5. When the balloon catheter is removed, a pressure dressing and/or a sandbag may be applied at the insertion site as per unit protocol. A large amount of blood may exsanguinate into the groin and upper thigh without any obvious evidence; therefore close monitoring is warranted. Watch for hematoma formation at the access site. Mark the site carefully with a skin marking pen and assess hourly for the first 4 hr and at least q4h thereafter to determine the magnitude of the hematoma.

Critical observations

Consult with the physician for the following:

1. Inability to maintain adequate augmentation
2. Accidental dislodgment or removal of catheter
3. Migration of balloon tip: decrease in urine output, changes in LOC, decrease or loss of pulse in an extremity
4. Excessive bleeding at access site
5. Balloon leak
6. Coagulation studies (PTT) out of range

PERCUTANEOUS TRANSLUMINAL CORONARY ANGIOPLASTY (PTCA)

Clinical Brief

The purpose of PTCA is to restore adequate blood supply to the myocardium by restoring the lumen diameter of a coronary artery. Indications for PTCA include documented myocardial ischemia unresponsive to medical management and emergently in select patients with acute myocardial infarction.

The procedure is similar to a cardiac catheterization. Once percutaneous access is established, a specially equipped catheter with a balloon tip is advanced to the affected area(s) of the coronary artery. The lesion is crossed with the catheter and the balloon is inflated, compressing the atherosclerotic plaque in an effort to increase the lumen diameter. Because the coronary artery distal to the balloon is occluded during inflation, the patient may experience angina. The patient receives anticoagulation therapy during the procedure with intravenous heparin. Intracoronary thrombolytic therapy may be administered to treat acute thrombus formation. Intracoronary nitroglycerin may also be administered to prevent or treat vasospasm. The restenosis rate for PTCA is 30% to 40%. Lasers, atherectomies, and stents may be treatment options to improve blood supply to the myocardium by restoring the lumen diameter of a coronary artery in patients with CAD. These procedures may be used with PTCA to treat complications of dilation and prevent restenosis. A catheter equipped with a laser, atherectomy device, or a loaded wire stent is used to vaporize or shave the atheromatous plaque or to mechanically support the coronary artery.

The laser may be used to burn a hole in the center of the plaque so that balloon angioplasty can be employed or the laser can be used to thermally seal the artery following angioplasty. Arterial perforation, embolization, and spasm are laser-related complications.

Transluminal atherectomy involves positioning the device at the lesion and shaving away the plaque. A balloon is inflated to stabilize the catheter, and the excised plaque is collected in a housing compartment and removed. Restenosis of the artery can occur following the atherectomy.

The intracoronary stent is a wire device designed to support the coronary artery and prevent acute stenosis following PTCA. A delivery system positions the stent at the lesion site, where it is released. The stent expands and improves the vessel's intraluminal diameter. However, acute closure secondary to thrombosis may occur; aggressive heparinization is required.

Patient selection

In general, patients who are candidates for PTCA include individuals with discrete lesions, preferably involving one or two vessels, and not at vessel bifurcations. The patient also should be a candidate for coronary artery bypass graft (CABG) surgery. Contraindications include <50% lesion, nonviable myocardium distal to the stenotic lesion, diffuse disease with distal vessels suitable for bypass grafting, and tortuous vessels.

In general, patients who are candidates for PTCA will be candidates for these new interventional procedures. Clinical studies are investigating the types of devices and techniques, as well as the safety and efficacy of the procedures.

▶ **Complications and related nursing diagnoses**

Acute occlusion/restenosis	Pain
Reaction to contrast agent	Decreased cardiac output Fluid volume excess Ineffective breathing pattern
Vasovagal reaction	Risk for injury: bradycardia
Reperfusion dysrhythmias	Risk for injury: heart blocks, ventricular ectopy/tachycardia, and/or accelerated idioventricular rhythm
Bleeding related to anticoagulation	Decreased cardiac output Risk for injury: bleeding
Hematoma formation at percutaneous access site	Pain in groin area secondary to hematoma Decreased cardiac output
Loss of peripheral pulses	Altered tissue perfusion: peripheral Pain in affected extremity

Patient Care Management Guidelines
Patient assessment

1. Assess vital signs q15min × 3, q30min × 3, q1h × 3, then per routine, if stable.
2. Assess cardiac rhythm continuously via bedside monitor. Note rate/rhythm and/or ST, T-wave changes.
3. Assess access site for oozing, ecchymosis, or hematoma formation with vital signs check. If a hematoma develops at the groin access site, the size should be monitored by outlining the borders with a skin marking pen. A large amount of blood may exsanguinate into the groin and upper thigh without necessarily an early drop in SBP or an increase in HR; therefore close observation of the access site is warranted.
4. Assess for comfort level q1 to 2h for 12 to 24 hours. if pain develops at the groin access site, assess for local hematoma formation.
5. Assess peripheral pulses (pedal and posttibial pulses) for strength and equality with vital signs check. A Doppler

device may be helpful in identifying peripheral pulses, especially if the patient is cool.

6. Monitor coagulation studies, especially PTT. The normal value for PTT is 30 to 45 sec.

Patient management

1. The patient should be instructed to promptly report any chest pain or SOB.
2. Low-flow oxygen therapy should be administered as per protocol.
3. The HOB should be elevated less than 30 degrees and the affected extremity should be kept straight to prevent dislodgement of the groin sheath.
4. Encourage fluids (if not contraindicated) to offset the effects of the hypertonic contrast.
5. Maintain hypercoagulated state as per protocol.
6. If the patient was sedated during the procedure and remains sedated, institute aspiration precautions until the patient is fully alert.
7. If the patient reports chest pain, intravenous or sublingual nitroglycerin may be ordered to relieve discomfort: sublingual, 1 tablet q5min × 3; IV, start with an infusion of 5 µg/min; titrate to desired response or to maintain SBP >90 mm Hg. Increase dosage q5 to 10min by 5 to 10 µg/min. If hypotension occurs, raise the patient's legs and stop the infusion.
8. If the patient becomes hypotensive, a fluid challenge may be ordered. If the patient is also bradycardic, administer atropine as per ACLS protocol.
9. If pain occurs at the groin access site, administer analgesics as per protocol.
10. If a hematoma forms at the access site, a pressure dressing should be applied.
11. If nausea and/or vomiting occur, administer antiemetics as per protocol.

SHEATH REMOVAL

1. Once the physician has ordered the sheath(s) removed, the patient should be informed of the forthcoming procedure.
2. The access site should be prepared as per protocol (local anesthesia, betadine prep, suture removal).
3. The sheath(s) should be removed and direct pressure applied until hemostasis is achieved. For an arterial

CV

sheath, apply pressure above the puncture site; for a venous sheath, apply pressure below the puncture site. Apply enough pressure to obtain hemostasis but not occlude the distal pulse. A mechanical device may be employed to establish hemostasis. If so, follow the manufacturer's directions.

4. Once the site is stable, a pressure dressing should be applied and the site and peripheral pulses should be monitored frequently.

Critical observations

Consult with the physician for the following:

1. Increase or onset of chest pain or angina symptoms
2. Hypotension and bradycardia
3. Significant oozing, bleeding, or hematoma formation
4. A change in quality or loss of peripheral pulses
5. Increased times in coagulation studies
6. The onset of dysrhythmias or ST, T-wave changes

PERCUTANEOUS VALVULOPLASTY (PV)

Clinical Brief

The purpose of PV is to restore normal blood flow through a previously stenotic cardiac valve. The procedure is similar to a cardiac catheterization. Percutaneous access is established and the patient receives anticoagulation therapy. For tricuspid, pulmonic, or mitral PV, a right-sided (venous) approach is used. Mitral PV requires an atrial transseptal approach and creates an increased risk for complications. For aortic PV, the most common form, a left-sided (arterial) approach, is used. Regardless of which valve is involved, a specially equipped balloon-tip catheter is used. Once the valve is crossed with the catheter, the balloon is inflated and the commissures are split or the calcium nodules are fractured. Indications for PV include a documented (via an echocardiogram or a ventriculogram) critical flow gradient across a valve. Because of the high restenosis rate, the procedure is used for patients who are high surgical risks. Contraindications include heavy calcification associated with the stenosis.

▶ **Complications and related nursing diagnoses**

Leaflet tearing, fragmentation of leaflets, annulus disruption	Decreased cardiac output Impaired gas exchange: pulmonary edema

Embolization to brain	Altered tissue perfusion: cerebral
Cardiac tamponade	Decreased cardiac output
Dyshythmias secondary to local edema resulting from balloon manipulation	Decreased cardiac output
Left to right shunt related to transseptal approach	Decreased cardiac output
Reaction to contrast agent	Decreased cardiac output Fluid volume excess Ineffective breathing pattern
Vasovagal reaction	Risk for injury: symptomatic bradycardia
Bleeding related to anticoagulation therapy	Risk for injury: bleeding
Hematoma formation at percutaneous access site	Pain in groin area secondary to hematoma
Loss of peripheral pulses related to thrombus formation at access site	Altered tissue perfusion: peripheral Pain in affected extremity

Patient Care Management Guidelines

Patient assessment

1. Assess vital signs q15min × 3, q30min × 3, q1h × 2, then per routine, if stable. Assess cardiac rhythm continuously via bedside monitor. Note rate/rhythm and/or ST, T-wave changes. The patient will most likely have central venous pressure (CVP) and pulmonary artery (PA) catheters in place, and these readings should be included in the cardiovascular assessment. Changes in CVP readings, PAP readings, and/or heart sounds may indicate acute valvular failure, cardiac tamponade, or exacerbation of left to right shunt resulting from the transseptal approach, requiring emergency surgery. Heart sounds should be auscultated and murmurs graded. Diastolic murmurs may develop as the procedure corrects the stenotic valve. The patient should also be monitored for dysrhythmias.

2. Assess access site for oozing, ecchymosis, or hematoma with vital signs check. If a hematoma develops at the groin access site, the size should be monitored by

outlining the borders with a skin marking pen. A large amount of blood may exsanguinate into the groin and upper thigh without an early drop in SBP or an increase in HR; close observation of the access site is warranted.

3. Assess for comfort level q1 to 2h for 12 to 24 hours. If pain develops at the groin access site, assess for local hematoma formation.

4. Assess peripheral pulses (pedal and posttibial pulses) for strength and equality with vital signs check. A Doppler device may be helpful in identifying peripheral pulses, especially if the patient is cool.

5. Monitor coagulation studies.

Patient management

1. Low-flow oxygen therapy should be administered.

2. The HOB should be elevated less than 30 degrees and the affected extremity should be kept straight to prevent dislodgement of the groin access sheath.

3. Maintain the hypercoagulated state as per protocol.

4. If the patient was sedated during the procedure and remains sedated, institute aspiration precautions until the patient is fully alert.

5. If the patient becomes hypotensive, place the patient flat and administer fluid challenges as ordered. If the patient is also bradycardic, administer atropine as per ACLS protocols.

6. If pain occurs at the groin access site, administer analgesics as per protocol.

7. If a hematoma forms at the access site, a pressure dressing should be applied.

8. If nausea and/or vomiting occur, administer antimetics as per protocol.

Sheath Removal

See PTCA, p. 607.

Critical observations

Consult with the physician for the following:

1. Significant changes in BP, CVP, and PA pressure readings

2. Muffling of heart sounds or development or changes in the quality of a murmur

3. Significant oozing, bleeding, or hematoma formation at the groin site

4. A change in quality or loss of peripheral pulses

PERIPHERAL ANGIOPLASTY OR LASER THERAPY
Clinical Brief
The purpose of angioplasty or laser therapy is to restore blood flow distal to the lesion. This is accomplished in the same manner as with PTCA or coronary artery laser therapy.

▶ Complications and related nursing diagnosis
See PTCA, p. 606.

Ischemia to organ system with reduced blood supply	Altered tissue perfusion: renal, GI, and/or peripheral

Patient Care Management Guidelines
Patient assessment
See PTCA, p. 606.
1. Monitor affected organ system for return of functioning or acute loss of function.

Patient management
See PTCA, p. 607.
Critical observations
See PTCA, p. 608.

PERIPHERAL VASCULAR SURGERY (PVS)
Clinical Brief
Peripheral arterial occlusive disease applies to any disease involving the aorta, its major branches, and the arteries. The cause of occlusive arterial disease may be (1) vasospastic, as in Raynaud's phenomenon; (2) inflammatory, as in thromboangiitis obliterans (Buerger's disease); or (3) atherosclerotic (arteriosclerosis obliterans), where an atheroma obstructs all or part of the lumen of the vessel. These conditions cause ischemia of the peripheral tissues resulting in pain and/or ultimately gangrene necessitating amputation.

Aortic aneurysms occur when there is an abnormal widening of the three layers of the aorta, resulting in increased aortic wall tension at the site. Rupture of this segment can occur. Aneurysms may be either fusiform, in which the entire circumference of the diseased segment has expanded, or saccular, in which there is an outpouching at the site of the diseased segment. The cause of aortic aneurysms may be atherosclerosis, cystic medial necrosis, trauma, or syphilis.

CV

Peripheral Vascular Surgeries

- *Type:* Thoracic Aortic Aneurysm Repair
  Indications: Aneurysms greater than 6 cm in diameter, dissecting aneurysms, or leaking aneurysms
  Description: Requires a sternotomy or thoracotomy approach and may require cardiopulmonary bypass (CPB). The aneurysm is excised and replaced by a synthetic graft. Any vessels that arise from the aneurysm are reanastomosed to the graft.
- *Type:* Abdominal Aortic Aneurysm Repair
  Indications: Same as above
  Description: Requires a large midline abdominal incision and groin incisions for distal anastomosis. Although CPB is not required, the surgical procedure is similar to thoracic repair.
- *Type:* Peripheral Bypass Surgery
  Indications: Rapid onset of decreasing ability to walk and peripheral ischemia resulting in ulcerative or gangrenous lesions
  Description: Requires abdominal, groin, or lower extremity incision depending on location of proximal and distal anastomosis sites. Areas of occlusion are either excised or bypassed and a synthetic graft is anastomosed in place.

The purpose of PVS is to bypass and/or remove occlusion and restore blood flow distal to the lesion. Common surgical procedures (see box above) include thoracic aortic aneurysm repair, abdominal aortic aneurysm repair, aortofemoral bypass, iliofemoral bypass, or femoropopliteal bypass.

▶ Complications and related nursing diagnoses

Increased afterload (relative)	Risk for injury: hypertension Altered tissue perfusion
Acute graft occlusion	Altered tissue perfusion Pain
Graft leakage	Decreased cardiac output
Respiratory insufficiency	Impaired gas exchange Ineffective breathing pattern
GI ileus	Altered tissue perfusion

Patient Care Management Guidelines
See Cardiac surgery, p. 591, for procedures requiring CPB.

Patient assessment

1. A thorough assessment should be completed upon patient arrival to the recovery area. The patient should be frequently assessed because of the instability often present in the early postoperative period.
2. The cardiovascular (CV) system should be assessed q15min until stable and then per unit protocol. The assessment should include VS, CVP, PA pressures, cardiac rhythm, and incisional dressing. Chest tube drainage (if present) and urine output should be monitored hourly. Hourly monitoring of peripheral pulses for presence and quality is necessary to detect early onset of graft occlusion. Adjunctive devices such as Dopplers are useful in detecting faint pulses. Mark pulse sites with a skin marking pen. Warming the extremity with thermal blankets may increase peripheral pulse amplitude.
3. A cardiac profile including CO, CI, and SVRI should be done on admission, q8h, and with any significant changes in hemodynamics.
4. Compare serial CBCs to detect significant blood loss requiring replacement with PRBCs.
5. Assess the patient's ability to take a deep breath. Auscultate lung sounds q2h and as clinically indicated for adventitious sounds that may indicate atelectasis/pneumonia.
6. Assess for return of bowel sounds postoperatively and check abdominal girth daily, if distention is a concern, for an increase in size. Mark the sites of measurement with a skin marking pen for consistency in assessments. Ileus is a common complication of PVS that includes a major abdominal incision.
7. Assess comfort level via interview, monitoring facial expression, and ability to take a deep breath.

Patient management

1. Nitroprusside may be ordered to maintain SBP <130 mm Hg, DBP <70 mm Hg, and SVRI in the normal range (1700 to 2600) to prevent leaking or rupture of anastomoses. Monitor MAP; a MAP of 70 is critical in preventing acute graft occlusion. Titrate IV infusion to maintain systolic BP to 100 mm Hg. Dose may range from 0.5 to 10 μg/kg/min. Do not administer more than 10 μg/kg/min or patient may exhibit signs and symptoms of cyanide toxicity: tinnitus, blurred vision, delirium, and muscle spasm.

2. Pain management is crucial in blood pressure control and the patient's ability to C & DB. Intravenous morphine sulfate or epidural analgesia is usually ordered in the immediate postoperative period. If managing pain with intravenous morphine sulfate, give IVP in 2 mg increments q5min to relieve symptoms. Dilute with 5 ml NS and administer over 4 to 5 minutes. Intramuscular and oral analgesia will be helpful later in postoperative course.

3. Encourage the patient to use the spirometry device and to C & DB. Instruct the patient on splinting with a pillow while coughing. IPPB may be helpful in preventing atelectasis.

4. Leave the NG tube in place until bowel sounds return to prevent vomiting and reduce the risk of aspiration. Early postoperative mobility may be the most important intervention in preventing an ileus. Metoclopramide may be used to stimulate return of gastric mobility. Administer 10 to 20 mg IV over 1 to 2 minutes as ordered.

Critical observations

Consult with the physician for the following:

1. Inability to control hypertension
2. Changes in intensity or quality of peripheral pulses
3. Signs of bleeding

RADIOFREQUENCY CATHETER ABLATION

Clinical Brief

Radiofrequency catheter ablation is a nonsurgical treatment used primarily for treatment of supraventricular tachycardias associated with WPW and AV nodal reentry. It has also been used in the treatment of ventricular tachycardia. The procedure is done in a cardiac catheterization laboratory.

Radiofrequency current (delivered by a catheter positioned in the heart) is used to destroy or ablate accessory pathway(s) or arrhythmogenic area(s) necessary to sustain a tachycardia. Heart block may occur if the area ablated is in close proximity to the AV node.

▶ **Complications and related nursing diagnosis**

See complications following Angiography, p. 437.

AV block   Decreased cardiac output

Patient Care Management Guidelines

See Angiography, p. 438.

TEMPORARY PACEMAKERS
Clinical Brief

The purpose of a temporary pacemaker is to provide an artificial stimulus to the myocardium when the heart is unable to initiate an impulse or the conduction system is defective. Types of pacemakers include temporary (external or internal) or permanent. Pacing modes can be asynchronous, in which the impulse is generated at a fixed rate despite the rhythm of the patient, or synchronous, in which the impulse is generated on demand or as needed according to the patient's intrinsic rhythm.

Indications for pacing include symptomatic or asymptomatic Mobitz type II AV block; complete heart block; sick sinus syndrome; symptomatic bradycardia; tachydysrhythmias such as SVT, atrial fibrillation, or atrial flutter with rapid ventricular response; and intermittent VT unresponsive to drug therapy.

The external temporary pacemaker (transcutaneous pacemaker) is used to emergently treat symptomatic bradydysrhythmias unresponsive to medications until more definitive treatment can be employed. The external pacemaker includes a pulse generator, pacing cable attached to large external electrodes, and an ECG cable for the demand mode. Place the pacing electrodes per the manufacturer's instructions. Usually one electrode is placed at V_3 or V_4 anteriorly and the other is placed in the left subscapular area. The mA setting necessary to achieve consistent capture will vary; an mA up to 200 may occasionally be necessary.

Temporary internal pacing can be accomplished via epicardial, transthoracic, or transvenous electrodes. Some PA catheters are designed to accommodate transvenous pacing electrodes. Epicardial electrodes are placed during cardiac surgery and exit through the chest wall. Transthoracic electrodes are inserted into the right ventricle via a cardiac needle using a subxyphoid approach. Transvenous electrodes are threaded into the right atrium or right ventricle using a venous approach. The mA setting necessary to achieve consistent capture with internal electrodes is much less than with external electrodes; often an mA of 5 to 10 will be adequate.

▶ Complications and related nursing diagnoses

Muscle twitching	Pain
Failure to place	Decreased cardiac output
Failure to capture	Decreased cardiac output

Failure to sense   Decreased cardiac output
                                  Risk for injury: life-threatening
                                      dysrhythmias

Patient Care Management Guidelines

Patient assessment

1. Monitor ECG for proper pacemaker functioning (e.g., evidence of "capture": pacer spike immediately followed by a P wave or wide QRS).
2. Assess sensorium, skin color and temperature, capillary refill, urine output, HR, and BP.

Patient management

1. Muscle twitching or chest wall discomfort occurs frequently with the use of external pacemakers. Sedation and/or analgesia are usually an effective treatment.
2. Failure to pace:
   a. Check the power supply (e.g., battery) and all connections between generator and patient.
   b. If the external pacemaker is in use, check the electrodes for adequate surface contact: excessive hair at the electrode placement should be trimmed; however, shaving may cause nicks and increase chest impedance. A displaced ECG lead, with subsequent flat line, will result in 100% pacing as the pacemaker interprets asystole. If the patient rolls onto the side, poor chest wall contact may result. Secure electrodes as necessary.
   c. With transvenous or epicardial pacing, lead displacement or fracture may cause failure to pace. If the situation cannot be quickly remedied, prepare to externally pace the patient until more definitive treatment can be rendered.
3. Failure to capture (Figure 7-5):
   a. The problem may arise from any of the problems mentioned in the previous section, and the same interventions are warranted.
   b. The problem may also be low voltage and may be corrected by increasing the mA.
   c. Repositioning the patient to the left side may also correct the problem.
4. Symptomatic hypotension may be a result of too slow a rate and may be corrected by merely increasing the rate.
5. If defibrillation is required, the pulse generator should be disconnected to prevent damage.

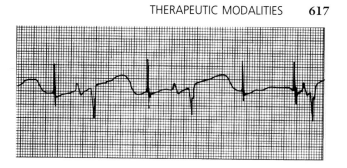

Figure 7-5 Failure to capture. (From Conover M: *Pocket guide to electrocardiography,* St Louis, 1990, Mosby.)

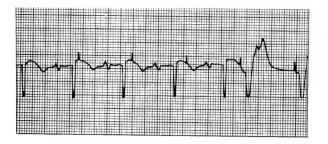

Figure 7-6 Failure to sense. (From Conover M: *Pocket guide to electrocardiography,* St Louis, 1990, Mosby.)

CV

6. Failure to sense (transvenous or epicardial pacemakers) (Figure 7-6):
   a. Failure to sense may be a result of catheter tip migration, sensitivity setting too low (e.g., asynchronous), or battery failure.
   b. Turn the patient to the left side, change the power source (battery), or increase the sensitivity of the generator.
   c. If failure to sense is creating pacer spikes that are dangerously close to the preceding QRS, then prepare to externally pace the patient and turn off the pacer.
   d. Sustained dysrhythmias should be treated as per ACLS protocol.

Critical observations
Consult with the physician for the following:
1. Failure to capture despite nursing interventions
2. Failure to pace despite nursing interventions
3. Failure to sense despite nursing interventions

THROMBOLYTIC THERAPY

Clinical Brief
The purpose of thrombolytic therapy is to lyse acutely formed thrombi in the coronary artery and restore blood flow to the myocardium. Thrombolytics may also be used in the treatment of pulmonary embolism and acute occlusion in peripheral vascular disease. Thrombolytic agents act as plasminogen activators and have an affinity for circulating plasminogen (non-clot-specific) or fibrin-bound plasminogen (clot-specific). Alteplase (activase) is clot-specific and has a half-life of 5 minutes. Streptokinase (SK), anisoylated plasminogen streptokinase activator complex (APSAC), and urokinase (UK) are non-clot-specific. In lower doses, APSAC is more clot-specific than SK. The half life of SK, APSAC and UK are 25, 90, and 15 minutes, respectively.

Traditional inclusion criteria for thrombolytic therapy include: chest pain or discomfort of ischemic nature lasting greater than 30 minutes, but less than 6 hours and unrelieved by nitroglycerin; ST segment elevation in two contiguous leads with or without Q waves.

Contraindications include active internal bleeding, history of hemorrhagic cerebrovascular disease, BP >200/120, major surgery or trauma within 2 weeks, recent head trauma or known intracranial neoplasm, history of intracranial or intraspinal surgery, pregnancy, hemorrhagic retinopathy, suspected aortic bisection, prolonged/traumatic CPR, or previous allergic reaction.

▶ Complications and related nursing diagnoses

Hematoma formation	Risk for injury: bleeding
	Decreased cardiac output
	Pain at puncture site
Acute reocclusion	Altered tissue perfusion: myocardial ischemia
	Pain: chest discomfort
Reperfusion dysrhythmias	Decreased cardiac output
Bleeding	Decreased cardiac output
	Fluid volume deficit

Altered tissue perfusion:
peripheral and/or cerebral

Pain: abdominal pain, back pain,
headache, and/or puncture
site pain

Allergic response
(SK, APSAC)

Decreased cardiac output
Ineffective breathing pattern
Impaired gas exchange

Patient Care Management Guidelines

NOTE: Refer to policy/procedure and pharmacy protocol.

Patient assessment

1. The cardiovascular (CV) system should be assessed on patient's arrival to the unit and q15min until the patient's condition is stable. This assessment should include P, RR, and BP and cardiac rhythm strip assessment. Carefully observe for and document rate, rhythm, and ST, T-wave changes. Urinary output should be monitored hourly.
2. Obtain a baseline ECG and monitor serial ECGs as ordered to determine the efficacy of therapy as evidenced by normalization of ST segments and T waves. Although the patient may continue to experience minimal residual discomfort, notify the physician of any change in the quality of pain.
3. Assess baseline neurological status and monitor for change in LOC or other functions that may indicate intracranial bleeding.
4. Assess the patient for bleeding. All recent puncture sites should be monitored for oozing or hematoma formation. Test all stools and emesis and dipstick urine for occult blood.

Patient management

1. Before the initiation of thrombolytic therapy, establish IV access via two, or preferably three, routes. If feasible, use double-lumen peripheral intravenous catheters. Avoid IM injections and unnecessary trauma (e.g., continuous-use automatic blood pressure cuffs). Insertion of a Foley catheter after therapy is initiated should be avoided.
2. Evaluate response to thrombolytic therapy by monitoring for pain relief, normalization of ST segments, and reperfusion dysrhythmias.
3. Nitroglycerin and/or morphine sulfate should be administered to treat angina. Recurrence of angina with documented ECG changes represents possible reocclusion,

CV

and the patient should be prepared for possible emergent cardiac catheterization, PTCA, or CABG surgery.

4. A wide variety of dysrhythmias occurs with thrombolytic therapy, including nonsustained VT, bradydysrhythmias, junctional escape rhythms, and idioventricular rhythms. If the rhythm is self-limiting and the patient is asymptomatic, no treatment is needed. Symptomatic dysrhythmias are treated per ACLS protocol.

5. All puncture sites should be compressed until hemostasis is assured.

6. Prophylactic antiulcer medication, such as IV cimetidine or ranitidine, and/or PO antacids may be ordered.

7. Monitor PTT and CBC for acute changes. PTT is generally kept 2½ times greater than normal during heparin therapy to prevent thrombus reformation.

Critical observations

Consult with the physician for the following:

1. Inability to achieve ordered PTT value
2. Signs of bleeding
3. Significant hematoma formation
4. New onset of chest pain
5. New changes in ECG after initial improvement
6. No change in ECG/pain level despite thrombolytic therapy
7. Neurological changes

VENTRICULAR ASSIST DEVICES (VAD)

Clinical Brief

The purpose of a VAD is to maintain systemic circulation and improve tissue perfusion in patients with severe ventricular dysfunction while allowing the ventricle(s) to recover. Examples of VADs include resuscitative devices (cardiopulmonary bypass, extracorporeal membrane oxygenation systems); external nonpulsatile devices (Biomedicus, Sarns); external pulsatile assist devices (Thoratec VAD, Abiomed BVS 5000); and implantable left ventricular assist systems (Novacor LVAD, Heartmate LVAD). Both right and left VADs can be used if needed to support ventricular function. Improvement is generally observed within 48 hours.

Indications for a VAD include profound cardiogenic shock refractory to medications and counterpulsation, and inability to wean from cardiopulmonary bypass. A VAD can also be used while the patient awaits cardiac transplantation. Contraindications include irreversible disease processes from which recovery is unlikely.

▶ Complications and related nursing diagnoses

Significant postoperative bleeding • Anticoagulation • Hemolysis	Decreased cardiac output Fluid volume deficit
Air embolus and thrombus • Cerebral • Peripheral • Renal • GI	Altered tissue perfusion
Ventricular failure of unassisted ventricle	Decreased cardiac output
Sepsis	Risk for infection
Mechanical failure	Decreased cardiac output

(Also see Complications following cardiac surgery, p. 591.)

Patient Care Management Guidelines

NOTE: Follow the guidelines detailed under Cardiac surgery (p. 594), as appropriate, in addition to the following.

Patient assessment

1. A thorough assessment should be completed on the patient on arrival to the recovery area. The patient should be frequently assessed because of the instability present in the early postoperative period. Careful assessment of patient, tubing, VAD, and blood flow should be performed q15min until stable and q1h thereafter.
2. The cardiovascular system should be assessed q15min until stable and then q1h. Include VS, CVP, PA pressures, cardiac rhythm, incision/dressing appearance, chest tube drainage, quality of the peripheral pulses, and urine output.
3. A cardiac profile including CO, CI, and SVRI should be done on admission and q1 to 2h. Note thermodilution CO/CI is accurate only with LVADs, not RVADs.
4. Monitor serial Hgb and Hct and coagulation profiles as ordered for evidence of bleeding and/or coagulopathy.
5. Monitor temperature q2h.

Patient management

1. Once vital signs are stable, turn the patient q2h unless contraindicated. Perform range of motion twice daily.
2. Avoid tension in the tubes; eliminating kinks in tubing will assist in preventing emboli or thrombi formation.

The use of heparin via a continuous IV infusion may be necessary, especially with continuous flow devices.

3. Monitor PA pressures and hemodynamics to maintain filling pressures. Maintain MAP >70 mm Hg and LAP 10 to 20 mm Hg.

4. RV failure may occur after initiation of LVAD use and may necessitate RVAD.

5. Chest tube drainage in excess of 150 to 200 ml/hr for 2 hours may indicate increased bleeding and may require emergent thoracic reexploration. Excess bleeding may also be a result of coagulopathy. Serum coagulation profiles (e.g., PT, PTT, platelet count, fibrinogen) may reveal deficits requiring replacement with fresh frozen plasma, platelets, cryoprecipitate, and clotting factors. Anemia associated with excess bleeding can lead to relative hypoxemia and requires prompt replacement with packed RBCs.

6. Prophylactic antibiotic therapy may be ordered.

7. If cardiac arrest occurs, internal cardiac massage and internal defibrillation should be substituted in the ACLS protocol.

Critical observations

Consult with the physician for the following:

1. Dislodgement of cannulas
2. Tubing obstruction
3. Inability to maintain MAP
4. Evidence of infection

GI INTUBATION

Clinical Brief

GI tubes are used to evacuate gastric contents, to decompress the stomach and intestines, to instill irrigants and/or medications, and to feed the patient. GI tubes are summarized in Table 7-9.

Contraindications for nasogastric tubes include patients with aneurysms or obstructive diseases of the throat or who have had a recent MI. Nasointestinal tubes should not be placed in patients with decreased intestinal motility or an obstruction of any kind, unless the tube is being used to decompress the intestines.

In addition to nasogastric and nasointestinal tubes, several types of tubes are available to tamponade (compress) the stomach and esophagus to temporarily control bleeding.

▶ Complications and related nursing diagnoses

General

Excessive removal of body fluids and electrolytes	Risk for injury: dysrhythmias Fluid volume deficit
Nares breakdown	Impaired skin integrity
Esophageal ulceration	Altered tissue perfusion
Esophageal rupture	Decreased cardiac output
Otitis media or parotitis	Pain
Incompetent gastroesophageal sphincter	Risk for aspiration
Inadequate airway clearance	Ineffective breathing pattern Impaired gas exchange
Epistaxis	Fluid volume deficit Impaired tissue integrity
Sinusitis	Altered tissue perfusion
Esophagitis	Altered tissue perfusion

TABLE 7-9 Summary of Gastrointestinal Tubes

Tube	Description
Nasogastric	
Levin	Single-lumen, no air vent; rubber or plastic; risk of mucosal damage when applied to suction
Salem sump	Double-lumen; air vent reduces risk of mucosal damage; clear plastic
Nutriflex	Feeding tube, weighted tip
Ewald	Large bore used to lavage clots or substances from the stomach; used for emergencies only
Esophageal	
Sengstaken-Blakemore	Triple-lumen, double balloon: one for esophageal compression and one for gastric compression; allows for gastric aspiration but not esophageal suction
Minnesota	Quadruple-lumen, double balloon for esophageal and gastric compression as well as gastric and esophageal suctioning
Linton	Triple-lumen, single balloon for gastric compression allows for gastric and esophageal suctioning
Nasointestinal	
Miller-Abbott	Double-lumen, one for suctioning, one to fill the distal balloon with mercury or air after insertion to decompress the small bowel
Cantor	Weighted with mercury before insertion; single-lumen
Harris	Weighted, single-lumen
Duotube (Entriflex, Dobhoff)	Feeding tubes, weighted, single-lumen; guidewire used to facilitate insertion

Nasogastric

Pharyngeal obstruction with Sengstaken-Blakemore tube	Ineffective breathing pattern
Esophageal/gastric erosion	Pain
	Decreased cardiac output
	Fluid volume deficit

General Patient Care Management Guidelines

Patient assessment

1. Prior to insertion, assess for history of nasal surgery, nasal fractures, or deviated septum. Notify physician if history positive.
2. Assess level of consciousness; patients with altered mentation may inadvertently remove the NG or NI tube.
3. Examine the naris daily for redness or skin breakdown.
4. Be alert for complications related to nasoenteric intubation.

Patient management

1. Once proper tube placement is confirmed, secure the tube per facility policy. Prevent movement at the nares to avoid skin irritation.
2. Attach to appropriate amount and type of suction as prescribed by the physician.
3. Provide meticulous mouth care: teeth brushing, mouthwash, lozenges if permitted. Mucous membranes should be kept moist; apply lip balm as needed.
4. Keep HOB elevated to prevent the possibility of aspiration.
5. Irrigate the tube as ordered to ensure patency. Validate tube irrigation with physician if the patient has undergone gastric surgery.
6. Check placement of the tube before administering anything down the tube. Flush before and after instillation of medications. Clamp tube for 30 to 45 minutes after the instillation of medications.
7. To obtain a gastric pH reading, have the patient lie on the left side; stop NG suction, and withdraw 10 to 15 ml discard fluid; use a second syringe to withdraw a sample for testing. Use pH paper with appropriate pH range. Do not use the syringe used for antacid administration to obtain the gastric sample. Generally gastric pH should be kept above 3.5 to decrease the chance for stress ulcers. An inability to raise pH >4 may indicate sepsis.
8. Record color, consistency, and amount of drainage.

GI

Nasogastric-tube patient care management

1. Check placement of tube in the stomach by aspirating with a syringe and testing pH of aspirate. Instill 10 to 30 ml of air into the tube and auscultate the gastric area: air rushing or gurgling will be heard if the tube is in the proper position.
2. See p. 635 for information on enteral feedings.

Nasointestinal-tube patient care management

1. If inserting an NI tube that requires a stylet to facilitate placement, never reinsert the stylet into the tube after it is placed in the patient.
2. Feeding tubes require radiographic verification of position before feedings can begin. Placing the patient in a right side-lying position may enhance tube advancement.
3. See information on p. 635 for enteral feedings.

Sengstaken-Blakemore/Minnesota tube patient care management

1. Intubation and sedation are recommended before insertion of a Sengstaken-Blakemore (Figure 7-7) or Minnesota tube.

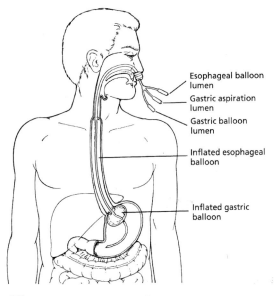

Esophageal balloon lumen

Gastric aspiration lumen

Gastric balloon lumen

Inflated esophageal balloon

Inflated gastric balloon

Figure 7-7 Sengstaken-Blakemore tube.

2. Tube placement is verified by air injection into the stomach or aspiration of gastric contents. A radiograph confirms the position of the gastric balloon against the cardia of the stomach.

3. After radiographic verification, the gastric balloon is inflated with 200 to 500 ml of air. Many institutions require a football helmet to be placed on the patient's head to secure the tractioned tube to the helmet. Be sure the helmet is a proper fit. A Salem sump is inserted into the esophagus to remove secretions if a Sengstaken-Blakemore tube is used, since the patient will not be able to swallow. A gastric aspirate port and Salem sump (or esophageal aspirate port) are connected to low suction.

4. The esophageal balloon is inflated only after radiographic confirmation of the position of the gastric balloon and if bleeding continues. Pressure in the esophageal balloon (usually 2 to 25 mm Hg) should be checked q2h to be sure it does not exceed 40 mm Hg. Esophageal balloon deflation should be done q4h for 10 minutes by physician's order only. The gastric balloon is never deflated while the esophageal balloon is inflated. Generally the tube is not left inflated for more than 48 hours.

5. Scissors should be kept at the bedside to cut the balloon ports in case of airway obstruction from upward migration of the tube.

6. All ports of the tube should be clearly labeled. Never inject fluids in the esophageal port. Normal saline irrigation may be needed to keep the gastric aspirate port patent.

7. If bleeding appears to have stopped, the esophageal balloon is slowly deflated. Traction is relaxed on the gastric balloon and gastric aspirate is monitored for recurrence of bleeding. All air from the esophageal and gastric balloon is aspirated before the tube is removed.

8. Hgb and Hct are usually monitored every 2 to 4 hours. A drop in hematocrit by 3% indicates 1 unit of blood lost.

9. An acute onset of abdominal or back pain may indicate esophageal rupture.

Critical observations

Consult with the physician for the following:

1. Fluid or electrolyte imbalance from prolonged gastric suctioning

2. Possible esophageal or gastric rupture and patient showing signs of shock

3. Respiratory distress from tube displacement or aspiration
4. Complaints of ear or neck pain associated with otitis media or parotitis
5. Increasing abdominal distention
6. Obstructed tube that will not irrigate
7. Inability to remove the tube
8. Gastric pH less than 3.5 or value specified by the physician

GI SURGERY

Clinical Brief

Surgical intervention may be required to control gastric bleeding if conservative medical therapy fails. The primary aim is to prevent the patient from bleeding to death with a secondary aim of preventing recurrence. Common surgical procedures may include laparoscopic vagotomy, pyloroplasty, and antrectomy accompanied by gastroduodenostomy with or without vagotomy. Common surgical procedures to treat duodenal ulcers may include vagotomy with antrectomy and either a gastroduodenostomy (Billroth I) or gastrojejunostomy (Billroth II). These procedures partially neutralize gastric acid and remove stimuli for acid secretion.

Esophageal varices can be corrected with (1) portacaval, (2) mesocaval, (3) splenorenal, and (4) gastric venacaval shunts or emergency staple transection. Shunts decrease venous blood flow through the portal system and consequently reduce portal hypertension.

▶ Complications and related nursing diagnoses

Gastric surgery

Hemorrhage	Decreased cardiac output
	Fluid volume deficit
	Altered tissue perfusion
Paralytic ileus/obstruction	Pain
	Ineffective breathing pattern
Respiratory distress	Ineffective breathing pattern
	Altered tissue perfusion
	Impaired gas exchange
Stump leakage/peritonitis	Hyperthermia
	Pain
Wound infection	Hyperthermia
	Impaired skin integrity
Dumping syndrome	Altered nutrition: less than body requirements

Fluid and electrolyte loss	Risk for injury
	Fluid volume deficit
Dehiscence	Risk for infection
	Pain
Acute gastric dilation	Ineffective breathing pattern
	Pain
	Constipation
Fistula	Altered nutrition: less than body requirements
	Diarrhea
Diarrhea	Fluid volume deficit

Shunt

Encephalopathy	Acute confusion
	Altered protection
GI bleed	Decreased cardiac output
	Altered tissue perfusion
Ascites	Ineffective breathing pattern
	Fluid volume deficit

Patient Care Management Guidelines

Patient assessment

1. Assess hemodynamic status: A HR >100 beats/min, SBP <90 mm Hg, CVP <2 mm Hg, and a PAWP <4 mm Hg are signs of hypovolemia. A MAP <60 mm Hg reflects inadequate tissue perfusion. Assess the surgical dressing for excessive bleeding or drainage. Review serial Hgb and Hct levels. Measure I & O hourly, including drainage from all tubes and drains. Urine output should be >30ml/hr; 50ml/hr is more desirable. Determine fluid balance q8h: output should approximate intake. Compare serial weights to evaluate rapid changes (0.5-1 kg/day indicates fluid imbalance; 1 kg ~ 1000 ml fluid). Note skin turgor on the inner thigh or forehead, the condition of buccal membranes, and development of edema or crackles. Gastric surgery: NG drainage may be bright red postoperatively but should become dark red or brown within 12 hours after surgery; drainage should normalize to green-yellow within 24 to 36 hours postoperatively.

2. Continuously monitor ECG for lethal dysrhythmias that may result from electrolyte imbalance, hypoxemia, hemorrhage.

GI

3. Assess respiratory status: Note depth, rate, and skin color q15min postoperatively until stable, then every 1 to 2 hours. Patients with abdominal surgery tend to take shallow breaths secondary to incisional pain.
4. Assess GI function: epigastric pain, tachycardia, and hypotension may signal gastric dilation; distention, rebound tenderness or rigidity may signal internal bleeding. Note any hiccups or complaints of fullness or gagging and auscultate abdomen for return of bowel sounds.
5. Determine level of comfort by using a visual analogue scale (VAS) or other pain-measuring tool. (See Figure 1-1.)
6. Record temperature and monitor for development of infection: assess incision, IV sites, and drain sites. Consider the urinary tract and lungs as potential sites of infection. Review serial WBC and culture reports (if available).
7. Assess neurological status, development of GI bleeding, and onset of ascites in patients undergoing portacaval shunts.

Patient management

1. Provide supplemental oxygen as ordered. (See p. 577 for information on mechanical ventilation.)
2. Administer IV fluids and/or blood products as ordered to correct intravascular volume and replace blood loss.
3. Monitor serum electrolytes and replace as ordered.
4. Use sterile procedure when manipulating gastrointestinal tubes, surgical dressings, and indwelling lines. Protect the integrity of the skin during frequent dressing changes by using Montgomery straps. Use an abdominal binder to protect against wound dehiscence.
5. Maintain patency of the NG tube to prevent undue pressure on suture line. Do not irrigate or reposition tubes without the physician's order. Provide good care of the nares and mouth. Test gastric secretions for blood and pH. Generally gastric pH is maintained between 3.5 and 5 to prevent further development of stress ulcers. Antacids may be prescribed.
6. Administer antiemetics to prevent vomiting and preserve the integrity of the suture line.
7. Administer nutritional supplements or support as ordered. Vitamin B_{12} will be ordered for patients undergoing a total gastrectomy to prevent pernicious anemia.

Oral feedings may not be instituted until bowel sounds have returned.

8. Administer analgesics as indicated, since abdominal pain may interfere with adequate ventilation; note RR before and after medication administration. If RR is <12/min, do not administer narcotics. Evaluate effectiveness of pain medication. (See p. 30 for information on pain.)

9. Assist patient with turning, coughing, and deep breathing at least q2h to maximize oxygenation and prevent atelectasis.

Critical observations

Consult with the physician for the following:

1. Signs of hypovolemia: increasing trend in heart rate; decreasing trend in urine output, CVP, PA pressures, and BP
2. Respiratory distress
3. Temperature elevation or signs of infection
4. An unusual amount of bright red blood that appears 24 hours after surgery, either through the NG/NI tube or on the dressings
5. Increasing abdominal distention
6. Absence of drainage from the NG/NI tube
7. Urine output less than 30 ml/hr
8. Wound dehiscence
9. Abnormal laboratory data
10. Uncontrolled pain

LIVER TRANSPLANTATION

Clinical Brief

Liver transplantation may be considered in patients with (1) end-stage liver disease with a life expectancy of less than one year, (2) a quality of life poor enough to justify the risks of transplant, and (3) liver-based metabolic disease that has lethal implications. The majority of liver transplants are done for cirrhosis (chronic hepatitis, primary and secondary biliary cirrhosis, Laennec's cirrhosis, postnecrotic cirrhosis secondary to viral, autoimmune or cryptogenic mechanisms). The selection criteria vary depending on the transplant center.

Absolute contraindications are extrahepatic malignancy, sepsis, multisystem disease, active use of hepatotoxic drugs, and HIV antibody positive. Relative contraindications include history of or active alcohol abuse, portal vein thrombosis, hepatitis B surface antigen, prior complex hepatobiliary disease, advanced chronic renal disease, or prior porta-caval shunt. One year survival is 75%; 5 year survival is 70% with best results in patients with cholestatic liver disease and poorest results in patients with hepatitis B and hepatobiliary malignancy. The most important determinant of survival is the patient's clinical condition.

▶ Complications and related nursing diagnoses

Rejection	Pain
	Hyperthermia
	Risk for injury
Post-op infection	Pain
	Hyperthermia
	Impaired skin integrity
Renal insufficiency	Risk for injury
Hemorrhage	Fluid volume deficit
	Decreased cardiac output
	Altered tissue perfusion
Respiratory failure	Impaired gas exchange
	Ineffective breathing pattern
Ascites	Ineffective breathing pattern
	Fluid volume deficit
Fluid and electrolyte loss	Risk for injury
	Fluid volume deficit
Coagulopathy	Altered tissue perfusion
	Risk for injury
Encephalopathy	Acute confusion
	Risk for injury
Thrombosis hepatic artery or portal vein	Altered tissue perfusion
	Increased cardiac output
	Hyperthermia
Bile leak	Pain
	Hyperthermia
Biliary obstruction	Hyperthermia
	Increased cardiac output
Bowel obstruction/ paralytic ileus	Pain
	Ineffective breathing pattern
Bowel perforation	Decreased cardiac output
	Pain

Patient Care Management Guidelines

Patient assessment

1. Assess hemodynamic status: CVP, PA pressures, CI, HR, BP. Patients in liver failure frequently have an

increased CI and decreased SVRI before surgery; this may continue into the early postoperative period. Fluid shifts frequently occur affecting circulating volume. Hemorrhage may also occur and Hgb and Hct should be monitored. Hypertension is frequently seen post-op.

2. Assess fluid status: measure intake and output hourly, including drainage from all tubes and drains. Urine output should be >30 ml/hr; 50 ml/hr is more desirable. Determine fluid balance q8h. Compare serial weights to evaluate rapid changes (0.5 to 1 kg/day indicates fluid imbalance). Note skin turgor on inner thigh or forehead, condition of buccal membranes, development of edema or crackles.

3. Assess tissue perfusion: note level of mentation, skin color and temperature, peripheral pulses, and capillary refill.

4. Continuously monitor ECG for dysrhythmias that may result from electrolyte imbalance, hypoxemia, and/or hemorrhage.

5. Assess temperature. Patients may be hypothermic on returning from surgery. Monitor for signs of infection: incision lines, T-tube site, drain tubes. Consider the urinary tract, lungs, and mucous membranes as potential sites of infection, especially because of immunosuppression. Review serial WBC and culture reports (if available).

6. Assess respiratory status: Note depth, rate, and skin color q15min postoperatively until stable, then every 1 to 2 hours. Monitor pulse oximetry continuously and ABGs as ordered. Patients with abdominal surgery tend to take shallow breaths secondary to incisional pain.

7. Assess GI function: reaccumulation of ascites, bowel sounds. Abdominal tenderness, nausea and vomiting, or abdominal distention may indicate ileus or a more significant event (e.g., bowel infarction, hemorrhage). Measure abdominal girth q shift.

8. Assess bile production: quality and quantity. Bile should be thick, viscous, and range from dark gold to brown. Variation from these findings may indicate a primary nonfunctioning graft.

9. Determine level of comfort by using a visual analogue scale (VAS) or other pain-measuring tool. (See Figure 1-1.)

10. Assess liver function: monitor coagulation times, potassium, and glucose and liver function tests closely. Normal coagulation times, decreased potassium, increased glucose, and decreased liver function tests indicate a

functioning liver. Decreased coagulation times, increased potassium, decreased glucose, and continued elevation of liver function tests are indicative of a non-functioning liver.

11. Monitor acid-base balance. Patients are frequently in a metabolic alkalosis in the first 24 to 48 hours due to the large citrate load, decreased potassium, diuretics, and large amounts of fresh frozen plasma.

12. Assess neurological status. Potential side effects of cyclosporine include confusion, cortical blindness, quadriplegia, encephalopathy, seizures, and coma

13. Assess renal function: monitor BUN and creatinine daily. Patients are at risk for renal insufficiency.

Patient management

1. Provide supplemental oxygen as ordered. See p. 577 for information on mechanical ventilation.

2. Administer IV fluids and/or blood products as ordered to correct intravascular volume and replace blood loss and coagulation factors.

3. Monitor serum electrolytes and replace as ordered.

4. Use sterile procedure when manipulating gastrointestinal tubes, surgical dressings, and indwelling lines. Protect the integrity of the skin during frequent dressing changes by using Montgomery straps.

5. Maintain patency of the NG tube to prevent undue pressure on suture line. Do not irrigate or reposition tubes without the physician's order. Provide good care of the nares and mouth.

6. Administer corticosteroids, azathioprine, cyclosporine, and/or OKT3 as ordered. Monitor for side effects.

7. Administer analgesics as indicated, since abdominal pain may interfere with adequate ventilation; note RR before and after medication administration. If RR is <12/min, do not administer narcotics. Evaluate effectiveness of pain medication.

8. Assist patient with turning, coughing, and deep breathing at least q2h once extubated to maximize oxygenation and prevent atelectasis.

9. Administer prophylactic antibiotics as ordered.

10. Administer meticulous skin and mouth care, using nystatin for oral care.

11. When the patient is able to eat, ensure a high calorie, high protein diet, as protein synthesis is decreased by liver damage and steroids have a catabolic effect.

Critical observations

Consult with the physician for the following:

1. Signs of hypovolemia: increasing trend in heart rate; decreasing trend in urine output, CVP, PA pressures, and BP
2. Signs of respiratory distress
3. Temperature elevation or signs of infection
4. Change in bile production or drainage
5. Increasing abdominal distention, tenderness
6. Increased potassium, decreased glucose, abnormal coagulation times, and increased liver function tests
7. Urine output <30 ml/hr; increasing BUN and creatinine
8. Uncontrolled pain

NUTRITION: ENTERAL FEEDINGS

Clinical Brief

Enteral feedings include liquid formula diets that are provided orally or via a tube placed down the esophagus into either the stomach or the intestines when the patient's voluntary intake does not meet at least two thirds of the patient's needs. Intermittent feedings infused by gravity are recommended when feedings are instilled into the stomach. If feedings are entering the duodenum or jejunum, continuous feeding via pump is recommended, which usually results in less bowel distention, less fluid and electrolyte imbalance, less aspiration, and improved patient tolerance of the product. When tube feedings are considered for long-term nutritional therapy (greater than 4 weeks), the tube is surgically placed in the patient (e.g., gastrostomy or jejunostomy). Blenderized feedings and commercially prepared dietary formulations are ordered by the physician based on GI tract ability to digest and absorb nutrients, the nutrient needs of the patient, and fluid and electrolyte restrictions.

Preparations

Generally all products contain carbohydrates, fats, protein, vitamins, minerals, and water but vary in the amounts and types of each nutrient. Complete (polymeric) formulas require digestion and thus an intact GI tract. Elemental (monomeric or oligomeric) formulas are predigested and can be absorbed in GI tracts with limited digestion. Specially designed products are also available in both forms for specific disease states or conditions.

Patients with hepatic encephalopathy may receive Travasorb-Hepatic or Hepatic Aid II, since they contain high quantities of branched-chain amino acids. Amin-Aid or Travasorb-Renal

GI

may be prescribed for patients in renal failure, since these formulas attempt to decrease the urea production. Patients who are burned or septic may be prescribed Stresstein, Criticare, or Traum-Aid, which attempt to stimulate protein synthesis and reduce proteolysis. Patients in respiratory failure having difficulty weaning from the ventilator may be prescribed Pulmocare or formulas with increased fat content, which attempt to reduce CO_2 production, oxygen consumption, and ventilatory requirements.

Most formulas are isotonic and provide about 45 g of protein per liter although hypertonic formulas are available. High-fiber (Jevity) and low-residue (Resource, Fortison) formulas are available, as are supplements that provide extra calories (Microlipid, Promod, MCT oil).

Isotonic formulas are usually administered at full-strength and the rate is increased as tolerated. Hypertonic formulas are initially administered either at full-strength at a slow rate (25 ml/hr) or half-strength at 50 ml/hr. Intolerance of hypertonic formulas may be indicated by severe diarrhea, electrolyte depletion, and dehydration.

Contraindications

Enteral feedings are not recommended in patients with persistent nausea and vomiting, intolerable postprandial abdominal pain or diarrhea, severe ileus, intestinal obstruction, GI bleeding, and acute pancreatitis.

▶ Complications and related nursing diagnoses

Aspiration	Ineffective airway clearance
	Impaired gas exchange
Diarrhea	Impaired skin integrity
	Fluid volume deficit
Abdominal distention	Pain
Hyperglycemic hyperosmolar nonketotic coma	Decreased cardiac output
	Fluid volume deficit
	Risk for injury: seizures
Hyponatremia/hypokalemia	Risk for injury

Patient Care Management Guidelines

Patient assessment

1. Assess nutritional status: prealbumin is considered the best indicator of nutrition status. Serum albumin <3.5% g/dl, transferrin <180 mg/dl, and lymphocyte <1500/µl

are indications of malnourishment. Skin anergy testing (negative response to antigen) represents malnutrition. Twenty-four-hour urinary urea nitrogen study measures nitrogen balance by subtracting the amount of nitrogen lost from the daily intake in either enteral or parenteral sources. Creatinine-height index measures the amount of creatinine excreted in a 24-hour period proportionately to the height of the patient and reflects muscle wasting. Anthropometric measurements of body size can be taken; tricep skinfold thickness <3 mm indicates severely depleted fat stores; a midarm circumference <15 cm means muscle wasting. Measure height and weight and compare with desired-weight tables. A decrease of 15% from ideal weight indicates impaired nutrition.

2. Assess GI tolerance: note nausea, vomiting, diarrhea or cramping, and any abdominal distention or absence of bowel sounds; the infusion rate may need to be reduced if these symptoms appear.

3. Monitor flow rates and volumes to ensure that the patient is actually receiving the prescribed amount of calories, since continuous feedings are often interrupted.

Patient management

1. Insufflation of air and aspiration of gastric contents do not confirm placement of nasoenteric tubes. Confirmation with radiography is necessary before feedings are initiated. Mark feeding tube at exit site once placement is confirmed.

2. With continuous feedings, elevate the HOB 30 degrees at all times to reduce the risk of aspiration. If the patient needs to be supine, turn off the feeding.

3. Small bowel feedings are generally initiated at 50 ml/hr with full-strength isotonic solution. A hypertonic formula can be diluted to quarter-strength or half-strength. Gradually increase the rate, usually 25 ml q8h, and strength of the formula; evaluate patient tolerance.

4. For intragastric feedings, generally, tube feedings are initiated with an isotonic formula and the nutrient requirements are achieved by increasing the rate over 1 to 2 days.

5. A small amount of food dye added to the formula will help assess the patient for possible aspiration. When suctioning or coughing produces sputum that matches the

GI

color of the formula, turn the feeding off. Check the sputum or tracheal aspirate for glucose with a glucose reagent strip if aspiration of formula is suspected. Have the placement of the feeding tube confirmed.

6. Check residual at least q4h for patients receiving continuous gastric feedings. If more than 100 ml or greater than 50% of the hourly rate, hold the feedings and check again for residual in 2 hours. Metoclopramide (Reglan) may be ordered to increase gastric motility. Small-bore feeding tubes often collapse when the nurse is aspirating for residuals. Observe the patient for the development of abdominal distention.

7. Administer the feeding as ordered, slowly and consistently. A feeding pump is recommended for more accurate administration. Time tape the bag if a pump is not readily available.

8. Flush the feeding tube with 50 to 150 ml of water or carbonated beverage q4h, before and after each intermittent feeding, or once a shift for continuous feeding. Flush the tube if the feeding has been stopped for any reason and after administration of medications via the tube. Carbonated beverages have been shown to unclog feeding tubes. Use a clear beverage (not cola) to accurately assess the gastric residual if GI bleeding is suspected. Other substances that have been used successfully to clear an obstructed tube include cranberry juice, meat tenderizer, and pancreatic enzymes.

9. Have medications changed to elixirs. If medications must be crushed, be certain they are finely ground and dissolved in water to prevent obstruction of the feeding tube. Sustained-release and enteric-coated medications must not be crushed. Flush the tube before and after medication administration.

10. Provide good oral care, since mouth breathing is common in patients who have a nasal tube present.

11. Limit bacterial growth by changing tube-feeding containers q24h or per hospital policy; generally formula should not hang longer than 4 hours.

12. Administer free-water supplements as ordered by the physician to prevent dehydration; as much as 0.5 ml for every 1 ml of feeding can be ordered.

13. When flushing or irrigating small-bore tubing, use the syringe size recommended by the manufacturer. A small

syringe can exert greater pressure with minimal effort and may rupture the tube.

14. If the patient develops diarrhea, consider the use of pre-mixed sterile bags of tube feeding and bulk-forming cathartics.

Critical observations

Consult with the physician for the following:

1. Gastric residual >50% of hourly delivery rate
2. Uncontrolled diarrhea
3. Increasing abdominal distention, N/V, absent bowel sounds
4. Elevated serum glucose
5. Dehydration: dry buccal membranes, nonelastic skin turgor, specific gravity >1.035
6. Tube displacement
7. Possible aspiration/respiratory distress
8. Mucosal damage from tube

NUTRITION: PARENTERAL

Clinical Brief

In the event the patient does not receive sufficient nutrition with enteral feedings or cannot functionally take substances through the stomach or bowel or when it is necessary to put the GI system to rest, parenteral nutrition (PN) containing the required water, nutrients, protein, carbohydrates, fats, electrolytes, vitamins, and minerals may be initiated. Parenteral nutrition may be administered peripherally or via a central line. Centrally, a hypertonic solution of as much as 50% dextrose may be administered. Amino acids, electrolytes, vitamins, and minerals can be tailored to meet the needs of the patient. Regular laboratory assessment (nutritional panel) and anthropometric measurements provide information to guard against underfeeding or overfeeding, conditions that can adversely affect pulmonary, renal, and hepatic functioning.

Peripheral parenteral nutrition can be initiated when the objective is to prevent starvation and not to treat malnutrition or when central venous access cannot be obtained. The glucose concentration is limited to 10% in peripheral parenteral nutrition, since sclerosis of the vein can occur with more hypertonic solutions. Other components include amino acids, vitamins, electrolytes, and trace elements. The prescribed solution is transfused through a dedicated peripheral line, eliminating the complications of central line insertion and maintenance.

Lipids

To avoid the excessive production of carbon dioxide that results when carbohydrates are used as the sole caloric source and to prevent essential endogenous fatty acid deficiency, lipids are administered in addition to PN. Lipids supply the essential fatty acids necessary for protein metabolism and cell function and should constitute 30% or more of total calories. Usually a 10% emulsion (500 ml) is administered 2 to 3 times a week.

▶ **Complications and related nursing diagnoses**

Sepsis	Decreased cardiac output Altered tissue perfusion
Glucose intolerance hyperglycemia	Risk for infection
Electrolyte imbalance	Risk for injury
Dehydration	Fluid volume deficit

Catheter-related complications can be found on p. 551.

Patient Care Management Guidelines

Patient assessment

1. Monitor temperature at least once each shift to evaluate the onset of infection. Unexplained fever may be related to central venous catheter sepsis.
2. Assess IV catheter insertion site for redness, drainage, or tenderness.
3. Check serum glucose as ordered to identify onset of hyperglycemia. Glucose homeostasis should be 120 to 180 mg/dl. Levels >220 mg/dl can impair phagocyte function. Acute hyperglycemia may signal sepsis.
4. Review laboratory results for metabolic abnormalities associated with PN therapy: serum glucose, electrolytes, CBC, platelet count, potassium, phosphate, calcium, magnesium, BUN, creatinine, alkaline phosphatase, bilirubin, PT, iron, uric acid, and AST (SGOT).
5. Monitor total lymphocyte count, serum albumin, and transferrin to determine efficacy of PN.
6. Assess fluid volume status: compare daily weights and record intake and output. Note signs and symptoms of dehydration or fluid overload.
7. If the patient is mechanically ventilated or has a history of CO_2 retention, assess CO_2 levels.

8. Central line placement must be confirmed via chest radiograph prior to administration of any solutions through the lines.

Patient management

1. Do not administer medications or blood products through the nutrition-dedicated line. If long-term parenteral nutrition is necessary, a long-term venous access device may be required. See p. 551 for information and venous access devices.

2. To prevent infection, use aseptic technique when performing dressing or tubing changes. Change dressing and tubing per hospital guidelines or if dressing becomes soiled or nonocclusive. Keep all solutions refrigerated, check expiration dates, and administer within 24 hours of preparation. Do not use the PN if the solution is cloudy or contains particulates. Luer lock all tubing connections to prevent inadvertent disconnection and a possible air embolus.

3. Validate correct nutritional components and infuse as ordered. Initial rate is usually 50 to 100 ml/hr and increased 25 to 50 ml/hr/day, depending on cardiovascular and renal status.

4. Do not stop PN abruptly, since hypoglycemia can result. If PN is not available, administer $D_{10}W$ at the PN rate until the solution is available. To avoid inconsistent delivery rates that may precipitate rebound hypoglycemia or hyperglycemia reactions, use an infusion pump to administer PN.

5. Insulin added to the PN solution or on a sliding scale is usually required to control hyperglycemia. Check glucose levels q6h.

6. Phytonadione may be given weekly to prevent coagulopathy associated with vitamin K deficiency.

7. Fat supplements may be prescribed. Initial therapy requires a slow infusion rate for the first 15 to 30 minutes (1 ml/min for a 10% emulsion; 0.5 ml/min for a 20% emulsion); monitor the patient for respiratory distress associated with hypoxemia and cyanosis. If no adverse effects occur initiate the prescribed infusion rate. Blood samples to measure serum triglyceride and liver function tests may be obtained to determine the patient's ability to utilize lipids.

Critical observations

Consult with physician for the following:

1. Temperature elevation
2. Catheter displacement or thrombosis

3. Fluid overload or dehydration
4. Hyperglycemia
5. Electrolyte imbalances
6. Adverse effects with lipid administration

PANCREAS TRANSPLANTATION

Clinical Brief

Pancreas transplantation may be considered in patients with (1) insulin-dependent diabetes mellitus, (2) evidence of secondary complications which are or will be more serious than the risks of major surgery and immunosuppression, (3) secondary complications not advanced enough to be self-perpetuating, (4) diabetes mellitus with end-stage renal disease who have or will receive a kidney transplant, and (5) imperfect metabolic control of exogenous insulin. The ideal patient will have no secondary lesions. Pancreas transplants can be performed (1) alone in the preuremic patient, (2) after successful kidney transplant, or (3) simultaneously with kidney transplant.

Contraindications include metastatic cancer, infection, psychosis, severe incapacitating neuropathies, inoperable peripheral vascular or cardiovascular disease, or overwhelming immunosuppressive disease.

► **Complications and related nursing diagnoses**

Rejection	Pain
	Hyperthermia
	Risk for injury
Thrombosis	Altered tissue perfusion
Infection	Pain
	Hyperthermia
	Impaired skin integrity
Hemorrhage	Fluid volume deficit
	Decreased cardiac output
	Altered tissue perfusion
Anastomotic leaks	Pain
	Hyperthermia
Graft pancreatitis	Pain
Urethritis (males)	Pain

Patient Care Management Guidelines

Patient assessment

1. Assess hemodynamic status: A HR >100 beats/min, SBP <90 mm Hg, CVP <2 mm Hg, and a PAWP

<4 mm Hg are signs of hypovolemia. Monitor MAP; a MAP <60 mm Hg reflects inadequate tissue perfusion.

2. Assess fluid status: measure intake and output hourly, including drainage from all tubes and drains. Urine output should be >30 ml/hr; 50 ml/hr is more desirable. Determine fluid balance q8h. Compare serial weights to evaluate rapid changes (0.5 to 1kg/day indicates fluid imbalance). Note skin turgor on inner thigh or forehead, condition of buccal membranes, and development of edema or crackles.

3. Assess tissue perfusion: note level of mentation, skin color and temperature, peripheral pulses, and capillary refill.

4. Continuously monitor ECG for dysrhythmias that may result from electrolyte imbalance, hypoxemia, or hemorrhage.

5. Assess temperature. Monitor for signs of infection. Consider the urinary tract, lungs, and mucous membranes as potential sites of infection, especially because of immunosuppression. Review serial WBC and culture reports (if available).

6. Assess respiratory status: Note depth, rate, and skin color q15min postoperatively until stable, then every 1 to 2 hours. Monitor pulse oximetry continuously and ABGs as ordered. Patients with abdominal surgery tend to take shallow breaths secondary to incisional pain.

7. Assess GI function: palpate graft site for pain, edema, and tenderness that might indicate rejection. Assess for bowel sounds.

8. Determine level of comfort by using a visual analogue scale (VAS) or other pain-measuring tool. (See Figure 1-1.) See p. 30 for information on pain.

9. Assess glucose q30min to 1h, urine amylase q6h, urine pH q6h and temperature q4h. Glucose is an indicator of graft perfusion. An upward trend in glucose and temperature and downward trend in urine amylase and urine pH indicate rejection. A *sudden* increase in serum glucose or *sudden* decrease in urine amylase may indicate thrombosis.

10. Assess acid-base balance. Metabolic acidosis may occur when urinary diversion is used for exocrine drainage.

11. Assess for signs of anastomotic leaks: lower abdominal pain, fever, leukocytosis, increased serum amylase and creatinine.

12. Assess for rejection (renal transplant): increased BUN and creatinine, decreased urine output, increased BP, increased weight, fever, graft tenderness. See p. 656 for information on renal transplant.

Patient management

1. Provide supplemental oxygen as ordered. See p. 577 for information on mechanical ventilation.
2. Administer IV fluids and/or blood products as ordered to correct intravascular volume and replace blood loss.
3. Monitor serum electrolytes and replace as ordered.
4. Use sterile procedure when manipulating gastrointestinal tubes, surgical dressings, and indwelling lines. Protect the integrity of the skin during frequent dressing changes by using Montgomery straps.
5. Maintain patient on bed rest without hip flexion on side of graft for 48 to 72 hours to prevent thrombosis of graft vessels.
6. Administer corticosteroids, azathioprine, cyclosporine, and antilymphocyte globulin (OKT3) as ordered.
7. Administer anticoagulants as ordered to decrease platelet aggregation and prevent thrombosis.
8. Administer bladder irrigation as ordered if simultaneous kidney transplant.
9. Maintain patency of the NG tube to prevent undue pressure on suture line. Do not irrigate or reposition tubes without the physician's order. Provide good care of the nares and mouth.
10. Administer analgesics as indicated, since abdominal pain may interfere with adequate ventilation; note RR before and after medication administration. If RR is <12/min, do not administer narcotics. Evaluate effectiveness of pain medication.
11. Administer prophylactic antibiotics as ordered.
12. Administer meticulous skin and mouth care, using nystatin for oral care.

Critical observations

Consult with the physician for the following:

1. Signs of fluid imbalance: decreasing systolic BP >20 mm Hg, increasing HR of >25 beats/min from baseline, decreasing trend in urine output, CVP, and PA pressures
2. Signs of respiratory distress

3. Temperature elevation or signs of infection
4. Upward trend in serum glucose or amylase, downward trend in urine amylase or urine pH
5. Urine output less than 30 ml/hr; increasing BUN and creatinine
6. Uncontrolled pain
7. Increasing abdominal distention, tenderness

TRANSJUGULAR INTRAHEPATIC PORTOSYSTEMIC SHUNT (TIPS)

Clinical Brief

Transjugular intrahepatic portosystemic shunt is used to treat patients with variceal hemorrhage not controlled by endoscopic or other nonoperative techniques, to stabilize patients awaiting liver transplant, and to treat patients with cirrhosis in which surgical decompression of portal hypertension is contraindicated. It is a nonsurgical procedure performed in interventional radiology to create a portosystemic shunt within the parenchyma of the liver. An expandable metal stent is inserted via the jugular vein into a tract created between the systemic and portal venous systems to redirect portal blood flow. The result is a decrease in portal venous pressure that decompresses varices and can relieve ascites.

▶ Complications and related nursing diagnoses

Stent stenosis/occlusion	Fluid volume deficit
	Altered tissue perfusion
Hemorrhage	Decreased cardiac output
	Altered tissue perfusion
Encephalopathy	Acute confusion
	Altered protection
Sepsis	Decreased cardiac output
	Altered tissue perfusion
Renal failure	Altered urinary elimination
	Fluid volume excess

Patient Care Management Guidelines

Patient assessment

1. Assess hemodynamic status: a HR >100 beats/min, SBP <90 mm Hg, CVP <2 mm Hg, PAWP <4 mm Hg, and cool, clammy skin may be signs of hemorrhage. Patient is

GI

at risk for hemorrhage due to damage to blood vessels and liver or inadvertent puncture of hepatic arteries. Recurrent esophageal bleeding may result from a stenotic or occluded stent.

2. Continuously monitor ECG for dysrhythmias.
3. Measure I & O hourly: urine output should be >30ml/hour. Determine fluid balance q8h; diuresis is desirable. Patient may receive Mannitol in radiology to aid in excretion of contrast media and prevent renal impairment.
4. Monitor respiratory status: depth, rate, and skin color q15min postprocedure until stable. Continuously monitor oxygen saturation via pulse oximetry.
5. Record temperature and monitor for development of infection.
6. Assess GI function: abdominal pain or abdominal distention, which may indicate hemorrhage, ascites, infection of the stent, or a stenotic or occluded stent. Recurrent esophageal bleeding may signal an occluded or stenotic stent.
7. Assess neurological status for signs of encephalopathy: personality changes, slurred or slow speech, decreased level of consciousness.

Patient management
1. Provide supplemental oxygen as ordered.
2. Administer IV fluids and/or blood products as ordered.
3. Administer antibiotics as ordered for prophylaxis.

Critical observations
Consult with the physician for the following:
1. Signs of hemorrhage
2. Change in level of consciousness
3. Urine output less than 30 ml/hr; increasing BUN and creatinine
4. Respiratory depression
5. Elevated temperature and signs of infection
6. Signs of hypovolemia: increasing trend in HR, decreasing trend in urine output, CVP, PA pressures, and BP

Renal Modalities

RENAL REPLACEMENT THERAPY

Clinical Brief

In all forms of renal replacement therapy, fluid is removed when a hydrostatic (hemodialysis and hemofiltration) or osmotic (peritoneal dialysis) pressure gradient is induced across a semipermeable membrane that contains the patient's blood. Solutes are removed by ultrafiltration (convection) or by diffusion (dialysis) across the semipermeable membrane.

There are various modes of renal replacement therapy, each having different advantages and disadvantages (Table 7-10).

Hemodialysis involves pumping the patient's heparinized blood through an extracorporeal filter composed of semipermeable membranes. Blood is removed from and returned to the body through a venous or an arteriovenous access in the form of femoral lines, a subclavian catheter, arteriovenous (AV) shunt, AV fistula, or AV graft.

Peritoneal dialysis involves introducing a hypertonic glucose solution (dialysate) into the peritoneal cavity through an abdominal catheter. The dialysate is left to dwell in the abdomen, allowing the exchange of solutes across the peritoneal membrane. The solution is then drained from the abdominal cavity.

Continuous renal replacement therapy (CRRT) is a continuous, slow form of hemofiltration that requires arteriovenous blood flow and extracorporeal filtration. The most basic form of CRRT is *slow continuous ultrafiltration (SCUF)*, also called *continuous arteriovenous ultrafiltration (CAVU)*, which is extracorporeal filtration with arteriovenous blood flow that does not use a blood pump or air detector as is done in hemodialysis (Figure 7-8). Blood flow through the CAVU circuit is primarily determined by the patient's mean arterial blood pressure, and an ultrafiltrate of plasma is removed (urea clearance is limited). Adding intravenous fluid replacement to the circuit, a process called *continuous arteriovenous hemofiltration (CAVH)*, improves fluid and solute removal. Hypertonic dialysate can also be run countercurrent to the

TABLE 7-10 Comparison of Renal Replacement Therapy Modes

	Peritoneal dialysis	Hemodialysis	CRRT*
Access	Peritoneal catheter	Arteriovenous or venous access	Arteriovenous or venous access
Membrane	Peritoneal	Extracorporeal filter	Extracorporeal filter
Advantages	Continuous, gentle fluid removal	Rapid, efficient fluid and waste removal	Continuous, slow, gentle fluid removal
Disadvantages	Protein loss, poor potassium removal	Hemodynamic instability, heparinization	Heparinization
Contraindications	Abdominal surgery, adhesions, or an undiagnosed acute condition of the abdomen; respiratory insufficiency	Hypotension, bleeding	Bleeding

*CRRT, continuous renal replacement therapy.

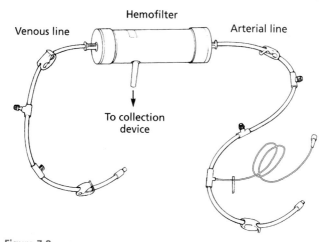

Figure 7-8 CAVH system. Venous blood flows through the hemofilter and returns through the arterial line. Various ports are available for fluid replacement, blood drawing, and heparinizing the system.

blood flow in a form of CRRT called *continuous arteriovenous hemodiafiltration (CAVHD)*. CAVHD combines the advantages of CAVH with improved clearance of BUN. *Continuous venovenous hemofiltration (CVVH)* is CRRT that utilizes a single double-lumen venous access and a blood pump. The advantages of CVVH are that it provides a constant blood flow rate, can be used in a patient with low blood pressure, and does not require femoral artery access. CVVH requires the use of venous pressure monitoring and an air detector.

▶ **Complications and related nursing diagnoses**

All forms of renal replacement therapy

Hypotension	Decreased cardiac output
	Fluid volume deficit
	Altered tissue perfusion
Infection	Risk for infection
	Hyperthermia
Electrolyte imbalances	Risk for injury

RENAL

Hemodialysis

Disequilibrium syndrome	Risk for injury
Air embolus	Decreased cardiac output
	Impaired gas exchange
	Pain
Hemolysis	Impaired gas exchange
	Altered tissue perfusion
Hemorrhage	Altered tissue perfusion
	Fluid volume deficit
	Decreased cardiac output

Continuous renal replacement therapy

Hemorrhage	Altered tissue perfusion
	Fluid volume deficit
	Decreased cardiac output
Clotting of filter	Risk for injury: thromboembolism

Peritoneal dialysis

Respiratory insufficiency	Ineffective breathing pattern
	Impaired gas exchange
Peritonitis	Risk for infection
	Hyperthermia

Patient Care Management Guidelines

HEMODIALYSIS
Patient assessment

1. Assess arteriovenous (AV) shunt, fistula, or graft for bruit and thrill each shift.
2. Assess for signs of infection, including redness, swelling, increased tenderness, and drainage at access site. Obtain temperature q4h and note any increase.
3. Assess hemodynamic and fluid volume status by monitoring:
   a. Hourly I & O.
   b. Vital signs and hemodynamic parameters (if available) q15min at the onset of treatment until stable, every half-hour during treatment once stable, and q4h when not being dialyzed.
   c. Breath sounds and heart sounds q4h.

   d. Weights daily if no dialysis is done; weights before, during, and after hemodialysis.

Patient management

1. Prevent infection by using good handwashing; initiating good hygiene; separating the patient from other patients with infections; aseptically caring for wounds and all invasive catheters; having the patient turn and C & DB; encouraging early ambulation; and providing good nutrition.

2. Post a sign in the patient's room informing all personnel not to draw blood or check blood pressure in limb with permanent vascular access device.

3. Keep two cannula clamps next to AV shunt at all times. If shunt becomes disconnected, apply clamps or direct pressure. Reconnect and assess for blood loss.

4. Aseptically clean insertion sites daily and before initiating dialysis. Change wet, soiled, or loose dressings immediately.

5. Consult with the physician regarding administration of antihypertensive, antiemetic, or narcotic agents before hemodialysis, since these agents induce hypotension.

6. Adjust schedule for administration of medications based on dialyzability of drug and time of dialysis. (See the box on p. 652 for common dialyzable medications.) Consult with the physician about administering a postdialysis supplemental dosage of any medication that is dialyzed out. Consult with the physician about obtaining drug levels of dialyzable medications to increase accuracy of dosing.

7. If the patient becomes hypotensive (SBP <90 mm Hg), place the patient flat. If SBP remains low, raise the patient's legs. Administer normal saline, replacement solution, or vasoactive medications as ordered. Assess for dysrhythmias and chest pain during hypotension.

8. If the patient experiences cramping in extremities, administer normal saline or hypertonic saline as ordered and decrease the rate of dialysis.

9. If the patient complains of popping or ringing in ears, dizziness, chest pain, and coughing or if the air is visible entering the patient's vascular return, suspect air embolus. Clamp all blood lines and place the patient in Trendelenberg position and on left side; administer oxygen.

RENAL

Common Dialyzable Medications

Aminoglycosides: Amikacin, gentamycin, kanamycin, neomycin, streptomycin, tobramycin, vancomycin

Cephalosporins: Cefazolin, cefuroxime, cefoxitin, ceftazidime, cephalothin, cephaloridine, cephalexin, cephapirin

Penicillins: Amoxicillin, ampicillin, carbenicillin, oxacillin, piparacillin, penicillin G, ticarcillin

Other antibiotics: Chloramphenicol, sulfonamides, trimethoprim

Cardiovascular agents: Procainamide, bretylium, nitroprusside, captopril, enalapril

Immunosuppressives/antineoplastics: Azathioprine, methylprednisolone, methotrexate

Miscellaneous: Acetaminophen, acetysalicylic acid, cimetidine, antituberculous drugs, librium, theophylline, phenobarbital, phenytoin, ranitidine, lorazepam

These medications often require increased dosing during dialysis or supplemental dosing after dialysis.
NOTE: Digoxin, propranolol, quinidine, lidocaine, furosemide, heparin, ibuprofen, and morphine are not removed by hemodialysis.

10. If the patient develops nausea, vomiting, confusion, headache, hypertension, or seizures, suspect disequilibrium syndrome. Reduce the dialysis rate and treat the symptoms.
11. If the patient's blood takes on a "cherry pop" appearance and the patient develops chest pain, dyspnea, burning at the access site, and cramping, suspect acute hemolysis. Clamp the blood line, monitor vital signs, and observe for dysrhythmias. Be prepared to manage a shock state.

Critical observations

Consult with the physician for the following:
1. Absent bruit or thrill
2. Infected dialysis access site
3. Suspected air embolus
4. Disequilibrium syndrome
5. Acute hemolysis
6. Shock

PERITONEAL DIALYSIS

Patient assessment

1. Assess for signs of infection, including redness, swelling, increased tenderness, and drainage at peritoneal access site. Obtain temperature q4h and note any increase.

2. Assess fluid volume status by monitoring:
   a. Weight
   b. Vital signs
   c. I & O (including dialysate infused and effluent drained) q4h or with each exchange
3. Assess the patient for abdominal pain and assess effluent for cloudiness, blood, and/or fibrin clots with each exchange.

Patient management

1. Prevent infection by using good handwashing; initiating good hygiene; separating patient from other patients with infections; aseptically caring for wounds and all invasive catheters; having patient turn and C & DB; encouraging early ambulation; and providing good nutrition.
2. Until the catheter exit site is healed, use sterile technique to clean around the exit site and change the dressing around catheter once per day or when wet. Once the exit site is healed, the patient may shower and should clean with betadine or apply a topical antibiotic ointment around the exit site at the end of the shower.
3. Use strict aseptic technique during exchanges. If the effluent is cloudy and peritonitis is suspected, obtain a sample of effluent before administration of antibiotics.
4. Before an exchange, warm the dialysate solution to body temperature.
5. If ordered, add medications to the dialysate and label the dialysate appropriately (Heparin is often used to prevent catheter obstructions by fibrin or blood clots; insulin is often used to control glucose in the diabetic patient; antibiotics may be administered in the dialysate to patients with peritonitis).
6. Instill the ordered amount and concentration of dialysate with medications (over 10 minutes) via the peritoneal catheter using aseptic technique. Allow fluid to dwell in the abdomen for physician-ordered time period. When dwell-time is over, drain the effluent from the abdomen by gravity over a 20- to 30-minute period.
7. Measure effluent volume by weighing or draining.
8. If difficulty is encountered in draining, check for kinks or clamps on tubing, turn the patient from side to side, sit the patient up in bed, reposition the drainage bag to the lowest possible position, and apply gentle pressure to the abdomen.

RENAL

9. If the patient develops tachypnea and dyspnea, place the patient in semi-Fowler's position and encourage deep breathing.
10. If a tubing spike becomes contaminated by touching an unclean surface, soak the spike in betadine for 5 minutes. If the spike becomes grossly contaminated (e.g., by touching clothing, the floor), clamp tubing; do not continue exchanges.
11. Change peritoneal dialysis tubing monthly using sterile technique.

Critical observations

Consult with the physician for the following:

1. Symptoms of peritonitis
2. Blood or fibrin clots noted in peritoneal effluent
3. Inability to drain effluent
4. Respiratory distress
5. Grossly contaminated tubing spike

CONTINUOUS RENAL REPLACEMENT THERAPY (CAVU, CAVH, CAVHD, OR CVVH)

Patient assessment

1. Assess for signs of infection, including redness, swelling, increased tenderness, and drainage at access site. Obtain a temperature q4h and note any increase.
2. Assess hemodynamic and fluid volume status by monitoring:
   a. Hourly I & O
   b. Vital signs, CVP, and PA pressures (if available), q15min at onset of treatment until stable, every half hour during treatment once stable, and q4h when not being dialyzed.
   c. Breath sounds and heart sounds q4h
   d. Weights three times per day
   e. Ultrafiltrate rate q15min until stable and then qh
   f. Activated clotting time (ACT) q15min until stable and then q4h.

Patient management

1. Prime filter and blood circuit with heparinized saline and administer a physician-ordered heparin bolus to the patient at the onset of therapy. Connect the hemofilter circuit to the patient's access sites, ensuring that all connections are secure.
2. For CAVHD, administer dialysate through the filter, countercurrent to blood flow. For CVVH, set blood

pump rate and apply air and venous pressure-detecting devices.

3. Infuse a heparin drip through the arterial side of the circuit and titrate the heparin infusion to achieve the desired ACT.

4. If ordered, infuse replacement solution, usually hourly, via the arterial side (predilutional) or the venous side (postdilutional) of the circuit. Adjust amount of replacement solution to obtain desired fluid balance. Replacements are based on ultrafiltration rate (UFR). If the UFR is high, volume depletion may occur.

5. If using a gravity drainage bag, keep the bag at least 16 inches below the filter. The ultrafiltration rate can be increased by lowering the bag or can be decreased by raising the collection bag (or by increasing the blood pump rate for CVVH).

6. If collecting ultrafiltrate using vacuum suction, keep suction set between 80 and 120 mm Hg.

7. If SBP <90 mm Hg, place the patient flat or in Trendelenberg position. Reduce the ultrafiltrate rate by lowering the bed, raising the collection bag, or decreasing suction (or by decreasing the blood pump rate for CVVH). Administer normal saline, replacement solution, or vasoactive medications as ordered. If hypotension continues or becomes extreme, clamp ultrafiltrate line.

8. If the amount of ultrafiltrate is reduced, check for kinks or clamps in the access site or tubing; check for changes in the blood flow rate (e.g., decreased cardiac output, hypovolemia); raise the bed, lower the collection bag, or increase the suction; and assess for a clotted filter.

9. Hematest ultrafiltrate q4h.

10. If the ultrafiltrate appears pink-tinged or the hematest result is positive, suspect a blood leak. Clamp the ultrafiltrate line.

11. If the ultrafiltrate rate decreases and the blood in the circuit is darkened (or venous pressure is increased for CVVH), suspect clotting in the filter. Adjust heparinization; be prepared to replace the circuit.

Critical observations

Consult with the physician for the following:

1. Cardiovascular collapse
2. Blood in ultrafiltrate
3. Clotted filter

RENAL

RENAL TRANSPLANTATION
Clinical Brief

Renal transplantation is indicated as a treatment for chronic renal failure. The procedure involves transplanting a tissue-matched kidney from a living-related or a cadaveric donor into the recipient's iliac fossa. Success of the transplant depends on avoiding rejection through the use of immuno-suppressive medications. Transplants are contraindicated if the patient has an underlying disease process that could be aggravated by immunosuppression, such as chronic infection or malignancy.

▶ Complications and related nursing diagnoses

Rejection	Altered urinary elimination
	Risk for fluid volume excess
Acute tubular necrosis (ATN)	Altered urinary elimination
	Risk for fluid volume excess
Infection	Risk for infection
Fluid overload	Fluid volume excess
Dehydration	Fluid volume deficit
	Decreased cardiac output
Hematoma/bleeding	Risk for fluid volume deficit
	Altered tissue perfusion

Patient Care Management Guidelines
Patient assessment

1. Monitor BP, HR, CVP q15min postoperatively until stable, then every hour.
2. Monitor urine flow q15min postoperatively until stable, then hourly. Diuresis is induced following the cold ischemic period; urine output as great as 600 ml/hr can result.
3. Assess for signs of hemorrhage or hematoma at the incisional site every hour for the first 8 hours postoperatively and then every shift. Monitor Hgb and Hct.
4. Assess for signs of urinary leak by assessing for urinary drainage from incisional site, decreased urine output, and for edema of the scrotum, labia, or thigh near the transplant site every hour for the first 8 hours postoperatively and then every shift.
5. Assess I & O hourly and weights each day to determine fluid volume status. Assess fluid volume status and

cardiac output to ensure adequate renal perfusion and to monitor for fluid volume excess.

6. Monitor electrolytes frequently and assess the patient for signs of electrolyte imbalances, especially cardiac dysrhythmias related to hypokalemia during large diuresis or hyperkalemia related to allograft dysfunction.

7. Assess weight, BUN, and creatinine daily to determine renal functioning.

8. Monitor for temperature elevation q4h and each shift for signs of infection. Assess lung sounds q4h; apnea monitoring may be used in the immediate postoperative period to continuously monitor respiratory status.

9. Monitor for signs of rejection, which include decreased urine output, weight gain, increased creatinine, hypertension, general malaise, fever, and graft pain, tenderness, or swelling.

Patient management

1. Anticipate diuresis in living-related donor transplants and cadaveric donor transplants with a short ischemic time.

2. Anticipate acute tubular necrosis in cadaveric donor transplants.

3. If ATN develops, educate the patient on clinical course of ATN, the need for dialysis, and difference between ATN and rejection. Frequently reinforce to the patient that ATN does not predict or affect graft survival.

4. Replace fluids according to urine output (usually milliliter for milliliter, based on the previous-hour urine output) and CVP to maintain normal fluid and electrolyte balance.

5. Anticipate blood in urine for first 24 to 48 hours.

6. If ordered, irrigate the bladder to prevent urinary catheter occlusion by blood clots.

7. If urine output suddenly drops, suspect catheter obstruction by a blood clot and gently irrigate the catheter using sterile technique. If the catheter is not obstructed, assess the patient for signs of dehydration and rejection.

8. Once the urinary catheter is removed, encourage frequent urination. Recatheterization may be required if the patient is unable to void within 6 hr.

9. Prepare the patient for a renal scan or biopsy if ordered.

10. Administer immunosuppressive medications as ordered. Corticosteroids (prednisone, methylprednisolone), azathioprine (Imuran), and cyclosporine (Sandimmune, CsA) are most frequently used. Some centers may use

RENAL

Tracrolimus (Prograf, FK506). Administer oral cyclosporine before meals by diluting it in juice or milk in a glass container. Monitor for side effects of immunosuppressive medications. Monitor cyclosporine and tacrolimus drug levels to ensure adequate immuno-suppression without causing toxic damage to the kid-ney. Hold azathioprine if WBC count is $<3 \times 10^3/\mu l$.

11. Prevent infection by using good handwashing tech-nique; initiating good hygiene; preventing contact with patients, staff, or visitors who have infectious diseases; aseptically caring for wound and all invasive catheters, including meticulous care of the urinary catheter; hav-ing the patient turn and C & DB; encouraging early ambulation; and providing good nutrition.

12. Encourage the physician to remove invasive lines at the earliest possible date to minimize the risk of infection.

13. During acute rejection, dosages of immunosuppressives are adjusted and high doses of intravenous steroids are usually administered for 3 days. Oral steroids are then administered, gradually tapering back toward mainte-nance doses.

14. During acute rejection, not responsive to steroids, muromonab-CD3 (Orthoclone OKT3) may be admin-istered. The recommended dose is 5mg or less per day by rapid IV bolus (less than 1 minute) for 10 to 14 days. If the patient does not respond, OKT3 may be administered at a dosage of 10 mg per day for 3 to 5 days. Ensure that the patient is not fluid overloaded before receiving OKT3. If it is ordered, premedicate the patient before the first dose with methylprednisolone and acetaminophen. If ordered, administer hydrocorti-sone after administering OKT3. Anticipate fever, chills, dyspnea, and malaise within the first 6 hours after the first dose of OKT3. With the first dose of OKT3, moni-tor VS q15min for 2 hours and then q30min until the patient is stable; monitor closely for pulmonary edema, especially in patients who are fluid overloaded.

15. Antilymphocyte globulin (ALG) and antithymocyte globulin (ATG) can also be used in acute rejection that is not responsive to high-dose steroids. Local or sys-temic allergic responses should be anticipated when administering these medications. If ordered, skin testing should be done before administering the first dose, and

premedication with acetaminophen and diphenhydramine hydrochloride (Benadryl) should be provided
before each dose. Administration through a central line
is preferred; if administration is through a peripheral
line, monitor for signs of thrombophlebitis.

16. Tracrolimus (Prograf), commonly known as FK506, is
being used in some facilities for immunosuppression
and/or for renal transplant rejection that is not responsive to high-dose steroids. FK506 can be administered
orally or intravenously. Oral dosage in 0.1 mg/kg
infused over 4 to 24 hours. Dosages should be reduced
in patients with hepatic dysfunction. Side effects include
nephrotoxicity, neurotoxicity, elevated blood glucose
levels, gastrointestinal distress, and hyperkalemia.
Administration of FK506 in conjunction with
cyclosporine greatly increases the risk of nephrotoxicity.

17. Maintain stringent infection control interventions during treatment with immunosuppressive medications.

Critical observations

Consult with the physician for the following:

1. Sudden increase in drainage from incision site
2. Hematoma formation at surgical site
3. Urinary drainage noted at the incision site or edema
   development in the scrotum, labia, or thigh areas
4. Decreased urine output despite nursing interventions
5. Signs of infection
6. WBC count below $3 \times 10^3/\mu l$
7. Onset of dyspnea during OKT3 infusion

REFERENCES

1. ACCP consensus statement on mechanical ventilation, *Respir Care* 38(12):1389-1417, 1993.
2. American Heart Association: Adjuncts for airway control, venti-lation, and oxygenation. In Cummins RO, ed: *Advanced cardiac life support,* Dallas, 1994, American Heart Association.
3. Barbiere C, Liberatore K: From emergent transvenous pace-maker to permanent implant and follow-up, *Crit Care Nurse* 13(2):39-44, 1993.
4. Bardy G et al: Implantable transvenous cardioverter-defibrillators, *Circulation* 87(4):1152-1168, 1993.
5. Bass PS, Bidon-Perler PA, Lewis RJ: Liver transplantation: the recovery phase, *Crit Care Nurs Q* 13(4):51-61, 1991.
6. Beckman NJ et al: Kidney transplantation: a therapy option, *AACN Clin Issues Crit Care Nurs* 3(3):570-584, 1992.

RENAL

7. Berry V: Wolff-Parkinson-White syndrome and the use of radio-frequency catheter ablation, *Heart Lung* 22(1):15-25, 1993.

8. Blanford NL: Renal transplantation: a case study of the ideal, *Crit Care Nurse* 13(1):46-55, 1993.

9. Boggs RL, Wooldridge-King M: *AACN procedure manual for critical care,* ed 3, Philadelphia, 1993, W.B. Saunders.

10. Bosworth C: SCUF/CAVH/CAVHD: critical differences, *Crit Care Nurs Q* 14(4):45-55, 1992.

11. Bremner S et al: A follow-up study of patients with implantable cardioverter defibrillators, *J Cardiovasc Nurs* 7(3):40-51, 1993.

12. Brown BJ, Kahan BD: Renal transplantation, *Surg Clin North Am* 74(5):1097-1116, 1994.

13. Burns D: Review of thrombolytic use in acute myocardial infarction, pulmonary embolism, and cerebral thrombosis, *Crit Care Nurs Q* 15(4):1-12, 1993.

14. Christianson D: Caring for a patient who has an implanted venous port, *AJN* 94(11):40-44, 1994.

15. Coleman J, Mendoza MC, Bindon-Perler PA: Liver diseases that lead to transplantation, *Crit Care Nurs Q* 13(4):41-50, 1991.

16. Cross J: Initiating temporary pacing. In Logston Boggs R, Wooldridge-King M, eds: *AACN procedure manual for critical care,* ed 3, Philadelphia, 1993, W.B. Saunders.

17. Cushieri A: Laparoscopic vagotomy: gimmick or reality? *Surg Clin North Am* 72(2):357-367, 1992.

18. Davidson J: Neuromuscular block: indications, peripheral nerve stimulation and other concurrent interventions, *New Horizons* 2(1):75-84, 1994.

19. Davidson T et al: Implantable cardioverter defibrillators: a guide for clinicians, *Heart Lung* 23(3):205-215, 1994.

20. Deelstra M: Coronary rotational ablation: an overview with related nursing interventions, *Am J Crit Care* 2(3):216-227, 1993.

21. Dirkes S: How to use the new CVVH renal replacement systems, *AJN* 94(5):67-73, 1994.

22. Doherty MM, Carver DK: Transjugular intrahepatic portosystemic shunt: new relief for esophageal varices, *AJN* 93(4):58-63, 1993.

23. Drew B, Tisdale L: ST segment monitoring for coronary artery reocclusion following thrombolytic therapy and coronary angioplasty: identification of optimal bedside monitoring leads, *Am J Crit Care* 2(4):280-292, 1993.

24. Duffy MM: Immunosuppressive medicine, *Dialysis Transplantation* 23(10):571-574, 1994.

25. Dunn SA: How to care for the dialysis patient, *AJN* 93(6):26-33, 1994.

26. Durbin CG: Sedation in the critically ill patient. *New Horizons* 2(1):64-74, 1994.

27. Evans NJ: The role of total parenteral nutrition in critical illness: guidelines and recommendations, *AACN Clin Issues Crit Care Nurs* 5(4):476-484, 1994.

28. Finkelmeier BA: *Cardiothoracic surgical nursing,* Philadelphia, 1995, J.B. Lippincott.

29. Fitzgerald C: Current perspectives on prosthetic heart valves and valve repair, *AACN Clin Issues Crit Care Nurs* 4(2):228-243, 1993.

30. Fleck AM, Wilkerson D: Pediatric extracorporeal membrane oxygenation, *Crit Care Nurse* 12(2):60-67, 1992.

31. Fletcher SM: Current status of renal transplantation, *Urol Clin North Am* 21(2):265-282, 1994.

32. Flynn J, Bruce N: *Introduction to critical care skills,* St Louis, 1993, Mosby.

33. Frazier O et al: Multicenter clinical evaluation of the Heartmate 1000 left ventricular assist device, *Ann Thorac Surg* 53(6):1080-1090, 1992.

34. Futterman L, Lemberg L: An alternative to pharmacologic management of atrial fibrillation: the maze procedure, *Am J Crit Care* 3(3):238-242, 1994.

35. Futterman L, Lemberg L: Radiofrequency catheter ablation for supraventricular tachycardias: part I, *Am J Crit Care* 2(6):500-505, 1993.

36. Futterman L, Lemberg L: Radiofrequency catheter ablation for supraventricular tachycardias: part II, *Am J Crit Care* 3(1):77-79, 1994.

37. Goodnough L, Bodner M, Martin J: Blood conservation and blood salvage, *J Intensive Care Med* 9(2):86-97, 1994.

38. Guzzetta C, Dossey B: *Cardiovascular nursing holistic practice,* St Louis, 1992, Mosby.

39. Handerhan B: Managing pericardial tamponade, *Nursing 93* 23(4):77-78, 1993.

40. Hendrix W: Dialysis therapies in critically ill children, *AACN Clin Issues Crit Care Nurs* 3(3):605-613, 1992.

41. Hinder RA: Duodenal switch: a new form of pancreaticobiliary diversion, *Surg Clin North Am* 72(2):487-499, 1992.

42. Jehle ED, Siewert JR, Blum AL: Sequelae of gastric surgery. In Misiewicz JJ, Pounder RE, Venables CW, eds: *Diseases of the gut and pancreas,* ed 2, Boston, 1994, Blackwell Scientific Publications.

43. Juban A, Khandelwal S: Weaning patients with COPD from mechanical ventilation, *J Resp Care Practitioners,* 67-72, October/November, 1994.

44. Kahan BD, Ghobrial R: Immunosuppressive agents, *Surg Clin North Am* 74(5):1029-1054, 1994.

45. Kinney M et al: *AACN's clinical reference for critical-care nursing,* ed 3, St Louis, 1993, Mosby.

46. Klein S, Flemin CR: Enteral and parenteral nutrition. In Sleisenger MH, Fordtran JS, eds: *Gastrointestinal disease: pathophysiology/diagnosis/management,* ed 5, Philadelphia, 1993, W.B. Saunders.

47. Lemmon P et al: Tissue plasminogen activator: the nurse's role, *Crit Care Nurse* 14(6):32-40, 1994.

48. Lynn-McHale D, McGrory J: Intraaortic balloon pump management, In Logston Boggs R, Wooldridge-King M, eds: *AACN procedure manual for critical care,* ed 3, Philadelphia, 1993, W.B. Saunders.

49. Macnaughton PD, Evans TW: Adult respiratory distress syndrome. In Mitchell DM, ed: *Recent advances in respiratory medicine,* New York, 1991, Churchill Livingstone.

50. Manolis A: Transvenous endocardial cardioverter defibrillator systems: is the future here? *Arch Intern Med* 154(6):617-622, 1994.

51. Manolis S et al: Fully transvenous cardioverter defibrillators: rare need for subcutaneous patch with two newer-generation systems, *Am Heart J* 128(4):808-815, 1994.

52. Maroney D, Reedy J: Understanding ventricular assist devices: a self-study guide, *J Cardiovasc Nurs* 8(2):1-15, 1994.

53. Martin M et al: Transjugular intrahepatic portosystemic shunt in the management of variceal bleeding: indications and clinical results, *Surgery* 114:719-727, 1993.

54. Meares C: PICC and MLC lines, *Nursing 92* 22(10):52-55, 1992.

55. Metheny N: Minimizing respiratory complications of nasoenteric tube feedings: state of the science, *Heart Lung* 22:213-223, 1993.

56. Morris PJ: *Kidney transplantation: principles and practice,* ed 4, Philadelphia, 1994, W.B. Saunders.

57. Moser S et al: Updated care guidelines for patients with automatic implantable cardioverter defibrillators, *Crit Care Nurse* 13(2):62-73, 1993.

58. Naber L, Jones G, Halm M: Epidural analgesia for effective pain control, *Crit Care Nurse* 14(5):69-83, 1994.

59. Nahum A, Marini JJ: Alternatives to conventional mechanical ventilation in acute respiratory failure. In Tierney DF, ed: *Current pulmonology,* vol 15, St Louis 1994, Mosby.

60. Ohler L et al: Cardiac transplantation: a review for critical care nurses, *J Intensive Care Med* 9(5):211-230, 1994.

61. Ozaki CF et al: Surgical complications of liver transplantation, *Surg Clin North Am* 74(5):1155-1167, 1994.

62. Ozaki CF et al: Surgical complications in solitary pancreas and combined pancreas-kidney transplantations, *Am J Surg* 164(5):546-551, 1992.

63. Parrillo JE, Bone RC, eds: *Critical care medicine: principles of diagnosis and management*, St Louis, 1995, Mosby.

64. Perel A, Stock MC: *Handbook of mechanical ventilatory support*, Philadelphia, 1992, Williams & Wilkins.

65. Peschman P: Acute hemodialysis: issues in the critically ill, *AACN Clin Issues Crit Care Nurs* 3(3):545-557, 1992.

66. Pettrey L, Leflar-DiLeva K: Preparing for cardiomyoplasty: a new horizon in cardiac surgery, *Dimens Crit Care Nurs* 13(5):226-236, 1994.

67. Pilbeam SP: *Mechanical ventilation physiological and clinical applications*, ed 2, St Louis, 1992, Mosby.

68. Posa PJ: Nutritional support strategies: a case study approach, *AACN Clin Issues Crit Care Nurs* 5(4):436-442, 1994.

69. Price CA: An update on continuous renal replacement therapies, *AACN Clin Issues Crit Care Nurs* 3(3):597-604, 1992.

70. Quaal S: *Comprehensive intraaortic balloon counterpulsation*, ed 2, St Louis, 1993, Mosby.

71. Rasmussen J, Mangan D: Third generation antitachycardia pacing implantable cardioverter-defibrillators, *Dimens Crit Care Nurs* 13(6):284-291, 1994.

72. Reedy J: Transfer of a patient with a ventricular assist device to a non-critical care area, *Heart Lung* 22(1):71-76, 1993.

73. Robertson RP, Sutherland DER: Pancreas transplantation as therapy for diabetes mellitus, *Ann Rev Med* 43:395-415, 1992.

74. Rossie M et al: The transjugular intrahepatic portosystemic stent-shunt procedure for variceal bleeding, *N Engl J Med* 330:165-171, 1994.

75. Ruppel G: *Manual of pulmonary function tests*, ed 6, St Louis, 1994, Mosby.

76. Ryan T et al: Guidelines for percutaneous transluminal coronary angioplasty, *J Am Coll Cardiol* 22(7):2033-2054, 1993.

77. Sax HC, Souba WW: Enteral and parenteral feedings: guidelines and recommendations, *Med Clin North Am* 77(4):863-880, 1993.

78. Seifert PC: *Cardiac surgery*, St Louis, 1994, Mosby.

79. Shinn A, Joseph D: Concepts of intraaortic balloon counterpulsation, *J Cardiovasc Nurs* 8(2):45-60, 1994.

80. Shuster MH: Enteral feeding of the critically ill, *AACN Clin Issues Crit Care Nurs* 5(4):459-475, 1994.

81. Sirowatka B: The implantable cardioverter defibrillator: patient and family education, *Dimens Crit Care Nurs* 12(6):328-334, 1993.

82. Smith JW, Brenna MF: Surgical treatment of gastric cancer, *Surg Clin North Am* 72(2):381-399, 1992.

83. Smith LJ: Peritoneal dialysis in the critically ill patient, *AACN Clin Issues Crit Care Nurs* 3(3):558-569, 1992.

84. Smith SL: *Tissue and organ transplantation: implications for professional nursing practice,* St Louis, 1990, Mosby.

85. Smith SL, Ciferni M: Liver transplantation for acute hepatic failure: a review of clinical experience and management, *Am J Crit Care* 2(2):137-144, 1993.

86. Sollinger HW, Geffner SR: Pancreas transplantation, *Surg Clin North Am* 74(5):1183-1195, 1994.

87. Stabile BE: Current surgical management of duodenal ulcers, *Surg Clin North Am* 72(2):335-356, 1992.

88. *Standards for blood banks and transfusion services,* ed 16, American Association of Blood Banks, 1994, Bethesda, MD.

89. Stark JL: Dialysis options in the critically ill patient: hemodialysis, peritoneal dialysis, and continuous renal replacement therapy, *Crit Care Nurs Q* 14(4):40-44, 1992.

90. Stehling L et al: Guidelines for blood utilization review, *Transfusion* 34(5):438-448, 1994.

91. Stewart J et al: Cardiomyoplasty: treatment of the failing heart using the skeletal muscle wrap, *J Cardiovasc Nurs* 7(2):23-31, 1993.

92. Thelan L et al: *Critical care nursing,* ed 2, St Louis, 1994, Mosby.

93. Thompson JM: Respiratory system. In Thompson JM et al, eds: *Mosby's clinical nursing,* ed 3, St Louis, 1993, Mosby.

94. Thompson S: Using a groshong central venous catheter, *Nursing 91* 21(10):58-60, 1991.

95. Tobin MJ: Mechanical ventilation, *N Engl J Med* 330(15):1056-1061, 1994.

96. Topulos G: Neuromuscular blockade in adult intensive care, *New Horizons* 1(3):447-462, 1993.

97. Trusler LA: Management of the patient receiving simultaneous kidney-pancreas transplantation, *Crit Care Nurs Clin North Am* 4(1):89-95, 1992.

98. Urban N et al: *Guidelines for critical care nursing,* St Louis, 1995, Mosby.

99. Wood RP et al: Liver transplantation: the last ten years, *Surg Clin North Am* 74(5):1133-1154, 1994.

100. Zaloga G, Ackerman MH: A review of disease-specific formulas, *AACN Clin Issues Crit Care Nurs* 5(4):421-435, 1994.

101. Zheng T et al: Early markers of pancreas transplant rejection, *American Surgeon* 58(10):630-633, 1992.

CHAPTER 8

Pharmacology: Emergency Drugs in the Adult Patient

ADENOSINE (ADENOCARD)

Classification
Antidysrhythmic

Effects
Adenosine restores normal sinus rhythm by slowing conduction time through the AV node.

Indications
Paroxysmal supraventricular tachycardia (PSVT), including PSVT associated with Wolff-Parkinson-White (W-P-W) syndrome

Contraindications
Hypersensitivity to adenosine, second- or third-degree AV heart block, sick sinus syndrome (unless functioning artificial pacemaker is present); not recommended in the treatment of atrial fibrillation, atrial flutter, and ventricular tachycardia (VT)

Administration
Dose
Administer 6 mg IV bolus over 1 to 2 seconds; follow with a saline flush to ensure that the drug reaches the circulation. Give 12 mg rapid IV bolus if the first dose fails to eliminate the PSVT within 1 to 2 minutes. Repeat the 12 mg dose a second time if needed. Doses greater than 12 mg are not recommended; the unused solution should be discarded.
Precautions
Use cautiously in patients with asthma; adenosine may produce bronchoconstriction. A short-lasting first-, second-, or

third-degree heart block may result. Patients developing high-level block after one dose of adenosine should not be given additional doses. New dysrhythmias may develop during conversion (e.g., PVCs, PACs, sinus bradycardia, sinus tachycardia, and AV blocks), but are generally self-limiting because the half-life of adenosine is <10 seconds. Higher degrees of heart block may result in patients taking carbamazepine. Smaller doses of adenosine may be required in patients taking dipyridamole, since dipyridamole potentiates the effects of adenosine. Larger doses may be required in patients taking theophylline or other methylxanthine products, since the effects of adenosine are antagonized by methylxanthines.

Patient Management
- Check patency of IV and flush IV after adenosine administration to ensure that the drug reaches the circulation.
- Evaluate heart rate (HR) and rhythm 1 to 2 minutes after administering adenosine and monitor for dysrhythmias during conversion; blood pressure (BP) is not adversely affected with the usual dose of adenosine, but larger doses may result in hypotension.
- Measure PR interval for development of AV block.
- Observe for adverse effects: nonmyocardial chest discomfort, hypotension, and dyspnea. Patients may complain of facial flushing, sweating, headache, lightheadedness, tingling in the arms, blurred vision, heaviness in arms, burning sensation, neck and back pain, numbness, metallic taste, tightness in throat, and pressure in groin.
- Individualize treatment for prolonged adverse effects (e.g., external pacemaker for prolonged third-degree block).

AMINOPHYLLINE
Classification
Bronchodilator

Effects
Aminophylline dilates bronchioles and pulmonary blood vessels. It is a central respiratory stimulant and has a potent effect on diaphragmatic contractility. It also increases cardiac output (CO), HR, and myocardial contractility. It decreases BP, increases urine output, and stimulates the CNS.

Indications

Prevention and treatment of bronchospasm; not very useful in treating an acute asthma attack; possible use as an adjunct in the treatment of Cheyne-Stokes respiration and pulmonary edema

Contraindications

Hypersensitivity to xanthine preparations such as caffeine; peptic ulcer

Administration
Dose

The dose must be individualized because it has a narrow therapeutic window. Lean body weight should be used for dosage determination. The loading dose of aminophylline is 6 mg/kg. IV infusion rate should not exceed 25 mg/min.

Rapid infusion can cause ventricular fibrillation (VF) or cardiac arrest. Serum theophylline levels are used to guide dosage adjustments.

Precautions

Adjust dose for patients with hepatic disease because the drug is metabolized in the liver. Use cautiously in patients with heart failure, preexisting cardiac dysrhythmias, and hyperthyroidism. Side effects are related to theophylline serum levels.

Patient Management

- Check serum theophylline levels; therapeutic drug level is 10 to 20 µg/ml.
- Monitor vital signs; tachycardia and hypotension can occur with rapid administration.
- Assess lungs for adventitious sounds, evaluating patient response to therapy.
- Maintain the ordered infusion rate, using an IV volume infusion-control pump.
- Observe for adverse effects: restlessness, dizziness, insomnia, convulsions, palpitations, tachycardia, hypotension, dysrhythmias, nausea and vomiting, anorexia, and epigastric pain.

AMRINONE (INOCOR)
Classification
Inotrope/vasodilator

Effects
Amrinone increases myocardial contractility and CO. It decreases afterload and preload.

Indications
Heart failure refractory to traditional therapies

Contraindications
Hypersensitivity to amrinone or bisulfites

Administration
Dose
The IV loading dose is 0.75 mg/kg over 2 to 3 minutes. Loading dose may be repeated in 30 minutes. The drug can be given undiluted. As an infusion, administer at 5 to 15 µg/kg/min.
Precautions
Avoid administration with disopyramide. Use cautiously in patients who have hepatic or renal disease. Outflow tract obstruction may worsen in patients with hypertrophic subaortic stenosis.

Patient Management
- Monitor BP, PAWP, MAP, SVRI, PVRI, CI, and HR during infusion.
- Monitor intake and output, electrolytes, and renal function.
- Observe for adverse effects: thrombocytopenia, hypotension, dizziness, dysrhythmias, chest pain, hypokalemia, nausea and vomiting, abdominal pain, anorexia, hepatic toxicity, and fever.

ATENOLOL (TENORMIN)
Classification
β-adrenergic blocking agent

Effects
Reduces heart rate, cardiac output, blood pressure, and myocardial oxygen consumption. Promotes redistribution of blood flow from adequately supplied areas of the heart to ischemic areas. Reduces incidence of recurrent myocardial infarction, size of the infarct, and incidence of fatal dysrhythmias.

Indications

Acute myocardial infarction

Contraindications

Sinus bradycardia, second- and third-degree heart block, cardiogenic shock, overt heart failure

Administration

Dose

Administer 5 to 10 mg IV over 5 min. Give 50 mg po 10 min after the IV bolus and repeat the oral dose in 12 hours. Maintenance: 100 mg po daily for 6 to 9 days or until discharged from hospital.

Precautions

Use cautiously in patients with heart failure, lung disease/bronchospasm. Abrupt withdrawal in patients with thyroid disease may precipitate thyroid storm. May mask tachycardia associated with hyperthyroidism or hypoglycemia.

Patient Management

- Monitor cardiac rhythm, HR, and BP; notify physician if bradycardia or hypotension develop.
- Assess cardiac output and signs of myocardial ischemia (e.g., angina, dysrhythmias, ST, T-wave changes).
- Assess patient for development of heart failure.
- Monitor blood glucose levels, especially in patients with diabetes.
- Observe for adverse effects: breathing difficulties, bradycardias, heart block, ventricular dysrhythmias, hypotension, cardiac failure.

ATRACURIUM (TRACRIUM)

Classification

Nondepolarizing neuromuscular blocking agent

Effects

Produces skeletal muscle paralysis but has no effect on consciousness or pain

Indications

Facilitation of endotracheal intubation and mechanical ventilation; to reduce metabolic demands, prevent ventilator asynchrony and stabilize cerebral blood flow in patients with increased ICP

Contraindications
Hypersensitivity to atracurium

Administration
Dose
Initial bolus is 0.4 to 0.5 mg/kg IV; maximum blockade occurs in 3 to 5 min. Infusion rates are adjusted according to the patient's response. Use lowest dosage that provides the desired level of paralysis.
Precautions
Use cautiously in patients with history of asthma or anaphylaxis; significant CV disease or neuromuscular disorders. Patients with burns may need increased doses. A peripheral nerve stimulator should be used to obtain baseline reading and to monitor neuromuscular transmission during the paralysis. Patients must have a patent airway and be mechanically ventilated. Patients are conscious but unable to communicate. Atracurium has no effect on pain and anxiety. Sedation and analgesia should be maintained during period of paralysis.

Patient Management
- Monitor HR, rhythm, BP, and respirations.
- Ensure patent airway and controlled mechanical ventilation.
- Analyze ABGs and monitor pulse oximetry for adequate oxygenation.
- Monitor exhaled volume with spirometer and end tidal CO_2 with capnograph.
- Use adjunctive therapy for pain control and sedation throughout the period of paralysis.
- Have emergency respiratory support available in case of accidental extubation or lack of endotracheal tube patency.
- Use a peripheral nerve stimulator to monitor neuromuscular suppression and recovery.
- Monitor serum electrolytes since abnormalities can affect neuromuscular transmission.
- Observe for adverse effects: hypotension, tachycardia, bradycardia, flushing allergic reactions, bronchospasm, seizures.
- See Neuromuscular blockade in the critically ill, p. 542.

ATROPINE

Classification
Anticholinergic

Effects
Atropine increases conduction through the AV node and increases the HR.

Indications
Symptomatic bradycardia and asystole

Contraindications
Adhesions between the iris and lens, advanced renal and hepatic impairment, asthma, narrow-angle glaucoma, obstructive disease of the GI and urinary tract, myasthenia gravis, and paralytic ileus

Administration
Dose
For bradycardia, administer 0.5 to 1 mg IV bolus every 3 to 5 minutes until adequate response or a total dose of 0.04 mg/kg mg is given. Doses of less than 0.5 mg can cause further bradycardia. For asystole, administer 1 mg IV; repeat once in 3 to 5 minutes if needed.

Atropine can be given undiluted IV push in emergency situations. Atropine may also be given via the endotracheal tube by diluting 1 to 2 mg in 10 ml sterile water or normal saline (NS) and followed by five forceful inhalations.

Precautions
In the presence of an acute infarction, atropine can increase cardiac irritability.

Patient Management
- Monitor HR for response to therapy (>60 is desirable); be alert for development of VF or VT.
- Excessive doses can result in tachycardia, flushed hot skin, delirium, coma, or death.
- Antidote for overdose is physostigmine salicylate.

BRETYLIUM (BRETYLOL)

Classification
Antidysrhythmic

Effects

Bretylium increases the refractory period without increasing HR. Initially it causes an increase in BP, HR, and myocardial contractility as a result of the norepinephrine release. This response is followed by hypotension, which is caused by neuronal blockade.

Indications

VF and VT, currently the second drug of choice (after lidocaine) in the treatment of refractory or recurrent VF

Contraindications

Digitalis-induced dysrhythmias, not effective in abolishing atrial dysrhythmias

Administration

Dose

Administer 5 mg/kg IV followed by defibrillation; increase dose to 10 mg/kg every 5 minutes if necessary. A maximum total dose of 30 to 35 mg/kg may be given. A continuous infusion of 1 to 2 mg/min may be given after a loading dose of 5 to 10 mg/kg diluted in 50 ml D_5W over 8 to 10 minutes for VF. (See drug dosage chart, p. 710.)

Precautions

Postural hypotension occurs regularly following administration of bretylium. Correct hypovolemia before administration. The dosage should be adjusted accordingly for patients with renal impairment. Pressor effects of catecholamines are enhanced by bretylium. Avoid simultaneous initiation of bretylium and digitalis therapy.

Patient Management

- Keep patient supine and monitor BP during infusion.
- Evaluate dysrhythmia control and CI.
- Observe for adverse effects: hypotension, vertigo, dysrhythmias, angina, syncope, and nausea and vomiting.

BUMETANIDE (BUMEX)

Classification

Diuretic

Effects

Bumetanide promotes the excretion of fluid and electrolytes and reduces plasma volume. It is 40 times more potent than furosemide (Lasix).

Indications

Edematous states: heart failure, pulmonary edema, and hepatic and renal disease

Contraindications

Hepatic coma, anuria, and hypersensitivity to sulfonamides

Administration

Dose

Administer 500 µg to 2 mg orally per day as a single dose. If a diuretic response is not achieved, a second or third dose may be given at 4 to 5 hour intervals. IV dose is 500 µg to 1 mg given undiluted over 1 to 2 minutes. May repeat at 2 to 3 hour intervals. Maximum is 10 mg.

Precautions

Profound electrolyte and water depletion can occur. Changes in electrolytes can precipitate hepatic encephalopathy and coma in patients with hepatic cirrhosis and ascites. Concurrent use with aminoglycosides or rapid injection may increase the risk for ototoxicity.

Patient Management

- Assess potassium level before administration; hypokalemia should be corrected before administration.
- Monitor for signs of electrolyte and water depletion.
- Monitor BP and HR during increased diuresis period.
- Assess serial weights and I & O to evaluate fluid loss (1 kg = 1000 ml fluid).
- Monitor patient receiving digitalis for digitalis toxicity secondary to diuretic-induced hypokalemia.
- Evaluate hearing and assess for ototoxicity.
- Monitor serial BUN and creatinine levels to assess renal function.
- Observe for adverse effects: volume depletion (e.g., dryness of the mouth, increased thirst, dizziness, and orthostatic

hypotension), headache, muscle cramps, nausea, transient deafness, glucose intolerance, and hepatic dysfunction.

CALCIUM CHLORIDE

Classification
Electrolyte replenisher

Effects
Calcium chloride replaces and maintains calcium in body fluids.

Indications
Hypocalcemia, hyperkalemia, magnesium toxicity, and calcium channel blocker overdose; possibly indicated during a cardiac resuscitation

Contraindications
VF, hypercalcemia, renal calculi, and digitalis toxicity

Administration
Dose
Give 500 mg to 1 g slowly IV, not to exceed 50 to 100 mg/min. When adding to parenteral fluids, monitor for a precipitate. One gram of calcium chloride is equivalent to 13.6 mEq of calcium.
Precautions
The dosage of calcium may need to be adjusted in patients with renal or cardiac disease. Cardiac dysrhythmias may be evidenced when calcium is administered to patients who are receiving digitalis glycosides or who have been digitalized. Severe necrosis and sloughing of tissues will occur with infiltration.

Patient Management
- Administer calcium through a central line.
- Assess patency of IV; note any precipitate.
- Monitor BP, since peripheral vasodilation will occur.
- Monitor serial serum calcium levels.
- Continuously monitor ECG for onset of dysrhythmias.

- Monitor for electrolyte imbalances.
- Observe for adverse effects: bradycardia, cardiac arrest, constipation, fatigue, venous irritation, depression, loss of appetite, and tingling.

DIAZEPAM (VALIUM)

Classification
Antianxiety agent, anticonvulsant, skeletal muscle relaxant

Effects
Diazepam depresses the CNS, suppresses the spread of seizure activity, and relaxes skeletal muscle.

Indications
Anxiety, status epilepticus, and preprocedure sedation

Contraindications
Shock, coma, acute alcohol intoxication, acute glaucoma, psychoses, and myasthenia gravis

Administration
Dose
Administer 2 to 10 mg orally three or four times daily. IV dose is 5 to 10 mg. The drug may be given IV push at a rate of 2 to 5 mg/min.

In status epilepticus, administer 5 to 10 mg IV; can be repeated every 10 to 15 minutes, up to 30 mg in 1 hour. Do not mix diazepam with other drugs.

Precautions
Dosage should be reduced in the elderly. Use cautiously in patients with blood dyscrasias, hepatic or renal damage, or depression and in those with diminished pulmonary function.

Patient Management
- Monitor respirations before and after the IV dose.
- Evaluate patient's response (e.g., decreased anxiety, absence of seizures).
- Observe for adverse effects: drowsiness, cardiovascular collapse, pain, phlebitis at injection site, and respiratory depression.

DIGOXIN (LANOXIN)

Classification
Cardiac glycoside

Effects
Digoxin increases myocardial contractility, decreases HR, and enhances CO, which improves renal blood flow and increases urinary output.

Indications
Patients with heart failure, cardiogenic shock, and atrial dysrhythmias such as atrial fibrillation, atrial flutter, and paroxysmal atrial tachycardia

Contraindications
Patients who demonstrate signs and symptoms of digitalis toxicity

Administration
Dose
Digitalizing and maintenance doses must be individualized. Usual loading dose is 1 to 1.25 mg IV or orally in divided doses over 24 hours. IV dose may be given undiluted over at least 5 minutes. Maintenance doses are based upon the percentage of the peak body stores lost each day.
Precautions
Use cautiously in the elderly and in patients with acute infarction or renal impairment. Administer IV digoxin with caution in the hypertensive patient because a transient increase in BP may occur. Patients with partial AV block may develop complete heart block. Patients with W-P-W may experience fatal ventricular dysrhythmias.

Patient Management
- Check potassium and magnesium levels before administration, since hypokalemia and hypomagnesemia are associated with increased risk of digitalis toxicity.
- Check calcium level since hypercalcemia can increase risk of digitalis toxicity and hypocalcemia can nullify the effects of digoxin.
- Take apical pulse before administration; if <60, consult with physician.
- Measure serial PR intervals for development of heart block.

Digibind

The dose of Digibind varies according to the amount of digoxin to be neutralized. Each vial (40 mg) will bind with 0.6 mg of digoxin. An average dose is 10 vials, administered over 30 minutes through a 0.22 μm filter. If the toxicity has not been reversed after several hours, readministration may be required. Monitor potassium levels because digibind can cause a rapid drop in potassium secondary to reversing the effects of digitalis. Monitor HR because the withdrawal of digoxin effects in patients with atrial fibrillation or atrial flutter may cause a return of rapid ventricular rate. Heart failure may worsen secondary to withdrawal of the inotropic effects of digitalis.

- Evaluate patient for controlled dysrhythmia (decreased ventricular response to atrial fibrillation or atrial flutter).
- Evaluate patient for resolution of heart failure.
- Be prepared to treat overdose with IV magnesium sulfate or digoxin immune fab (Digibind) if patient has severe, life-threatening refractory dysrhythmias (see the box above).
- Observe for digitalis toxicity: nausea and vomiting, anorexia, epigastric pain, unusual fatigue, diarrhea, dysrhythmias, excessive slowing of HR, blurred or yellow vision, irritability or confusion, ST segment sagging, or prolonged PR interval.

DILTIAZEM (CARDIZEM)

Classification
Calcium channel blocker

Effects
Depresses impulse formation and conduction velocity. Dilates coronary arteries and arterioles.

Indications
Temporary control of rapid ventricular response in atrial fibrillation or flutter; conversion of paroxysmal supraventricular tachycardia

Contraindications
Ventricular tachycardia, atrial fibrillation, or flutter when associated with an accessory bypass tract (W-P-W, short PR

syndrome), second- or third-degree heart block, severe hypotension, cardiogenic shock, heart failure, sick sinus syndrome unless functioning pacemaker in place, patients receiving IV beta-adrenergic blocking agents within 2 to 4 hours

Administration
Dose
Initially, administer 0.25 mg/kg IV over 2 min; in 15 min give 0.35 mg/kg if needed. If an infusion is required, initial rate is 10 mg/hr; maximum dose is 15 mg/hr. Infusion not recommended greater than 24 hrs.

Precautions
Life-threatening tachycardia with severe hypotension in atrial fibrillation or flutter in patients with an accessory bypass tract can occur; periods of asystole can occur in patients with sick sinus syndrome. Use cautiously in patients with preexisting impaired ventricular function; condition may exacerbate. May cause AV block. For short-term use only.

Patient Management
- Evaluate dysrhythmia control.
- Monitor HR, rhythm, and blood pressure. Notify physician if hypotension or bradycardia develop.
- Measure PR interval for onset of AV block.
- Monitor cardiac output and assess for signs of heart failure.
- Observe for adverse effects: dysrhythmias, hypotension, flushing, heart block, chest pain, heart failure, dyspnea, edema.

DOBUTAMINE (DOBUTREX)
Classification
Inotrope, adrenergic-stimulating agent

Effects
Dobutamine increases myocardial contractility and increases CO without significant change in BP. It increases coronary blood flow and myocardial oxygen consumption.

Indications
Heart failure and cardiogenic shock

Contraindications

Idiopathic hypertrophic stenosis

Administration

Dose

IV infusion is 2 to 20 µg/kg/min titrated to desired patient response. A dose of 250 mg/250 ml 250 D_5W yields 1 mg/ml. Concentration of solution should not exceed 5 mg/ml of dobutamine. (See drug dosage chart, p. 708.)

Precautions

Hemodynamic monitoring is recommended for optimal benefit when dobutamine is administered. Fluid deficits should be corrected before infusion of dobutamine. At doses greater than 20 µg/kg/min, an increase in HR may occur. Dobutamine facilitates conduction through the AV node and can cause a rapid ventricular response in patients with inadequately treated atrial fibrillation. Concurrent use with general anesthetics may increase the potential for ventricular dysrhythmias.

Patient Management

- Use large veins for administration; an infusion pump should be used to regulate flow rate.
- Check BP and HR every 2 to 5 minutes during initial administration and during titration of the drug.
- Monitor CI, PAWP, and urine output continuously during administration.
- Observe for adverse effects: tachycardia, hypertension, chest pain, and cardiac dysrhythmias.

DOPAMINE (INTROPIN)

Classification

Sympathomimetic, vasopressor

Effects

Dopamine in low doses (1 to 2 µg/kg/min) increases blood flow to the kidneys, glomerular filtration rate, urine flow, and sodium excretion. In low to moderate doses (2 to 10 µg/kg/min), it increases myocardial contractility and CO. In high doses (10 to 20 µg/kg/min), it increases peripheral resistance and renal vasoconstriction.

Indications

Shock state, septicemia, myocardial infarction, and renal failure

Contraindications

Uncorrected tachydysrhythmias, pheochromocytoma, VF

Administration

Dose

For IV infusion, administer 2 to 20 µg/kg/min up to 50 µg/kg/min, titrated to effect and/or renal response. A dose of 400 mg/500 ml D_5W yields 800 µg/ml. (See drug dosage chart, p. 709.)

Precautions

Concurrent use with β blockers may antagonize the effect of dopamine. Use with caution in patients receiving monoamine oxidase (MAO) inhibitors because the drug may cause a hypertensive crisis. Use cautiously in patients with occlusive vascular disease, arterial embolism, and diabetic endarteritis. Correct hypovolemic states before administering dopamine. Extravasation may cause necrosis and sloughing of surrounding tissue.

Patient Management

- Use large vein; check vein frequently for blanching/pallor, which may indicate extravasation.
- Notify physician if extravasation occurs. Treat with phentolamine (5 to 10 mg in 10 to 15 ml NS) via local infiltration as soon as possible.
- Do not use the proximal port of a pulmonary artery (PA) catheter to infuse the drug if CO readings are being obtained.
- Monitor BP and HR every 2 to 5 minutes initially and during titration of the drug.
- Measure urine output hourly to evaluate renal function.
- Determine pulse pressure, since a decrease indicates excessive vasoconstriction.
- Taper infusion gradually to avoid sudden hypotension.
- Observe for adverse effects: tachycardia, headache, dysrhythmias, nausea and vomiting, hypotension, chest pain, shortness of breath, and vasoconstriction (numbness, tingling, pallor, cold skin, decreased pulses, decreased cerebral perfusion, and decreased urine output).

- Report the drug's inability to maintain a desired response despite increased dosage.

EDROPHONIUM (TENSILON)

Classification
Cholinesterase inhibitor

Effects

Edrophonium produces vagal stimulation, which results in a decreased HR.

Indications

Diagnosis of myasthenic crisis and treatment of PSVT

Contraindications

Hypersensitivity to anticholinesterase agents, bronchial asthma, or intestinal or urinary obstruction

Administration

Dose
For patients with myasthenia gravis, administer 1 mg IV; if no response, repeat dose in 1 minute. Increased muscular strength confirms myasthenic crisis, and no increase confirms cholinergic crisis, at which point atropine sulfate (0.4 to 0.5 mg) needs to be given. For patients with supraventricular tachyarrhythmias, administer 5 to 10 mg IV; repeat in 10 minutes if needed. The drug is administered undiluted.

Precautions
Use cautiously in patients with cardiac dysrhythmias, those who are receiving digitalis, and those with hypotension and bradycardia.

Patient Management

- Have atropine available to counteract cholinergic reactions.
- Monitor HR and respirations; observe for signs of respiratory distress and bradycardia.
- Observe for adverse effects: muscle weakness, shortness of breath, bradycardia, fatigue and weakness, bronchospasm, cardiac arrest, convulsions, diarrhea, increased lacrimation, laryngospasm, ptosis, urinary frequency, vomiting, and perspiration.

EPINEPHRINE (ADRENALINE)

Classification
Bronchodilator, vasopressor, cardiac stimulant

Effects
Epinephrine increases myocardial contractility, HR, systolic BP, and CO. It also relaxes bronchial smooth muscle.

Indications
Cardiac arrest, hypersensitivity reactions, anaphylaxis, and acute asthma attacks

Contraindications
Acute narrow-angle glaucoma and coronary insufficiency

Administration

Dose
For patients in cardiac arrest, give 1 mg IV or 2 to 2.5 mg endotracheally every 3 to 5 minutes. As a vasopressor, administer as an IV infusion, at 2 µg/min and titrate to desired response; 1 mg/250 ml D_5W yields 4 µg/ml. (See drug dosage chart, p. 710.)

For bronchospasm/anaphylaxis, give 0.1 to 0.5 ml of 1:1000 solution subcutaneously and repeat every 10 to 20 minutes. If using an IV route, give 0.1 to 0.25 ml of 1:1000 solution.

Precautions
Use cautiously in elderly patients and patients with angina, hypothyroidism, hypertension, psychoneurosis, and diabetes. Epinephrine should be administered cautiously in patients with long-standing bronchial asthma and emphysema who have developed degenerative heart disease. Do not administer concurrently with isoproterenol—death may result. Repeated local injections can cause necrosis at the site.

Patient Management
- Monitor BP and HR every 2 to 5 minutes during the initial infusion and during drug titration.
- Use an infusion device; validate correct drug and infusion rate.
- Do not use the proximal port of a PA catheter for infusing epinephrine if CO readings are being obtained.
- Evaluate patient's response; monitor CI.

- Observe for adverse effects: chest pain, dysrhythmias, headache, restlessness, dizziness, nausea and vomiting, weakness, and excessive vasoconstriction.
- Report the drug's inability to maintain a desired effect despite increased doses.

ESMOLOL (BREVIBLOC)

Classification
β-adrenergic blocking agent

Effects

Esmolol decreases HR, BP, contractility, and myocardial oxygen consumption.

Indications

Supraventricular tachycardia and hypertension

Contraindications

Sinus bradycardia, heart block greater than first degree, cardiogenic shock, and overt heart failure

Administration
Dose

Administer 500 µg/kg/min IV for 1 minute; give 50 µg/kg/min for 4 minutes. Repeat loading dose and increase infusion to 100 µg/kg/min if desired response is not achieved in 5 minutes. Continue same loading dose but increase maintenance dose by 50 µg/kg/min until desired response is achieved or hypotension occurs. Do not exceed 200 µg/kg/min. A dose of 5 g/500 ml D_5W yields 10 mg/ml.

Discontinue infusion: Infusion dose can be reduced by 50% 30 minutes after the first dose of an alternate antidysrhythmic agent is given. If the patient remains stable an hour after the second dose of the alternative agent is administered, esmolol may be discontinued.

Precautions

Use cautiously in patients with impaired renal function, diabetes, or bronchospasm.

Patient Management

- Monitor BP every 2 minutes during titration. Hypotension can be reversed by decreasing the dose or by discontinuing the infusion.
- Evaluate dysrhythmia control.

- Monitor ECG for bradycardia or heart block.
- Evaluate patient for heart failure.
- Monitor blood glucose levels, especially in patients with diabetes.
- Observe for adverse effects: hypotension, pallor, light-headedness, paresthesias, urinary retention, nausea and vomiting, bronchospasm, and inflammation at the infusion site.
- Report signs of overdose: tachycardia/bradycardia, dizziness/fainting, difficulty in breathing, bluish color on palmar surface of hands, seizures, cold hands, fever, sore throat, or unusual bleeding.

FUROSEMIDE (LASIX)

Classification
Diuretic

Effects
Furosemide promotes the excretion of fluid and electrolytes and reduces plasma volume.

Indications
Edematous states: heart failure, pulmonary edema, hepatic and renal disease, and hypertension

Contraindications
Sensitivity to furosemide or sulfonamides

Administration
Dose
Oral dose is 20 to 80 mg in the morning, followed by a second dose 6 to 8 hours later if necessary. IV dose is 20 to 40 mg given undiluted over 1 to 2 minutes; additional doses may be given until the desired outcome is achieved.
Precautions
Profound electrolyte and water depletion can occur.

Patient Management
- Check potassium level before administering furosemide; hypokalemia should be corrected before administering the drug.
- Evaluate hearing and assess for ototoxicity.
- Monitor urine output to evaluate drug effectiveness.

- Monitor serial BUN and creatinine levels to assess renal function.
- Assess patient for volume depletion and electrolyte imbalance.
- Monitor BP and I & O and assess serial weights (1 kg = 1000 ml fluid) to evaluate fluid loss.
- Monitor patient receiving digitalis for digitalis toxicity secondary to diuretic-induced hypokalemia.
- Advise patient to report ringing in ears, severe abdominal pain, or sore throat and fever. These symptoms may indicate furosemide toxicity.
- Observe for adverse effects: volume depletion, orthostatic hypotension, electrolyte imbalance, transient deafness, glucose intolerance, and hepatic dysfunction.

ISOPROTERENOL (ISUPREL)

Classification
Sympathomimetic, β-adrenergic agonist

Effects
Isoproterenol increases CO, coronary blood flow, and stroke volume; decreases MAP; and relaxes bronchial smooth muscle.

Indications
Bronchial asthma, obstructive pulmonary disease, bronchospasm, heart block, atropine refractory bradycardia, and shock states

Contraindications
Digitalis-induced tachycardia or patients receiving β blockers

Administration
Dose
In hemodynamic significant bradycardia, the IV infusion rate is 2 to 10 μg/min; titrate to desired response. A dose of 1 mg/250 ml D_5W yields 4 μg/ml. (See drug dosage chart, p. 710.)
Precautions
Volume deficit should be corrected before initiating isoproterenol. Administer cautiously in patients with hypertension, coronary artery disease, hyperthyroidism, and diabetes. The drug is not indicated in cardiac arrest. Do not use concurrently with epinephrine. VF and VT may develop.

Patient Management

- If the HR exceeds 110 bpm, the dose may need to be decreased. If the HR exceeds 130 bpm, ventricular dysrhythmias may be induced.
- Monitor BP, MAP, central venous pressure (CVP), and urinary output.
- An infusion pump should be used to administer the infusion.
- Observe for adverse effects: headache, tachycardia, anginal pain, palpitations, flushing of the face, nervousness, sweating, hypotension, and pulmonary edema.

LABETALOL (NORMODYNE, TRANDATE)

Classification

β-adrenergic blocking agent

Effects

Labetalol decreases BP and renin secretion and can decrease HR and CO.

Indications

Hypertension

Contraindications

Bronchial asthma, cardiac failure, heart block, cardiogenic shock, and bradycardia

Administration

Dose

Oral dose is 100 mg twice daily. IV dose is 20 mg given undiluted over 2 minutes, and additional doses of 40 to 80 mg every 10 minutes up to 300 mg may be required for the desired effect. IV infusion is 2 mg/min titrated to desired response; 200 mg/160 ml D_5W yields 1 mg/ml.

Precautions

Use cautiously in patients with heart failure, hepatic impairment, chronic bronchitis, emphysema, preexisting peripheral vascular disease, and pheochromocytoma.

Patient Management

- Check HR and BP before administering labetalol and 10 minutes after an IV dose.

- Monitor BP every 5 minutes during infusion; avoid rapid BP drop because cerebral infarction or angina can occur.
- Have patient remain supine immediately following injection.
- Assess patient for heart failure development.
- Monitor blood glucose levels especially in patients with diabetes.
- Observe for adverse effects: dizziness, orthostatic hypotension, fatigue, nasal stuffiness, edema, paresthesias, dysrhythmias, and wheezing.

LIDOCAINE

Classification
Antidysrhythmic

Effects
Lidocaine suppresses the automaticity of ectopic foci.

Indications
Ventricular dysrhythmias

Contraindications
Patients with Adams-Stokes syndrome and severe heart block without a pacemaker

Administration
Dose
The loading dose is 1 to 1.5 mg/kg IV; repeat with 0.5 to 1.5 mg/kg every 5 to 10 minutes. Maximum is 3 mg/kg. IV infusion is 2 to 4 mg/min. A dose of 2 g/500 ml D_5W yields 4 mg/ml. (See drug dosage chart, p. 710.)

Precautions
Concurrent use with phenytoin can produce excessive cardiac depression. Use with β blockers or cimetidine may slow hepatic metabolism of lidocaine. Elderly patients are more susceptible to adverse effects. Do not use lidocaine solutions containing epinephrine.

Patient Management
- Evaluate dysrhythmia control.
- Measure serial PR intervals.
- Evaluate CI.

- Assess for CNS effects such as twitching and tremors, which may precede seizures.
- Observe for adverse effects: dizziness, restlessness, confusion, twitching, paresthesias, dysarthria, convulsions, drowsiness, bradycardia, itching, rash, anxiety, respiratory depression, blurred vision, tinnitus, vomiting, and malignant hyperthermia.

LORAZEPAM (ATIVAN)

Classification
Sedative, hypnotic, anticonvulsant

Effects
Lorazepam produces sedation and amnesia, relieves anxiety, and suppresses the spread of seizure activity.

Indications
Anxiety, agitation, preprocedure sedation, and status epilepticus

Contraindications
Acute narrow-angle glaucoma

Administration
Dose
Oral dose is 2 to 6 mg/day in divided doses. Maximum is 10 mg daily. IV or IM dose is 0.05 mg/kg or 2 mg (whichever is the lower dose). The drug may be given 2 mg/min as an IV injection. Dilute with equal volume of solution for IV injection.
Precautions
Administer cautiously in patients with organic brain syndrome, myasthenia gravis, and renal or hepatic impairment. Concurrent use with other CNS depressants will result in increased CNS depression.

Patient Management
- Ensure bed rest 3 hours after IV injection.
- Monitor for respiratory depression; maintain patent airway.
- Observe for adverse effects: excessive drowsiness, lethargy, blurred vision, delirium, hallucinations, transient hypotension, and abdominal discomfort.
- See Sedation of the critically ill, p. 545.

MAGNESIUM SULFATE

Classification
Electrolyte replenisher

Effects
Magnesium sulfate replaces and maintains magnesium levels in body fluids. It depresses the CNS, producing anticonvulsant effects.

Indications
Seizures associated with eclampsia and preeclampsia, hypomagnesemia, and torsades de pointes

Contraindications
Heart block, myocardial damage, and renal failure; also contraindicated for the pregnant patient within 2 hours of expected delivery

Administration
Dose

For seizures, give 1 to 4 g as a 10% solution. Administer 1.5 ml of a 10% solution IV over 1 minute. As an infusion of 4 g/250 ml D_5W, do not exceed a rate of 4 ml/min.

For hypomagnesemia, give an infusion of 5 g/1000 ml D_5W over 3 hours (rate not to exceed 3 ml/min).

For torsades de pointes, administer 2 g IV over 1 to 2 minutes.

Precautions

Use cautiously in patients with renal disease and in the presence of heart failure or myocardial damage. CNS effects are potentiated when the drug is administered with other CNS depressants. If magnesium toxicity occurs in a digitalized patient requiring calcium to treat the toxicity, heart block may occur. Magnesium crosses the placenta and can produce adverse effects on the baby.

Patient Management
- Evaluate presence of patellar reflexes before each dose. If they are absent, magnesium should not be given until they return.
- Monitor respirations: respirations must be at least 16/min before a dose can be given to reduce the risk for respiratory arrest.

- Monitor renal status: urine output should be at least 25 ml/hr.
- Monitor for signs of heart block and hypotension.
- Have emergency equipment available in case of respiratory/cardiac arrest.
- Calcium 5 to 10 mEq can be given to reverse respiratory depression and heart block.
- Observe for adverse effects: absent patellar reflex; flushing; hypotension; sweating; flaccid paralysis; prolonged PR, QRS, and QT intervals; respiratory depression; and cardiac arrest.

METOPROLOL (LOPRESSOR)

Classification
β-adrenergic blocking agent

Effects
Reduces incidence of recurrent myocardial infarction, size of the infarct, and incidence of fatal dysrhythmias.

Indications
Acute myocardial infarction

Contraindications
Severe bradycardia, second- and third-degree heart block, cardiac failure, hypotension (SBP <100 mm Hg), first-degree heart block (PR >0.24)

Administration
Dose
Administer 5 to 10 mg IV at 5 min intervals to a total of 15 mg. Fifteen min after the last IV bolus, give 50 mg po q6h for 48 hrs. Maintenance: 100 mg po BID. Oral dosage is dependent on degree of intolerance to IV dose. Patients who are not treated early should be started on 100 mg po BID as soon as their condition allows. Therapy may be continued for months or years.
Precautions
Use cautiously in patients in heart failure, lung disease/bronchospasm. May mask tachycardia associated with hyperthyroidism or hypoglycemia.

Patient Management

- Monitor cardiac rhythm, HR, and BP. Notify physician if hypotension and bradycardia develop.
- Evaluate patient for development of heart failure.
- Monitor blood glucose levels, especially in patients with diabetes.
- Observe for adverse effects: breathing difficulties, bradycardias, heart block, hypotension, cardiac failure.

MIDAZOLAM (VERSED)

Classification
Sedative, hypnotic

Effects

Midazolam relieves anxiety and produces sedation and amnesia.

Indications

To produce sedation, relieve anxiety, and impair memory of painful or other experiences

Contraindications

Acute narrow-angle glaucoma, shock, coma

Administration

Dose
For short-term sedation, administer 0.5 to 2.5 mg IV over 2 min. Titrate in small increments to slurred speech. Dilute with NS to permit slow titration. Infusion: 0.05 to 0.1 mg/kg/hr after a bolus of 0.05 to 0.1 mg/kg.

Precautions
Reduce dosage in presence of narcotic or other CNS depressants. Use cautiously in patients in heart failure, chronic obstructive pulmonary disease.

Patient Management

- Monitor cardiac rhythm, HR, BP.
- Assess patient for respiratory embarrassment; maintain patent airway and monitor respiratory rate.
- Monitor blood glucose levels, especially in patients with diabetes.

- Observe for adverse effects: breathing difficulties, brady-cardia, cardiac or respiratory arrest, dysrhythmias, hypotension.

MILRINONE (PRIMACOR)

Classification
Inotrope and vasodilator

Effects
Arterial vasodilation and increase in myocardial contractility

Indications
Treatment of heart failure

Contraindications
Hypersensitivity to milrinone

Administration
Dose
Loading dose is 50 mcg/kg IV slowly over 10 min. Usual maintenance: 0.5 mcg/kg/min.
Precautions
Outflow tract obstruction may worsen in patients with obstructive aortic or pulmonic valve disease or hypertrophic subaortic stenosis. Ventricular dysrhythmias may develop. Infusion rates should be reduced in patients with renal function impairment.

Patient Management
- Monitor HR and rhythm, MAP, SVRI PVRI, CI, PAWP.
- Monitor intake and output, creatinine and BUN, and serum electrolytes.
- Titrate infusion to maximum hemodynamic effect.
- Reduce infusion rate if hypotension occurs.
- Observe for adverse effects: dysrhythmias, hypotension, angina, hypokalemia, thrombocytopenia.

NALOXONE (NARCAN)

Classification
Narcotic antagonist

Effects

Naloxone competes with narcotics for receptor sites in the CNS. It has no pharmacological activity of its own.

Indications

Patients with known or suspected narcotic-induced respiratory depression

Contraindications

None

Administration

Dose

Administer 0.4 to 2 mg IV over 15 seconds; dose may be repeated every 2 to 3 minutes.

Precautions

Use cautiously in patients with cardiac irritability and narcotic addiction.

Drug is not effective in respiratory depression caused by anesthetics, barbiturates, or other nonnarcotic agents.

Patient Management

- Monitor respiratory depth and rate continuously; duration of narcotic may exceed that of naloxone, and the patient may lapse into respiratory depression.
- Provide O_2 and artificial ventilation as necessary.
- Observe for adverse effects: nausea and vomiting, sweating, tachycardia, hypertension, pulmonary edema, VT, and VF.

NIFEDIPINE (ADALAT, PROCARDIA)

Classification

Calcium channel blocker

Effects

Nifedipine dilates coronary arteries and arterioles. It has less effect on decreasing HR and myocardial contractility than other calcium channel blockers.

Indications

Chronic angina and hypertension

Contraindications

Aortic stenosis, cardiogenic shock, and acute angina attacks

Administration

Dose

Give 10 mg orally three times daily. Maximum is 180 mg. Single doses should not exceed 30 mg. Nifedipine should be decreased gradually if it is to be discontinued. The liquid in the oral capsule can be withdrawn by puncturing the capsule with a needle and administering 10 to 20 mg sublingually or bucally. Maximal effects can be achieved by chewing and swallowing the capsules. The extended-release preparation (Procardia XL) should never be crushed, chewed, or administered sublingually.

Precautions

Use with β blockers may cause profound hypotension and heart failure. Use cautiously in elderly patients, patients with heart failure or hypotension, and patients with impaired renal or hepatic function. Gradually taper calcium channel blocker to avoid rebound angina.

Patient Management

- Monitor for increased/decreased anginal episodes.
- Measure serial PR intervals.
- Check HR and BP before administration; if systolic blood pressure (SBP) <90 or HR <50, notify physician.
- Monitor CI and assess patient for development of heart failure.
- Monitor serum potassium levels frequently.
- Assess for signs of peripheral edema (pedal edema is dose related).
- Observe for adverse effects: dizziness, lightheadedness, flushing, headache, and nausea.

NITROGLYCERIN (TRIDIL, NITROL)

Classification

Vasodilator

Effects

Nitroglycerin decreases venous return, preload, myocardial oxygen demand, BP, MAP, CVP, PAWP, PVRI, and SVRI. It improves coronary artery blood flow and oxygen delivery.

Indications

Angina, hypertension, and heart failure in acute myocardial infarction

Contraindications

Patients with hypersensitivity to nitrites; patients with head trauma, cerebral hemorrhage, severe anemia, pericardial tamponade, or constrictive pericarditis; and those with hypertrophic cardiomyopathy who are experiencing chest pain

Administration

Dose

IV infusion is 5 μg/min; increase by 5 μg every 3 to 5 minutes and titrate to desired response. A dose of 50 mg/500 ml D_5W yields 100 μg/ml. No fixed maximum dose has been established. (See drug dosage chart, p. 710.)

Precautions

Use with tricyclic antidepressants may result in additive hypotension. Orthostatic hypotension may be potentiated with antihypertensives or vasodilators. Correct volume deficit to prevent profound hypotension. Tolerance may develop with prolonged use of nitroglycerin.

Patient Management

- Monitor HR; a 10 bpm increase suggests adequate vasodilation.
- Monitor BP every 2 to 5 minutes while titrating.
- Stop infusion and lift patient's lower extremities if SBP <90 or if patient complains of dizziness/lightheadedness.
- Calculate coronary perfusion pressure (CPP); monitor PAWP, SVRI, and PVRI; and evaluate CI.
- Observe for adverse effects: headache, dizziness, dry mouth, blurred vision, orthostatic hypotension, tachycardia, angina, flushing, palpitations, nausea, and restlessness.
- Report unrelieved angina and signs and symptoms of overdose: cyanotic lips and palmar surface of hands, extreme dizziness, pressure in head, dyspnea, fever, seizure, and weak/fast HR.

NITROPRUSSIDE (NIPRIDE)

Classification

Vasodilator, antihypertensive

Effects

Nitroprusside decreases BP and peripheral resistance and usually increases CO.

Indications

Hypertension

Contraindications

Coarctation of aorta

Administration

Dose

IV infusion is 0.5 to 10 μg/kg/min. Maximum is 10 μg/kg/min. A dose of 50 mg/250 ml D_5W yields 200 μg/ml. (See drug dosage chart, p. 711.)

Precautions

Use cautiously in patients with hypothyroidism or hepatic or renal disease and in those receiving antihypertensive agents. Infusion rates greater than 2 mcg/kg/min are associated with increased risk of cyanide toxicity.

Patient Management

- Monitor BP every 2 to 5 minutes; if hypotension develops, discontinue IV nitroprusside.
- Use an IV infusion device; validate concentration/dosage.
- Protect solution from light; it normally is brownish.
- Assess patient for chest pain, dysrhythmias, and fluid retention.
- Observe for adverse effects: headache, dizziness, excessive sweating, nervousness, restlessness, ataxia, delirium, loss of consciousness, ringing in the ears, abdominal pain, retrosternal discomfort, bradycardia, tachycardia, and increased intracranial pressure.
- Tolerance to nipride may indicate toxicity. Monitor thiocyanate levels. Thiocyanate levels of greater than 100 μg/ml indicate toxicity.
- Assess for signs of toxicity: profound hypotension, metabolic acidosis, dyspnea, headache, loss of consciousness, and vomiting.

NOREPINEPHRINE (LEVOPHED)

Classification

Sympathomimetic, vasopressor

Effects
Norepinephrine produces vasoconstriction, increases myocardial contractility, and dilates coronary arteries.

Indications
Hypotensive states caused by trauma, shock, and myocardial infarction

Contraindications
Mesenteric or peripheral vascular thrombosis, pregnancy, profound hypoxia, hypercarbia, hypotension from volume deficit, or with cyclopropane or halothane anesthesia

Administration
Dose
IV infusion is 0.5 to 1 µg/min; titrate to desired BP. A dose of 4 mg/250 ml D_5W yields 16 µg/ml. (See drug dosage chart, p. 712.)
Precautions
Concurrent administration with MAO inhibitors increases the risk of hypertensive crisis. When the drug is administered with tricyclic antidepressants, severe hypertension may result. Use cautiously in patients with hypertension, hyperthyroidism, and severe cardiac disease. Correct fluid volume deficit before administering norepinephrine.

Patient Management
- Monitor BP every 2 to 5 minutes.
- Evaluate CI.
- Assess patency of IV site and observe for extravasation; blanching may indicate extravasation. If extravasation occurs, stop the infusion and call the physician. Be prepared to infiltrate the area with phentolamine 5 to 10 mg in 10 to 15 ml NS.
- Use an infusion pump to regulate flow.
- Assess for signs and symptoms of excessive vasoconstriction: cold skin, pallor, decreased pulses, decreased cerebral perfusion, and decreased pulse pressure.
- Report decreased urinary output.
- Taper medication gradually and monitor vital signs.
- Observe for adverse effects: headache, VT, bradycardia, VF, decreased urinary output, metabolic acidosis, restlessness, and hypertensive state.

PANCURONIUM (PAVULON)

Classification

Nondepolarizing neuromuscular blocking agent

Effects

Pancuronium causes skeletal muscle paralysis but has no effects on consciousness or pain.

Indications

Facilitation of controlled mechanical ventilation

Contraindications

Hypersensitivity to bromides, preexisting tachycardia, and conditions in which an increase in HR is undesirable

Administration

Dose

A dose of 0.04 to 0.1 mg/kg IV may be given undiluted; a single dose may be given over 1 to 2 minutes. Subsequent doses are repeated as required and usually start at 0.01 mg/kg for continued muscle relaxation. As a constant infusion, titrate the dose to patient response.

Precautions

The dose needs to be adjusted when aminoglycosides are being administered. Use with quinidine can result in increased neuromuscular blockage. Use cautiously in elderly or debilitated patients and those with renal, hepatic, or pulmonary impairment; myasthenia gravis; dehydration; thyroid disorders; collagen disease; electrolyte disturbances; hyperthermia; and cardiac dysrhythmias. Patients with cardiovascular disease and edematous states may experience a delay in onset; drug dosage should not be increased.

Patients must have a patent airway and be artificially ventilated. Patients are conscious but unable to communicate and should be sedated. Pancuronium has no effect on pain; analgesics should be administered for pain.

Patient Management

- Ensure patent airway and controlled mechanical ventilation.
- Monitor the rhythm, BP, and respirations.
- Analyze arterial blood gases (ABGs) and pulse oximetry for adequate oxygenation.

- Monitor exhaled volume with spirometer and end tidal CO_2 with capnograph.
- See Neuromuscular blockade, p. 542.
- Monitor serum electrolyte levels since abnormalities can affect neuromuscular transmission.
- Use adjunctive therapy for pain control and sedation throughout the period of paralysis.
- Use a peripheral nerve stimulator to monitor neuromuscular suppression and recovery.
- Have emergency respiratory equipment readily available in case of accidental extubation or lack of endotracheal tube patency.
- Observe for adverse effects: tachycardia, hypertension, and malignant hyperthermia.

PHENOBARBITAL

Classification
Anticonvulsant, sedative, hypnotic

Effects
Phenobarbital depresses the CNS and increases the threshold for seizure activity.

Indications
Seizures and need for sedation

Contraindications
Barbiturate hypersensitivity, porphyria, hepatic dysfunction, respiratory disease, nephritis, and lactation

Administration
Dose
IV dose is 1 to 3 mg/kg/day. IV loading dose of 15 to 20 mg/kg is recommended for the treatment of patients with status epilepticus. Do not give faster than 60 mg/min intravenously.
Precautions
Use with other CNS depressants can result in excessive CNS depression. There may be a potentiated barbiturate effect when the drug is given concurrently with MAO inhibitors. Rifampin may decrease the barbiturate levels. Primidone and valproic acid may cause phenobarbital levels to be elevated. Diazepam and phenobarbital given together may result in an

increased effect of both drugs and should be used cautiously. Use cautiously in patients with hyperthyroidism, diabetes mellitus, or anemia and in elderly or debilitated patients.

Rapid infusion of phenobarbital may cause respiratory depression.

Patient Management

- Monitor vital signs hourly, including respiratory rate; ensure patent airway.
- Check phenobarbital level; therapeutic level is 15 to 40 µg/ml.
- Evaluate patient response (e.g., absence of seizure activity).
- Observe for adverse effects: drowsiness, lethargy, nausea and vomiting, hypotension, apnea, and hypothermia.

PHENYTOIN (DILANTIN)

Classification
Anticonvulsant

Effects
Phenytoin depresses seizure activity.

Indications
Generalized seizure control and digitalis-induced dysrhythmias

Contraindications
Bradycardia, SA and AV block, and Adams-Stokes syndrome

Administration
Dose
Anticonvulsant IV loading dose is 10 to 15 mg/kg followed by a maintenance dose of 100 mg orally or IV q6 to 8 hours.

Antidysrhythmic dose is 50 to 100 mg IV every 10 to 15 minutes, until desired effects are obtained. The dose should not exceed a total dose of 15 mg/kg. Do not exceed a rate of 50 mg/min. An in-line filter is recommended to administer the diluted phenytoin. Before and after each dose of phenytoin, the line should be flushed with normal saline.

Precautions
The effects of phenytoin may be decreased with barbiturates and folic acid. The effects of phenytoin can be increased when used with chloramphenicol, cimetidine, disulfiram, iso-

niazid, or sulfonamides. Use with antidysrhythmics may result in an additive cardiac depressant effect. Oral contraceptives and phenytoin may result in decreased contraceptive reliability and/or loss of seizure control. Use cautiously in patients with hepatic or renal dysfunction, hypotension, myocardial insufficiency, or respiratory depression and in elderly or debilitated patients.

Patient Management

- Assess patency of IV; follow each injection with NS. Extravasation of phenytoin is damaging to the tissues.
- Monitor BP, HR, and respiratory rate with administration of IV phenytoin; bradycardia, cardiac arrest, and respiratory arrest can occur.
- Monitor blood levels; therapeutic level is 10 to 20 µg/ml.
- Observe for adverse effects: nystagmus, skin rash, blurred vision, double vision, unusual bleeding, jaundice, drowsiness, gum hyperplasia, and hypotension.

PROCAINAMIDE (PRONESTYL)

Classification
Antidysrhythmic

Effects
Procainamide depresses cardiac automaticity, excitability, and conductivity.

Indications
Premature ventricular complexes, ventricular tachycardia, and atrial dysrhythmias

Contraindications
Second- or third-degree heart block, hypersensitivity to procaine, myasthenia gravis, torsades de pointes, and lupus erythematosus.

Administration
Dose
Administer 20 mg/min IV until the dysrhythmia is abolished, hypotension occurs, QRS widens by 50%, or a total of 17 mg/kg has been given. IV infusion is 1 to 4 mg/min; a dose of 2 g/500 ml D_5W yields 4 mg/ml. (See drug dosage chart, p. 710.)

Precautions

Concurrent administration with cimetidine, beta blockers, ranitidine, or amiodarone may result in increased procainamide blood levels. Use cautiously in patients with conduction delays, hepatic or renal insufficiency, and heart failure. Patients with atrial fibrillation and atrial flutter may develop tachycardia.

Patient Management

- Monitor BP and ECG every 2 to 5 minutes during IV titration.
- Measure PR, QT, and QRS intervals.
- Assess for heart failure development.
- Evaluate CI.
- Observe for adverse effects: hypotension, agranulocytosis, neutropenia, joint pain, fever, chills, bradycardia, VT, VF, nausea and vomiting, anorexia, diarrhea, bitter taste, maculopapular rash, and lupus erythematosus-like syndrome.

PROPOFOL (DIPRIVAN)

Classification
Sedative, hypnotic

Effects
Produces sedation or anesthesia

Indications
Continuous sedation and control of stress response in intubated mechanically ventilated patients

Contraindications
Hypersensitivity to propofol or its components (e.g., soybean oil, egg lecithin, glycerol)

Administration
Dose
Initially, 5 mcg/kg/min; increase in increments of 5 to 10 mcg/kg/min over 5 to 10 minutes until desired level of sedation is attained. Allow 5 minutes between dose adjustments. Do not bolus propofol.
Precautions
Propofol injection does not contain preservatives and is capable of supporting rapid growth of microorganisms. Discard

tubing and unused portions after 12 hours. Do not use if there is separation of the emulsion. Patients must be intubated and mechanically ventilated. Use cautiously in patients with increased serum triglycerides (diabetic hyperlipemia, pancreatitis, hyperlipoproteinemia). Patients who have been medicated with opioids may require reduced dosages. Other drugs may need to be decreased when propofol is begun (e.g., beta-blockers, vasodilators).

Patient Management

- Evaluate level of sedation and assess neurological function daily.
- To awaken the patient, taper the infusion rate in 5 to 10 mcg/kg/min at 10 to 15 min intervals until the desired level of light sedation is achieved. Do not awaken the patient abruptly. Once the patient is oriented, discontinue the infusion and assess the patient's neuro and respiratory function. To titrate to a deeper level of sedation, increase the infusion rate 5 to 10 mcg/kg/min at 10 to 15 min intervals.
- Monitor BP, HR, CI, and PAWP (if available) for cardiovascular depression.
- Assess oxygenation and ventilation with ABG results and pulse oximetry.
- Monitor serum triglycerides.
- Provide pain medication as prescribed; propofol is not an analgesic.
- To wean the patient from the ventilator, the infusion rate should be decreased until the patient is awake, can follow commands, and has no evidence of hypoventilation. If extubation criteria are met, discontinue the propofol 10 to 15 minutes before extubation.
- Observe for adverse effects: decrease in cardiac output, bradycardia, hypotension, hyperlipidemia, respiratory acidosis.

See Sedation in the critically ill, p. 545.

PROPRANOLOL (INDERAL)

Classification
β-adrenergic blocking agent, antidysrhythmic

Effects
Propranolol decreases cardiac oxygen demand, HR, BP, and myocardial contractility.

Indications

Angina, MI, cardiac dysrhythmias, hypertension, migraine or vascular headache, and pheochromocytoma

Contraindications

Diabetes mellitus, asthma, chronic obstructive pulmonary disease (COPD), allergic rhinitis, sinus bradycardia, heart block greater than first degree, cardiogenic shock, and right ventricular failure secondary to pulmonary hypertension

Administration

Dose

Oral dose is 10 to 60 mg three or four times daily. IV dose is 1 to 3 mg; drug may be given undiluted at a rate of 1 mg/min. After 3 mg have been administered, wait 2 minutes and give 3 mg (1 mg at a time, if needed). Subsequent doses may not be given for at least 4 hours, regardless of route to be administered.

Precautions

Additive effects may result when the drug is administered with diltiazem or verapamil. Use with digoxin may result in excessive bradycardia with potential for heart block. Concurrent use with epinephrine may result in significant hypertension and excessive bradycardia. Propranolol may mask certain symptoms of developing hypoglycemia. Use cautiously in patients with heart failure or respiratory disease and in patients taking other antihypertensive drugs. The dosage should be adjusted in elderly patients.

Patient Management

- Continuously monitor ECG with IV administration; if bradycardia develops, do not administer propranolol.
- Monitor BP and other hemodynamic parameters (e.g., CVP, PAWP) frequently during IV administration; if SBP <90, notify physician.
- Assess patient for development of heart failure.
- Monitor blood glucose levels, especially in patients with diabetes.
- Do not abruptly withdraw medication.
- Observe for adverse effects: bradycardia, heart failure, intensification of AV block, nausea and vomiting, abdominal cramps, hypoglycemia, and difficulty in breathing.

SODIUM BICARBONATE

Classification

Alkalizer, antacid, electrolyte replenisher

Effects

Sodium bicarbonate increases the plasma bicarbonate, buffers excess hydrogen ion concentration, and increases blood pH.

Indications

Metabolic acidosis and need to alkalinize the urine

Contraindications

Metabolic or respiratory acidosis, hypocalcemia, not recommended in cardiac arrest unless other interventions have been instituted and specific clinical circumstances exist (e.g., pre-existing metabolic acidosis)

Administration

Dose

If used in cardiac arrest, the IV dose is 1 mEq/kg initially, then 0.5 mEq/kg in 10 minutes if indicated by arterial pH and P_{CO_2}. IV infusion is 2 to 5 mEq/kg; drug may be administered over 4 to 8 hours in less acute acidosis.

Precautions

Rapid administration of sodium bicarbonate may result in severe alkalosis. Tetany or hyperirritability may occur with increased alkalosis.

Patient Management

- Assess patency of IV; extravasation may cause necrosis or sloughing of tissue.
- Obtain arterial blood pH, P_{O_2}, and P_{CO_2} results before administering sodium bicarbonate.
- Flush line before and after administration of sodium bicarbonate.
- Observe for adverse effects: restlessness, tetany, hypokalemia, alkalosis, and hypernatremia.

VECURONIUM (NORCURON)

Classification

Nondepolarizing neuromuscular blocking agent

Effects

Vecuronium produces skeletal muscle paralysis but has no effect on consciousness or pain.

Indications

Facilitation of endotracheal intubation, need for skeletal muscle relaxation during surgery or mechanical ventilation, and adjunct to general anesthesia

Contraindications

Hypersensitivity to bromides

Administration

Dose

Administer 0.08 to 0.10 mg/kg IV; the drug may be given over 1 minute. Maintenance doses of 0.010 to 0.015 mg/kg may be required to prolong the muscle relaxant effects. Maintenance doses may be repeated as necessary.

Precautions

Neuromuscular blockade may be potentiated by administration of aminoglycoside antibiotics. Patients with cardiovascular disease and edematous states may experience a delay in onset; drug dosage should not be increased. Patients must have a patent airway and be mechanically ventilated. Patients are conscious but unable to communicate. Vecuronium has no effect on pain and analgesics should be administered for pain.

Patient Management

- Ensure patent airway and controlled mechanical ventilation.
- Monitor HR rhythm, BP, and respiration.
- Analyze ABGs and pulse oximetry for adequate oxygenation.
- Use adjunctive therapy for pain control and sedation throughout the period of paralysis.
- Use a peripheral nerve stimulator to monitor neuromuscular suppression and recovery.
- Monitor exhaled volume with spirometer and end tidal CO_2 with capnograph.
- Monitor serum electrolytes since abnormalities can affect neuromuscular transmission.
- See Neuromuscular blockade, p. 542.

- Have emergency respiratory support available in case of accidental extubation or lack of endotracheal tube patency.
- Observe for adverse effects: malignant hyperthermia, respiratory depression, apnea.

VERAPAMIL (CALAN, ISOPTIN)

Classification
Calcium channel blocking agent

Effects
Verapamil decreases myocardial contractility, dilates coronary arteries and arterioles, decreases BP, and decreases HR.

Indications
Angina, atrial dysrhythmias, hypertension, and migraine headache prophylaxis

Contraindications
Advanced heart failure, heart block, cardiogenic shock, aortic stenosis, W-P-W syndrome, and severe hypotension

Administration
Dose
To treat SVT, IV dose is 2.5 to 5 mg given undiluted over 2 minutes. Repeat doses of 5 to 10 mg to a maximum of 20 mg in 15 to 30 minutes if no response.
Precautions
Concurrent administration with β blockers, disopyramide, or verapamil may produce profound cardiac depressant effects. Use caution in patients with myocardial infarction, advanced heart block, heart failure, and atrial tachydysrhythmias.

Patient Management
- Monitor ECG continuously in patients receiving verapamil intravenously.
- Measure serial PR intervals and HR.
- Assess for development of heart failure.
- Monitor BP and HR before administration; if SBP <90 or HR <50, notify the physician.
- Evaluate CI and efficacy of therapy (e.g., BP control, dysrhythmia control, angina control).
- Observe for adverse effects: transient hypotension, dizziness, heart failure, and constipation.

Dobutamine: 250 mg/250 ml*
CONCENTRATION: 1000 µg/ml

Weight (kg)	45	50	55	60	65	70	75	80	85	90	95	100
µg/kg/min	Flow rate (ml/hr)											
5	14	15	17	18	20	21	23	24	26	27	29	30
7.5	20	23	25	27	29	32	34	36	38	41	43	45
10	27	30	33	36	39	42	45	48	51	54	57	60
12.5	34	38	41	45	49	53	56	60	64	68	71	75
15	41	45	50	54	59	63	68	72	77	81	86	90
17.5	47	53	58	63	68	74	79	84	89	95	100	105
20	54	60	66	72	78	84	90	96	102	108	114	120

*Dobutamine—ACLS: patient weight in kg × 15 determines the amount of dobutamine (mg) to be added to 250 ml of IV fluid. The rate set on the infusion pump = µg/kg/min.

Dopamine: 400 mg/500 ml*
CONCENTRATION: 800 µg/ml

Weight (kg)	45	50	55	60	65	70	75	80	85	90	95	100
µg/kg/min	Flow rate (ml/hr)											
1	3	4	4	5	5	6	6	6	6	7	7	8
2	7	8	8	9	10	11	11	12	13	14	14	15
3	10	11	12	14	15	16	17	18	19	20	21	23
5	17	19	21	23	24	26	28	30	32	34	36	38
7	24	26	29	32	34	37	39	42	45	47	50	53
10	34	38	41	45	49	53	56	60	64	68	71	75
13	44	49	54	59	63	68	73	78	83	88	93	98
15	51	56	62	68	73	79	84	90	96	101	107	113
20	68	75	83	90	98	105	113	120	128	135	143	150
25	84	94	103	113	122	131	141	150	159	167	178	188
30	101	113	124	135	146	158	169	180	191	203	214	225

*Dopamine—ACLS: patient weight in kg × 15 determines the amount of dopamine (mg) to be added to 250 ml of IV fluid. The rate set on the infusion pump = µg/kg/min.

Lidocaine, Bretylium, Procainamide: 2 g/500 ml
CONCENTRATION: 4 mg/ml

Dose (mg/min)	Rate (ml/hr)
1	15
2	30
3	45
4	60

Isoproterenol, Epinephrine: 1 mg/250 ml
CONCENTRATION: 4 µg/ml

Dose (µg/min)	Rate (ml/hr)
1	15
2	30
3	45
4	60

Nitroglycerin: 50 mg/500 ml
CONCENTRATION: 100 µg/ml

Dose (µg/min)	Rate (ml/hr)
5	3
10	6
15	9
20	12
25	15
30	18
35	21
40	24
45	27
50	30

Nitroprusside: 50 mg/250 ml
CONCENTRATION: 200 µg/ml

Weight (kg)	45	50	55	60	65	70	75	80	85	90	95	100
µg/kg/min	Flow rate (ml/hr)											
1	14	15	16	18	20	21	23	24	26	27	29	30
2	27	30	33	36	39	42	45	48	51	54	57	60
4	54	60	66	72	78	84	90	96	102	108	114	120
6	81	90	99	108	117	126	135	144	153	162	171	180
8	108	120	132	144	156	168	180	192	204	216	228	240

Norepinephrine: 4 mg/250 ml
CONCENTRATION: 16 µg/ml

Weight (kg)	45	50	55	60	65	70	75	80	85	90	95	100
µg/kg/min	Flow rate (ml/hr)											
0.1	17	19	21	23	24	26	28	30	32	34	36	38
0.2	34	38	41	45	49	53	56	60	64	68	71	75
0.3	51	56	62	68	73	79	84	90	96	101	107	113
0.4	68	75	82	90	98	105	112	120	128	135	142	150
0.5	85	94	103	113	122	132	141	150	160	169	178	188
0.6	101	113	124	135	146	158	168	180	191	203	214	225
0.7	118	132	144	158	171	184	197	210	223	237	249	263
0.8	135	150	165	180	195	210	225	240	255	270	285	300
0.9	152	169	185	203	220	237	253	270	287	304	320	338
1.0	169	188	206	225	244	263	281	300	319	338	356	375

Norepinephrine: 4 mg/250 ml
CONCENTRATION: 16 µg/ml

Dose (µg/ml)	Rate (ml/hr)
1	4
2	8
3	11
4	15
5	19

CALCULATIONS

The critical care environment requires that nurses be able to calculate infusion drips to determine the amount of drug that is being administered. Medications are frequently administered as continuous IV infusions and titrated to achieve the desired response.

Drug Concentration in mg/ml or µg/ml

$$1 \text{ mg} = 1000 \text{ µg}$$

$$1 \text{ g} = 1000 \text{ mg}$$

To determine the amount of drug in one ml, divide the amount of drug in solution by the amount of solution (ml).

Example: 200 mg of drug in 500 ml
Determine mg/ml:

$$\frac{200 \text{ mg}}{500 \text{ ml}} = 0.4 \text{ mg/ml}$$

Determine µg/ml:
First change mg to µg:

$$200 \text{ mg} \times 1000 \text{ µg/mg} = 200,000 \text{ µg}$$

Then divide µg by ml of solution:

$$\frac{200,000 \text{ µg}}{500 \text{ ml}} = 400 \text{ µg/ml}$$

Calculating µg/kg/min

Drug dosages are often expressed in µg/kg/min. Three parameters must be known to determine the amount of medication the patient is receiving:
1. Patient weight in kg (1 kg = 2.2 lb)
2. Infusion rate (ml/hr)
3. Drug concentration

The drug concentration is multiplied by the infusion rate and divided by the patient weight × 60 min/hr:

$$\mu g/kg/min = \frac{\mu g/ml \times ml/hr}{kg \times 60 \ min/hr}$$

Example: A patient weighing 75 kg is receiving dobutamine at 20 ml/hr. There is 250 mg of dobutamine in 250 ml D_5W.
1. The patient weight is 75 kg
2. The infusion rate is 20 ml/hr
3. The drug concentration needs to be determined in µg/ml:

First change mg to µg:

$$250 \ mg = 250,000 \ \mu g$$

Next, divide the dosage by the amount of solution:

$$\frac{250,000 \ \mu g}{250 \ ml} = 1000 \ \mu g/ml$$

Since all three parameters are known, now determine µg/kg/min:

$$\mu g/kg/min = \frac{\mu g/ml \times ml/hr}{kg \times 60 \ min/hr}$$
$$= \frac{1000 \times 20}{75 \times 60}$$
$$= \frac{20,000}{4500}$$
$$= 4.44 \ \mu g/kg/min$$

Calculating the Amount of Fluid to Infuse (ml/hr)

Three parameters must be known to determine the infusion rate for the IV pump:
1. The patient weight in kg (1 kg = 2.2 lb)

2. The dose ordered by the physician in µg/kg/min
3. The drug concentration in µg/min

Multiply the dose ordered by the patient weight × 60 min and divide by the drug concentration:

$$ml/hr = \frac{\mu g/kg/min \ ordered \times kg \times 60 \ min}{\mu g/ml}$$

Example: A patient weighing 70 kg is to receive dopamine at 6 µg/kg/min. There is 400 mg of dopamine in 250 ml D$_5$W.
1. The patient weight is 70 kg
2. The dose ordered is 6 µg/kg/min
3. The drug concentration needs to be determined in µg/ml:
First change mg to µg:

$$400 \ mg \times 1000 \ \mu/mg = 400,000 \ \mu g$$

Next, divide the dosage by the amount of solution:

$$\frac{400,000 \ \mu g}{250 \ ml} = 1600 \ \mu g/ml$$

Since all three parameters are known, determine ml/hr:

$$ml/hr = \frac{\mu g/kg/min \ ordered \times kg \times 60 \ min}{\mu g/ml}$$

$$= \frac{6 \times 70 \times 60}{1600}$$

$$= \frac{25,200}{1600}$$

$$= 16 \ ml/hr$$

REFERENCES

1. Emergency Cardiac Care Committee and Subcommittees, American Heart Association: Guidelines for cardiopulmonary resuscitation and emergency cardiac care, *JAMA* 268(16):2171-2250, 1992.
2. *Facts and comparisons,* St Louis, 1995, J.B. Lippincott.
3. Gahart B: *Intravenous medications,* ed 11, St Louis, 1995, Mosby.
4. Kinney MR, Packa DR, Dunbar SB: *AACN's clinical reference for critical-care nursing,* ed 3, St Louis, 1993. Mosby.

ACLS Algorithms*

UNIVERSAL ALGORITHM FOR ADULT EMERGENCY CARDIAC CARE

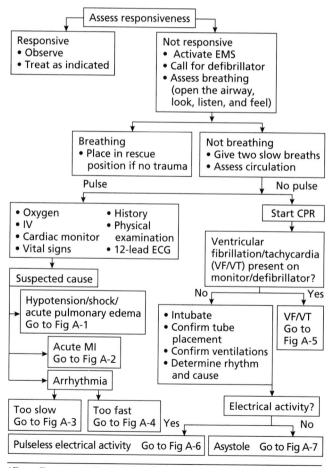

*From Emergency Cardiac Care Committee and Subcommittees, American Heart Association: *JAMA* 286(16):2216-2230, 1992.

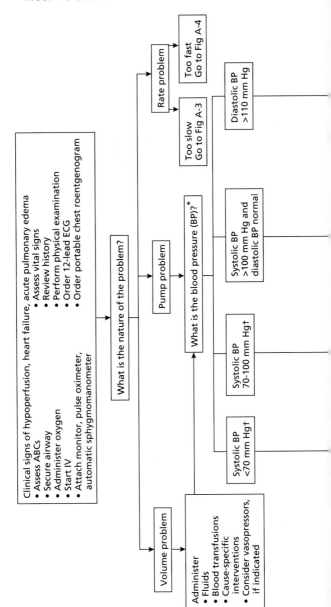

Clinical signs of hypoperfusion, heart failure, acute pulmonary edema
- Assess ABCs
- Secure airway
- Administer oxygen
- Start IV
- Attach monitor, pulse oximeter, automatic sphygmomanometer
- Assess vital signs
- Review history
- Perform physical examination
- Order 12-lead ECG
- Order portable chest roentgenogram

What is the nature of the problem?

Volume problem

Administer
- Fluids
- Blood transfusions
- Cause-specific interventions
- Consider vasopressors, if indicated

Pump problem

What is the blood pressure (BP)?*

Systolic BP <70 mm Hg†

Systolic BP 70-100 mm Hg†

Systolic BP >100 mm Hg and diastolic BP normal

Rate problem

Too slow
Go to Fig A-3

Too fast
Go to Fig A-4

Diastolic BP >110 mm Hg

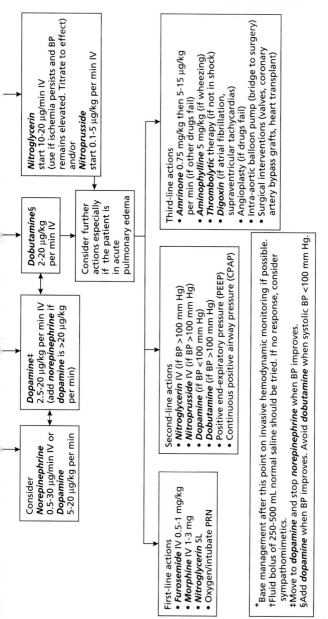

First-line actions
• **Furosemide** IV 0.5–1 mg/kg
• **Morphine** IV 1–3 mg
• **Nitroglycerin** SL
• Oxygen/intubate PRN

Second-line actions
• **Nitroglycerin** IV (if BP >100 mm Hg)
• **Nitroprusside** IV (if BP >100 mm Hg)
• **Dopamine** (if BP <100 mm Hg)
• **Dobutamine** (if BP >100 mm Hg)
• Positive end-expiratory pressure (PEEP)
• Continuous positive airway pressure (CPAP)

Third-line actions
• **Amrinone** 0.75 mg/kg then 5–15 µg/kg per min (if other drugs fail)
• **Aminophylline** 5 mg/kg (if wheezing)
• **Thrombolytic** therapy (if not in shock)
• **Digoxin** (if atrial fibrillation, supraventricular tachycardias
• Angioplasty (if drugs fail)
• Intra-aortic balloon pump (bridge to surgery)
• Surgical interventions (valves, coronary artery bypass grafts, heart transplant)

Consider further actions especially if the patient is in acute pulmonary edema

Nitroglycerin start 10–20 µg/min IV (use if ischemia persists and BP remains elevated. Titrate to effect) and/or
Nitroprusside start 0.1–5 µg/kg per min IV

Dobutamine§ 2–20 µg/kg per min IV

Dopamine‡ 2.5–20 µg/kg per min IV (add **norepinephrine** if **dopamine** is >20 µg/kg per min)

Consider **Norepinephrine** 0.5–30 µg/min IV or **Dopamine** 5–20 µg/kg per min

* Base management after this point on invasive hemodynamic monitoring if possible.
† Fluid bolus of 250–500 mL normal saline should be tried. If no response, consider sympathomimetics.
‡ Move to **dopamine** and stop **norepinephrine** when BP improves.
§ Add **dobutamine** when BP improves. Avoid **dobutamine** when systolic BP <100 mm Hg.

Figure A-1 Algorithm for hypotension, shock, and acute pulmonary edema.

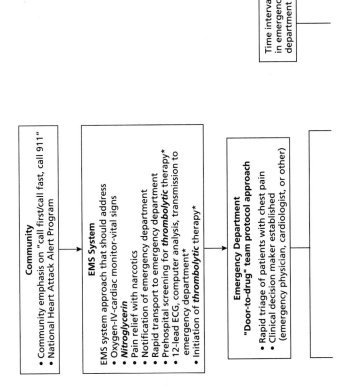

Community
- Community emphasis on "call first/call fast, call 911"
- National Heart Attack Alert Program

EMS System

EMS system approach that should address
- Oxygen–IV–cardiac monitor–vital signs
- *Nitroglycerin*
- Pain relief with narcotics
- Notification of emergency department
- Rapid transport to emergency department
- Prehospital screening for *thrombolytic* therapy*
- 12-lead ECG, computer analysis, transmission to emergency department*
- Initiation of *thrombolytic* therapy*

Emergency Department
"Door-to-drug" team protocol approach
- Rapid triage of patients with chest pain
- Clinical decision maker established (emergency physician, cardiologist, or other)

Time interval in emergency department

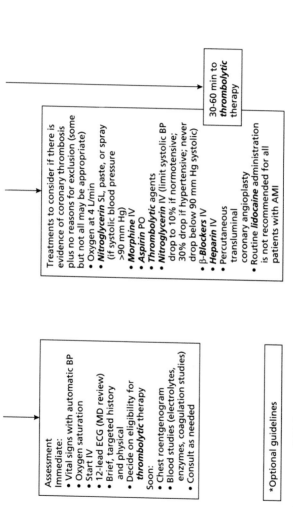

Assessment
Immediate:
• Vital signs with automatic BP
• Oxygen saturation
• Start IV
• 12-lead ECG (MD review)
• Brief, targeted history and physical
• Decide on eligibility for *thrombolytic* therapy
Soon:
• Chest roentgenogram
• Blood studies (electrolytes, enzymes, coagulation studies)
• Consult as needed

Treatments to consider if there is evidence of coronary thrombosis plus no reasons for exclusion (some but not all may be appropriate)
• Oxygen at 4 L/min
• *Nitroglycerin* SL, paste, or spray (if systolic blood pressure >90 mm Hg)
• *Morphine* IV
• *Aspirin* PO
• *Thrombolytic* agents
• *Nitroglycerin* IV (limit systolic BP drop to 10% if normotensive; 30% drop if hypertensive; never drop below 90 mm Hg systolic)
• *β-Blockers* IV
• *Heparin* IV
• Percutaneous transluminal coronary angioplasty
• Routine *lidocaine* administration is not recommended for all patients with AMI

30–60 min to *thrombolytic* therapy

*Optional guidelines

Figure A-2 Acute myocardial infarction (AMI) algorithm. Recommendations for early treatment of patients with chest pain and possible AMI.

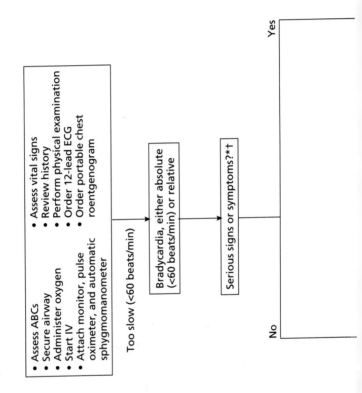

- Assess ABCs
- Secure airway
- Administer oxygen
- Start IV
- Attach monitor, pulse oximeter, and automatic sphygmomanometer
- Assess vital signs
- Review history
- Perform physical examination
- Order 12-lead ECG
- Order portable chest roentgenogram

Too slow (<60 beats/min)

Bradycardia, either absolute (<60 beats/min) or relative

Serious signs or symptoms?*†

No   Yes

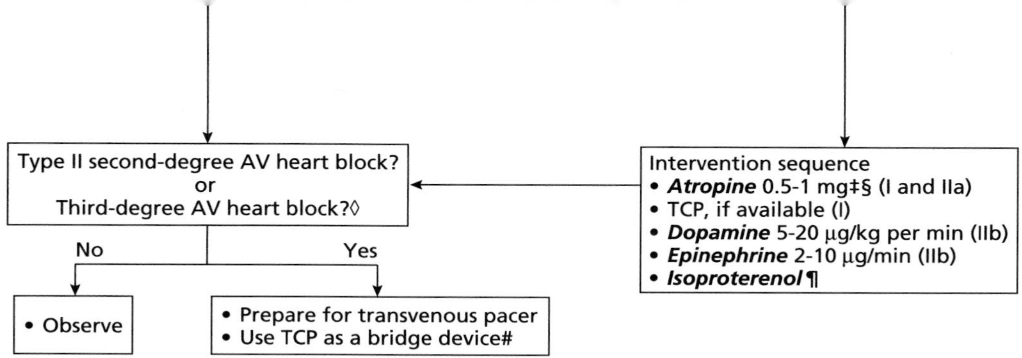

Figure A-3 Bradycardia algorithm (with the patient not in cardiac arrest).

Intervention sequence
- **Atropine** 0.5-1 mg‡§ (I and IIa)
- TCP, if available (I)
- **Dopamine** 5-20 µg/kg per min (IIb)
- **Epinephrine** 2-10 µg/min (IIb)
- **Isoproterenol**¶

Type II second-degree AV heart block?
or
Third-degree AV heart block?◊

No — • Observe

Yes — • Prepare for transvenous pacer
• Use TCP as a bridge device#

* Serious signs or symptoms must be related to the slow rate. Clinical manifestations include: *symptoms* (chest pain, shortness of breath, decreased level of consciousness) and *signs* (low BP, shock, pulmonary congestion, HF, acute MI).

† Do not delay TCP while awaiting IV access or for *atropine* to take effect if patient is symptomatic.

‡ Denervated transplanted hearts will not respond to *atropine*. Go at once to pacing, *catecholamine* infusion, or both.

§ *Atropine* should be given in repeat doses every 3-5 min up to a total of 0.04 mg/kg. Consider shorter dosing intervals in severe clinical conditions. It has been suggested that *atropine* should be used with caution in atrioventricular (AV) block at the His-Purkinje level (type II AV block and new third-degree block with wide QRS complexes) (Class IIb).

◊ Never treat third-degree heart block plus ventricular escape beats with *lidocaine*.

¶ *Isoproterenol* should be used, if at all, with extreme caution. At low doses it is a Class IIb (possibly helpful); at higher doses it is Class III (harmful).

Verify patient tolerance and mechanical capture. Use analgesia and sedation as needed.

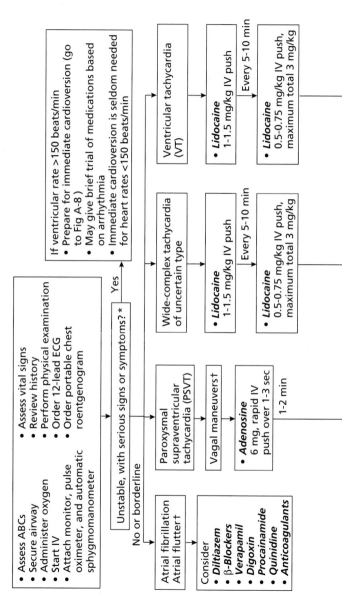

- Assess ABCs
- Secure airway
- Administer oxygen
- Start IV
- Attach monitor, pulse oximeter, and automatic sphygmomanometer
- Assess vital signs
- Review history
- Perform physical examination
- Order 12-lead ECG
- Order portable chest roentgenogram

Unstable, with serious signs or symptoms? *

No or borderline

Yes

If ventricular rate >150 beats/min
- Prepare for immediate cardioversion (go to Fig A-8)
- May give brief trial of medications based on arrhythmia
- Immediate cardioversion is seldom needed for heart rates <150 beats/min

Atrial fibrillation
Atrial flutter†

Consider
- *Ditiazem*
- β*-Blockers*
- *Verapamil*
- *Digoxin*
- *Procainamide*
- *Quinidine*
- *Anticoagulants*

Paroxysmal supraventricular tachycardia (PSVT)

Vagal maneuvers†

- *Adenosine* 6 mg, rapid IV push over 1-3 sec
1-2 min

Wide-complex tachycardia of uncertain type

- *Lidocaine* 1-1.5 mg/kg IV push
Every 5-10 min
- *Lidocaine* 0.5-0.75 mg/kg IV push, maximum total 3 mg/kg

Ventricular tachycardia (VT)

- *Lidocaine* 1-1.5 mg/kg IV push
Every 5-10 min
- *Lidocaine* 0.5-0.75 mg/kg IV push, maximum total 3 mg/kg

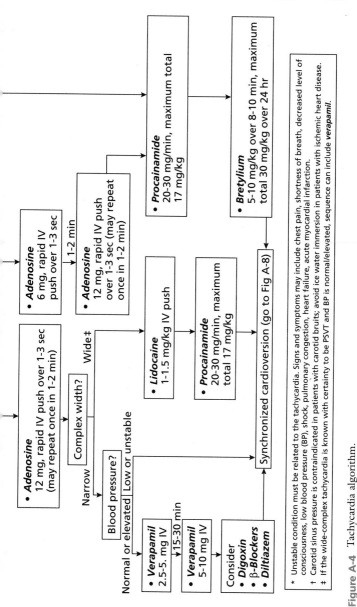

Figure A-4 Tachycardia algorithm.

* Unstable condition must be related to the tachycardia. Signs and symptoms may include chest pain, shortness of breath, decreased level of consciousness, low blood pressure (BP), shock, pulmonary congestion, heart failure, acute myocardial infarction.

† Carotid sinus pressure is contraindicated in patients with carotid bruits; avoid ice water immersion in patients with ischemic heart disease.

‡ If the wide-complex tachycardia is known with certainty to be PSVT and BP is normal/elevated, sequence can include *verapamil.*

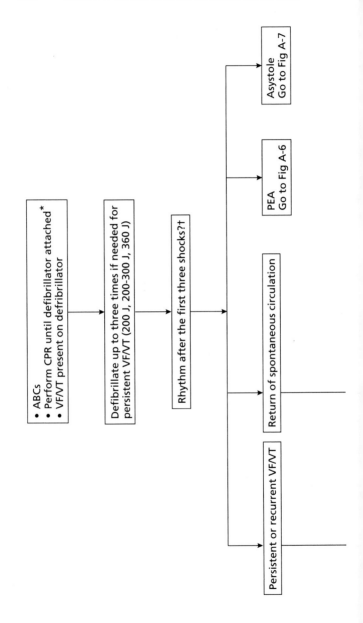

- ABCs
- Perform CPR until defibrillator attached *
- VF/VT present on defibrillator

Defibrillate up to three times if needed for persistent VF/VT (200 J, 200-300 J, 360 J)

Rhythm after the first three shocks?†

Persistent or recurrent VF/VT

Return of spontaneous circulation

PEA
Go to Fig A-6

Asystole
Go to Fig A-7

Class I: definitely helpful
Class IIa: acceptable, probably helpful
Class IIb: acceptable, possibly helpful
Class III: not indicated, may be harmful

* Precordial thump is a Class IIb action in witnessed arrest, no pulse, and no defibrillator immediately available.

† Hypothermic cardiac arrest is treated differently after this point. See section on hypothermia.

‡ The recommended dose of **epinephrine** is 1 mg IV push every 3-5 min. If this approach fails, several Class IIb dosing regimens can be considered:
- intermediate: **epinephrine** 2-5 mg IV push, every 3-5 min
- escalating: **epinephrine** 1 mg-3 mg-5 mg IV push, (3 min apart)
- high: **epinephrine** 0.1 mg/kg IV push, every 3-5 min

§ **Sodium bicarbonate** (1mEq/kg) is Class I if patient has known preexisting hyperkalemia.

◊ Multiple sequenced shocks (200 J, 200-300 J, 360 J) are acceptable here (Class I), especially when medications are delayed.

¶ • **Lidocaine** 1.5 mg/kg IV push. Repeat in 3-5 min to total loading dose of 3 mg/kg; then use
- **Bretylium** 5 mg/kg IV push. Repeat in 5 min at 10 mg/kg
- **Magnesium sulfate** 1-2g IV in torsades de pointes, or suspected hypomagnesemic state, or severe refractory VF.
- **Procainamide** 30 mg/min in refractory VF (maximum total 17 mg/kg)

Sodium bicarbonate (1 mEq/kg IV):
Class IIa
- if known preexisting bicarbonate-responsive acidosis
- if overdose with tricyclic antidepressants
- to alkalinize the urine in drug overdoses
Class IIb
- if intubated and continued long arrest interval
- upon return of spontaneous circulation after long arrest interval
Class III
- hypoxic lactic acidosis

- Assess vital signs
- Support airway
- Support breathing
- Provide medications appropriate for blood pressure, heart rate, and rhythm

- Continue CPR
- Intubate at once
- Obtain IV access

- **Epinephrine** 1 mg IV push‡§ repeat every 3-5 min

- Defibrillate 360 J within 30-60 sec◊

- Administer medications of probable benefit (Class IIa) in persistent or recurrent VF/VT¶#

- Defibrillate 360 J, 30-60 sec after each dose of medication◊
- Pattern should be drug-shock, drug-shock

Figure A-5 Algorithm for ventricular fibrillation and pulseless ventricular tachycardia (VF/VT).

PEA includes
- Electromechanical dissociation (EMD)
- Pseudo-EMD
- Idioventricular rhythms
- Ventricular escape rhythms
- Bradyasystolic rhythms
- Postdefibrillation idioventricular rhythms

- Continue CPR
- Intubate at once
- Obtain IV access
- Assess blood flow using Doppler ultrasound

Consider possible causes
(Parentheses = possible therapies and treatments)
- Hypovolemia (volume infusion)
- Hypoxia (ventilation)
- Cardiac tamponade (pericardiocentesis)
- Tension pneumothorax (needle decompression)
- Hypothermia (see Fig A-9)
- Massive pulmonary embolism (surgery, *thrombolytics*)
- Drug overdoses such as tricyclics, digitalis, β-blockers, calcium channel blockers
- Hyperkalemia*
- Acidosis†
- Massive acute myocardial infarction (go to Fig A-2)

- **Epinephrine** 1 mg IV push,*‡ repeat every 3-5 min

- If absolute bradycardia (<60 beats/min) or relative bradycardia, give **atropine** 1 mg IV
- Repeat every 3-5 min up to a total of 0.04 mg/kg§

Class I: definitely helpful
Class IIa: acceptable, probably helpful
Class IIb: acceptable, possibly helpful
Class III: not indicated, may be harmful

* **Sodium bicarbonate** 1 mEq/kg is Class I if patient has known preexisting hyperkalemia.

† **Sodium bicarbonate** 1 mEq/kg:
  Class IIa
  • if known preexisting bicarbonate-responsive acidosis
  • if overdose with tricyclic antidepressants
  • to alkalinize the urine in drug overdoses
  Class IIb
  • if intubated and long arrest interval
  • upon return of spontaneous circulation after long arrest interval
  Class III
  • hypoxic lactic acidosis

‡ The recommended dose of **epinephrine** is 1 mg IV push every 3-5 min. If this approach fails, several Class IIb dosing regimens can be considered.
  • intermediate: **epinephrine** 2-5 mg IV push, every 3-5 min
  • escalating: **epinephrine** 1 mg-3 mg-5 mg IV push, (3 min apart)
  • high: **epinephrine** 0.1 mg/kg IV push, every 3-5 min

§ Shorter **atropine** dosing intervals are possibly helpful in cardiac arrest (Class IIb).

Figure A-6   Algorithm for pulseless electrical activity (PEA) (electromechanical dissociation [EMD]).

Class I: definitely helpful
Class IIa: acceptable, probably helpful
Class IIb: acceptable, possibly helpful
Class III: not indicated, may be harmful

* TCP is a Class IIb intervention. Lack of success may be due to delays in pacing. To be effective TCP must be performed early, simultaneously with drugs. Evidence does not support routine use of TCP for asystole.

† The recommended dose of *epinephrine* is 1 mg IV push every 3-5 min. If this approach fails, several Class IIb dosing regimens can be considered:
- intermediate: *epinephrine* 2-5 mg IV push, every 3-5 min
- escalating: *epinephrine* 1 mg–3 mg–5 mg IV push (3 min apart)
- high: *epinephrine* 0.1 mg/kg IV push, every 3-5 min

‡ *Sodium bicarbonate* 1 mEq/kg is Class I if patient has known preexisting hyperkalemia.

§ Shorter *atropine* dosing intervals are Class IIb in asystolic arrest.

◊ *Sodium bicarbonate* 1 mEq/kg:
  Class IIa
  - if known preexisting bicarbonate-responsive acidosis
  - if overdose with tricyclic antidepressant
  - to alkalinize the urine in drug overdoses
  Class IIb
  - if intubated and continued long arrest interval
  - upon return of spontaneous circulation after long arrest interval
  Class III
  - hypoxic lactic acidosis

¶ If patient remains in asystole or other agonal rhythms after successful intubation and initial medications and no reversible causes are identified, consider termination of resuscitative efforts by a physician. Consider interval since arrest.

- Continue CPR
- Intubate at once
- Obtain IV access
- Confirm asystole in more than one lead

Consider possible causes
- Hypoxia
- Hyperkalemia
- Hypokalemia
- Preexisting acidosis
- Drug overdose
- Hypothermia

Consider immediate transcutaneous pacing (TCP)*

- *Epinephrine* 1 mg IV push,†‡ repeat every 3-5 min

- *Atropine* 1 mg IV, repeat every 3-5 min up to a total of 0.04 mg/kg§◊

Consider
- Termination of efforts¶

Figure A-7 Asystole treatment algorithm.

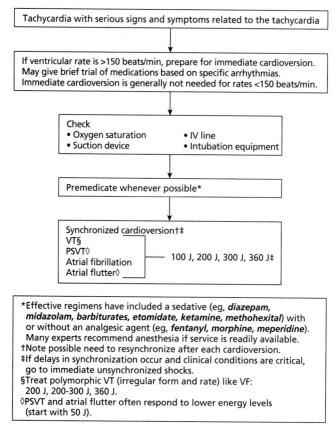

Tachycardia with serious signs and symptoms related to the tachycardia

↓

If ventricular rate is >150 beats/min, prepare for immediate cardioversion.
May give brief trial of medications based on specific arrhythmias.
Immediate cardioversion is generally not needed for rates <150 beats/min.

↓

Check
- Oxygen saturation
- Suction device
- IV line
- Intubation equipment

↓

Premedicate whenever possible*

↓

Synchronized cardioversion†‡
VT§
PSVT◊   — 100 J, 200 J, 300 J, 360 J‡
Atrial fibrillation
Atrial flutter◊

*Effective regimens have included a sedative (eg, *diazepam,
 midazolam, barbiturates, etomidate, ketamine, methohexital*) with
 or without an analgesic agent (eg, *fentanyl, morphine, meperidine*).
 Many experts recommend anesthesia if service is readily available.
†Note possible need to resynchronize after each cardioversion.
‡If delays in synchronization occur and clinical conditions are critical,
 go to immediate unsynchronized shocks.
§Treat polymorphic VT (irregular form and rate) like VF:
 200 J, 200-300 J, 360 J.
◊PSVT and atrial flutter often respond to lower energy levels
 (start with 50 J).

Figure A-8   Electrical cardioversion algorithm (with the patient not in
cardiac arrest).

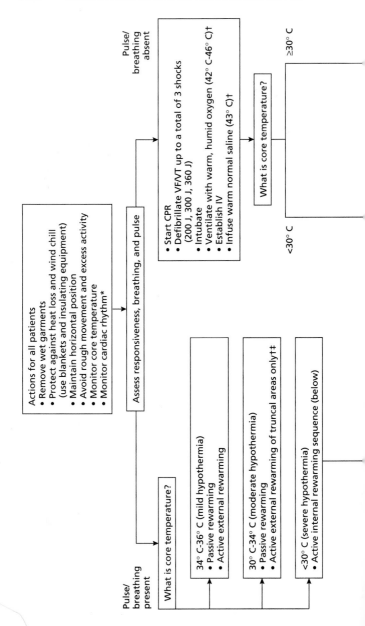

Actions for all patients
- Remove wet garments
- Protect against heat loss and wind chill (use blankets and insulating equipment)
- Maintain horizontal position
- Avoid rough movement and excess activity
- Monitor core temperature
- Monitor cardiac rhythm*

Assess responsiveness, breathing, and pulse

Pulse/breathing present

What is core temperature?

34° C-36° C (mild hypothermia)
- Passive rewarming
- Active external rewarming

30° C-34° C (moderate hypothermia)
- Passive rewarming
- Active external rewarming of truncal areas only‡

<30° C (severe hypothermia)
- Active internal rewarming sequence (below)

Pulse/breathing absent

- Start CPR
- Defibrillate VF/VT up to a total of 3 shocks (200 J, 300 J, 360 J)
- Intubate
- Ventilate with warm, humid oxygen (42° C-46° C)†
- Establish IV
- Infuse warm normal saline (43° C)†

What is core temperature?

<30° C   ≥30° C

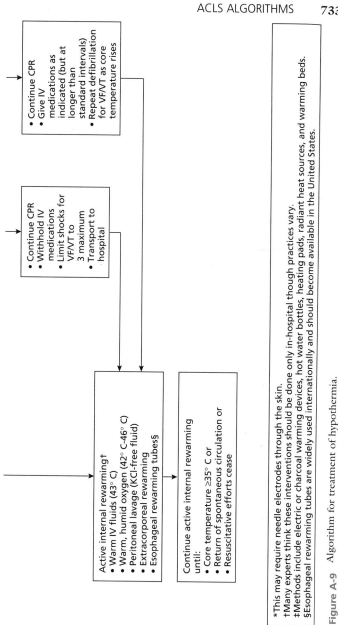

Continue CPR
• Give IV
  medications as
  indicated (but at
  longer than
  standard intervals)
• Repeat defibrillation
  for VF/VT as core
  temperature rises

• Continue CPR
• Withhold IV
  medications
• Limit shocks for
  VF/VT to
  3 maximum
• Transport to
  hospital

Active internal rewarming†
• Warm IV fluids (43° C)
• Warm, humid oxygen (42° C-46° C)
• Peritoneal lavage (KCl-free fluid)
• Extracorporeal rewarming
• Esophageal rewarming tubes§

Continue active internal rewarming
until:
• Core temperature ≥35° C or
• Return of spontaneous circulation or
• Resuscitative efforts cease

*This may require needle electrodes through the skin.
†Many experts think these interventions should be done only in-hospital though practices vary.
‡Methods include electric or charcoal warming devices, hot water bottles, heating pads, radiant heat sources, and warming beds.
§Esophageal rewarming tubes are widely used internationally and should become available in the United States.

Figure A-9 Algorithm for treatment of hypothermia.

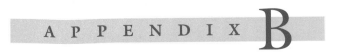

Laboratory Values

COMPLETE BLOOD COUNT

RBC . . . . 4.25-5.5 × 10⁶/μl (males)
. . . . 3.6-5 × 10⁶/μl (females)
WBC . . . . 5-10 × 10³/μl
Hgb . . . . 13.5-17.5 g/dl (males)
. . . . 12-16 g/dl (females)
Hct. . . . . 40%-54% (males)
. . . . 37%-47% (females)

COAGULATION

Plts . . . . 150-350 × 10³/μl
PT . . . . 10-14 sec
PTT . . . . 30-45 sec
APTT . . . . 16-25 sec
ACT . . . . 92-128 sec
FSP. . . . . <10 μg/dl

CHEMISTRY

Albumin . . . . 3.5-5 g/dl
Alkaline phosphatase . . . . . 25-97 U/L
Alanine aminotransferase
(ALT/SGPT) . . . . 4.35 U/L
Ammonia . . . . 18-54 μmll/L (males)
. . . . 12-50 μmol/L (females)
Amylase. . . . . 4-25 U/ml
Anion gap . . . . 8-16 mEq/L
Aspartate aminotransferase
(AST/SGOT) . . . . 8-33 U/L
Bilirubin
   Direct . . . . 0-0.2 mg/dl
   Total. . . . . 0.2-1 mg/dl
   Indirect. . . . . Total—direct
BUN. . . . . 10-20 mg/dl
BUN:Cr ratio 10:1-15:1

Calcium . . . . 8.5-10.5 mg/dl
Cholesterol . . . . 120-200 mg/dl
   HDL. . . . . 26-63 mg/dl (males)
   . . . . 39-92 mg/dl (females)
   LDL . . . . 70-180 mg/dl
   . . . . <130 is desirable
   LDL/HDL ratio . . . . . . <3
   Cholesterol/HDL ratio . <4.5
Chloride . . . . 98-106 mEq/L
CO_2 . . . . 24-32 mEq/L
Creatinine . . . . 0.7-1.3 mg/dl (males)
   . . . . 0.6-1.2 mg/dl (females)
Glucose. . . . . 70-110 mg/dl
Iron . . . . 50-150 µg/dl
Lactate . . . . 0.5-2.2 mEq/L
Lactic dehydrogenase
(LDH) . . . . 70-250 U/L
Lipase . . . . 4-24 U/L
Magnesium . . . . 1.3-2.1 mEq/L
Osmolality. . . . . 275-295 mOsm/kg
Potassium . . . . 3.5-5 mEq/L
Phosphorus . . . . 2.5-4.5 mg/dl
Protein . . . . 6-8 g/dl
Sedimentation rate. . . . . . . 0-10 mm/hr (males)
   . . . . . . 0-15 mm/hr (females)
Sodium . . . . 135-145 mEq/L
T_3. . . . . 0.8-1.1 µg/dl
T_4. . . . . 4.5-11.5 µg/dl
Triglyceride . . . . 46-316 mg/dl (males, 30-40 yr)
   . . . . 75-313 mg/dl (males >50 yr)
   . . . . 37-174 mg/dl (females, 30-40 yr)
   . . . . 52-280 mg/dl (females >50 yr)
Uric acid . . . . 3.5-8 mg/dl

CARDIAC PROFILE

SGOT (AST). . . . . 6-18 U/L (females)
   . . . . 7-21 U/L (males)
   With MI
      Onset . . . . 12-18 hr
      Peak . . . . 24-48 hr
      Duration . . . . 3-4 days
CK . . . . 96-140 U/L (females)
   . . . . 38-174 U/L (males)

With MI
    Onset . . . . 4-6 hr
    Peak . . . . 12-24 hr
    Duration . . . . 3-4 days
CK-MB. 0%
  With MI
    Onset . . . . 4-6 hr
    Peak . . . . 12-24 hr
    Duration . . . . 2-3 days
LDH . . . . 70-180 mg/dl
  With MI
    Onset . . . . 24-48 hr
    Peak . . . . 3-6 days
    Duration . . . . 7-10 days
LDH_1 . . . . 17.5%-28.3% of total LDH
LDH_2 . . . . 30.4%-36.4% of total LDH
  With MI
  $LDH_1 > LDH_2$
    Onset . . . . 12-24 hr
    Peak . . . . 48 hr
    Duration . . . . Variable

URINE ELECTROLYTES

Na . . . . 40-220 mEq/day
K . . . . 25-125 mEq/day
Cl. . . . . 110-250 mEq/day

CSF

Pressure (initial). . . . . 70-180 mm H_2O
Albumin . . . . 11-48 mg/dl
Cell count. . . . . 0-5 mononuclear cells
Chloride . . . . 120-130 mEq/L
Glucose. . . . . 50-75 mg/dl
IgG. . . . . 0-8.6 mg/dl
Protein . . . . 15-45 mg/dl

DRUG LEVELS

Digoxin. . . . . 1-2 ng/ml
Phenytoin . . . . 10-20 µg/ml
Theophylline. . . . . 10-20 µg/ml
Barbiturate coma . . . . 10 mg/dl

Gentamicin
    Trough . . . . 1-2 µg/ml
    Peak . . . . 6-8 µg/ml
Lidocaine . . . . 1.5-5 µg/ml
Tobramycin
    Trough . . . . 1-2 µg/ml
    Peak . . . . 6-8 µg/ml
Vancomycin
    Trough . . . . 5-10 µg/ml
    Peak . . . . 30-40 µg/ml

BLOOD GASES

Arterial

O_2 sat 95%
Po_2 . . . . 80-100 mm Hg
Pco_2 . . . . 35-45 mm Hg
pH 7.35-7.45
HCO_3 . . . . 22-26 mEq/L

Venous

O_2 sat 60%-80%
Po_2 . . . . 35-45 mm Hg
Pco_2 . . . . 41-51 mm Hg
pH 7.31-7.41
HCO_3 . . . . 22-26 mEq/L

Organ/Tissue Donation

Organs including the kidneys, heart, pancreas, and liver can be donated for transplantation. A heart-beating, brain-dead cadaver is mandatory, and blood type is required.

Tissues including skin, bone, eye, ear, heart valves, and soft tissues can also be transplanted. Tissue donation does not require a heart-beating cadaver because the tissues are avascular when transplanted. Organs and tissues may also be donated for medical research.

Potential Donor Identification
a. Brain-dead patients (see p. 12 for brain-death criteria)
b. No active infection
c. No history of transmissible disease
d. No previous disease of the organ/tissue (e.g., renal disease, insulin-dependent diabetes mellitus, rheumatoid arthritis, malignancy [except brain tumor], bone disease)
e. Any age (physiological age is considered)
f. Anyone, regardless of medical history or age, is eligible for eye donation, and donation of organs and tissues for biomedical research.

Resources Available
a. Contact your local organ-procurement organization
b. International Institute for Advancement of Medicine (donation for research): 610-363-3600
c. National Disease Research Interchange (donation for research): 215-557-7361

General Guidelines: Care of the Donor*
Respiratory function
OUTCOME CRITERIA
- pH   7.35-7.45
- PaO$_2$ 70-100 mm Hg

*Organ-specific protocols are used—contact your local organ-procurement agency.

- Paco$_2$ 40-45 mm Hg
- O$_2$ sat   ≥95%
- Absence of peripheral cyanosis
- Absence of adventitious lung sounds

INTERVENTIONS
- Regulate ventilator settings as needed.
- Monitor peak inspiratory pressure and suction prn.
- Avoid PEEP levels >5 cm H$_2$O and high Fio$_2$ levels.
- Assess nail beds.
- Auscultate lung fields.
- Turn patient frequently, if appropriate.
- Assess chest wall excursion.
- Prevent or aggressively treat pneumothorax.

Cardiovascular function

OUTCOME CRITERIA
- SBP   ≥100 mm Hg
- DBP   <100 mm Hg
- CVP   2-6 mm Hg

INTERVENTIONS
- Administer crystalloids/colloids to keep SBP ≥100 mm Hg.
- Administer sodium nitroprusside if SBP >200 mm Hg or DBP >100 mm Hg
- Administer PRBCs if Hct <30%.
- Administer dopamine to keep SBP ≥100 mm Hg, if necessary.
- Monitor fluid losses.
- Monitor for fluid overload (CVP, PAP).
- Monitor CO/CI and SVRI.

Renal function

OUTCOME CRITERIA
- Urine output   ~100 ml/hr
- CVP   2-6 mm Hg
- K   3.5-4.5 mEq/L
- BUN   10-20 mg/dl
- Creatinine   0.6-1.2 mg/dl

INTERVENTIONS
- Administer fluids such as Ringer's lactate, hespan, plasmanate to maintain CVP.
- Administer dopamine if necessary to increase renal perfusion.
- Administer diuretics (mannitol, furosemide) to increase urine output if patient is hydrated and BP stable.
- Monitor BP, CVP, urine output qlh.
- Monitor kidney function (BUN, Cr) and electrolytes.

If diabetes insipidus occurs:
- Administer aqueous pitressin as an infusion and titrate to keep urine output between 150 and 300 ml/hr.
- Replace urine output ml for ml.
- Administer additional fluids as necessary.

Thermal regulatory function

OUTCOME CRITERION
- T 36-38.3° C

INTERVENTIONS
- Monitor temperature qlh.
- Use warming blanket, heat shields.
- Avoid unnecessary exposure of patient.
- Warm blood products and IV fluids if T < 35° C.
- Administer tylenol suppository as ordered for T > 38.3° C.

Guidelines for Avascular Tissues

Cornea
- Apply ophthalmic saline solution to eyes; tape eyes closed.
- Apply cold compresses to eyes.
- Elevate HOB.

Skin
- Turn patient frequently.
- Assess for skin breakdown/infection.

REFERENCES

1. Albert P: Overview of the organ donation process, *Crit Care Nurs Clin North Am* 6(3):553-565, 1994.
2. Flynn J, Bruce N: *Introduction to critical care skills*, St Louis, 1993, Mosby.
3. Kozlowski L: Case study in identification and maintenance of an organ donor, *Heart Lung* 17(4):366-371, 1988.
4. Norris MK: How to manage tissue donation, *Am J Nurs* 89(10):1300-1302, 1989.
5. Snyder L, Peter N: How to manage organ donation, *Am J Nurs* 89(10):1294-1298, 1989.

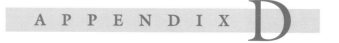
Scoring Tools

TRAUMA SCORE

Assessment parameter		Trauma score
Glasgow coma scale score	14-15	5
	11-13	4
	8-10	3
	5-7	2
	3-4	1
Respiratory rate	10-24	4
	25-35	3
	>35	2
	1-9	1
	0	0
Respiratory expansion	Normal	1
	Shallow	0
	Retractive	0
Systolic blood pressure	>90	4
	70-90	3
	50-69	2
	1-49	1
No carotid pulse	0	0
Capillary refill	Normal	2
	Delayed	1
	None	0

From Champion HR, Gainer PS, Yackee E: A progress report on the trauma score in predicting a fatal outcome, *J Trauma* 26:927-931, 1988; and Champion HR et al: Trauma score, *Crit Care Med* 9(9):672-676, 1981.

TRAUMA SCORE

Projected estimate of survival	
Trauma score	Percentage survival
16	99
15	98
14	96
13	93
12	87
11	76
10	60
9	42
8	26
7	15
6	8
5	4
4	2
3	1
2	0
1	0

THERAPEUTIC INTERVENTION SCORING SYSTEM (TISS)

4 Points

a. Cardiac arrest and/or countershock within past 48 hr*
b. Controlled ventilation with or without PEEP*
c. Controlled ventilation with intermittent or continuous muscle relaxants*
d. Balloon tamponade of varices*
e. Continuous arterial infusion*
f. Pulmonary artery catheter
g. Atrial and/or ventricular pacing*
h. Hemodialysis in unstable patient*
i. Peritoneal dialysis
j. Induced hypothermia*
k. Pressure-activated blood infusion*
l. G-suit
m. Intracranial pressure monitoring
n. Platelet transfusion
o. IABA (intraaortic balloon assist)
p. Emergency operative procedures (within past 24 hr)*
q. Lavage of acute GI bleeding
r. Emergency endoscopy or bronchoscopy
s. Vasoactive drug infusion (>1 drug)

2 Points

a. CVP (central venous pressure)
b. Two peripheral IV catheters
c. Hemodialysis—stable patient
d. Fresh tracheostomy (less than 48 hr)
e. Spontaneous respiration via endotracheal tube or tracheostomy (T-piece or trach mask)
f. GI feedings
g. Replacement of excess fluid loss*
h. Parenteral chemotherapy
i. Hourly neuro vital signs
j. Multiple dressing changes
k. Pitressin infusion IV

*For table footnote, see p. 745.

Continued.

THERAPEUTIC INTERVENTION SCORING SYSTEM (TISS)—cont'd

3 Points

a. Central IV hyperalimentation (includes renal, cardiac, hepatic failure fluid)
b. Pacemaker on standby
c. Chest tubes
d. Intermittent mandatory ventilation (IMV) or assisted ventilation*
e. Continuous positive airway pressure (CPAP)
f. Concentrated K^+ infusion via central catheter
g. Nasotracheal or orotracheal intubation*
h. Blind intratracheal suctioning
i. Complex metabolic balance (frequent I & O)*
j. Multiple ABG, bleeding, STAT studies (>4/shift)
k. Frequent infusions of blood products (>5 units/24 hr)
l. Bolus IV medication (nonscheduled)
m. Vasoactive drug infusion (one drug)
n. Continuous antiarrhythmia infusions
o. Cardioversion for arrhythmia (not defibrillation)
p. Hypothermia blanket
q. Arterial line
r. Acute digitalization—within 48 hr
s. Measurement of cardiac output by any method

1 Point

a. ECG monitoring
b. Hourly vital signs
c. One peripheral IV catheter
d. Chronic anticoagulation
e. Standard intake and output (q24h)
f. STAT blood tests
g. Intermittent scheduled IV medications
h. Routine dressing changes
i. Standard orthopedic traction
j. Tracheostomy care
k. Decubitus ulcer*
l. Urinary catheter
m. Supplemental oxygen (nasal or mask)
n. Antibiotics IV (two or less)
o. Chest physiotherapy
p. Extensive irrigations, packings, or debridement of wound, fistula, or colostomy
q. GI decompression
r. Peripheral hyperalimentation/intralipid therapy

t. Active diuresis for fluid overload or cerebral edema
u. Active Rx for metabolic alkalosis
v. Active Rx for metabolic acidosis
w. Emergency thoracentesis, paracentesis, pericardiocentesis
x. Active anticoagulation (initial 48 hr)*
y. Phlebotomy for volume overload
z. Coverage with more than 2 IV antibiotics
aa. Rx of seizures, metabolic encephalopathy (48 hr of onset)
bb. Complicated orthopedic traction*

*Therapeutic Intervention Scoring System explanation code:
4-Point Interventions: (a) Point score for 2 days after most recent cardiac arrest. (b) Does not mean intermittent mandatory ventilation (3-point intervention). Means that regardless of the internal plumbing of ventilator, the full ventilatory needs are being supplied by the machine. Whether the patient is ineffectively breathing around the ventilator is irrelevant as long as it is providing the needed minute ventilation. (c) For example, d-tubocurarine chloride, pancuronium (Pavulon), metocurine (Metubine). (d) Use Sengstaken-Blakemore or Linton tube for esophageal or gastric bleeding. (e) Pitressin infusion via IMA, SMA, gastric artery catheters for control of gastrointestinal bleeding, or other intraarterial infusion. Does not include standard 3 ml/hr heparin flush to maintain catheter patency. (g) Active pacing even if a chronic pacemaker. (h) Include first two runs of an acute dialysis. Include chronic dialysis when medical situation renders dialysis unstable. (j) Continuous or intermittent cooling to achieve temperature <33° C. (k) Use of a blood pump or manual pumping in those requiring rapid blood replacement. (p) May be the initial emergency procedure—precludes diagnostic tests.
3-Point Interventions: (d) The patient is supplying some ventilatory needs. (g) Not a daily point score. Patient must have been intubated in the ICU (elective or emergency) within previous 24 hr. (i) Measurement of intake/output above normal 24-hr routine. Frequent adjustment of intake according to total output. (x) Includes Rheomacrodex. (bb) For example, Stryker frame, CircOlectric.
2-Point Interventions: (g) Replacement of clear fluids over and above the ordered maintenance level.
1-Point Intervention: (k) Must have a decubitus ulcer. Does not include preventive therapy.
From Keene AR, Cullen DJ: Therapeutic intervention scoring system: update 1983, *Crit Care Med* 11(1):2, 1983.

APACHE III SCORING

An APACHE III score consists of points assigned to the following components: age, presence of chronic health, physiology/laboratory data, and neurological function.

Age	Points
≤44	0
45-59	5
60-64	11
65-69	13
70-74	16
75-84	17
≥85	24

Chronic Health	Points
Cirrhosis	4
Immunosuppression	10
Leukemia/multiple myeloma	10
Metastatic cancer	11
Lymphoma	13
Hepatic failure	16
AIDS	23

Acid-Base Points

pH	Paco$_2$	Points
<7.2	<50	12
<7.2	≥50	4
7.2-<7.35	<30	9
7.2-<7.3	30-<40	6
7.2-<7.3	40-<50	3
7.2-<7.3	≥50	2
7.35-<7.5	<30	5
7.3-<7.45	30-<45	0
7.3-<7.45	≥45	1
7.45-<7.5	30-<35	0
7.45-<7.5	35-<45	2
7.45-<7.5	>45	12
7.5-≥7.65	≥40	12
7.5-<7.6	<40	3
≥7.6	<25	0
≥7.6	25-<40	3

Neurological Scoring*

	Oriented, converses	Confused speech	Inappropriate words and incoherent sounds	No response
Obeys verbal command	0	3	10	15 16†
Localizes pain	3	8	13	15 16†
Flexion withdrawal/ decorticate rigidity	3	13	24 24†	24 33†
Decerebrate rigidity/no response	3	13	29 29†	29 48†

*Points assigned if eyes open spontaneously or to painful/verbal stimulation.
†Points assigned if eyes do not open spontaneously or to painful/verbal stimulation.

Physiological Scoring for Vital Signs and Laboratory Tests

Pulse 0 (50-99 beats/min)

Score	8	5	0	1	5	7	13	17
Range	≤39	40-49	50-99 beats/min	100-109	110-119	120-139	140-154	≥155

Mean BP 0 (80-99 mm Hg)

Score	23	15	7	6	0	4	7	9	10
Range	≤39	40-59	60-69	70-79	80-99 mm Hg	100-119	120-129	130-139	≥140

Temp 0 (36°C-39.9°C)

Score	20	16	13	8	2	0	4
Range	≤32.9	33-33.4	33.5-33.9	34-34.9	35-35.9	36°C-39.9°C	≥40

Respiratory rate* 0 (14-24 breaths/min)

Score	17	8	7	0	6	9	11	18
Range	≤5	6-11*	12-13	14-24 breaths/min	25-34	35-39	40-49	≥50

PaO_2† 0 (≥80 mm Hg)

Score	15	5	2	0
Range	≤49	50-69	70-79	≥80 mm Hg

$A\text{-}aDO_2$† 0 (<100)

Score	0	7	9	11	14
Range	<100	100-249	250-349	350-499	≥500

Hct 0 (41%-49%)

Score	3	0	3
Range	≤40.9	41%-49%	≥50

WBCs 0 (3-19.9/mm³)

Score	19	5	0	1	5
Range	<1	1-2.9	3-19.9/mm³	20-24.9	≥25

Cr† 0 (44-132 µmol/dl / 0.5-1.4 mg/dl)

Score	3	0	4	7
Range	<43 / 0.4	44-132 µmol/dl / 0.5-1.4 mg/dl	133-171 / 1.5-1.94	≥172 / ≥1.95

Creatinine (Cr§)

0	10
0-132 μmol/dl	≥133
0-1.4 mg/dl	≥1.5

Urine output (u/o)

15	8	7	5	4	0	1
≤399	400-599	600-899	900-1499	1500-1999	2000-3999 ml/day	≥4000

BUN

0	2	7	11	12
≤6.1 mmol/L	6.2-7.1	7.2-14.3	14.4-28.5	≥28.6
≤16.9 mg/dl	17-19	20-39	40-79	≥80

Na

0	3	2	4
135-154 mmol/L	≤119	120-134	≥155
135-154 mEq/L	≤119	120-134	≥155

Albumin

0	11	6	4
25-44 g/L	≤19	20-24	≥45
2.5-4.4 g/dl	≤1.9	2.0-2.4	≥4.5

Bilirubin

0	5	6	8	16
≤34 μmol/L	35-51	52-85	86-135	≥136
≤1.9 mg/dl	2-2.9	3-4.9	5-7.9	≥8.0

Glucose

0	8‖	9‖	3	5
3.4-11.1 mmol/dl	≤2.1	2.2-3.3	11.2-19.3	≥19.4
60-199 mg/dl	≤39	40-59	200-349	≥350

BP, blood pressure; Temp, temperature; PaO_2, arterial oxygen tension or partial pressure; A-aDO_2, alveolar-arterial oxygen gradient; Hct, hematocrit; WBCs, white blood cells (count); Cr, creatinine; u/o, urine output; BUN, blood urea nitrogen; Na, sodium.

* For patients on mechanical ventilation, no points are given for respiratory rates 6-12.

† Only use A-aDO_2 for intubated patients with FIO_2 ≥0.5. Do not use PaO_2 weights for these patients.

‡ Creatinine without acute renal failure (ARF). ARF is defined as creatinine ≥1.5 dl/day and urine output <410 ml/day and no chronic dialysis.

§ Creatinine with ARF.

‖ Glucose ≤39 mg/dl is lower weight than 40-59.

Modified from Knaus WA et al: The APACHE III prognostic system, *Chest* 100:1619-1636, 1991.

BSA Nomogram

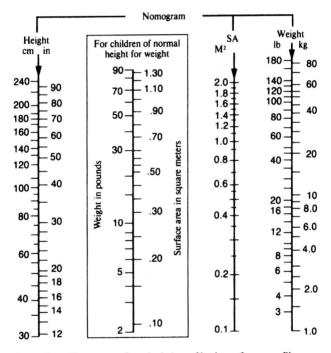

Figure E-1 Nomogram for calculation of body surface area. Place a straight edge from the patient's height in the left column to the weight in the right column. The point of intersection on the body surface area column indicates the body surface area. (From Behrman RE, Vaughn VC, eds: *Nelson's textbook of pediatrics,* ed 12, Philadelphia, 1983, W.B. Saunders.)

Formulas

Cardiopulmonary Parameters

Coronary perfusion pressure (CPP)

CPP is the driving pressure influencing coronary blood flow. Coronary blood flow ceases when CPP reaches 40 mm Hg.

EQUATION: CPP = DBP – PAWP (LVEDP)

NORMAL: 60-80 mm Hg

Pulse pressure (PP)

PP reflects stroke volume and arterial compliance. Widened PP is associated with a decrease in peripheral resistance and/or increase in stroke volume. Narrowed PP is associated with an increase in peripheral resistance and/or decrease in stroke volume.

EQUATION: PP = SBP – DBP

NORMAL: 30-40 mm Hg

Rate pressure product (RPP)

RPP is also known as double product (DP); it is an indirect measurement of myocardial oxygen demand. Activities performed at lower heart rates and systolic blood pressures are better tolerated by individuals with coronary artery disease.

EQUATION: RPP = HR × SBP

NORMAL: <12000

Mean arterial pressure (MAP)

MAP is a measure of the average arterial perfusion pressure, which determines blood flow to the tissues.

EQUATION: MAP = 1/3 PP + DBP or $\dfrac{2(DBP) + SBP}{3}$

NORMAL: 70-105 mm Hg

Cardiac output (CO)

CO is the measurement of the amount of blood ejected by the ventricles each minute. It reflects pump efficiency and is a determinant of tissue perfusion.

$$EQUATION:\ CO = HR \times SV$$

$$NORMAL:\ 4\text{-}8\ \text{L/min}$$

Cardiac index (CI)

CI is a measurement of the cardiac output adjusted for body size. It is a more precise measurement of pump efficiency than CO.

$$EQUATION:\ CI = \frac{CO}{BSA}$$

$$NORMAL:\ 2.5\text{-}4.0\ \text{L/min/m}^2$$

Stroke volume (SV)

SV represents the volume of blood ejected from the ventricle with each cardiac contraction. It is influenced by preload, afterload, and contractility.

$$EQUATION:\ SV = \frac{CO\ (ml/min)}{HR}$$

$$NORMAL:\ 60\text{-}120\ \text{ml/beat}$$

Stroke index (SI)

SI is a measurement of SV adjusted for body size.

$$EQUATION:\ SI = \frac{SV}{BSA}\ or\ \frac{CI\ (ml/min)}{HR}$$

$$NORMAL:\ 30\text{-}65\ \text{ml/beat/m}^2$$

Systemic vascular resistance (SVR)

SVR is a measurement of left ventricular afterload. A diseased aortic valve and resistance in the systemic arterial circulation increase left ventricular afterload.

$$EQUATION:\ SVR = \frac{MAP - CVP}{CO} \times 80$$

$$NORMAL:\ 900\text{-}1400\ \text{dynes/sec/cm}^{-5}$$

Systemic vascular resistance index (SVRI)

SVRI is a measurement of left ventricular afterload, adjusted for body size.

$$\text{EQUATION:} \quad \text{SVRI} = \frac{\text{MAP} - \text{CVP}}{\text{CI}} \times 80$$

NORMAL: 1700-2600 dynes/sec/cm^{-5}/m^2

Pulmonary vascular resistance (PVR)
PVR is a measurement of right ventricular afterload. A diseased pulmonic valve and resistance in pulmonary arterial circulation increase right ventricular afterload.

$$\text{EQUATION:} \quad \text{PVR} = \frac{\text{PAM} - \text{PAWP}}{\text{CO}} \times 80$$

NORMAL: 100-250 dynes/sec/cm^{-5}
PAM = pulmonary artery mean pressure

Pulmonary vascular resistance index (PVRI)
PVRI is a measurement of right ventricular afterload, adjusted for body size.

$$\text{EQUATION:} \quad \text{PVRI} = \frac{\text{PAM} - \text{PAWP}}{\text{CI}} \times 80$$

NORMAL: 200-450 dynes/sec/cm^{-5}/m^2
PAM = pulmonary artery mean pressure

Left ventricular stroke work index (LVSWI)
LVSWI is a measurement of amount of work the left ventricle does per cardiac contraction, adjusted for body size. It is an indirect method of measuring myocardial contractility.

EQUATION: LVSWI = SI × (MAP − PAWP) × 0.0136

NORMAL: 45-60 g-m/m^2

Right ventricular stroke work index (RVSWI)
RVSWI is a measurement of amount of work the right ventricle does per cardiac contraction, adjusted for body size. It is an indirect method of measuring myocardial contractility.

EQUATION: RVSWI = SI × (PAM − CVP) × 0.0136

NORMAL: 7-12 g-m/m^2

Ejection fraction (EF)
EF is a measurement of the ratio of the amount of blood ejected from the ventricle to the amount of blood remaining in the ventricle at end diastole. It is an indirect measurement of contractility.

$$EQUATION:\ EF = \frac{SV}{EDV} \times 100$$

NORMAL: 60% or greater

EDV = End diastolic volume

Alveolar air equation (P_{AO_2})

P_{AO_2} is a measurement of alveolar partial pressure of oxygen.

$$EQUATION:\ P_{AO_2} = F_{IO_2}\,(Pb - PH_2O) - \frac{P_{ACO_2}}{0.8}$$

Pb = Barometric pressure

PH_2O = Water vapor pressure

$Pb - PH_2O$ = 713

NORMAL: 100 mm Hg

Expected P_{aO_2} (P_{aO_2})

P_{aO_2} is a measurement of lung function when the expected P_{aO_2} is compared with the actual P_{aO_2}. For persons older than 60 years of age, subtract 1 mm Hg for each year over 60.

$$EQUATION:\ P_{aO_2} = F_{IO_2} \times 5$$

Alveolar-arterial oxygen gradient ($P[A\text{-}a]O_2$) or (A-a gradient)

$P(A\text{-}a)O_2$ is a measurement of the difference between partial pressure of oxygen in the alveoli and arterial blood and an indication of oxygen transfer in the lung. However, supplemental oxygen and age can affect the gradient in individuals who do not have an acute condition of the lung.

$$EQUATION:\ P(A\text{-}a)O_2 = P_{AO_2} - P_{aO_2}$$

NORMAL: <15 mm Hg (room air) 10-65 mm Hg (100% O_2)

Arterial-alveolar oxygen tension ratio ($P[a/A]O_2$ ratio)

$P(a/A)O_2$ ratio is a measurement of the efficiency of gas exchange in the lung. Supplemental oxygen does not affect the ratio. A value less than 0.75 can indicate ventilation-perfusion (V/Q) inequalities, shunt abnormalities, or diffusion problems.

$$EQUATION:\ \frac{P_{aO_2}}{P_{AO_2}}$$

NORMAL: 0.75-0.90

Arterial oxygen content (Cao$_2$)

Cao$_2$ is a measurement of oxygen content in arterial blood, including oxygen bound to hemoglobin and oxygen dissolved in blood. A decreased value may indicate a low Pao$_2$, Sao$_2$, and/or hemoglobin (Hgb).

EQUATION: Cao$_2$ = (Sao$_2$ × Hgb × 1.34) + (Pao$_2$ × 0.003)

NORMAL: 18-20 ml/100 ml

Venous oxygen content (Cvo$_2$)

Cvo$_2$ is a measurement of oxygen content in venous blood. It takes into account Svo$_2$, Pvo$_2$, and hemoglobin; thus any change in these indices affects the Cvo$_2$.

EQUATION: Cvo$_2$ = (Svo$_2$ × Hgb × 1.34) + (Pvo$_2$ × 0.003)

NORMAL: 15.5 ml/100 ml

Arteriovenous oxygen content difference (C[a-v]o$_2$)

C(a-v)o$_2$ is a measurement that reflects oxygen uptake at the tissue level. An increased value indicates inadequate cardiovascular functioning. A decrease in CO results in more O$_2$ extracted, thus reducing the O$_2$ content of venous blood. A decreased value indicates poor tissue utilization of oxygen.

EQUATION: C(a-v)o$_2$ = Cao$_2$ – Cvo$_2$

NORMAL: 4-6 ml/100 ml

Arterial oxygen delivery (Ḋo$_2$) or oxygen transport

Ḋo$_2$ is a measurement of volume of O$_2$ delivered to tissues every minute. A decrease in Ḋo$_2$ may be due to a decrease in oxygen content (Pao$_2$, Sao$_2$, Hgb) or decrease in cardiac output.

EQUATION: Ḋo$_2$ = CO × 10 × Cao$_2$

NORMAL: 900-1200 ml/min

Arterial oxygen delivery index (Ḋo$_2$I)

Ḋo$_2$I is a measurement of Ḋo$_2$ adjusted for body size.

EQUATION: Ḋo$_2$I = CI × 10 × Cao$_2$

NORMAL: 500-600 ml/min/m^2

Oxygen consumption ($\dot{V}o_2$)

$\dot{V}o_2$ is a measurement of volume of oxygen used by tissues every minute, and determines the amount of oxygen delivered to the cells. A decreased value may indicate that metabolic needs of tissues are not being met, usually as a result of inadequate O_2 transport.

EQUATION: $\dot{V}o_2 = CO \times 10 \times C(a\text{-}v)o_2$

NORMAL: 200-250 ml/min

Oxygen consumption index ($\dot{V}o_2I$)

$\dot{V}o_2I$ is a measurement of $\dot{V}o_2$ adjusted for body size.

EQUATION: $\dot{V}o_2I = CI \times 10 \times C(a\text{-}v)o_2$

NORMAL: 115-165 ml/min/m^2

Oxygen utilization coefficient or oxygen extraction ratio (ERo_2)

ERo_2 is a measurement that indicates the balance between oxygen supply and demand. It is the fraction of available O_2 that is utilized by the tissues. Values greater than 25% indicate that cellular oxygenation is threatened.

EQUATION: $ERo_2 = \dfrac{C(a\text{-}v)o_2}{Cao_2}$ or $\dfrac{\dot{V}o_2}{\dot{D}o_2}$

NORMAL: 25%

Physiological shunt (Qs/Qt)

Qs/Qt is a measurement of the efficiency of the oxygenation system. It reflects the portion of venous blood that is not involved in gas exchange. High values are indicative of lung dysfunction (e.g., atelectasis or pulmonary edema).

EQUATION: $Qs/Qt = \dfrac{Cco_2 - Cao_2}{Cco_2 - Cvo_2}$

NORMAL: 0%-8%

$Cco_2 = O_2$ content in capillary blood

$Cco_2 = (Hgb \times 1.34) + (Pao_2 \times 0.003)$

Qs/Qt approximation

$$EQUATION: \quad \frac{Pao_2}{Fio_2}$$

$$VALUES: \quad 500 = 10\%$$

$$300 = 15\%$$

$$200 = 20\%$$

Dynamic compliance

Dynamic compliance is a measure of maximum airway pressure required to deliver a given tidal volume. It reflects lung elasticity and airway resistance during the breathing cycle. A low value reflects a reduced compliance (bronchospasm, secretions in airway).

$$EQUATION: \quad \frac{V_T}{PIP - PEEP}$$

$$NORMAL: \text{33-55 ml/cm } H_2O$$

V_T = Tidal volume; PIP = peak inspiratory pressure;
PEEP = positive end-expiratory pressure

Static compliance

Static compliance is a measurement of airway pressure required to hold the lungs at end inspiration (after a tidal volume has been delivered and no air flow is present). It reflects only lung elasticity not affected by gas flow. A low value reflects lung stiffness.

$$EQUATION: \quad \frac{V_T}{\text{Plateau pressure} - PEEP}$$

$$NORMAL: \text{50-100 ml/cm } H_2O$$

Neurological Parameters

Cerebral perfusion pressure (CPP)

CPP is a measurement of the pressure necessary to provide adequate cerebral blood flow. A value <60 mm Hg is associated with cerebral ischemia.

$$EQUATION: \text{CPP = MAP – ICP}$$

$$NORMAL: \text{60-100 mm Hg}$$

Metabolic Parameters

Anion gap (GAP) or delta

GAP is a measurement of excess unmeasurable anions used to differentiate the mechanisms of metabolic acidosis. GAP will remain normal in metabolic acidosis resulting from bicarbonate loss.

EQUATION: GAP = Na − (HCO$_3$ + Cl)

NORMAL: 8-16 mEq/L

Basal energy expenditure (BEE) or Harris-Benedict equation

BEE is a measurement of basal energy expenditure required to support vital life functions.

EQUATION: Men: = (66.47 + 13.7W + 5H) − (6.76A)
Women: = (655.1 + 9.56W + 1.8H) − (4.68A)
W = wt(kg); H = ht(cm); A = age

Total energy expenditure (TEE) = BEE × AF × IF
AF = Activity factor (bed rest = 1.2; ambulatory = 1.3)
IF = Injury factor (surgery = 1.2; trauma = 1.35; sepsis = 1.6; burn = 2.1)

Respiratory quotient (RQ)

RQ is a measurement of the state of nutrition. The relationship of oxygen consumption and carbon dioxide production reflects the oxidative state of the cell and energy consumption.

$$EQUATION: RQ = \frac{CO_2 \text{ production}}{O_2 \text{ consumption}}$$

VALUES: 0.8-1 (normal)
0.7 = Lipolysis or starvation
0.8 = Protein is primary source of energy
0.85 = Carbohydrates, protein, and fat are energy sources
1 = Carbohydrate is primary source of energy
>1 = Lipogenesis; state of being overfed

Renal Parameters
Glomerular filtration rate (GFR)

GFR is a measurement of amount of blood filtered by glomeruli each minute. GFR is affected by blood pressure and glomerular capillary membrane permeability. A decreased value may indicate renal disease or decreased perfusion to the kidneys.

EQUATION: Male: $\dfrac{(140 - age) \times wt\ (kg)}{75 \times serum\ Cr}$

Female: $\dfrac{(140 - age) \times wt\ (kg)}{85 \times serum\ Cr}$

NORMAL: 80-120 ml/min

Osmolality

Osmolality is a measurement of solute concentration per volume of solution. An increased value is associated with dehydration, a decreased value with overhydration. Renal concentrating ability can be assessed with simultaneous urine and serum osmolality measurements.

EQUATION: $(2Na) + K + \dfrac{BUN}{3} + \dfrac{Glucose}{18}$

NORMAL: 275-295 mOsm (serum)

Glossary

afterload The force the ventricles must overcome to eject blood

angioedema Giant wheal; reaction of the subcutaneous or submucosal tissue resulting in localized edema

antrectomy The surgical excision of the pyloric part of the stomach

anuria Absence of urine formation, usually <75 ml/day

areflexia Absence of reflexes

asterixis Flapping tremor, usually a sign of neurological irritation

atelectasis Collapse of alveoli that results in a loss of surface area available for gas exchange

autoregulation The body's ability to control blood flow despite changes in arterial blood pressure

azotemia Presence of nitrogen compounds in the blood (elevated BUN level)

Brudzinski's sign Flexion of the knee and hip in response to bending the patient's head toward the chest; a sign of meningeal irritation

cardiovert Application of electrical current synchronized to the QRS complex to terminate a tachydysrhythmia

carpopedal The wrist (carpal) and foot (pedal)

Chvostek's sign Spasm of facial muscles elicited on tapping the area over the facial nerve; sign of tetany

circumoral Around the mouth; circumoral pallor or cyanosis refers to paleness or bluish color around the mouth

colloid Solutions that cannot pass through semipermeable membranes (e.g., dextran, albumin); usually retained in the intravascular space and used to restore volume

contractility Ability of the cell to shorten and lengthen its muscle fiber

contralateral Pertaining to the opposite side

crystalloid Solutions that can pass through semipermeable membranes (e.g., D_5W, NS)

decerebrate   Bilateral extension, internal rotation, and wrist flexion; bilateral extension, internal rotation, and plantar flexion of lower extremities

decorticate   Bilateral adduction of shoulders; extension, internal rotation, and plantar flexion of lower extremities; pronation and flexion of elbows and wrists

defibrillate   Application of nonsynchronized electrical current to the myocardium to terminate a life-threatening dysrhythmia

dehiscence   Separation or splitting open of a surgical wound

dermatome   Area of skin supplied by nerve fibers

distal   Farthest from the point of origin

dysesthesia   Impaired sensation (out of proportion to the stimulus)

dysphasia   Impairment of speech (e.g., inability to arrange words in the proper order)

dysrhythmia   Any disorder of rate, rhythm, electrical impulse origin, or conduction within the heart

ecchymosis   Nonraised, purplish hemorrhagic spot larger than a petechia

ectopy   Arising from an abnormal site (e.g., ectopic beats are impulses arising outside the normal electrical conduction system of the heart)

empyema   Pus accumulation in a body cavity

encephalopathy   Degeneration of the brain caused by several conditions or diseases

endocardial   Layer of cells that line the cavity of the heart

escharotomy   Surgical incision of the burned body part to reduce pressure on tissues and restore blood flow

eupnea   Normal respiration

flaccid   Weak muscles

gastroduodenostomy   Surgical connection of the duodenum and stomach (Billroth I procedure)

gastroenterostomy   Surgical connection of the stomach and intestine

gastrojejunostomy   Surgical connection of the stomach and jejunum (Billroth II procedure)

gastroparesis   Paralysis of the stomach

gavage   Feeding through a tube

hemianopsia   Blindness in half of the visual field

hemoptysis   Blood in sputum; coughing up of blood

hypercapnea   Elevated carbon dioxide in the blood

hypercarbia   Elevated carbon dioxide in the blood

hyperpyrexia   Elevated temperature, fever, hyperthermia

hypertonic   An osmolality greater than fluids it is being compared to (i.e., hypertonic IV fluids such as D_5NS and $D_{10}W$ refer to an osmolality >300 and, if infused, can cause cells to shrink and cause circulatory overload)

hypokinesia   Decreased movement or motion (e.g., a hypokinetic ventricle refers to decreased contraction [motion] of the ventricle)

hypotonic   An osmolality less than fluids it is being compared to (i.e., hypotonic IV fluids such as 0.45NS refer to an osmolality <300 and, if infused, can cause cells to swell, hypotension, and fluid depletion)

hypoxemia   Deficient oxygenation in the blood

hypoxia   Reduced oxygen availability to the tissues

inotropic   Pertaining to the force or strength of muscular contraction

ipsilateral   Pertaining to the same side

isotonic   The same osmolality of fluid it is being compared to (i.e., isotonic IV fluids such as 0.9NS and lactated Ringers refer to solutions that do not affect flow of water across the cell membranes)

Kernig's sign   Inability to completely extend the leg when the thigh is flexed on the abdomen

Kussmaul's sign   A rise, instead of a fall, in the venous pressure during inspiration

lateralizing   Pertaining to one side

lavage   Irrigation of a cavity or organ such as the stomach

leukocytosis   Increase in number of leukocytes (basophils, eosinophils, neutrophils, monocytes, lymphocytes)

leukopenia   Decrease in number of leukocytes (usually <5000/μl)

myoglobinuria   Presence of myoglobin (globulin from muscle) in the urine

nuchal rigidity   Stiff neck

oliguria   Urine volume <400 ml/day

otorrhea   Discharge from the ear

papilledema   Edema of the optic disk

paraplegia   Paralysis of the lower extremities

parenchyma   The essential elements of an organ

petechia   Nonraised, round, purplish spots caused by intradermal or submucous hemorrhages

pheochromocytoma A tumor of the adrenal medulla that secretes epinephrine and norepinephrine, resulting in severe hypertension, increased metabolism, and hyperglycemia

photophobia Intolerance to light

polydipsia Excessive thirst

polyuria Excessive urination

postictal Following a seizure

preload Volume of blood in the ventricles at the end of diastole

proprioception Pertaining to the position of the body; involves balance, coordination, and posture

proximal Closest or nearest to the point of origin

pyloroplasty Surgery involving the pylorus, usually to enlarge the communication between the stomach and duodenum

quadriplegia Paralysis of all four extremities

rhabdomyolysis Skeletal muscle injury that results in release of substances such as myoglobin that are potentially toxic to the kidney

rhinorrhea Discharge from the nose

stomatitis Inflammation of the oral mucosa

thrombocytopenia Reduction in the number of platelets

tonic-clonic Involuntary muscular contraction and relaxation in rapid succession

Trendelenberg Position in which the patient is supine and the head is down

Trousseau's sign Carpal spasm on compression of the upper arm; sign of tetany

urticaria Hives; vascular reaction that results in wheals and itching (pruritus)

vagotomy The surgical interruption of the vagus nerve, usually performed to reduce gastric secretions in the treatment of ulcers

ventilation Movement of air between the lungs and environment

Index

Cardiopulmonary Parameter Values

on	Parameter name	Normal
Ig)	Pulmonary artery systolic	15-30
Hg)	Pulmonary artery diastolic	5-15
Hg)	Pulmonary artery mean	10-20
Hg)	Pulmonary artery wedge	4-12
Hg)	Central venous pressure	2-6
Hg)	Mean arterial pressure	70-105
g)	Pulse pressure	30-40
)	Cardiac output	4-8
/m^2)	Cardiac index	2.5-4.0
t)	Stroke volume	60-120
t/m^2)	Stroke index	30-65
m/m^2)	Stroke work index, left ventricular	45-60
m/m^2)	Stroke work index, right ventricular	7-12
s/sec/cm^{-5})	Pulmonary vascular resistance	100-250
es/sec/cm^{-5}/m^2)	Pulmonary vascular resistance index	200-450
s/sec/cm^{-5})	Systemic vascular resistance	900-1400
s/sec/cm^{-5}/m^2)	Systemic vascular resistance index	1700-2600
00 ml)	Oxygen content, arterial	18-20
00 ml)	Oxygen content, venous	15.5
nl/100 ml)	Oxygen content, arteriovenous difference	4-6
in)	Oxygen consumption	200-250
nin/m^2)	Oxygen consumption index	115-165
in)	Oxygen delivery	900-1200
nin/m^2)	Oxygen delivery index	500-600
	Oxygen extraction ratio	25%

Abbrevia

PAS (mm
PAD (mn
PAM (mm
PAWP (m

CVP (mm
MAP (mr
PP (mm

CO (L/n
CI (L/m

SV (ml/b
SI (ml/bc
LVSWI (g

RVSWI (g

PVR (dyr

PVRI (dy

SVR (dyr

SVRI (dy

CaO_2 (ml
CvO_2 (ml
$C(a\text{-}v)O_2$

$\dot{V}O_2$ (ml/
$\dot{V}O_2I$ (ml/
$\dot{D}O_2$ (ml/
$\dot{D}O_2I$ (ml
ERO_2

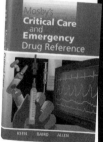

Cardiopulmonary Parameter Values

Abbreviation	Parameter name	Normal
PAS (mm Hg)	Pulmonary artery systolic	15-30
PAD (mm Hg)	Pulmonary artery diastolic	5-15
PAM (mm Hg)	Pulmonary artery mean	10-20
PAWP (mm Hg)	Pulmonary artery wedge	4-12
CVP (mm Hg)	Central venous pressure	2-6
MAP (mm Hg)	Mean arterial pressure	70-105
PP (mm Hg)	Pulse pressure	30-40
CO (L/min)	Cardiac output	4-8
CI (L/min/m^2)	Cardiac index	2.5-4.0
SV (ml/beat)	Stroke volume	60-120
SI (ml/beat/m^2)	Stroke index	30-65
LVSWI (g-m/m^2)	Stroke work index, left ventricular	45-60
RVSWI (g-m/m^2)	Stroke work index, right ventricular	7-12
PVR (dynes/sec/cm^{-5})	Pulmonary vascular resistance	100-250
PVRI (dynes/sec/cm^{-5}/m^2)	Pulmonary vascular resistance index	200-450
SVR (dynes/sec/cm^{-5})	Systemic vascular resistance	900-1400
SVRI (dynes/sec/cm^{-5}/m^2)	Systemic vascular resistance index	1700-2600
Cao$_2$ (ml/100 ml)	Oxygen content, arterial	18-20
Cvo$_2$ (ml/100 ml)	Oxygen content, venous	15.5
C(a-v)o$_2$ (ml/100 ml)	Oxygen content, arteriovenous difference	4-6
$\dot{V}$o$_2$ (ml/min)	Oxygen consumption	200-250
$\dot{V}$o$_2$I (ml/min/m^2)	Oxygen consumption index	115-165
$\dot{D}$o$_2$ (ml/min)	Oxygen delivery	900-1200
$\dot{D}$o$_2$I (ml/min/m^2)	Oxygen delivery index	500-600
ERo$_2$	Oxygen extraction ratio	25%